AF509217

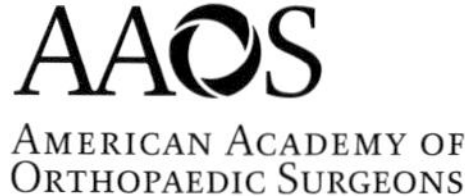

American Academy of Orthopaedic Surgeons

Pathophysiology of Orthopaedic Diseases
Volume 2

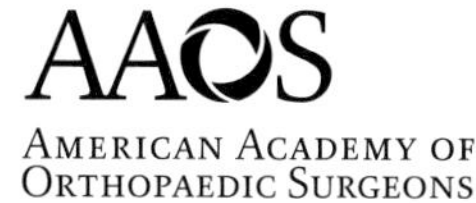

American Academy of Orthopaedic Surgeons

Pathophysiology of Orthopaedic Diseases
Volume 2

Henry J. Mankin, MD

Published 2009 by the
American Academy of Orthopaedic Surgeons
6300 North River Road
Rosemont, IL 60018

Copyright 2009
by the American Academy of Orthopaedic Surgeons

The material presented in *Pathophysiology of Orthopaedic Diseases, Volume 2* has been made available by the American Academy of Orthopaedic Surgeons for educational purposes only. This material is not intended to present the only, or necessarily best, methods or procedures for the medical situations discussed, but rather is intended to represent an approach, view, statement, or opinion of the author(s) or producer(s), which may be helpful to others who face similar situations.

Some drugs or medical devices demonstrated in Academy courses or described in Academy print or electronic publications have not been cleared by the Food and Drug Administration (FDA) or have been cleared for specific uses only. The FDA has stated that it is the responsibility of the physician to determine the FDA clearance status of each drug or device he or she wishes to use in clinical practice.

Furthermore, any statements about commercial products are solely the opinion(s) of the author(s) and do not represent an Academy endorsement or evaluation of these products. These statements may not be used in advertising or for any commercial purpose.

ISBN: 978-0-89203-635-6
Printed in the USA

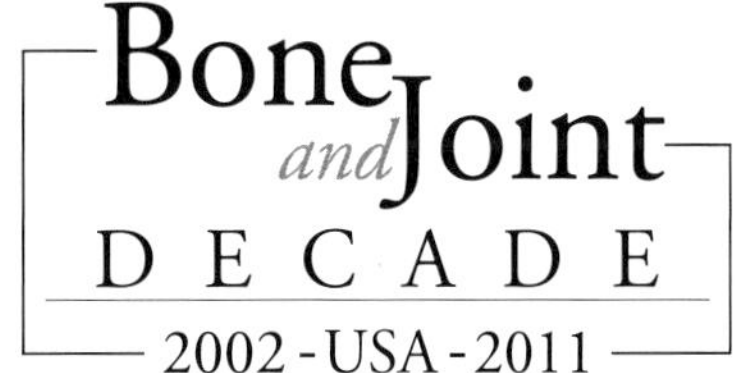

Table of Contents

Preface

This is Volume 2 of *Pathophysiology of Orthopaedic Diseases,* and it is clearly somewhat different from Volume 1. As I look over the 33 chapters, it is evident that I have extended my view of the chosen disease states. Volume 1 included more common disorders that the orthopaedists and particularly the residents or students are likely to encounter fairly frequently. Volume 2 is different, since I have included some unusual malignant and benign tumors, some mucopolysaccharidoses and a rather extensive collection of unusual genetic disorders that not only cause alterations in body structure and function but also materially affect the skeletal system.

In volume 2, I am committed to describing the historical data in fairly great detail, and spending even more time and space on the biologic problems of these entities, particularly when the genetic error has been identified. I have provided information about the diagnostic features, including the patient's physical presentation, their imaging studies, laboratory data, and a description of the histologic picture on tissue specimens. Less time has been spent on treatment, principally because of my commitment to deal with the pathophysiology of these disorders rather than their clinical management.

The purpose of all of this is to provide the interested reader with some background data related to the disorders, and with some understanding and perhaps even enthusiasm for approaching diseases biologically. As all of us know, much of orthopaedic education is currently devoted to aspects of clinical presentation and medical, and especially surgical, management of disease states. All of that is certainly essential for the purpose of satisfying our patients and, indeed, ourselves. Regrettably, it does not allow us to further define and identify the clinical entities or more importantly visualize and understand the possible biologic treatment protocols, which are now beginning to appear. As I have indicated in Volume 1, understanding biology and pathophysiology may be a key to the future of orthopaedic science and will allow our students and practitioners to more clearly understand the diseases, their nature, and indeed the new approaches to management.

Once again, I must emphasize the importance of education in our specialty. It is essential for teachers and students to view orthopaedic disorders not just as skeletal and structural deformities, but as sometimes extraordinary biologic abnormalities that can be more clearly understood and more effectively treated than by the application of our current protocols. As we all know, teaching our students is a major function in our lives, and we can do that much more successfully if we have them see our diseases as science rather than simply problems solved mechanically.

I must once again acknowledge the sources of the information included in both our volumes and express my sincere and deep appreciation for the way it was obtained. First, it should be apparent that many of the illustrations are from the Jaffe collection. As I indicated in Chapter 1 of Volume 1, I am deeply indebted to Henry Jaffe for teaching me, and many others, bone and connective tissue pathology and, more importantly, emphasizing the critical importance of education. In 1979, he willed his enormous pathology collection to me and I must admit that in some ways it changed my life. In terms of the Jaffe collection, I have worked with Carol Trahan, our great administrator and very talented computer person, for the last several years to put over 10,000 images from 2,000 from the collection into digital images. I have also utilized our Orthopaedic Oncology Computer system, which now contains clinical data on over 19,000 patients that we have seen since 1972, and the 16,000 2 × 2 slides from these patients in my personal collection. I remain deeply appreciative of the contributions of my wife Carole Mankin, a talented research librarian who not only helped to obtain the references for the chapters, but also reviewed the presentations and helped make them more readable.

I am deeply indebted to the American Academy of Orthopaedic Surgeons Publications Department and especially Marilyn Fox, PhD who helped me to develop an acceptable approach to my effort. One of the most important contributors to the educational material is Sharon O'Brien, a superb editor who has helped me to improve the quality of the chapters and make them much more readable. Courtney Astle, an outstanding member of the Academy publishing group, has been committed and very helpful in organizing the text and illustrations and I wish to thank them all...I could never have put all of this together without them!

Henry J. Mankin, MD

Chapter 1

Chondrosarcomas of Bone

Chondrosarcomas are the second most common malignant tumor of bone and are only about 15% less frequent in occurrence than osteosarcomas. All of the tumors appear to arise from cartilage and form abnormal chondroid tissue as their principal pathologic component. The tumors usually occur in older adults and are rarely seen in children. The severity of the disease in terms of local destruction and risk of metastases differs considerably according to the tumor grade (1 through 3), the anatomic site (tumors of the pelvis are more malignant than those of acral parts), the presence of a genetic disorder (Ollier's disease, Maffucci syndrome, or hereditary multiple osteocartilaginous exostosis), or the type of tumor (intramedullary, extramedullary, dedifferentiated, clear cell, or mesenchymal). Some chondrosarcomas can be very destructive locally and yet not metastasize, while others can be small and appear bland on imaging studies but metastasize early in their course. The tumors do not seem to respond to either radiation or standard chemotherapy. Regardless of all of these factors, chondrosarcomas have a lower overall death rate than either osteosarcomas or Ewing's tumors. Nevertheless, they still represent major problems for the patient, the surgeon, and the oncologist.

History of Malignant Cartilage Tumors

The history of the discovery of chondrosarcomas of bone is quite complex, partly because the tumors are relatively rare and also because they are sometimes difficult to distinguish from other types of lesions. The earliest descriptions of connective tissue tumors and more specifically those within or arising from the bone were those of Rudolf Virchow in his remarkable three-volume work published in the 1860s.[1] Although the majority of the cases presented in his collection were osteosarcomas and giant cell tumors, some of them were described as arising from or consisting of cartilage. In 1879, Samuel Gross[2] published a study in which he described 165 tumors arising from bone. Ten of these seemed to contain cartilage. In 1922, James Ewing,[3] a famous pathologist with an interest in bone disease, established a classification system for bone sarcomas that included those containing cartilage as a special group. It was Keiller,[4] however, who in 1925 was the first to identify tumors of bone that contained cartilaginous elements as their principal neoplastic tissue. Shortly thereafter, Dallas Phemister[5] described another series that not only contained cartilage, but clearly arose from it. In 1935, Roberg[6] defined the relationship of degree of malignancy to anatomic site for tumors that contained cartilage. In 1943, Louis Lichtenstein and Henry Jaffe[7] introduced the name "chondrosarcoma" for these malignant tumors, and these observations were extended by Thomson and Turner-Warwick in 1955.[8] Beginning in 1973, a multicenter study known by the term SEER (Surveillance, Epidemiology, and End Results) provided a 1 to 3 grading system for chondrosarcomas.[9,10] Only 10% of most series of cartilage tumors are grade 3 and hence have a high risk of metastasis. This clearly distinguished the low rate of metastasis for most chondrosarcomas as a major difference from the other two major malignant bone tumors, osteosarcoma and Ewing's sarcoma. Another type of tumor, the clear-cell chondrosarcoma, was first described in 1976 by Kristan Unni and associates.[11] These tumors have an extraordinary histologic appearance and are also generally benign. Another type of cartilage tumor, the juxtacortical chondrosarcoma, was described by Cooper,[12] and a subsequent study by Fritz Schajowicz[13] indicated its relatively benign nature. Lichtenstein and Bernstein[14] first described a rare tumor known as mesenchymal chondrosarcoma in 1959, and it was subsequently further described and actually named by Goldman.[15] Both articles defined it as a highly malignant tumor with a mortality rate of well over 60%. In 1971, Dahlin and Beabout[16] first identified another cartilaginous entity that they named dedifferentiated chondrosarcoma. This tumor appears to be a highly malignant tumor with a very poor survival history.

Forms of Chondrosarcoma

Intraosseous Chondrosarcoma

This is the standard or "classical" form of chondrosarcoma and is the most frequently encountered. A series of early cases were well described in 1952 by O'Neal and Ackerman,[17] and in the 1960s by Henderson and Dahlin[18] and Barnes and Catto.[19] The tumors are located inside the bone and are often centrally placed. They expand or sometimes thicken the cortices.[6,9,20-25] The lesions are sometimes associated with Ollier's disease or Maffucci syndrome.[9,20,24,26] The tumor is usually seen in the shaft of the femur, tibia, pelvis, or humerus but may be present in the spine, sternum, ribs, hands, or feet.[9,20,21,24,26] The architecture is lobular and frequently calcification is present within the tumor, sometimes resembling "popcorn balls".[20,24] Based on the histology and, to some extent, the degree of cortical destruction and presence of a soft-tissue extension, the tumors are graded 1, 2, or 3.[9,10,22,23,27-32] Grade 1 tumors are "benign" in the sense that they resemble enchondromas but, rather than remaining unchanged over time, they continue to slowly grow and expand. They only rarely metastasize. Grade 2 tumors are more aggressive, larger in size, and show either cortical destruction or coarse thickening of the cortical bone. Metastasis is uncommon. Grade 3 chondrosarcomas are believed to be highly malignant, often occurring in the pelvis and markedly expanding and destroying the cortical bone and extending into the soft tissues. Metastases occur with a frequency almost equivalent to osteosarcoma.[9,20,26,29]

Exostotic Chondrosarcoma

These lesions arise from the surface of the bone and resemble abnormal apophyseal structures.[9,12,13,20,24,26] The lesions often share a cortex with the subjacent bone and have an expanded bony base, which is deep to the chondrosarcomatous element. The lesions closely resemble benign osteocartilaginous exostoses, such as occur in patients with hereditary multiple osteocartilaginous exostoses, and the chondrosarcomas often occur in relation to that genetic disorder.[9,12,20] Some of these tumors are heavily calcified.[26] The majority of these lesions are grade 1, and the metastasis rate is very low.[9,12,13,20,24,26] Survival is almost 100%.[29]

Dedifferentiated Chondrosarcoma

These tumors are all stage 3 and very aggressive in imaging and histologic studies.[9,16,20,26,33-38] The tumors are very likely to metastasize and to recur locally if treated by surgical excision.[9,16,20,29,34,35,37,38] The survival rate for these uncommon tumors is only about 10%. The tumors are very destructive and have as a characteristic a soft-tissue mass that is generally heavily calcified.[9,20,26] The tumors occur most frequently in the pelvis and proximal femur.[9,16,20,33,35]

Clear-Cell Chondrosarcoma

Clear-cell chondrosarcoma is defined as a low-grade malignant cartilage lesion in which the tumor cells contain a large amount of glycogen, which results in an extraordinary histologic "clear-cell" appearance for the cells.[26,39-42] The tumors account for less than 5% of all chondrosarcomas and usually occur in young adults, with a male predominance. The tumors are located at the ends of long tubular bone, and most often in the proximal femur, humerus, or tibia. The lesions are relatively small, often heavily calcified, and are not as a rule very destructive.[9,20,26,40-44] The tumors grow slowly and have a low metastatic and death rate.

Mesenchymal Chondrosarcoma

This lesion is an extremely rare tumor, accounting for less than 2% of the total chondrosarcoma population.[9,15,20,38,45] The peak incidence is in the third decade; the maxilla and mandible are frequently affected, along with the vertebrae, ribs, pelvis, and humerus.[9,26,45-48] The tumors are often very destructive, expand the cortex, and present with only small amounts of calcification.[9,20,47,49] Mesenchymal chondrosarcoma may also present as extraskeletal lesions.[9] The tumors histologically consist of spindled primitive mesenchymal cells that resemble Ewing's sarcoma or myeloma but are surrounded by cells with cartilage differentiation.[9,20,26,45,49] The lesions are believed to be very aggressive and have a high rate of metastasis and death.[45,47,49,50] The tumors can be distinguished from other round-cell lesions such as Ewing's sarcoma, lymphoma, and myeloma by study of immunohistochemical markers, which are quite definitive for the other round-cell entities and differ from those of mesenchymal chondrosarcomas.[9,26,50]

Biochemistry and Pathophysiology

A 1980 study by Mankin and associates[30,31] described the structure of chondrosarcomas and provided the view that chondrosarcomas have biochemical features quite similar to those of articular cartilage. The tissue contains principally type II collagen and has molecular structures consistent with the aggrecan molecules.[30] Chondroitin and keratan sulfate glycosaminoglycans are present but appear to be altered in concentration, possibly related to the grade of disease.[9,30,31] The presence of type II collagen is particularly noticeable in clear-cell chondrosarcoma and distinguishes it from other lesions such as the chondroblastoma.[43,51,52] Two recent studies showed that chondrosarcomas have a high concentration of cyclooxygenase-2 (COX-2), a material that is not present in normal cartilage or enchondromas and may be an indicator of malignant behavior.[53,54]

Most chondrosarcomas appear to be positive for S100 protein and vimentin.[9,55] The S100 protein may be reduced in grade 3 intraosseous or dedifferentiated chondrosarcomas.[55] DNA ploidy flow cytometric studies have shown that almost all grade 1 chondrosarcomas are diploid, while almost all grade 2 or grade 3 tumors are aneuploid.[29,56-59] The presence of aneuploidy seems to correlate with local recurrence and metastasis.[29,56,57,59] Increased numbers of cells in the S-phase of flow cytometric studies also seem to correlate with malignancy.[58] Chromosomal analysis shows that high-grade lesions have complex aberrations with nonreciprocal translocations and deletions of numerous chromosomes.[9,60,61] Most frequently these are associated with chromosome 12. The rearrangement of 1p and 4, 5, 9, and 20 may also play a role in the biology of the tumors.[61-63] Accumulation of p53 appears to occur in high-grade lesions and may be a marker for malignancy.[52,64,65] The mesenchymal chondrosarcomas show a reciprocal translocation (11;22)(q24;q12), which resembles the

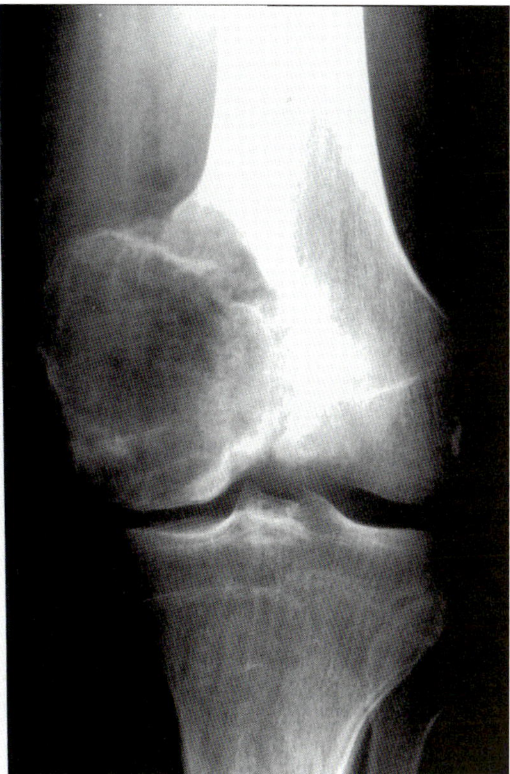

Figure 1

Radiograph of the distal femur showing an expansile destructive lesion arising from the lateral condyle.

findings seen in tumors with small round cells.[9,63,66] The mesenchymal cells also appear to be negative for S100.[9,55]

Imaging Studies

Radiographic studies of all forms of intramedullary chondrosarcoma usually show the lesions to be within the bone and essentially radiolucent and expansile[9,25,32,67,68] (Figure 1). The lesions cause thinning of the cortex, either of the entire segment of bone or, slightly more commonly, eccentrically placed (Figure 2). With grade 1 lesions, the tumor is very limited in its destructive element and has no extension into the soft tissues.[9,32] With grade 2 or 3 lesions, the tumors may show regions of thickening and distortion of the cortex and sometimes a soft-tissue mass outside the bone[9,32] (Figure 3). Of remarkable frequency in all of these lesions, calcified nodular elements appearing as "popcorn balls" are present and sometimes form dense masses with irregular contours.[9,20,26,32] The lesions have a similar appearance on CT, which is sometimes helpful in defining margins and planning surgi-

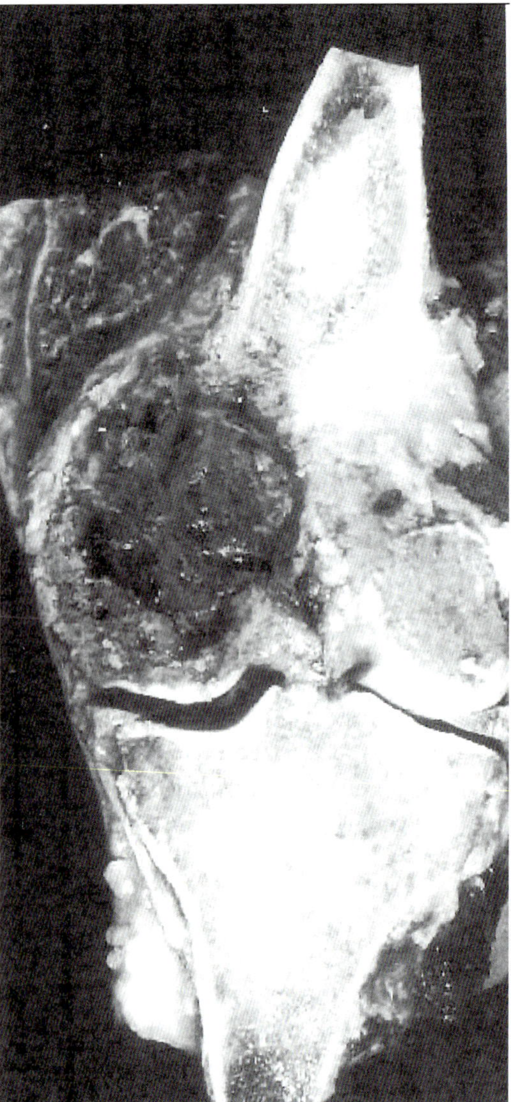

Figure 2
Photograph of the specimen obtained after resection of the lesion arising from the lateral condyle seen in Figure 1. Note the thinned cortex, the bony destruction, and the soft-tissue extension of the lesional tissue.

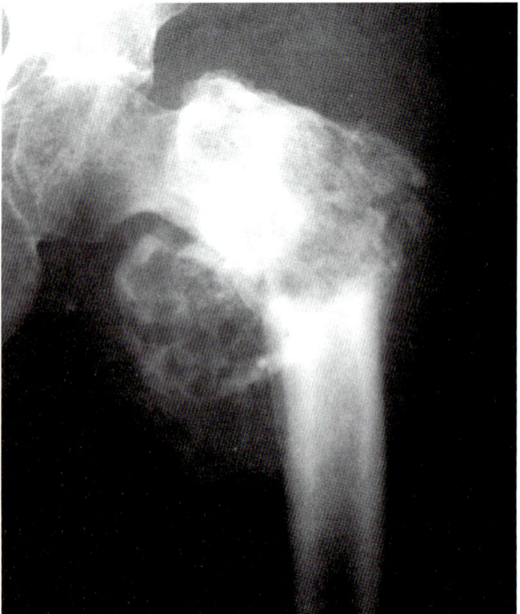

Figure 3
Radiograph of a high-grade chondrosarcoma arising from the proximal femur. The lesion is destructive, has caused a fracture, and has extended into the soft tissues.

cal resection. MRI is also very helpful in arriving at a diagnosis. Classically, the signal is low on T1 and high on T2-weighted images.[9,32,69] MRI is useful in defining the extent of the lesion and more clearly assessing the presence of cortical disruption and the presence or absence of a soft-tissue component outside the bone.[9,32,68,69] The tumors, even those that are grade 1, are virtually always intensely active on bone scan.

Imaging of exostotic chondrosarcoma is also quite characteristic.[9,12,70] The lesions arise from the surface of the bone, often with cortical continuity with the shaft (Figure 4). There is often a segment of bone providing an apophyseal relationship to the shaft, not unlike the osteocartilaginous exostosis. The cartilage cap is often heavily calcified, sometimes in an irregular fashion. There may also be small calcified masses present, particularly in the soft-tissue region adjacent to the tumor.

Clear-cell chondrosarcomas usually lie close to the joint in the epiphyseometaphyseal region, particularly in the proximal femur or proximal tibia.[39,41-44] The lytic lesion is rounded and sometimes quite regular in contour, resembling a chondroblastoma.[9,39,42,43] The tumor may be radiolucent or calcified, sometimes with tiny masses of calcified cartilage simulating the chondroblastoma.[9,39,42,43]

Mesenchymal chondrosarcoma appears radiographically as a radiolucent lesion with varying degrees of matrix calcification, often stippled in nature.[9,45,47,49] Extensions into the soft tissues seen best by MRI or CT can be observed in more than 50% of the cases.[9,20,49]

Histologic Findings

All of the chondrosarcomatous lesions by definition arise from cartilage, and most of the cellular elements resemble aspects of

Table 1. | Chondrosarcoma Histologic Grading System

Grade	Matrix	Cells	Replicative Activity
1	Abundant	Uniform size, small Dark, round nuclei Little nuclear detail	Rare binucleate form
2	Uneven distribution and staining	Slight pleomorphism Nuclear detail evident Well-defined nucleoli Mild atypism	Common binucleate forms
3	Less matrix, unevenly distributed	Marked pleomorphism Large cells with large, hyperchromatic nuclei Marked atypism	Many binuclear forms Many mitoses present
Dedifferentiated	Minimal matrix present	Marked pleomorphism Hyperchromatic nuclei Bizarre forms, giant cells	Abundant bizarre mitotic activity

epiphyseal or articular cartilage. The intramedullary or classical form of the disease is most common and provides the histologic characteristics used for grading[9,18-21,24,26-28,31,32,67] (Table 1). The cells resemble normal chondrocytes and lie in lacunar spaces embedded with cartilaginous biochemical materials including type II collagen and proteoglycans (Figure 5). The material at times is myxoid or contains islands of calcified matrix. At the margins, lobules of cartilage appear to be surrounding bone segments, permeating the marrow spaces or attached to the cortex. Deposition of new bone can be seen in areas of cortical disruption (Figure 6). Small islands of calcification may be present and in some sites, the cartilaginous tissue is heavily calcified (Figure 7).

Grade 1 tumors show increased cellularity as compared with articular cartilage or enchondroma, and the cells are larger, with plump nuclei and an occasional double nucleus. No atypism or mitotic figures are present. Grade 2 chondrosarcoma has increased cellularity, either evenly distributed or in clusters. The cells are plump and have enlarged nuclei with distinct nucleoli present in many of them. Foci of myxoid matrix are noted. Atypism and pleomorphism are common and double nuclei are present in many of the cells. Occasional mitotic figures are noted. Grade 3 tumors are characterized by increased cellularity, marked pleomorphism, cellular atypism, and presence of double nuclei. A high percentage of cells display mitotic figures, which are sometimes quite bizarre in structure[9,18-21,24,26-28,30,32,67] (Table 1).

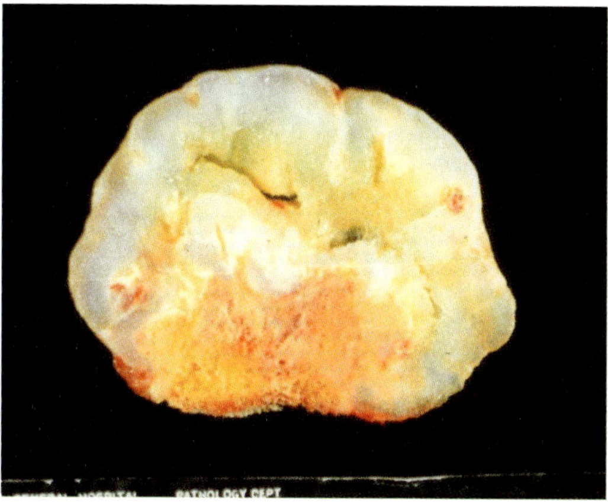

Figure 4
An exostotic chondrosarcoma arising from the posterior aspect of the tibia. The lesion is not present within the bone but seems to arise from the subjacent cortex.

Clear-cell chondorsarcomas show a large number of cells with clear cytoplasm, presumably related to the presence of glycogen in the cell matrix.[9,20,39,41,43,44] Nuclear atypia is commonly seen and the cells have prominent nucleoli. Multinucleated cells are sometimes present and these resemble osteoclasts. Mitotic activity is uncommon.

The microscopic findings for mesenchymal chondrosarcomas are quite extraordinary.[9,20,26,45,49] The cell types are mesenchymal and closely resemble those seen in hemangiopericytomas, myelomas, or Ewing's tumors. There are also multiple vascular spaces. The tumor would not be considered cartilaginous in origin except that there are numerous foci of chondrocytes and areas containing classical chondroid matrix

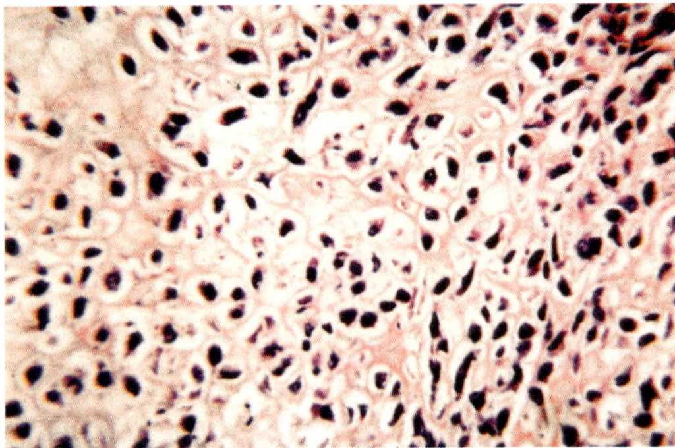

Figure 5
Histologic pattern of a chondrosarcoma, showing the atypical cartilage cells with dense nuclei in a sometimes markedly distorted cellular structure.

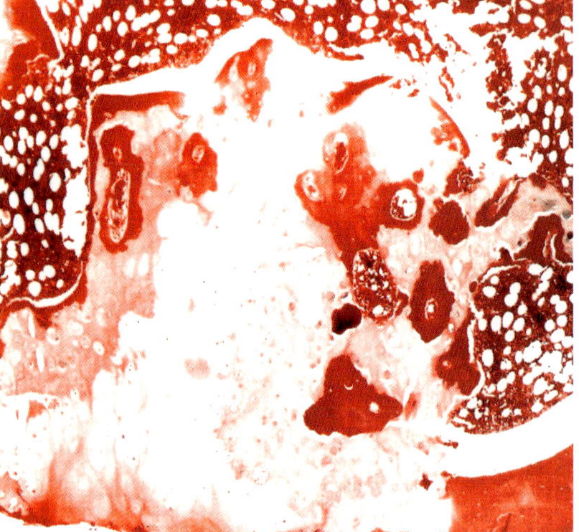

Figure 6
Chondrosarcomas may invade the bone and produce destructive sites within the shaft of a long bone. These may result in fracture.

that is sometimes calcified. Cellular atypism is present as are occasional mitotic figures.[9,20,26,45,49]

Treatment

It is essential to establish a method for the clinical assessment of the cartilage neoplasms, as the treatment protocols for the various tumors may vary greatly based on their likelihood of local recurrence and metastasis. The following eight-point assessment protocol provides the information required:

1. Patient's age
2. Presence or absence of pain at the site of the tumor.
3. Presence of genetic disorders such as Ollier's disease, Maffucci syndrome, or hereditary multiple osteocartilaginous exostosis
4. Anatomic site of the tumor
5. Tumor size
6. Histologic grade of the tumor
7. Based on biopsy, the diagnosis of exostotic, dedifferentiated, clear-cell, or mesenchymal chondrosarcoma
8. Bone scan activity

Each of the following factors is essential to determine the nature, aggressiveness, and potential malignity for a tumor-containing cartilage.

1. Age—Chondrosarcomas rarely occur before the age of 15 years.[9,20,26,29]
2. Pain—Almost all of the chondrosarcomas have pain as their presenting complaint. Absence of pain suggests that the lesion is benign.
3. Ollier's or Maffucci disorders are associ-

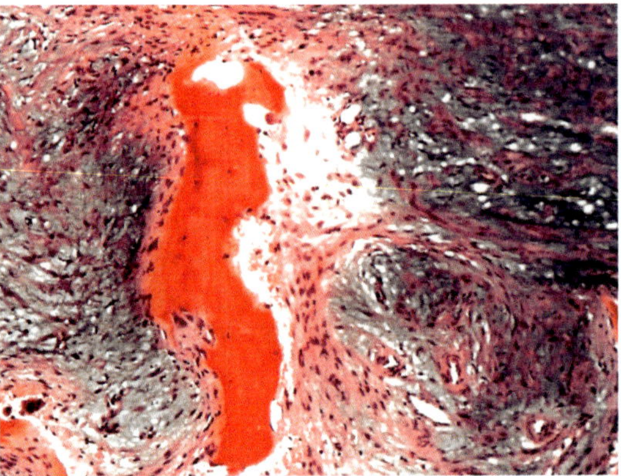

Figure 7
Calcification and bone formation are commonly present in chondrosarcomas and produce irregular patterns on imaging and structural abnormalities on histologic study.

ated with central chondrosarcomas, and malignant lesions are frequently present with Maffucci syndrome. Hereditary multiple osteocartilaginous exostosis has occasional exostotic chondrosarcoma but these rarely metastasize.[9,20,24,26]

4. Anatomic site—This factor is critical because lesions of the acral parts, and particularly the hands and feet, very rarely metastasize, while those of the pelvis, spine, proximal femur, or proximal humerus not only have a high rate of metastasis but poor survival.[6,29,71-75]
5. Size of tumor—It should be evident that large tumors are more dangerous and threatening than small ones and patients

whose tumors have broken out of the bone are at higher risk.[29]

6. Grade—Grade 1 lesions have a low rate of metastasis (less than 5%); grade 2 lesions, a medium rate (20%); and grade 3, a high rate (60 + %).[9,18,20,23,26-29,76]

7. Type of tumor—Exostotic and clear-cell tumors are relatively benign, while dedifferentiated or mesenchymal tumors are highly malignant.[9,26,29,34,37,41,42,49]

8. Bone scan—If the bone scan is negative, the likelihood of the tumor being a chondrosarcoma or certainly one of high grade is very limited.

Based on this formula, a 7-year-old child without genetic disorders who presents with a small, painless lesion of the foot with a negative bone scan is unlikely to have a true chondrosarcoma and, even if the child did, the risk is minimal. On the other hand, a 50-year-old person with Maffucci syndrome and a large, painful lesion of the pelvis that is positive on bone scan and grade 3 on biopsy is almost surely at great risk for metastasis and poor survival.

Imaging studies must be performed to help define the extent of the tumor and its character. The studies should include a CT scan of the chest. A biopsy is essential for these tumors and fine-needle biopsy may be helpful.[77] Often, however, an open biopsy is necessary to be certain that the diagnosis is correct. This will also allow accurate grading of the lesion.[9,20,26,32] Low-grade lesions such as those in the hand or foot can be treated with cryosurgery or curettage, phenolization, and implantation of bone chips or polymethylmethacrylate.[20,25,40,41,78,79] Higher-grade lesions require wider resection and replacement with allograft transplant or with metallic devices.[9,20,29] Amputation is occasionally required.[9,20,22,25,38,74] Radiation and chemotherapy have little effect on chondrosarcomas, but it is possible that they will be of value to patients with intralesional or marginal resection or those with recurrences or with lung metastases.[9,20,29]

Discussion

Cartilage tumors in general, and especially chondrosarcomas, are not easy to diagnose or treat. Because of the large numbers of different tumor types, the required grading, and the seeming insensitivity of the tumors to adjuvant therapy, the surgeon and the patient stand alone in diagnosing, planning, and executing appropriate care. Fortunately, many of the tumors are unlikely to metastasize or threaten the patient's life and a large number of the more aggressive tumors respond to surgical care and reconstruction of the part after wide resection. It would nevertheless be of great advantage to find ways of treating the high-grade lesions with agents that negate or interfere with the biologic character of the lesions and diminish the likelihood of local recurrence or metastasis after therapy. The future will hopefully hold some new approaches, which include COX-2 inhibitors, antibodies transforming growth factor-beta and insulin-like growth factors, and inhibitors of appropriate matrix metalloproteinases.

References

1. Virchow R: *Die Krankhaften Gewulste*. Berlin, Hirschwalst, 1863-1867.

2. Gross SW: Sarcoma of the long bones: Based on the study of one hundred and sixty-five cases. *Am J Med Sci* 1879;78:17-57, 338-377.

3. Ewing J: A review and classification of bone sarcomas. *Arch Surg* 1922;4:485-533.

4. Keiller VH: Cartilaginous tumors of bone. *Surg Gynecol Obstet* 1925;40:510-521.

5. Phemister DB: Chondrosarcoma of bone. *Surg Gynecol Obstet* 1930;50:216-233.

6. Roberg OT: Chondrosarcoma: Relation of structure and location to the clinical course. *Surg Gynecol Obstet* 1935;61:68-82.

7. Lichtenstein L, Jaffe HL: Chondrosarcoma of bone. *Am J Pathol* 1943;19:553-589.

8. Thomson AD, Turner-Warwick RT: Skeletal sarcomata and giant cell tumour. *J Bone Joint Surg Br* 1955;37:266-303.

9. Dorfman HD, Czerniak B: *Bone Tumors*. St. Louis, MO, Mosby, 1998, pp 353-440.

10. Dorfman HD, Czerniak B: Bone cancers. *Cancer* 1995;75(1 Suppl):203-210.

11. Unni KK, Dahlin DC, Beabout JW, Sim FH: Chondrosarcoma: Clear cell variant. A Report of sixteen cases. *J Bone Joint Surg Am* 1976;58:676-683.

12. Cooper RR: Juxtacortical chondrosarcoma. *J Bone Joint Surg Am* 1965;47:524-528.

13. Schajowicz F: Juxtacortical chondrosarcoma. *J Bone Joint Surg Br* 1977;59:473-480.

14. Lichtenstein L, Bernstein D: Unusual benign and malignant chondroid tumors of bone. *Cancer* 1959;12:1142-1147.

15. Goldman RL: "Mesenchymal" chondrosarcoma, a rare malignant chondroid tumor usually primary in bone: Report of a case arising in extraskeletal soft tissue. *Cancer* 1967;20:1494-1498.

16. Dahlin DC, Beabout JW: Dedifferentiation of low-grade chondrosarcoma. *Cancer* 1971;28:461-466.

17. O'Neal LW, Ackerman LV: Chondrosarcoma of bone. *Cancer* 1952;5:551-557.

18. Henderson ED, Dahlin DC: Chondrosarcoma of bone: A study of two-hundred and eighty-eight cases. *J Bone Joint Surg Am* 1963;45:1450-1458.

19. Barnes R, Catto M: Chondrosarcoma of bone. *J Bone Joint Surg Br* 1966;48:729-764.

20. Campanacci M: *Bone and Soft Tissue Tumors*, ed 2. New York, NY, Springer Verlag, 1999, pp 283-379.

21. Campanacci M, Guernelli N, Leonessa C, Boni A: Chondrosarcoma: A study of 133 cases, 80 with long term followup. *Ital J Orthop Traumatol* 1975;1:387-414.

22. Eriksson AL, Schiller A, Mankin HJ: The management of chondrosarcoma of bone. *Clin Orthop Relat Res* 1980;153:44-66.

23. Gitelis S, Bertoni F, Picci P, Campanacci M: Chondrosarcoma of bone: The experience of the Istituto Ortopedico Rizzoli. *J Bone Joint Surg Am* 1981;63:1248-1257.

24. Jaffe HL: *Tumors and Tumorous Conditions of the Bones and Joints*. Philadelphia, PA, Lea and Febiger, 1958, pp 314-340.

25. Marcove RC: Chondrosarcoma: Diagnosis and treatment. *Orthop Clin North Am* 1977;8:811-820.

26. Schajowicz F: *Tumors and Tumorlike Lesions of Bone and Joints*. New York, NY, Springer Verlag, 1981, pp 160-204.

27. Evans HL, Ayala AG, Romsdahl MM: Prognostic factors in chondrosarcoma of bone: A clinico-pathologic analysis with emphasis on histologic grading. *Cancer* 1977;40:818-831.

28. Ishida T, Kikuchi F, Machinami R: Histological grading and morphometric analysis of cartilaginous tumors. *Virchows Arch A Pathol Anat Histopathol* 1991;418:149-155.

29. Lee FY, Mankin HJ, Fondren G, et al: Chondrosarcoma of bone: An assessment of outcome. *J Bone Joint Surg Am* 1999;81:326-338.

30. Mankin HJ, Cantley KP, Lippiello L, Schiller AL, Campbell CJ: The biology of human chondrosarcoma: I. Description of the cases, grading and biochemical analysis. *J Bone Joint Surg* 1980;62:160-176.

31. Mankin HJ, Cantley KP, Schiller AL, Lippiello L: The biology of human chondrosarcoma II: Variation in chemical composition among types and subtypes of benign and malignant cartilage tumors. *J Bone Joint Surg Am* 1980;62:176-188.

32. Rosenthal DI, Schiller AL, Mankin HJ: Chondrosarcoma: Correlation of radiologic and histologic grade. *Radiology* 1984;150:21-26.

33. Bertoni F, Present D, Bacchini P, et al: Dedifferentiated peripheral chondrosarcomas: A report of seven cases. *Cancer* 1989;63:2054-2059.

34. Bruns J, Fiedler W, Werner M, Delling G: Dedifferentiated chondrosarcoma: A fatal disease. *J Cancer Res Clin Oncol* 2005;131:333-339.

35. Capanna R, Bertoni RF, Bettelli G, et al: Dedifferentiated chondrosarcoma. *J Bone Joint Surg Am* 1988;70:60-69.

36. Dickey ID, Rose PS, Fuchs B, et al: Dedifferentiated chondrosarcoma: The role of chemotherapy with updated outcomes. *J Bone Joint Surg Am* 2004;86:2412-2418.

37. Frassica FJ, Unni KK, Beabout JW, Sim FH: Dedifferentiated chondrosarcoma: A report of the clinicopathological features and treatment of seventy-eight cases. *J Bone Joint Surg Am* 1986;68:1197-1205.

38. Mitchell AD, Ayoub K, Mangham DC, et al: Experience in the treatment of dedifferentiated chondrosarcoma. *J Bone Joint Surg Br* 1980;82:55-61.

39. Bjornsson J, Unni KK, Dahlin DC, et al: Clear cell chondrosarcoma of bone: Observations in 47 cases. *Am J Surg Pathol* 1984;8:223-230.

40. Itala A, Leerapun T, Inwards C, Collins M, Scully SP: An institutional review of clear cell chondrosarcoma. *Clin Orthop Relat Res* 2005;440:209-212.

41. Kumar R, David R, Cierney G III: Clear cell chondrosarcoma. *Radiology* 1985;154:45-48.

42. Leggon RE Jr, Unni KK, Beabout JW, Sim FH: Clear-cell chondrosarcoma. *Orthopedics* 1990;13:593-596.

43. Collins MS, Koyama T, Swee RG, Inwards CY: Clear cell condrosarcoma: Radiographic, computed tomographic and magnetic resonance findings in 34 patients with pathologic correlation. *Skeletal Radiol* 2003;32:687-694.

44. Weiss A-PC, Dorfman HD: Clear-cell chondrosarcoma: A report of ten cases and review of the literature. *Surg Pathol* 1988;1:123-129.

45. Bertoni F, Picci P, Bacchini P: Mesenchymal chondrosarcoma of bone and soft tissues. *Cancer* 1983;52:533-541.

46. Ranjan A, Chacko G, Joseph T, Chandi SM: Intraspinal mesenchymal chondrosarcoma: Case report. *J Neurosurg* 1994;80:928-930.

47. Salvador AH, Beabout JW, Dahlin DC: Mesenchymal chondrosarcoma: Observation on 30 new cases. *Cancer* 1971;28:605-615.

48. Takahashi K, Sato K, Kanazawa H, Wang XL, Kimura T: Mesenchymal chondrosarcoma of the jaw: Report of a case and review of 41 cases in the literature. *Head Neck* 1993;15:459-464.

49. Nakashima Y, Unni KK, Shifves TC, Swee RG, Dahlin DC: Mesenchymal chondrosarcoma of bone and soft tissue: A review of 111 cases. *Cancer* 1986;57:2444-2453.

50. Swanson PE, Lillemoe TJ, Manivel JC, Wick MR: Mesenchymal chondrosarcoma: An immunohistochemical study. *Arch Pathol Lab Med* 1990;114:943-948.

51. Soder S, Oliveira AM, Inwards CY, Muller S, Aigner T: Type II collagen, but not aggrecan expression distinguishes clear cell chondrosarcoma and chondroblastoma. *Pathology* 2006;38:35-38.

52. Sreekantaiah C, Leong SP, Davis JR, Sandberg AA: Cytogenetic and flow cytometric analysis of a clear cell chondrosarcoma. *Cancer Genet Cytogenet* 1991;52:193-199.

53. Endo M, Matsumura T, Yamaguchi T, et al: Cyclooxygenase –2 overexpression associated with a poor prognosis in chondrosarcomas. *Hum Pathol* 2006;37:471-476.

54. Sutton KM, Wright M, Fondren G, Towle CA,

Mankin HJ: Cyclooxygenase-2 expression in chondrosarcoma. *Oncology* 2004;66:275-280.

55. Weiss AP, Dorfman HD: S-100 protein in human cartilage lesions. *J Bone Joint Surg Am* 1986;68:521-526.

56. Alho A, Connor JF, Mankin HJ, Schiller AL, Campbell CJ: Assessment of malignancy of cartilage tumors using flow cytometry: A preliminary report. *J Bone Joint Surg Am* 1983;65:779-785.

57. Alho A, Skjeldal S, Melvik JE, Pettersen EO, Larsen TE: The clinical importance of DNA synthesis and aneuploidy in bone and soft tissue tumours. *Anticancer Res* 1993;13:2383-2387.

58. Kreicsbergs A, Boquist L, Borssen B, Larsson SE: Prognostic factors in chondrosarcoma: A comparative study of cellular DNA content and clinicopathologic features. *Cancer* 1982;50:577-583.

59. Mankin HJ, Fondren G, Hornicek FJ, Gebhardt MD, Rosenberg AE: The use of flow cytometry in assessing malignancy in bone and soft tissue tumors. *Clin Orthop Relat Res* 2002;397:95-105.

60. Mandahl N, Heim S, Arheden K, et al: Chromosomal rearrangements in chondromatous tumors. *Cancer* 1990;65:242-248.

61. Terek RM: Recent advances in the basic science of chondrosarcoma. *Orthop Clin North Am* 2006;37:9-14.

62. Ozusik YY, Meloni AM, Peier A, et al: Cytogenetic findings in 19 malignant bone tumors . *Cancer* 1994;74:2268-2275.

63. Sandberg AA: Genetics of chondrosarcoma and related tumors. *Curr Opin Oncol* 2004;16:342-354.

64. Dobashi Y, Sugimura H, Sato A, et al: Possible association of p53 overexpression and mutation with high-grade chondrosarcoma. *Diagn Mol Pathol* 1993;2:257-16.

65. Simms W, Ordonez N, Johnston D, Ayala AG, Czerniak B: p53 expression in dedifferentiated chondrosarcoma. *Cancer* 1995;76:223-227.

66. Rozeman LB, Szuhai K, Schrage YM, et al: Array-comparative genomic hybridization of central chondrosarcoma: Identification of ribosomal protein S6 and cyclin-dependent kinase 4 as candidate target genes for genomic aberrations. *Cancer* 2006;107:380-388.

67. Crim JR, Seeger LL: Diagnosis of low-grade chondrosarcoma. *Radiology* 1993;189:503-504.

68. Hudson TM, Manaster BJ, Springfield DS, et al: Radiology of medullary chondrosarcoma: Preoperative treatment planning. *Skeletal Radiol* 1983;10:69-78.

69. Exner GU, von Hochstetter AR, Augustiny N, von Schulthess GL: Magnetic resonance imaging in malignant bone tumors. *Int Orthop* 1990;14:49-55.

70. Lindblom A, Soderberg G, Spjut JH: Primary chondrosarcoma of bone. *Acta Radiol* 1961;55:81-96.

71. Donati D, El Ghoneimy A, Bertoni F, DiBella C, Mercuri M: Surgical treatment and outcome of conventional pelvic chondrosarcoma. *J Bone Joint Surg Br* 2005;87:1527-1530.

72. Pachter MR, Alpert M: Chondrosarcoma of the foot skeleton. *J Bone Joint Surg Am* 1964;46:601-607.

73. Patil S, de Silvas MV, Crossan J, Reid R: Chondrosarcoma of the small bones of the hand. *J Hand Surg [Br]* 2003;28:602-608.

74. Shives TC, McLeond RA, Unni KK, Schray MF: Chondrosarcoma of the spine. *J Bone Joint Surg Am* 1989;71:1158-1165.

75. Zeytoonjian T, Mankin HJ, Gebhardt MC, Hornicek FJ: Distal lower extremity sarcomas: Frequency of occurrence and patient survival rate. *Foot Ankle Internat* 2004;25:325-330.

76. Kristensen JB, Sunde LM, Jensen OM: Chondrosarcoma: Increasing grade of malignancy in local recurrence. *Acta Pathol Microbiol Immunol Scand A* 1986;94:73-77.

77. Dodd LG: Fine needle aspiration of chondrosarcoma. *Diagn Cytopathol* 2006;34:413-418.

78. Ahlmann ER, Menendez LR, Fedenko AN, Learch T: Influence of cryosurgery on treatment outcome of low-grade chondrosarcoma. *Clin Orthop Relat Res* 2006;451:201-207.

79. Marcove RC, Stovell PB, Huvos AG, Bullough PG: The use of cryosurgery in the treatment of low and medium grade chondrosarcoma. *Clin Orthop Relat Res* 1977;122:147-155.

Chapter 2

Central Osteosarcoma

Although relatively rare by standards of other malignant tumors, central osteosarcoma is the most common primary malignancy of bone.[1-6] The tumor most often affects young people between 10 and 25 years of age and the most frequent sites are the metaphyseal regions of the distal femur and proximal tibia.[3,4,7] Fewer than 1,500 new cases are seen annually in the United States.[4,7] There are several disorders that resemble the standard central osteosarcoma and these should be ruled out before the definitive diagnosis is established. Parosteal osteosarcoma arises from the periosteum of long bones and is a much more benign lesion with a high survival rate.[3,7,8] Metachronous osteosarcoma also seems to have a higher survival rate.[9] Paget's sarcoma has the clinical and histologic appearance of central osteosarcoma but occurs in patients with diffuse Paget's disease.[3,4,7,10] The prognosis is much worse than for central osteosarcoma, with almost all patients dying of disease in less than 5 years. Radiation-induced osteosarcoma, although a rare event today, occurred with high frequency among the "Radium Girls," who in the early part of the 20th century used their fingers and tongues (to wet paintbrushes) to put radium into watch dials.[7,10-12]

Furthermore, in terms of the histologic appearance, pathologists have introduced the terms chondroblastic, fibroblastic, and telangiectatic and, with perhaps the exception of the last mentioned, the lesions do not seem to differ greatly in prognosis.[3,7,13,14]

Historical Data

The earliest description of malignant connective tissue neoplasms was by Abernethy[15] in 1804, who described a malignant bone tumor and was the first to introduce the term "sarcoma" to describe it. Shortly thereafter, in 1805, Dupuytren[16] described a similar tumor arising from bone and alluded to its aggressiveness and the likelihood of metastasis. The more extensive description of connective tissue tumors and, more specifically, those within or arising from the

bone were those of Rudolf Virchow,[17] in his remarkable three-volume series published from 1863 to 1867. The majority of the cases presented in his collection were osteosarcomas and giant cell tumors. Virchow was considered to be the father of bone pathology and indicated that although these tumors were a problem for patients, they were much rarer than carcinomas.[17] In 1845, Hermann Lebert[18] published an illustrated atlas titled *Physiologie Pathologique*, in which he used artist renderings of cut sections of tumors arising from bone to identify them and distinguish them from other forms of cancer. It was not until 1879, however, that osteosarcoma was clearly described by Samuel Gross[19] as a highly malignant bone-forming neoplasm. In his series of 165 cases, 28 were central osteosarcomas and a high percentage of these metastasized to the lungs. In 1922, Ernest Amory Codman[20] first described the tumor as an osteogenic sarcoma, and in 1925, along with James Ewing and Joseph Bloodgood, he established a Bone Tumor Registry that included a large number of patients from the eastern part of the United States with osteosarcomas.[21,22] Codman is also responsible for describing "Codman's triangle," which on radiographs appeared as a benign collection of periosteal new bone at the margin of distal femoral or proximal tibial osteosarcomas[7,20] (Figure 1). In 1936, Charles Geschickter and Murray Copeland[23] published *Tumors of Bone (Including the Jaws and Joints)*, which further described the disease. In 1950, Coley and Harrold[24] reported an 11% survival for patients with osteosarcoma from the Sloan Kettering Cancer Memorial Hospital in New York City, and in the mid-1950s, Henry Jaffe,[25] Louis Lichtenstein,[26] and Beller and Stein[27] all stated that only 10% of patients with osteosarcoma are likely to survive. In 1957, Coventry and Dahlin[28] defined the 10-year survival rate for patients with osteosarcoma treated at the Mayo Clinic to be 15%. In 1962, Weinfeld and Dudley[29] reported a follow-up study on 94 patients treated at Massachusetts General Hospital (MGH) and

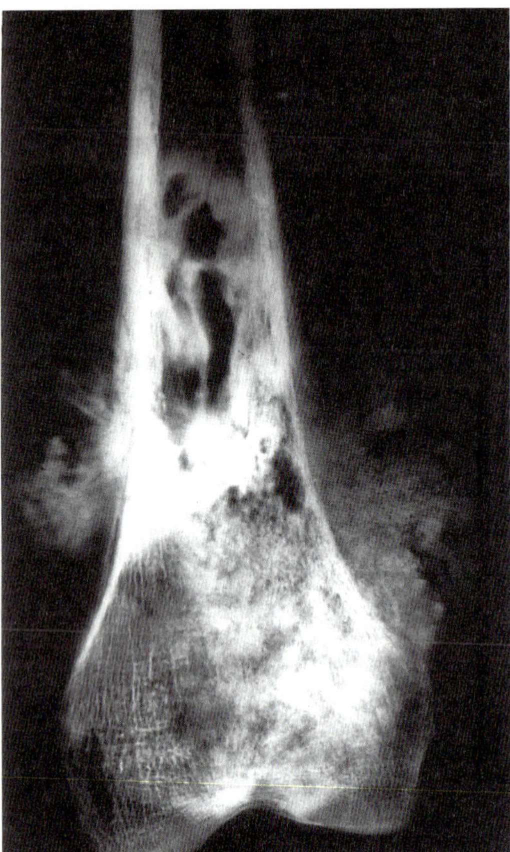

Figure 1
Radiograph of a distal femoral osteosarcoma showing the destruction of the cortex, moderate expansion of the bone, and periosteal new bone adjacent to the site (Codman's triangles).

stated that the 5-year and 10-year survival rates were 14% and 9%, respectively. Even with amputation, the prognosis for patients with these tumors was considered among the worst for connective tissue lesions.[2,4,5,14,20,23,24,28,30] In 1893, W. B. Coley[31] introduced a treatment protocol described as "Coley's Toxin," which was a material derived from the bacterial disorder, erysipelas; in 1905, he also attempted to treat the tumors with radiation.[32] Neither of these approaches was considered to be successful.

Physiology

Central osteosarcoma is most often encountered in the distal femur or proximal tibia in patients 10 through 25 years of age and is thought to be slightly more common in males than females.[1-8,25,28,30,33-36] It is also common in large dogs, namely Great Danes, Saint Bernards, and German Shepherds.[37]

Although no clear genetic error is associated with the entity in either humans or animals,[7,37] the disease is known to have a relationship with retinoblastoma in the Li Fraumeni syndrome.[7,38-41] Another lesion associated with osteosarcoma is the Rothmund-Thomson syndrome, an autosomal recessive disorder consisting of congenital bone defects, hair and skin dysplasias, hypogonadism, and cataracts.[7,42-45] Some of the more aggressive central osteosarcoma lesions show a greater degree of aneuploidy on flow cytometry[4,46,47] or germ cell alterations in p53 or c-fos.[48-54] In addition, investigators have recently described gene and enzyme factors including MDM2[49,51,53] and HER2/erb-2,[55-57] cyclooxygenase-2,[58] proliferating cell nuclear antigen (PCNA),[49] P-glycoprotein,[53,59-61] and bone morphogenetic proteins.[62] Some of these factors, especially p53 and MDM2, are believed to indicate an increased malignancy of the tumor.

Some of the rarer special forms of central osteosarcoma include telangiectatic, fibrohistiocytic, chondroblastic, and metachronous osteosarcomas,[7,9,13,14] but only the last two seem to have a better outcome than the rest.

Imaging, Histologic, and Laboratory Studies

Imaging studies of osteosarcoma are an essential part of the diagnostic and prognostic studies. Lesions are almost always centrally placed and very destructive on radiography and frequently contain large quantities of irregular bony and calcified structures[2-8,30,63] (Figure 1). Most of the tumors appear to have broken out of the bone by the time of discovery and have a soft-tissue mass that is often heavily ossified (or calcified) on one side or sometimes surrounding the bone.[3,7,8,63] The periosteum distal or proximal to the lesion usually shows displacement from the bone, with small amounts of normal-looking bone placed subjacently (Figure 2). These are called Codman's triangles.[3,7,20,21] Occasionally, the tumors break into the joint and may extend into the adjacent bone. Lesions of the pelvis or scapula and even of the proximal humerus are frequently considerably larger than those of the distal femur or proximal tibia, and lesions of the foot or hand bones are generally smaller in size and believed to be considerably less malignant.[1,3,6,7,64-66]

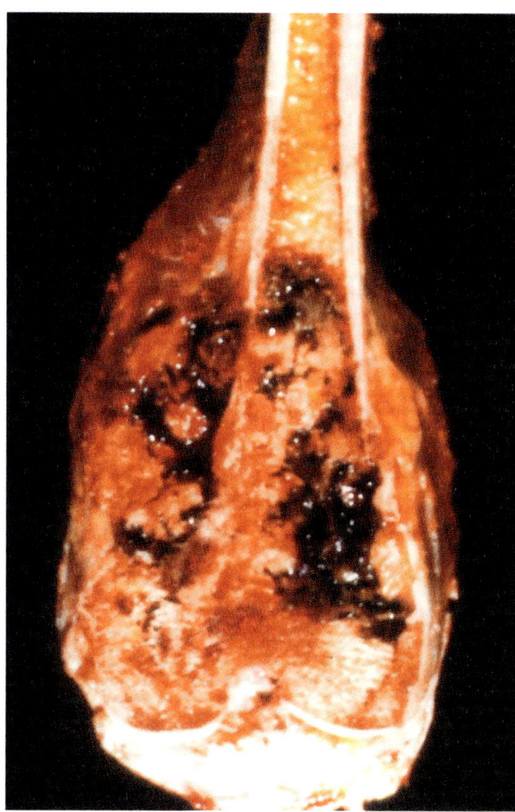

Figure 2
A photograph of the gross specimen of the tumor seen as a radiographic image in Figure 1. The tissue shows expansion, and there is a marked cortical destruction and irregular ossification and tissue substances within and outside the bone.

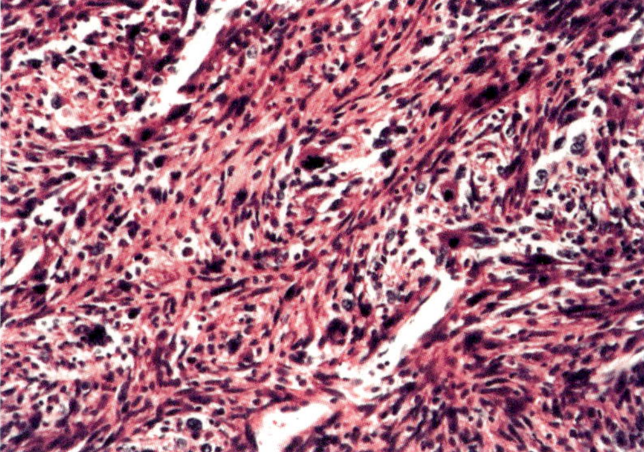

Figure 3
Histologic picture of the tumor shown in Figures 1 and 2. The tissue shows marked cellular atypism and contains many multinucleated cells and some with mitotic figures.

Bone scans are always positive and sometimes disclose the presence of tumors at different sites in the shaft of the affected bone or in other bony parts.[3,7,67] Computed tomography studies are helpful in planning surgery, in the sense that they show the extent of the lesion in the bone, and MRI is very valuable in assessing the degree of the soft-tissue extension.[3,4,7,68,69] These studies are particularly valuable for lesions arising from the pelvis and the spine.[3,7,64] A CT scan of the chest is an essential part of the study initially, and regularly in the post-treatment and postoperative periods; it should be done as often as every 3 to 6 months after treatment and less frequently after the first 2 years.[3,4,7] Studies using positron emission topography scanning may be helpful in identifying the presence of metastases in sites such as the liver, brain, kidneys, lymph nodes, or in other bones.

The biopsy is essential to establish the diagnosis and plan for treatment. Open biopsies may cause problems with wound healing or increase the extent of the subsequent surgery. Recently, CT-guided core biopsies have been introduced and are more easily performed and less likely to cause complications.[4,7] The tissue obtained will often show hypercellularity with marked cellular atypism, pleomorphism, atypical spindle cells, clusters of giant cells, and sometimes bizarre mitotic figures in a telangiectatic vascular bed[3,7,8] (Figure 3). Abnormal cartilage or fibrous tissue may be present and both sometimes calcify. Within the tumor are areas of small or medium irregular islands of woven bone production, sometimes dense and sclerotic in nature[3,7,8,63] (Figure 4). Tumors may be graded by the Musculoskeletal Tumor Society (MSTS) grading system and hence may be considered as low grade (IA or IB), high grade (IIA, IIB), or already metastatic at the time of discovery (III).[70]

Of the available laboratory studies, the alkaline phosphatase is almost always increased, as is the erythrocyte sedimentation rate. Liver and renal studies should also be performed as part of the initial workup.

Treatment Protocols and Results

Survival data for patients with central osteosarcoma until the early 1970s were very poor and approximated only 10% to 15%. In a classic article by Goorin and associates,[71] published in the *New England Journal of Medicine* in 1985, the authors described the changes, which occurred over the previous 15 years, that led to an increase in the survival rate from 10% to approximately 70%. Although Coley had introduced his toxin in

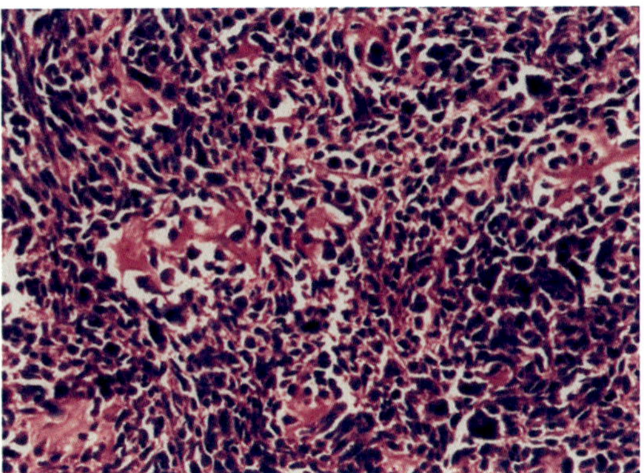

Figure 4

Another higher power histologic picture of the tissue from the specimen shown in Figure 1. The cells are osteoblastic in character and are making segments of new bone. The cells show marked atypism.

1893 and radiation in 1905, both were ineffective. The new era began in 1973, with a spectacular contribution by Jaffe and associates,[72] who reported the successful use of methotrexate with citrovorum rescue for patients with osteosarcoma. The subsequent introduction of doxorubicin by Cores and associates,[73] and ifosfamide, cisplatinum, and cyclophosphamide by others, led to a marked diminution in the frequency and growth rates of metastatic deposits for patients with osteosarcoma.[3,7,34-36,41,74-78] The introduction of neoadjunctive therapy by Rosen and his associates was a major contribution that markedly reduced the patient's metastasis rate.[7,76,79-89] Current studies suggest that in the last decade, the overall rate for patient survival approximates 70%.[1,3,4,7,33-35,51,74,76,80,85,88,90,91]

Surgical procedures initially consisted of amputation,[7,25,30] but with the advent of chemotherapy and the possibility that radiation could further reduce the size of the lesion,[3,7,92,93] it was possible to perform limb-sparing procedures. These included resection, metallic implant, or allograft. Initially the metallic devices were specifically designed and constructed for each patient, but this became unnecessary with technical improvements in the devices.[1,2,4,7,34,35,71,77,80,91,94,95] The systems now consist of modular devices, often with attached joint arthroplasty systems for hip, femur, tibia, and humerus.[80,95] The other technique, which was used for patients after wide resections of the lesion, was allograft

implantation, originally introduced for high-grade tumors in the late 1960s.[4,96] Several studies have been performed that have demonstrated the efficacy of such devices; although the complication rate remains somewhat high, the procedures are often successful in returning the patient to excellent function.[4,96] Other techniques include turn-up plasty and turn-about techniques.[2-4,7,51] In both of these, most of or sometimes the entire femur may be removed and replaced by either a "turned up" or a "turned about" tibia, which then continues to grow in the immature patient.

In a recent study performed by the orthopaedic oncology team at MGH on 648 patients with central osteosarcoma treated before June 2001, 438 are alive (68%) at a mean duration of follow-up of 6 years with a range up to 23 years.[4] Two hundred ten of the patients (32%) have died of disease. There was no difference in the survival rate for males and females. Patient age, however, had a significant effect. The survival rate for the patients younger than 20 years of age was 78%, while that for those from 20 to 40 years of age was 70%. Older patients had a much lower survival rate; this was especially noticeable in 89 patients older than 55 years of age, for whom the survival rate dropped to 39%. This finding concurs with the result reported by Carsi and Rock in 2002.[90] A study of MSTS stage showed that 463 of the patients were classified as stage IIA or stage IIB and their survival rate was 71%. The survival rate for the 48 patients with stage IA or IB was 79%, and that for 78 stage III patients was 50%.

In terms of anatomic site, the frequencies of tumors about the knee, proximal humerus, proximal femur, and pelvic sites found in this series were essentially the same. The survival rate for the 146 patients with osteosarcomas of the lumbar spine, pelvis, and proximal and mid-femur was significantly different from that for the 331 patients with tumors of the distal femur or proximal tibia.[3,7,64] Two hundred ninety-one patients had an allograft replacement as part of their surgical management system. Although the survival rate for these patients was 71%, the success rate of the surgical procedure itself was 64%. Forty-nine patients had an amputation either initially or subsequent to some procedure that failed. The number of patients who died in this group was 18, for a survival rate of 63%. This value was not statistically different from the ones for the allograft or metallic implant procedures.[3,7,95,96]

Effect of Chemotherapy

Adjuvant chemotherapy for osteosarcoma evolved over the time span of this patient experience. In the period from 1972 to 1980, 22 patients from the MGH series received a relatively low dose of methotrexate and doxorubicin chemotherapy, which at the time was reported to be an effective treatment of osteosarcoma. These patients had a survival rate of only 41%. In the next decade, 214 patients received much larger doses of adjuvant chemotherapy for at least 6 months, often with the addition of cisplatinum. The survival rate for this group of patients was 57%. In the period from 1990 to 2000, the intensity of chemotherapy was increased, neoadjuvant treatment was used for all patients who could tolerate it, and higher doses of doxorubicin and cisplatinum became the norm. For poor responders, according to examination of the specimen for percent kill, ifosfamide plus etoposide with or without carboplatin were added to the postoperative regimen. The survival rate for this group of 320 patients was 72%. Still of some concern are the poorer rates of survival of patients with pelvic tumors, those who are older than age 40 years,[90] and those who have a local recurrence after surgical resection.[3,4,6,33,82,97,98] In addition, pre- and postoperative radiation have been used in the MGH and other series for patients with poor surgical margins.[3,7,92,93] Metastatic and locally recurrent tumors are very troublesome but can be treated with radiation, chemotherapy, and surgical resections.[3,4,7,88] The survival rate is poor, however.[4,7,43,88]

Discussion

Several studies have provided similar data to those reported by MGH Orthopaedic Oncology. Of some importance was a study performed in the late 1980s by a cooperative group, in which patients with osteosarcoma were randomly assigned to either receive chemotherapy or to have no systemic treatment.[75] The projected 6-year survival for the chemotherapy group was 67%, while that for the no-treatment patients was only 14%.[75] A 1999 report on 136 patients with stage II osteosarcoma from the University of Muenster defined the average patient survival to be 78%,[91] and in 2000, a Hungarian group study showed a value of 72% for 96 patients of all MSTS stages.[94] In 2001, the Rizzoli Institute reported a 67% success rate for 140 patients,[79] and in 2002, a cooperative group in Germany and the Netherlands showed a 60% survival rate for 570 patients.[1,36] Similar results were shown in studies reported from Scandinavia.[33,83]

The data obtained during more than 20 years of follow-up for the MGH series show that the anatomic site of the tumor, the MSTS stage, the age of the patient, the use of chemotherapy, the size of the lesion, and the percent kill of the specimen after adjuvant chemotherapy all had significant predictive effects on the outcome in terms of survival. Based on these data, it is possible to predict that a young patient with a small lesion located below the knee or elbow, which is an MSTS stage I or II, whose specimen after neoadjuvant treatment has a percent kill of 90% is highly likely to survive, while an older patient with a large stage II or III pelvic, proximal, or midfemoral or proximal humeral tumor whose percent kill after neoadjuvant therapy is less than 90% has a high risk of metastases developing and death within a 3-year period.

The most important aspect of this study is the challenge. Jaffe[25] and Lichtenstein[26] separately reported a 10% survival rate for patients with osteosarcoma treated in the early 1950s, and the values were not really greatly improved until the introduction of chemotherapy and improved imaging technology in the 1970s. Neoadjuvant chemotherapy further increased survival.

In their remarkable review in the *New England Journal of Medicine*, Goorin and associates[71] indicated that in the preceding 15 years, the use of neoadjuvant chemotherapy and improvement in surgical technology had brought the survival rate up to 65% to 75%. The question is whether it will be possible for someone to write another article about the 15 years between 1985 and 2000 and demonstrate that we have significantly increased our rate of survival for patients with central osteosarcoma. The data really do not support that as yet, which suggests that the MGH statistic seems to be stable over the past 10+ years.

Some questions arise that may, if answered, help our patients conquer this terrible disease. Can we discover markers, which will define the virulence of the tumor more effectively than current studies or the ones described in this chapter? Recent studies have proposed a number of these, which may help to assess the likelihood of increased risk of metastasis or death. Controversy exists regarding whether P-glycoprotein may be a prognostic factor for the response to chemotherapy and clinical disease progression for patients with osteosarcoma. As in breast cancer, HER2/neu expression in patients with osteosarcoma seems to be associated with an increased risk of metastasis and may define a subset of patients with a more aggressive tumor phenotype, but some additional studies are less supportive. The clinical value of MDM2 protein in osteosarcoma is as yet unresolved, as is the value of the expression of bone morphogenetic proteins in patients with osteosarcomas.

Are there new drugs available that may help to limit the likelihood of metastasis or local recurrence? Are there ways of decreasing the rate of metastasis by introducing agents to the tumor or the patient? Will antiangiogenesis factors or materials that enhance the rate of apoptotic activity or agents, which decrease the capacity of the tumor to destroy collagen and invade blood vessels, be added to our therapeutic regimen? Will any or all of these bring the rate of success above the current just barely acceptable level?

That is the challenge, and it is hoped that using these technologies will help us arrive at some means or methods of improving the life and survival status of our patients.

References

1. Bielack SS, Kempf-Bielack B, Delling G, et al: Prognostic factors in high-grade osteosarcoma of the extremities or trunk: An analysis of 1,702 patients treated on neoadjuvant cooperative osteosarcoma study group protocols. *J Clin Oncol* 2002;20:776-790.

2. Campanacci M, Cervellati C: Osteosarcoma: A review of 345 cases. *Ital J Orthop Traumatol* 1975;1:5-22.

3. Campanacci M: *Bone and Soft Tissue Tumors*. New York, NY, Springer, 1999, pp 463-516.

4. Mankin HJ, Hornicek FJ, Rosenberg AE, Harmon DC, Gebhardt MC: Survival data for 648 patients with osteosarcoma treated at one institution. *Clin Orthop Relat Res* 2004;429:286-291.

5. Sweetnam R: Osteosarcoma. *Ann R Coll Surg Engl* 1969;44:38-58.

6. Unni KK: *Dahlin's Bone Tumors: General Aspects and Data on 11,087 Cases*, ed 5. Philadelphia, PA, Lippincott Raven, 1996, pp 143-184.

7. Dorfman HD, Czerniak B, eds: *Bone Tumors*. St Louis, MO, Mosby, 1998, pp 128-252.

8. Jaffe HL: *Tumors and Tumorous Conditions of the Bones and Joints*. Philadelpha, PA, Lea and Febiger, 1958, pp 256-278.

9. Rodriguez EK, Hornicek FJ, Gebhardt MC, Mankin HJ: Metachronous osteosarcoma: A report of five cases. *Clin Orthop Relat Res* 2003;411:227-235.

10. Frassica FJ, Sim SH, Frassica DA, Wold LE: Survival and management considerations in post irradiation osteosarcoma and Paget's osteosarcoma. *Clin Orthop Relat Res* 1991;270:120-127.

11. Clark C: *Radium Girls: Women and Industrial Health Reform, 1910-1935*. Chapel Hill, NC, University of North Carolina Press, 1997.

12. Hatcher CH: The development of sarcoma in bone subjected to roentgen or radium irradiation. *J Bone Joint Surg* 1945;27:179-195.

13. Mervak TR, Unni KK, Pritchard DJ, McLeod RA: Telangiectatic osteosarcoma. *Clin Orthop Relat Res* 1991;270:135-139.

14. McKenna RJ, Schwinn CP, Soong KY, Higinbotham NL: Sarcoma of the osteogenic series (osteosarcoma, fibrosarcoma, chondrosarcoma, periosteal osteosarcoma and sarcomata arising in abnormal bone): An analysis of 552 cases. *J Bone Joint Surg Am* 1966;48:1-26.

15. Abernethy J: *Surgical Observations on Tumors*. London, England, Longman and Rees, 1804.

16. Dupuytren G: Tumors of bone. *Bull Ecole Med de Paris* 1805;2:13-24.

17. Virchow R: *Die Krankhaften Gewulste*. Berlin, Germany, Hirschwald, 1863-1867 (3 volumes).

18. Lebert J: *Physiologie Pathologique*. Paris, France, JB Balliere, 1845.

19. Gross SW: The classic: Sarcoma of the long bones. Based upon a study of one hundred and sixty-five cases: 1879. *Clin Orthop Relat Res* 2005;438:9-14.

20. Codman EA: The registry of cases of bone sarcoma. *Surg Gynecol Obstet* 1922;34:335-343.

21. Codman EA: *Bone Sarcoma: An Interpretation of the Nomenclature Used by the Committee on the Registry of Bone Sarcoma of the American College of Surgeons*. New York, NY, Paul B. Hoeber, 1925.

22. Ewing J: A review and classification of bone sarcomas. *Arch Surg* 1922;4:485-533.

23. Geschickter CF, Copeland MM: *Tumors of Bone (Including the Jaws and Joints)*, ed 2. New York, NY, American Journal of Cancer, 1936.

24. Coley BL, Harrold CC Jr: An analysis of 59 cases of osteogenic sarcoma with survival for 5 years or more. *J Bone Joint Surg Am* 1950;32:307-310.

25. Jaffe HL: Osteogenic sarcoma of bone. *Clin Orthop Relat Res* 1956;7:27-40.

26. Lichtenstein L: *Bone Tumors*. St Louis, MO, CV Mosby Company, 1959, pp 191-214.

27. Beller ML, Stein I: Osteogenic sarcoma of bone. *Clin Orthop* 1956;7:41-46.

28. Coventry MB, Dahlin DC: Osteogenic sarcoma: A critical analysis of 430 cases. *J Bone Joint Surg Am* 1957;39:741-758.

29. Weinfeld MS, Dudley HR Jr: Osteogenic sarcoma: A follow-up study of the ninety-four cases observed at the Massachusetts General Hospital from 1920 to 1960. *J Bone Joint Surg Am* 1962;44:269-276.

30. Dahlin DC, Coventry MB: Osteogenic sarcoma: A study of six hundred cases. *J Bone Joint Surg Am* 1967;49:101-110.

31. Coley WB: The treatment of malignant tumors by repeated inoculations of erysipelas: With a report of ten original cases. 1893. *Clin Orthop Relat Res* 1991;202:3-11.

32. Coley WB: I: Final results in the X-ray treatments of cancer, including sarcoma. *Ann Surg* 1905;42:161-184.

33. Brosjö O: Surgical procedure and local recurrence in 223 patients treated between 1982-1997 according to two osteosarcoma chemotherapy protocols: The Scandinavian Sarcoma Group experience. *Acta Orthop Scand Suppl* 1999;285:58-61.

34. Ogihara Y, Sudo A, Fujinami S, Sato K, Miura T: Current management, local management, and survival statistics of high grade osteosarcoma: Experience in Japan. *Clin Orthop Relat Res* 1991;270:72-78.

35. Smeland S, Müller C, Alvegard TA, et al: Scandinavian Sarcoma Group Osteosarcoma Study SSG VIII: Prognostic factors for outcome and role of replacement salvage chemotherapy for poor histological responders. *Eur J Cancer* 2003;39:488-494.

36. Veth RP: IIB osteosarcoma: Current management, local control and survival statistics. The Netherlands. *Clin Orthop Relat Res* 1991;270:67-71.

37. Withrow SJ, Powers BE, Straw RC, Wilkins RM: Comparative aspects of osteosarcoma: Dog versus man. *Clin Orthop Relat Res* 1991;270 :159-168.

38. Draper GJ, Sanders BM, Kingston JE: Second primary neoplasms in patients with retinoblastoma. *Br J Cancer* 1986;53:661-671.

39. Li FP, Fraumeni JF Jr, Mulvihill JJ, et al: A cancer family syndrome in twenty-four kindreds. *Cancer Res* 1988;48:5358-5362.

40. Potepan P, Luksch R, Sozzi G, et al: Multifocal osteosarcoma as second tumor after childhood retinoblastoma. *Skeletal Radiol* 1999;28:415-421.

41. Stine KC, Saylors RL, Saccente S, Becton DL: Long-term survival in osteosarcoma patients following retinoblastoma use doxorubicin, cisplatin and methotrexate. *Med Pediatr Oncol* 2003;41:77-78.

42. Anbari KK, Ierardi-Curto LA, Silber JS, et al: Two primary osteosarcomas in a patient with Rothmund-Thomson syndrome. *Clin Orthop Relat Res* 2000;378:213-223.

43. Cumin I, Cohen JY, David A, Méchinaud F, Avet-Loiseau H, Harousseau JL: Rothmund Thomson syndrome and osteosarcoma. *Med Pediatr Oncol* 1996;26:414-416.

44. Dick DC, Morley WN, Watson JT: Rothmund Thomson syndrome and osteogenic sarcoma. *Clin Exp Dermatol* 1982;7:119-123.

45. Pujol LA, Erickson RP, Heidenreich RA, Cunniff C: Variable presentation of Rothmund-Thomson syndrome. *Am J Med Genet* 2000;95:204-207.

46. Alho A, Connor JF, Mankin HJ, Schiller AL, Campbell CJ: Assessment of malignancy of cartilage tumors using flow cytometry: A preliminary report. *J Bone Joint Surg Am* 1983;65:779-785.

47. Mankin HJ, Gebhardt MC, Springfield DS, Litwak GJ, Kusazaki K, Rosenberg AE: Flow cytometric studies of human osteosarcoma. *Clin Orthop Relat Res* 1991;270:169-180.

48. Gokgoz N, Wunderf JS, Mousses S, Eskandarian S, Bell RS, Andrulis IL: Comparison of p53 mutations in patients with localized osteosarcoma and metastatic osteosarcoma. *Cancer* 2001;92:2181-2189.

49. Kakar S, Mihalov M, Chachalani NA, Ghosh L, Johnstone H: Correlation of c-fos, p53 and PCNA expression with treatment outcome in osteosarcoma. *J Surg Oncol* 2000;73:125-126.

50. Kawaguchi K, Oda Y, Sakamoto A, et al: Molecular analysis of p53, MDM2 and H-ras genes in osteosarcoma and malignant fibrous histiocytoma of bone in patient older than 40 years. *Mod Pathol* 2002;15:878-888.

51. Marina N, Gebhardt M, Teot L, Gorlick R: Biology and therapeutic advances for pediatric osteosarcoma. *Oncologist* 2004;9:422-441.

52. Park HR, Jung WW, Bertoni F, et al: Molecular analysis of p53, MDM2 and H-ras genes in low-grade central osteosarcoma. *Pathol Res Pract* 2004;200:439-445.

53. Park YB, Kim HS, Oh JH, Lee SH: The co-expression of p53 protein and P-glycoprotein is correlated to a poor prognosis in osteosarcoma. *Int Orthop* 2001;24:307-310.

54. Yokoyama R, Schneider-Stock R, Radig K, Wex T, Roessner A: Clinicopathologic implications of MDM2, p53 and K-ras alterations in osteosarcomas: MDM2 amplification and p53 mutations found in progressive tumors. *Pathol Res Pract* 1998;194:615-621.

55. Gorlick R, Huvos AG, Heller G, et al: Expression of HER2/erbB-2 correlates with survival in osteosarcoma. *J Clin Oncol* 1999;17:2781-2788.

56. Maitra A, Wanzer D, Weinberg AG, Ashfaq R: Amplification of the HER-2/neu oncogene is uncommon in pediatric osteosarcomas. *Cancer* 2001;92:677-683.

57. Zhou H, Randall RL, Brothman AR, Maxwell T, Coffin CM, Goldsby RE: Her-2/neu expression in osteosarcoma increases risk of lung metastasis and can be associated with gene amplification. *J Pediatr Hematol Oncol* 2003;25:27-32.

58. Dickens DS, Kozielski R, Leavey PJ, Timmons C, Cripe TP: Cyclooxygenase-2 expression does not correlate with outcome in osteosarcoma or rhabdomyosarcoma. *J Pediatr Hematol Oncol* 2003;25:282-285.

59. Hornicek FJ, Gebhardt MC, Wolfe MW, et al: P-glycoprotein levels predict poor outcome in patients with osteosarcoma. *Clin Orthop Relat Res* 2000;373:11-17.

60. Pakos EE, Ioannidis JP: The association of P-glycoprotein with response to chemotherapy and clinical outcome in patients with osteosarcoma: A meta-analysis. *Cancer* 2003;98:581-589.

61. Serra M, Scotlandi K, Reverter-Branchat G, et al:

Value of P-glycoprotein and clinicopathologic factors as the basis for new treatment strategies in high-grade osteosarcoma of the extremities. *J Clin Oncol* 2003;21:536-542.

62. Sulzbacher I, Birner P, Tirieb K, Pichlbauer E, Lang S: The expression of bone morphogenetic proteins in osteosarcoma and its relevance as a prognostic measure. *J Clin Pathol* 2002;55:381-385.

63. Phemister DB: A study of the ossification in bone sarcoma. *Radiology* 1926;7:17-23.

64. Fahey M, Spanier SS, Vander Griend RA: Osteosarcoma of the pelvis: A clinical and histopathological study of twenty-five patients. *J Bone Joint Surg Am* 1992;74:321-330.

65. Ozaki T, Flege S, Kevric M, et al: Osteosarcoma of the pelvis: Experience of the Cooperative Osteosarcoma Study Group. *J Clin Oncol* 2003;21:334-341.

66. Zeytoonjian T, Mankin HJ, Gebhardt MC, Hornicek FJ: Distal lower extremity sarcomas: Frequency of occurrence and patient survival rate. *Foot Ankle Int* 2004;25:325-330.

67. Malmud LS, Charkes ND: Bone scanning: Principles, techniques and interpretation. *Clin Orthop Relat Res* 1975;107:112-122.

68. Hounsfield GN: Computerized transverse axial scanning (tomography): 1. Description of system. *Br J Radiol* 1973;46:1016-1022.

69. Schima W, Amann G, Stiglbauer R, et al: Preoperative staging of osteosarcoma: Efficacy of MR imaging in detecting joint involvement. *AJR Am J Roentgenol* 1994;163:1171-1175.

70. Enneking WF, Spanier SS, Goodman MA: Current concepts review: The surgical staging of musculoskeletal sarcoma. *J Bone Joint Surg Am* 1980;62:1027-1030.

71. Goorin AM, Abelson HT, Frei E III: Osteosarcoma: Fifteen years later. *N Engl J Med* 1985;313:1637-1643.

72. Jaffe N, Paed D, Farber S, et al: Favorable response of osteogenic sarcoma to high-dose methotrexate with citrovorum rescue and radiation therapy. *Cancer* 1973;31:1367-1373.

73. Cores EP, Holland JF, Wang JJ, Sinks LF: Doxorubicin in disseminated osteosarcoma. *JAMA* 1972;221:1132-1138.

74. Lewis IJ, Weeden S, Machin D, Stark D, Craft AW: Received doses and dose-intensity of chemotherapy and outcome in nonmetastatic extremity osteosarcoma: European Osteosarcoma Intergroup. *J Clin Oncol* 2000;18:4028-4037.

75. Link MP, Goorin AM, Horowitz M, et al: Adjuvant chemotherapy of high-grade osteosarcoma of the extremity: Updated results of the Multi-Institutional Osteosarcoma Study. *Clin Orthop Relat Res* 1991;270:8-14.

76. Provisor AJ, Ettinger LJ, Nachman JB, et al: Treatment of nonmetastatic osteosarcoma of the extremity with preoperative and postoperative chemotherapy: A report from the Children's Cancer Group. *J Clin Oncol* 1997;15:76-84.

77. Rosen G, Tan C, Sanmaneechai A, Beattie EJ Jr, Marcove R, Murphy ML: The rationale for multiple drug chemotherapy in the treatment of osteogenic sarcoma. *Cancer* 1975;35:936-945.

78. Sutow WW: Multidrug chemotherapy in osteosarcoma. *Clin Orthop Relat Res* 1980;153:67-72.

79. Bacci G, Ferrari S, Longhi A, et al: Relationship between dose-intensity of treatment and outcome for patients with osteosarcoma of the extremity treated with neoadjuvant chemotherapy. *Oncol Rep* 2001;8:883-888.

80. Bacci G, Picci P, Ruggieri P, et al: Primary chemotherapy and delayed surgery (neoadjuvant chemotherapy) for osteosarcoma of the extremities: The Istituto Rizzoli Experience in 127 patients treated preoperatively with intravenous methotrexate (high versus moderate doses) and intraarterial cisplatin. *Cancer* 1990;65:2539-2553.

81. Berend KR, Pietrobon R, Moore JO, Dibernardo L, Harrelson JM, Scully SP: Adjuvant chemotherapy for osteosarcoma may not increase survival after neoadjuvant chemotherapy and surgical resection. *J Surg Oncol* 2001;78:162-170.

82. Ferrari S, Bacci G, Picci P, et al: Long term follow-up and post-relapse survival in patients with non-metastatic osteosarcoma of the extremity treated with neoadjuvant chemotherapy. *Ann Oncol* 1997;8:765-771.

83. Ferrari S, Smeland S, Mercuri M, et al: Neoadjuvant chemotherapy with high-dose Ifosfamide, high-dose methotrexate, cisplatin and doxorubicin for patients with localized osteosarcoma of the extremity: A joint study by the Italian and Scandinavian Sarcoma Groups. *J Clin Oncol* 2005;23:8845-8852.

84. Machak GN, Tkachev SI, Solvoyev YN, et al: Neoadjuvant chemotherapy and local radiotherapy for high-grade osteosarcoma of the extremities. *Mayo Clin Proc* 2003;78:147-155.

85. Rosen G: Preoperative (neoadjuvant) chemotherapy for osteogenic sarcoma: A ten year experience. *Orthopedics* 1985;8:659-664.

86. Rosen G, Caparos B, Huvos AG, et al: Preoperative chemotherapy for osteogenic sarcoma: Selection of postoperative adjuvant chemotherapy based on the response of the primary tumor to preoperative chemotherapy. *Cancer* 1982;49:1221-1230.

87. Rosen G, Marcove RC, Caparros B, Nirenberg A, Klosloff C, Huvos AG: Primary osteogenic sarcoma: The rationale for preoperative chemotherapy and delayed surgery. *Cancer* 1979;43:2163-2177.

88. Thompson RC Jr, Cheng EY, Clohisy DR, Perentesis J, Manivel C, Le CT: Results of treatment for metastatic osteosarcoma with neoadjuvant chemotherapy and surgery. *Clin Orthop Relat Res* 2002;397:240-247.

89. Wanebo HJ, Temple WJ, Popp MB, Constable W, Aron B, Cunningham SL: Preoperative regional therapy for extremity sarcoma: A tricenter update. *Cancer* 1995;75:2299-2306.

90. Carsi B, Rock MG: Primary osteosarcoma in adults older than 40 years. *Clin Orthop Relat Res* 2002;397:53-61.

91. Lindner NJ, Ramm O, Hillmann A, et al: Limb salvage and outcome of osteosarcoma: The University of Muenster experience. *Clin Orthop Relat Res* 1999;358:83-89.

92. DeLaney TF, Park L, Goldberg SI, et al: Radiotherapy for local control of osteosarcoma. *Int J Radiat Oncol Biol Phys* 2005;61:492-498.

93. Dinçbas FO, Koca S, Mandel NM, et al: The role of preoperative radiotherapy in nonmetastic high-

grade osteosarcoma of the extremities for limb-sparing surgery. *Int J Radiat Oncol Biol Phys* 2005;62:820-828.

94. Szendroi M, Pápai Z, Koós R, Illés T: Limb-saving surgery, survival and prognostic factors for osteosarcoma: The Hungarian experience. *J Surg Oncol* 2000;73:87-94.

95. Zeegen EN, Aponte-Tinao LA, Hornicek FJ, Gebhardt MC, Mankin HJ: Survivorship analysis of 141 modular metallic endoprostheses at early followup. *Clin Orthop Relat Res* 2004;420:239-250.

96. Mankin HJ, Friedlaender GE, Tomford WW: Massive allograft transplantation following tumor resection, in Friedlaender GE, Mankin HJ, Goldberg VM (eds): *Bone Grafts and Bone Graft Substitutes*. Rosemont, IL, American Academy of Orthopaedic Surgeons, 2006, pp 39-47.

97. Ferrari S, Briccoli A, Mercuri M, et al: Postrelapse survival in osteosarcoma of the extremities: Prognostic factors for long-term survival. *J Clin Oncol* 2003;21:710-715.

98. Weeden S, Grimer RJ, Cannon SR, Taminiau AH, Uscinska BM, European Osteosarcoma Intergroup: The effect of local recurrence on survival in resected osteosarcoma. *Eur J Cancer* 2001;37:39-46.

Chapter 3

Chordomas of the Sacrum, Coccyx, or Spine

Chordomas are rare tumors that take origin from a persisting ectopic remnant of the notochord and are sometimes variable in presentation. The principal sites of presentation for chordomas are the base of the skull in the region of the clivus (sphenooccipital synchondrosis) and the sacrococcygeal region of the spine. The lesions are rare; 30% appear in the clivus and approximately 50% are seen in the sacrum. In general, sacrococcygeal tumors are difficult to treat and the outcomes for these patients are considerably poorer than for tumors in the clivus. Histologically, the tissue of the chordoma consists of large round cells, some of which are enormously distended by vacuoles and are described as "physaliphorous cells," the presence of which is considered to be a diagnostic feature for the tumor. Because of the orthopaedic orientation of this chapter, most of the discussion will be based on chordomas of sacral, coccygeal, or spinal origin.

Nomenclature and History

The majority of sacrococcygeal chordomas are considered to be malignant lesions that are aggressive, destructive, and can metastasize.[1-8] The most severe forms are known as "dedifferentiated" or malignant chordomas, which often resemble malignant fibrous histiocytomas histologically.[1,3,8-12] Benign forms of chordoma are sometimes known as intraosseous benign notochordal cell tumors (BNCTs), embryonic chordomas, or ectopic benign notochordal remnants.[3,4,8,13] Extra-axial chordomas are known as chordoma periphericum, parachordoma, or ecchordosis physaliphora.[8,14-17] Some lesions that seem to partly convert to cartilage are known as chondroid chordomas.[1,3,8,18]

In 1857, Hubert von Luschka[19] described bizarre lesions arising in the clivus, and in 1858, Müller[20] introduced the name "chordoma," based on the lesions proximity to notochordal remnants. Late in the century, Ribbert[21] suggested that the lesions in the clivus were of notochordal origin. He also attributed their identification to Virchow, but both of them chose to call them ecchondroses physalifora, based on the characteristic and quite striking histologic pattern.[22] A malignant form of the disease was described by Albert in 1915.[23] Stewart and associates[24,25] defined and clearly described the characteristics of the lesions of the clivus and, a few years later, the tumors in the sacrum, calling them both chordomas. The name chordoma is now used for all lesions, even when they are atypically located or structurally altered. Over the many years that followed the initial discoveries, numerous reports were presented describing patients with sacrococcygeal chordomas; these helped to establish the clinical nature, histologic resemblance to notochordal tissue, and, perhaps most strikingly, the difficulty with surgical treatment.[4,6,8,26-33] The disease is not restricted to humans, as several reports have described chordomas occurring in the sacrococcygeal location in dogs.[34,35]

Origin and Biology

In the developing embryo, the notochord is formed by a proliferation of cells from the cephalic end of the primitive posterior body structure.[3,4,13,36-41] It first appears as a midsagittal rod of cells lying ventral to the neural tube to which its dorsal surface is in contact. The cell collection then closes ventrally to form an elongated cylinder that retains its contact with the neural tube posteriorly and the gut anteriorly. At the fetal age of approximately 3 weeks, the formed notochord is present as a longitudinal, nonsegmented rod of cells, extending along the midaxis from the region of Rathke's pouch to the most caudal posterior segment. The notochord and neural tube become surrounded by a sheath of mesoderm, which initially becomes chondrified and then ossified, forming the basiocciput and basisphenoid bones and, below that level, the vertebral column.

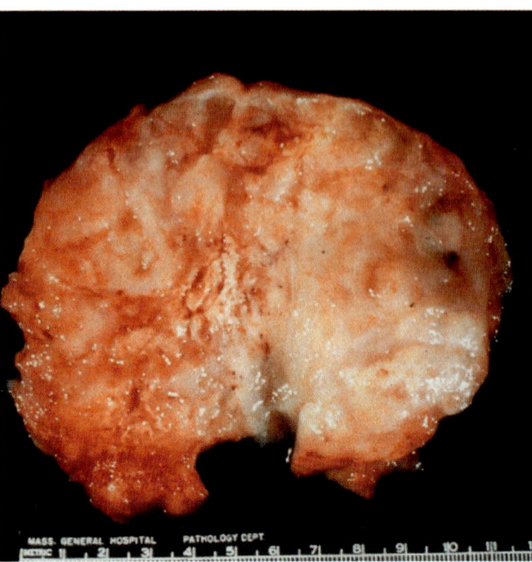

Figure 1

Gross appearance of a chordoma removed from the sacrum. The tissue appears compressed, resembles chondroid lesions, and has little evident vascularity.

The notochord begins to disappear as these structures are formed. By the second month of fetal life, notochordal tissue is no longer present, with two exceptions—in the nucleus pulposus of the vertebral segments, and in the cranium in the sphenooccipital synchondrosis.[4,5] In the sacrococcygeal region, the notochord is continued into the tail end of the embryo but also disappears with time, except as a sometimes prominent portion of the coccygeal structure.[4]

Although a small number of cases of chordoma have been described as being familial, there is very limited evidence to suggest that the tumors are genetic.[1,3,6,8,42,43] Several studies have related some of the tumors to the 1p36.13 chromosome,[44-46] and others have suggested an abnormality in chromosome 7[47] or chromosome 10.[48] Another marker is CD24, which may be found in most chordomas.[3,49] Still another is the brachyury transcription factor, which is an essential part of the notochordal development.[41] This agent may provide a means of differentiating chordomas from other similar tumors, such as those arising from cartilage or from metastatic tumors.[41] Still another recently described test is for galectin-3, which appears to be related to the extent of the disease.[50] Both chordomas and fragments of notochord stain heavily for S100, which aids in distinguishing the tumors from metastatic carcinoma.[1,3] In addi-

tion, P53 is found in most chordomas and the concentration may be an indicator of malignancy and a poor prognosis.[3,51] According to the Musculoskeletal Tumor Society staging system,[52] almost all of the tumors are classified as IA or, less commonly, IB.[1,2,5,6] Flow cytometric analysis of DNA structure and apoptotic activity shows that half of the tumors show aneuploidy, but this does not seem to correlate with metastasis or survival.[53,54] Parachordoma cells do not show a significant difference in immunochemistry from sacrococcygeal tumors.[34]

Gross, Histologic, and Imaging Characteristics

Spinal chordomas seem to originate within bone and almost always have a component that is strikingly located in the midline of the sacral, coccygeal, or vertebral segments.[1,3,4,6,8,55] The tumor itself is lobulated and appears to be encapsulated.[1,3] It extends into the marrow cavity of the affected bone and expands the cortex of the sacrum or the vertebral segment.[2,3,6,55] The surface is gray or bluish-white with extensive gelatinous translucent areas, sometimes alternating with cystic or hemorrhagic foci[2,4,8] (Figure 1). Occasional calcified zones are observed.[1,6,8] The gross pattern is similar to that seen for chondroid tumors.[4,8] Parachordomas have identical features.[17]

Histologic examination shows a characteristic lobular arrangement with a framework of fibrous trabeculae of varying sizes and shapes, containing thin-walled blood vessels.[1,3,4,8] The tumor cells vary in shape and size and have an eosinophilic cytoplasm. The cells resemble epithelial cells and are associated with abundant amounts of intercellular mucin that characteristically increases the size of the lobules[1,4,7,8,28] (Figure 2). A prominent and characteristic finding is the presence of intracellular cytoplasmic, mucin-containing vacuoles that vary in size and number and often displace the nuclei.[3,8] These are designated as physaliphorous cells and are considered to be diagnostic elements.[1,3,4,6,8,13,28,29,39,56] The cells to some extent resemble some types of chondroid or chondrosarcomatous tumors; one type of chordoid tumor that is difficult to separate from these is the chondroid chordoma, which has cartilaginous elements within the histologic structure.[7,18]

22

Chordoma cells tend to stain positively with periodic acid-Schiff (PAS) stain; the matrix stains with mucicarnine and Alcian blue, and metachromatically with toluidine blue.[1,3,44,54] Electron microscopic studies show desmosomal attachments and prominent mucinous vacuoles.[15,37,44,57] The malignant variant often shows tissue indistinguishable from malignant fibrous histiocytosis.[3,9,11]

Imaging studies using plain radiographs show the lesion to be destructive, causing cortical thinning and bony expansion.[1,3,6,8,21,55,58] As noted above, the lesion is almost always centrally placed in the bone, related to the site of origin of the notochordal tissue. The tumors may be massive, with a large soft-tissue component and calcification, both of which are more frequently located in the periphery.[1,3,6,58] The expansion is more frequently located anterior to the sacrum or coccyx rather than posterior.[58] Lesions that arise in the vertebral bodies are also centrally placed and may have extension into the ventral region.[2,3,26,59] They may invade the lateral elements and have soft-tissue masses extending from them. They rarely involve the adjacent intervertebral disks or vertebrae.

CT is valuable in identifying the extent of the soft-tissue mass and the degree of destruction, but in recent years, MRI using T1- and T2-weighted sequences with or without gadolinium has become the major diagnostic tool.[1,3,60,61] Most chordomas exhibit low signal on T1 and high signal on T2, and the gadolinium is of great value in demonstrating lobulated areas with a honeycomb appearance and clear definition of the borders[60,61] (Figure 3). Bone scan is almost always positive in relation to spinal or sacrococcygeal lesions; a recent report suggests that positron emission tomography may be helpful in identifying metastases.[62] However, benign chondromas and some chondrosarcomas have a similar appearance on imaging studies.

It is sometimes difficult to distinguish the various forms of chordoma from primary tumors, including enchondroma, chondrosarcoma, lymphoma, aneursymal bone cyst, giant cell tumor, chondromyxoid fibroma, and several others. Metastatic lesions from the prostate, kidney, uterus, and bowel are also problems in diagnostic distinction, on imaging studies and sometimes histologically.

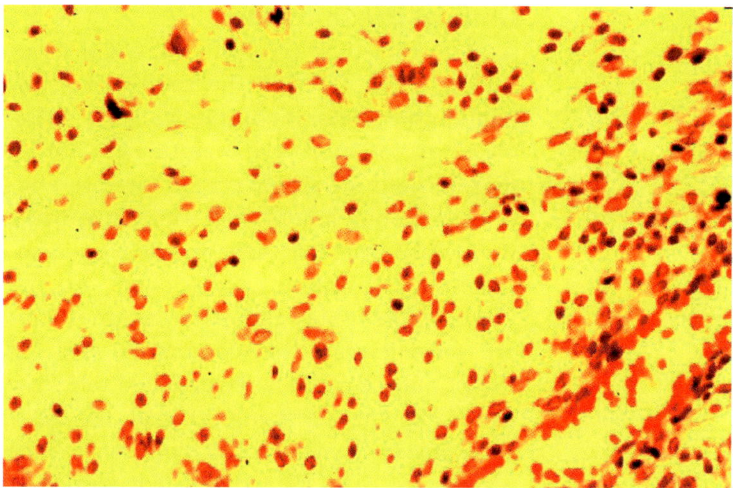

Figure 2

Histologic appearance of a chordoma from the sacrum. The cells are small and round and stain darkly in hematoxylin and eosin. A prominent and characteristic finding is the presence of intracellular mucin-containing vacuoles that vary in size and number and often displace the nuclei. These are designated as physaliphorous cells.

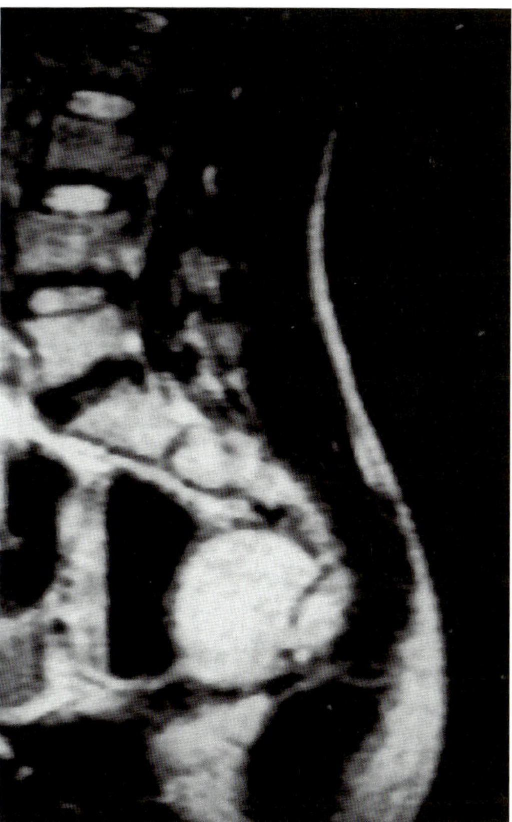

Figure 3

Lateral MRI study of the sacrum showing an enormous chordoma that not only extends into the abdominal space but also affects the canal, frequently causing damage to the sacral nerves.

Clinical Presentation

As determined by combining the data from several series,[1,6-8,27,55] the average age for patients with sacral chordomas is 56 years, 46 years for those with vertebral chordomas. Lesions are rarely encountered in children or young adults, and males are more frequently affected than females (approximately 2:1). Ethnic assessments in the United States show that African Americans are considerably less commonly affected than Caucasians.[3] The course is often slow and somewhat obscure, so that the time from onset of symptoms to diagnosis can be as long as 10 to 12 months. For sacral lesions, the presenting complaints are those of back pain, usually mild initially but progressing slowly to become incapacitating.[1-3,6-8,28,33] With advancing disease, the sacral nerves become involved and lower extremity pain, sensory loss, and motor weakness become significant problems.[1,3,6,8] Late in the course, the pain can become associated with urinary obstruction or incontinence and rectal dysfunction.[1,3,5,6,8] About half of the patients have a palpable mass on rectal examination, even early in the course.[5,8]

Only about 10% to 15% of patients with chordomas have axial spinal tumors. These patients usually present with back pain and, early in the course, show evidence of root or even spinal cord entrapment, leading to weakness and numbness either locally or in the lower extremities.[1,8,26,59] Patients with chordomas in the cervical region may present with hoarseness, dysphagia, and occasionally pharyngeal bleeding.[63]

Another very rarely encountered tumor is the parachordoma, a term introduced in 1977 by Dabska.[14] Patients have classical chordomas in nonspinal anatomic sites such as the ribs, clavicles, and extremities.[8,14-17] They show similar problems in management, but it is often much easier to resect the chordomas without risk to vascular, neural, or abdominal structures.

Treatment

Patients who present with the complaints and findings described above must be fully evaluated by physical examination, imaging studies (preferably MRI with gadolinium), and a biopsy.[1,3] Fine needle aspiration or a core biopsy under CT guidance are the most appropriate.[60] Once the diagnosis is made, the physical findings and tumor imaging studies should be assessed to determine if the lesion can be resected surgically and, perhaps equally important, whether the resection will result in serious pelvic and lower extremity deficits. If surgical resection of the total mass can be done with only limited neural and urogenital or rectal functional loss, it should be very carefully performed with wide margins.[5,6,31,55,64-66] Radiation may be helpful if the margins are marginal or intralesional. Total sacrectomy from both front and rear has been suggested as a treatment,[55] but has many complications including sensory, motor, and urogenital malfunction. Many patients require bowel resection and colostomy,[5,6,31,65,67,68] and others are urinary catheter–dependent. Reconstruction after these types of surgery is sometimes very difficult, requiring metallic devices to avoid further injury to nerves and vascular systems.[64,66,68] One recent study suggested that sacral resection in which only the S2 roots are retained has a high incidence of bladder and bowel malfunction.[5] For young people, retaining one S3 root is helpful in decreasing the severity of these complications, and retention of both S3 roots seems to markedly diminish the problem.

The danger with sacral and spinal tumors is the frequency of local recurrence after marginal surgery. The incidence of metastasis after local recurrence is high, and the death rate for such patients ranges from 20% to 50%.[1-3,5,6,27,64,68] If the lesion cannot be resected completely or if the patient is elderly or otherwise incapacitated, radiation can be the primary treatment. In recent years, the proton beam system has been the most popular choice, particularly as it is less likely to further affect function and seems to be effective in eliminating the tumor and reducing the frequency of local recurrence.[2,55,69,70]

Over the past several years, several chemotherapeutic agents have been introduced; although their value currently appears to be limited, they may be helpful in preventing metastases in patients with local recurrences.[55] In addition to standard chemotherapeutic agents, these materials include ifosfamide, doxorubicin, vincristine, decarbazine, and cisplatin.[55] In addition, reports suggest the value of imatinib mesylate, an inhibitor of platelet-derived growth factor receptor-β;[71] 9-nitro-camptothecin;[72] and cetuximab/gefitinib.[73] In general, there seems to be only limited success with any of these agents, and patients with local recurrence and metastatic disease often die early in their course.

Conclusions

Sacrococcygeal and spinal chordomas are puzzling entities. They are difficult to diagnose, to distinguish benign from malignant forms, and most of all to treat. The tumors are rare and there are a broad range of entities, including benign forms, malignant tumors, dedifferentiated chordomas, parachordomas, and chondroid chordomas. The differential diagnosis from chondromatous tumors, aneurysmal bone cyst, lymphoma, and metastatic carcinoma from the prostate, colon, bladder, or even kidney is difficult on imaging studies and sometimes even on biopsy. Perhaps the most problematic issue is treatment. Surgical procedures must be wide because patients with local recurrences have a high rate of metastasis and ultimate death from disease. Wide surgery may be devastating in terms of motor loss, bladder and bowel malfunction, and damage to adjacent structures. Radiation, especially proton beam, is helpful but probably not in itself curative, and chemotherapy has very limited success. Orthopaedic oncologists, radiologists, and radiation and medical oncologists view this strange lesion as a curse in their practices and hope that the future holds improvement in diagnostic systems and especially therapeutic regimens to improve the lives of their patients.

References

1. Campanacci M: Chordoma, in *Bone and Soft Tissue Tumors: Clinical Features, Imaging, Pathology and Treatment*, ed 2. New York, NY, Springer-Verlag, 1999, pp 689-706.

2. Cheng EY, Ozerdemoglu RA, Tranfeldt EE, Thompson RC Jr: Lumbosacral chordoma: Prognostic factors and treatment. *Spine* 1999;24:1639-1645.

3. Dorfman HD, Czerniak B: Chordoma, in *Bone Tumors*. St Louis, MO, Mosby, 1998, pp 974-999.

4. Jaffe HL: Chordoma, in *Tumors and Tumorlike Lesions of Bone and Joints*. Philadelphia, PA, Lea and Febiger, 1958, pp 451-463.

5. Mankin HJ: Sacral chordoma: Treatment by posterior resection, in Harsh G (ed): *Chordomas and Chondrosarcomas of the Skull Base and Spine*. New York, NY, Thieme, 2003, pp 277-286.

6. Mindell ER: Chordoma. *J Bone Joint Surg Am* 1981;63:501-505.

7. Rich TA, Schiller A, Suit HD, Mankin HJ: Clinical and pathologic review of 48 cases of chordoma. *Cancer* 1985;56:182-187.

8. Schajowicz F: Chordoma, in *Tumor and Tumor-like Lesions of Bone and Joints*. New York, NY, Springer-Verlag, 1981, pp 387-393.

9. Belza MG, Urich H: Chordoma and malignant fibrous histiocytoma: Evidence for transformation. *Cancer* 1986;58:1082-1087.

10. Chalmers J, Coulson WF: A metastasizing chordoma. *J Bone Joint Surg Br* 1960;42:556-559.

11. Choi YJ, Kim TS: Malignant fibrous histiocytoma in chordoma: Immunohistochemical evidence for transformation from chordoma to malignant fibrous histiocytoma. *Yonsei Med J* 1994;35:239-243.

12. McPherson CM, Suki D, McCutcheon IE, et al: Metastatic disease from spinal chordoma: A 10 year experience. *J Neurosurg Spine* 2006;5:277-280.

13. Yamaguchi T, Suzuki S, Ishiiwa H, Ueda Y: Benign notochordal cell tumors: A comparative histological study of benign notochordal cell tumors, classic chordomas, and notochordal vestiges of fetal intervertebral discs. *Am J Surg Pathol* 2004;28:756-761.

14. Dabska M: Parachordoma: A new clinicopathologic entity. *Cancer* 1977;40:1586-1592.

15. Niezabitowski A, Limon J, Wasilewski A, et al: Parachordoma: A clinicopathologic, immunohistochemical, electron microscopic, flow cytometric and cytogenetic study. *Gen Diagn Pathol* 1995;141:49-55.

16. Scolyer RA, Bonar SF, Palmer AA, et al: Parachordoma is not distinguishable from axial chordoma using immunohistochemistry. *Pathol Int* 2004;54:364-370.

17. Van Akkooi AC, van Geel AN, Bessems JH, den Bakker MA: Extra-axial chordoma. *J Bone Joint Surg Br* 2006;88:1232-1234.

18. Rosenberg AE, Brown GA, Bhan AK, Lee JM: Chondroid chordoma: A variant of chordoma. A morphologic and immunohistochemical study. *Am J Clin Pathol* 1994;101:36-41.

19. von Luschka H: Über gallertartige Auswüchse am clivus blumenbachii. *Virchows Arch* 1857;11:8-12.

20. Müller H: Über das vorkommen von resten der chorda dorsalis bei menschen nach der geburt und über ihr verhältnis zu den gallertgeschwülsten am clivus. *Z Rationelle Med* 1858;2:202-229.

21. Ribbert H: Über die ecchondrosis physalifora spheno-occipitalis. *Zentralb Allg Pathol* 1894;5:457-461.

22. Ribbert H, Virchow R : Chordoma. *Proc R Soc Med* 1959;52:1088-1100.

23. Albert H: Chordoma, with the report of a malignant case from the sacrococcygeal region. *Surg Gynecol Obstet* 1915;21:766-770.

24. Stewart MJ, Burrow JLF: Ecchordrosis physaliphora sphenooccipitalis. *J Neurol Psychopathol* 1923;4:218-220.

25. Stewart MJ, Morin JE: Chordoma: A review with report of a new sacrococcygeal case. *J Pathol Bacteriol* 1926;29:41-60.

26. Baker HW, Coley BL: Chordoma of the lumbar vertebra. *J Bone Joint Surg Am* 1953;35:403-408.

27. Dahlin DC, MacCarty CS: Chordoma. *Cancer* 1952;5:1170-1178.

28. Fletcher EM, Woltman HW, Adson AW: Sacrococcygeal chordomas: A clinical and pathologic study. *Arch Neurol Psychiat* 1935;33:283-299.

29. Friedmann I, Harrison DFN, Bird ES: The fine structure of chordoma with particular reference to the physaliphorous cell. *J Clin Pathol* 1962;15:116-125.

30. Graf L: Sacrococcygeal chordoma with metastases. *Arch Pathol* 1944;37:136-139.

31. Localio SA, Francis KC, Rossano PG: Abdominosacral resection of sacrococcygeal chordoma. *Ann Surg* 1967;166:394-402.

32. Mabrey RE: Chordoma: A study of 150 cases. *Am J Cancer* 1935;25:501-517.

33. MacCarty CS, Waugh JM, Coventry MB, O'Sullivan DC: Sacrococcygeal chordomas. *Surg Gynecol Obstet* 1961;113:551-554.

34. Munday JS, Brown CA, Weiss R: Coccygeal chordoma in a dog. *J Vet Diagn Invest* 2003;15:285-288.

35. Pease AP, Berry CR, Mott J, et al: Radiographic, computed tomographic and histopathologic appearance of a presumed spinal chordoma in a dog. *Vet Radiol Ultrasound* 2002;43:338-342.

36. Horten BC, Montague SR: Human ecchordosis physaliphora and chick embryonic notochord: A comparative electron microscopic study. *Virchows Arch A Pathol Ana Histol* 1976;371:295-303.

37. Murad TM, Murthy MS: Ultrastructure of a chordoma. *Cancer* 1970;25:1204-1215.

38. Salisbury JR: The pathology of the human notochord. *J Pathol* 1993;171:253-255.

39. Salisbury JR, Deverell MH, Cookson MJ, Whimster WF: Three-dimensional reconstruction of human embryonic notochords: Clue to the pathogenesis of chordoma. *J Pathol* 1993;171:59-62.

40. Taylor JR: Persistence of the notochordal canal in vertebrae. *J Anat* 1972;111:211-217.

41. Vujovic S, Henderson S, Presneau N, et al: Brachyury, a crucial regulator of notochordal development is a novel biomarker for chordomas. *J Pathol* 2006;209:157-165.

42. Bhadra AK, Casey ATH: Familial chordoma: A report of two cases. *J Bone Joint Surg Br* 2006;88:634-636.

43. Parry DM, Patronas N, Glenn GM, et al: Autosomal dominant transmission of chordoma in three successive generations. *Am J Hum Genet* 1997;61:72-77.

44. Bridge JA, Pickering D, Neff JR: Cytogenetic and molecular cytogenetic analysis of sacral chordoma. *Cancer Genet Cytogenet* 1994;75:23-25.

45. Miozzo M, Dalpra L, Riva P, et al: A tumor suppressor locus in familial and sporadic chordoma maps to 1p36. *Int J Cancer* 2000;87:68-72.

46. Riva P, Crosti F, Orzan F, et al: Mapping of candidate region for chordoma development to 1-36.13 by LOH analysis. *Int J Cancer* 2003;107:493-497.

47. Brandal P, Bjerkehagen B, Danielsen H, Heim S: Chromosome 7 abnormalities are common in chordomas. *Cancer Genet Cytogenet* 2005;160:15-21.

48. Tallini G, Dorfman H, Brys P, et al: Correlation between clinicopathological features and karyotype in 100 cartilaginous and chordoid tumours: A report from the Chromosomes and Morphology (CHAMP) Collaborative Study Group. *J Pathol* 2002;196:194-203.

49. Fujita N, Miyamoto T, Imai J, et al: CD24 is expressed specifically in the nucleus pulposus of intervertebral discs. *Biochem Biophys Res Commun* 2005;338:890-896.

50. Juliao SF, Rand N, Schwartz HS: Galectin-3: A biologic marker and diagnostic aid for chordoma. *Clin Orthop Relat Res* 2002;397:70-75.

51. Naka T, Boltze C, Kuester D, et al: Alterations of G1-S checkpoint in chordoma: The prognostic impact of p53 overexpression. *Cancer* 2005;104:1255-1263.

52. Enneking WF, Spanier SS, Goodman MA: Current concepts review: The surgical staging of musculoskeletal sarcoma. *J Bone Joint Surg Am* 1980;62:1027-1030.

53. Berven S, Zurakowski D, Mankin HJ, et al: Clinical outcome in chordoma: Utility of flow cytometry in DNA determination. *Spine* 2002;27:374-379.

54. Kilgore S, Prayson RA: Apoptotic and proliferative markers in chordomas: A study of 26 tumors. *Ann Diagn Pathol* 2002;6:222-228.

55. Harsh G: *Chordomas and Chondrosarcomas of the Skull Base and Spine*. New York, NY, Thieme, 2003.

56. Gui X, Siddiqi NH, Guo M: Physaliphorous cells in chordoma. *Arch Pathol Lab Med* 2004;128:1457-1458.

57. Spjut H, Luse SA: Chordoma: An electron microscopic study. *Cancer* 1964;17:643-656.

58. Utne JR, Pugh DG: The roentgenologic aspects of chordoma. *Am J Roentgenol Radium Ther Nucl Med* 1955;74:593-608.

59. Bjornsson J, Wold LE, Ebersold MJ, Laws ER: Chordoma of the mobile spine: A clinicopathologic analysis of 40 patients. *Cancer* 1993;71:735-740.

60. Rosenthal DI, Scott JA, Mankin HJ, et al: Sacrococcygeal chordoma: Magnetic resonance imaging and computed tomography. *AJR Am J Roentgenol* 1985;145:143-147.

61. Sung MS, Lee GS, Kang H, et al: Sacrococcygeal chordoma: MR imaging in 30 patients. *Skeletal Radiol* 2005;34:87-94.

62. Lin CY, Kao CH, Liang JA, Hsieh TC, Yen KY, Sun SS: Chordoma detected on F-18 FDG PET. *Clin Nucl Med* 2006;31:506-507.

63. Murali R, Rovit RL, Benjamin MV: Chordoma of the cervical spine. *Neurosurgery* 1981;9:253-256.

64. Fuchs B, Dickey ID, Yazemski MJ, Inwards CY, Sim FH: Operative management of sacral chordoma. *J Bone Joint Surg Am* 2005;87:2211-2216.

65. Gallia GL, Haque R, Garonzik I, et al: Spinal pelvic reconstruction after total sacrectomy for en bloc resection of a giant sacral chordoma: Technical note. *J Neurosurg Spine* 2005;3:501-506.

66. Samson IR, Springfield DS, Suit HD, Mankin HJ: Operative treatment of sacrococcygeal chordoma: A review of 21 cases. *J Bone Joint Surg Am* 1993;75:1476-1484.

67. Gunterberg B: Effects of major resection of the sacrum: Clinical studies on urogenital and anorectal function and a biomechanical study on pelvic strength. *Acta Orthop Scand Suppl* 1976;162:1-38.

68. Hulen CA, Temple HT, Fox WP, et al: Oncologic and functional outcome following sacrectomy for sacral chordoma. *J Bone Joint Surg Am* 2006;88:1532-1539.

69. Park L, DeLaney F, Liebsch NJ, et al: Sacral chordomas: Impact of high-dose proton/photon-beam radiation therapy combined with or without surgery for primary versus recurrent tumor. *Int J Radiat Oncol Biol Phys* 2006;65:1514-1521.

70. Rutz HP, Weber DC, Sugahara S, et al: Extracranial chordoma: Outcome in patients treated with function-preserving surgery followed by spot-scanning proton beam irradiation. *Int J Radiat Oncol Biol Phys* 2007;67:512-520.

71. Casali PG, Messina A, Stacchiotti S, et al: Imatinib mesylate in chordoma. *Cancer* 2004;101:2086-2097.

72. Chugh R, Dunn R, Zalupski MM, et al: Phase II study of 9-nitro-camptothecin in patients with advanced chordoma or soft tissue sarcoma. *J Clin Oncol* 2005;23:3597-3604.

73. Hof H, Welzel T, Debus J: Effectiveness of cetuximab/gefitinib in the therapy of a sacral chordoma. *Onkologie* 2006;29:572-574.

Chapter 4

Ewing's Sarcoma

In 1921, James Ewing[1] first described a destructive tumor of bone that he called "diffuse endothelioma of bone." There was considerable disagreement about the nature of this lesion because of a proposed array of possible endothelial, hematologic, neurologic, or lymphatic origins. In 1958, the great pathologist Henry Jaffe[2] finally solved the problem by calling the tumor "Ewing's sarcoma," a name that has remained in use ever since. The tumor is principally located in the lower extremities, most frequent in children between 5 and 15 years of age, and slightly more prevalent in males. The frequency is far less than osteosarcoma or chondrosarcoma but it remains the third most frequently encountered primary tumor in bone. Until relatively recently, the survival rate was poor with metastatic disease often present at the time of discovery of the primary lesion. Current treatment systems have led to a surprising survival rate for what is considered to be a very aggressive tumor.

History

James Ewing was a remarkable and accomplished person. He was born in Pittsburgh, Pennsylvania, in 1866. At the age of 14, he developed osteomyelitis of the femur and spent almost 2 years in bed; during this time, he learned to use a microscope. After completing his education in college and medical school, he became interested in pathology, and in 1899 he was named a Professor of Clinical Pathology at Cornell. In 1913, he founded the American Society for the Control of Cancer and, along with Ernest Amory Codman and Joseph Bloodgood, started the Registry of Bone Tumors. He was elected President of the medical board and subsequently the Director of Research for Memorial Sloan-Kettering Hospital. In 1921, he described a "diffuse endothelioma of bone," noted in the introductory paragraph above.[1] Despite considerable effort, the origin of the tumor still remains an enigma. For that reason, in 1958 Henry Jaffe[2] added Ewing's name to the tumor, and he will forever remain the father of "Ewing's sarcoma of bone."

In 1926, Connor[3] studied a large number of these tumors and distinguished three types: an angioendothelioma, a diffuse endothelioma, and a reticular form of tumor. Oberling[4] expanded on these types and tried to establish a relationship to reticulosarcoma of lymph nodes, introducing the term "reticulosarcoma of the bone marrow." In 1939, Parker and Jackson[5] suggested that the tumor was a primary reticulum cell sarcoma of bone. Colville and Willis[6,7] decided there was no such lesion and that the tumors seen were really metastatic from various sites. Many other clinicians and scientist have studied Ewing's sarcomas over the years, contributing to our understanding of the nature of the lesion, its structure, and the relationship to primitive neuroectodermal tumor, and providing imaging studies and outcome data.[8-21]

Tumor Origin and Nomenclature

Unlike many connective tissue tumors such as chondrosarcoma (cartilage) or osteosarcoma (bone), the tissue of origin for Ewing's sarcoma is still not clearly known and continues to be the subject of sometimes heated discussion since Ewing's original description in 1921.[1] Ewing's original suggestion was that the tumor was an endothelioma, but others suggested that the lesion was of neurologic, lymphogenous, or hematopoietic origin.[2,3,20] The similarity to myeloma has also been introduced.[2,13,20] On the basis of some biologic characteristics, it is evident that Ewing's tumor is closely related to a lesion known as a primitive neuroectodermal tumor (PNET) and could be a slightly less aggressive form of that entity.[10-13,15,20]

Pathophysiology

Although there are some peculiar genetic characteristics, it is apparent that Ewing's sarcoma and PNET are not familial. There are some ethnic differences in that the tumors are rare in Africans and African-Americans, but family transmission is almost unknown. As noted above, Ewing's tumor and PNET have some similar biologic characteristics. Almost all Ewing's tumors and PNETs are positive for vimentin.[10] An overexpression of p53 is commonly observed and appears to play a role in predicting the survival outcome.[22-25] A reciprocal translocation between chromosomes 11 and 22 involving bands q24 and q12, t(11;22)(q24;q12), occurs most frequently and is seen in approximately 90% of both Ewing's sarcomas and PNETs[10,12,13,15,20,26,27] The "t" encodes an EWS/FLI1 fusion oncoprotein, which serves as an aberrant transcription factor.[9,27-31] This may be a major factor in the development of Ewing's sarcoma cells from other types of mesenchymal progenitor cells and may constitute the initiating event for the development of Ewing's sarcoma or PNET.[9,13,27,31] In addition, Ewing's sarcoma cells overexpress vascular endothelial growth factor isoform 165 (VEGF165), which is critical for the migration of CD34+ cells from the bone marrow into the tumor and may also serve as a prognostic factor for greater survival.[32,33] Another feature of the tumor is the presence of CD99^{MIC2}, a 32 kDa surface glycoprotein involved in cell-cell adhesion and apoptosis.[10,13,34] In terms of definition of disease, it has become evident that FLI-1 and CD99^{MIC2} are both excellent immunohistochemical markers for the diagnosis of both Ewing's sarcoma and PNET.[9,10,26,28,30,31,34]

Clinical Aspects

Ewing's sarcoma principally occurs from age 5 through 15 years.[2,10,11,13-16,20,21] Although it is the third most frequently occurring primary tumor of bone, following osteosarcoma and chondrosarcoma, it is still considered to be a rare lesion, with only 5 to 10 cases per 1,000,000 children in the United States.[13,20,21] It is slightly more frequent in males than females and very rare in Africans and African-Americans.[10,11,13,16,20,21] As noted above, although there are clearly some genetic characteristics to the disease, it is not familial and is almost never encountered in the families of patients with the disease.[10,13,20]

The locations for Ewing's sarcomas are almost always in long bones, and most often the metaphyseal or diaphyseal sites of the fe-

mur, tibia, fibula, and humerus.[2,11,13,14,16,20] It is also found in the pelvis, where these lesions are very difficult to treat.[35] The tumors are rarely present in the calvarium, clavicle, hands, or feet and are almost never epiphyseal in location.[11,13] Involvement of the ribs ands spine rarely occurs but may be more common in a more benign form of PNET known as Askin's tumor.[36]

Patients with Ewing's sarcoma, even with small lesions, are almost always symptomatic. The site is painful, tender to touch, and may in some children produce local swelling and redness of the skin.[11,13,16,20] Pathologic fractures can occur and cause marked deformity and vascular or nerve damage.[10,11,13,20] Not surprisingly, approximately 10% of the patients have metastases, usually in the lungs, present at the time of initial presentation.[11,20,21] Chemistry studies for lactic dehydrogenase often show an increase, and the erythrocyte sedimentation rate is almost always elevated.[13,20] Flow cytometric studies of Ewing's sarcomas rarely show aneuploidy, which differs considerably from osteosarcoma or other high-grade connective tissue cancers.[37]

Imaging Studies

The most frequent presentation of Ewing's sarcoma is a poorly defined, permeative lesion of the medullary space with expansion and destruction of the cortices[2,11,13,20] (Figure 1). Lesions are sometimes symmetric in that both cortices are equally involved and a soft-tissue mass may be seen on all sides of the affected bone. Cortices above or below the center of the lesion may show thickening and occasionally Codman's triangles can be observed. Although Ewing's tumors are almost always purely lytic, the cortical abnormalities may provide a suggestion of "sunburst" bone formation.[11,13,20] CT and MRI are very useful in defining the extent of the lesion and the size and distribution of the soft-tissue mass[11,13,16,20,21,38] (Figure 2). A CT scan of the chest is an essential part of the initial studies and must not only be done at the time of presentation but at regular intervals during treatment and for a considerable period following. Virtually all lesions are very active on bone scan in contrast with myeloma, in which the bone scan fails to show approximately 25% of the lesions.[11,13] Positron emission tomography

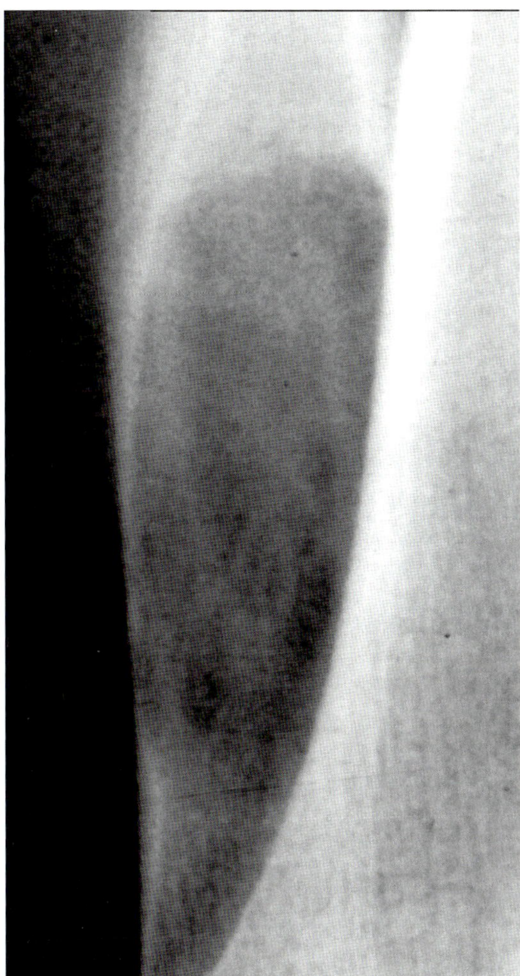

Figure 1
A destructive lesion of the distal portion of the fibula. The bone is expanded.

(PET) scans are very useful in not only defining the extent of the original tumor, but also in detecting metastases or multicentric primary sites.[39,40]

Ewing's sarcoma on plain radiographs, and even sometimes on examination of biopsy specimens, may be difficult to distinguish from some other types of osseous lesions. The differential diagnoses include osteomyelitis, non-Hodgkin's lymphoma, and metastatic neuroblastoma (in children younger than 8 years of age). Somewhat less commonly, the tumors can be confused with Langerhans cell histiocytosis, small cell osteosarcoma, mesenchymal chondrosarcoma, and even adamantinoma of the tibia.[11,13,20]

Histology

The primary cell type in Ewing's sarcoma is a nonhematologic, small, round cell that

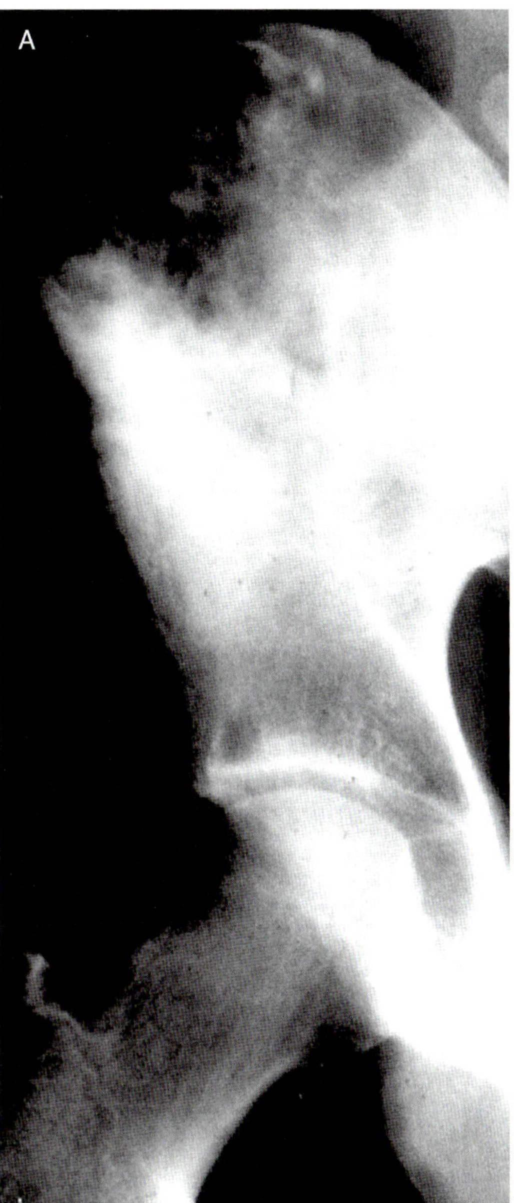

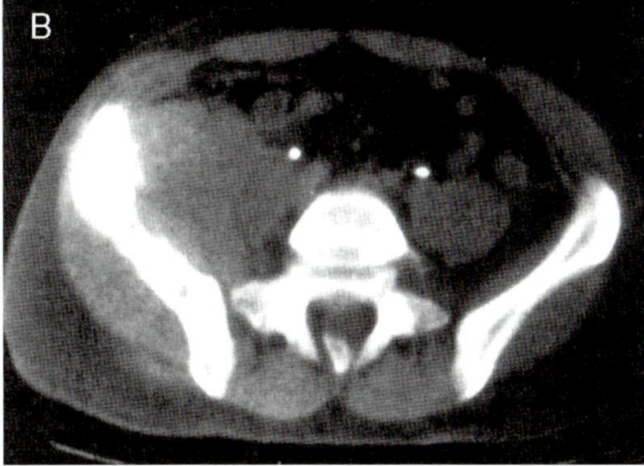

Figure 2
A, A highly destructive lesion of the ilium with a soft-tissue mass. **B,** The large soft-tissue mass is evident on CT scan.

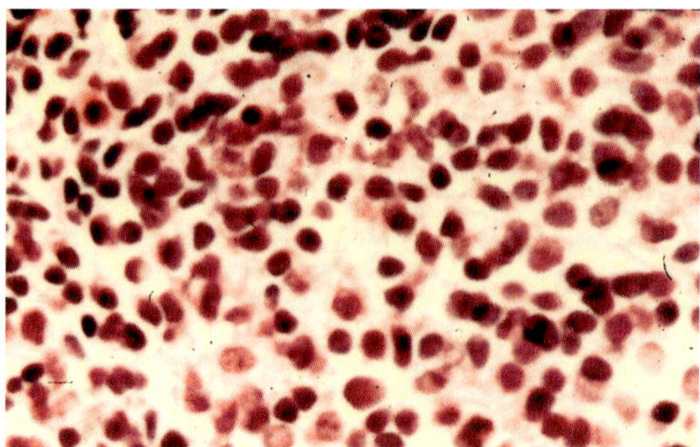

Figure 3
Classical appearance of Ewing's sarcoma cells. They are round with dark staining nuclei.

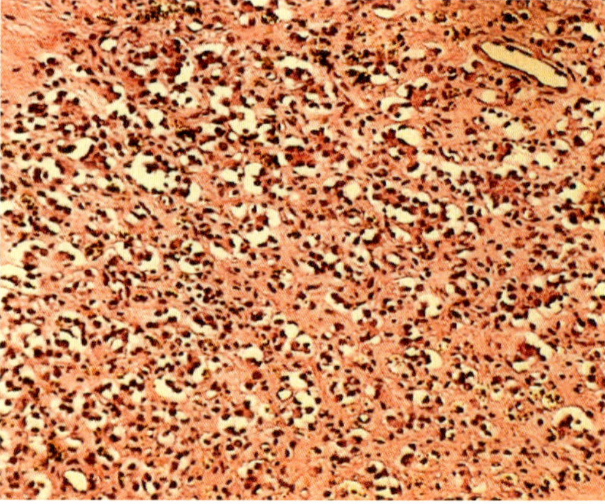

Figure 4
Histologic appearance of a Ewing's tumor with typical cells within a matrix structure. The cells are irregular, and some show atypism.

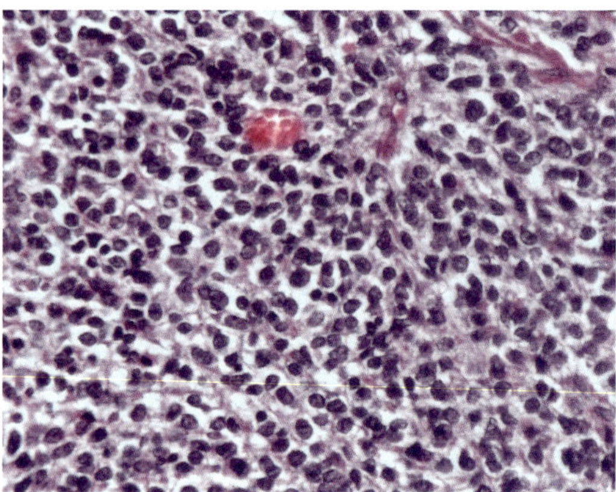

Figure 5
Dark staining of the cells and matrix are believed to indicate the presence of apoptotic activity.

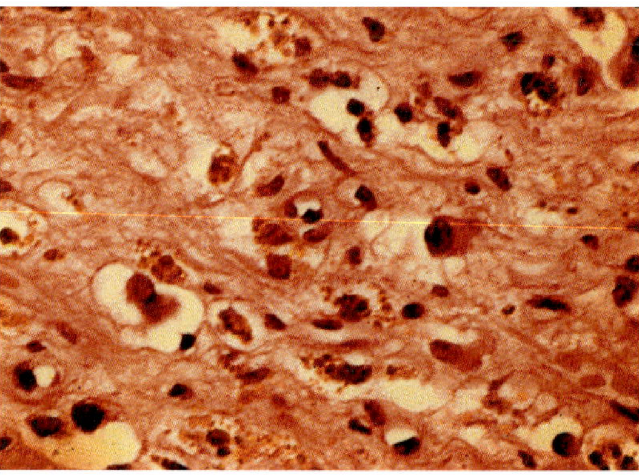

Figure 6
If bone repair related to fractures is present, considerable cell atypia and other abnormalities associated with bone formation may be observed.

closely resembles mesenchymal cells[11,13,20] (Figure 3). The cells are closely packed as sheets, without matrix components (known as a "blue tumor"), and tend to fill bony defects.[11] The cells have round, centrally located nuclei that are larger than those of lymphocytes[13,20] (Figure 4). There are usually several nucleoli within the nucleus, which vary in size. Mitotic figures are rarely encountered,[13,20] but the cells may be dark in color, believed to indicate that they are undergoing apoptosis[13] (Figure 5). The cells sometimes form a "rosette pattern," described as having the nuclei at the periphery and the cytoplasmic projections toward the center. Rosettes are more common in PNETs than in Ewing's tumors and may be a more classical form described as a "Homer Wright" abnormality.[11,13,20,21] Special stains will quite frequently demonstrate glycogen in the cytoplasm.[11,13,20] Inflammatory cell infiltrates are uncommon, and vascular formation is usually limited and thin in size. Occasionally, however, the vessels are large and thick-walled. Focal areas of spindle cells are sometimes present and if a fracture has occurred, there may be evidence of attempts at osseous repair[13] (Figure 6). Necrosis of cells is commonly encountered and when that occurs, leukocyte infiltration may suggest osteomyelitis.[11]

PNET Characteristics

PNET occurs considerably less often than Ewing's sarcoma, with approximately the same distribution of lesional sites.[11-13,15,20,21] Patients with PNET are older (15 to 40 or more years) and males are still more often affected than females. The tumor itself has most of the biologic characteristics of Ewing's sarcoma but has considerably more resemblance to neural tissue and specifically shows the presence of a large number of Homer Wright rosettes on histologic study.[11,13,20] The outcome data for PNET show it to be slightly more malignant, with poorer survival statistics. Most authors now agree that the two lesions are related, but that the PNET is possibly a more aggressive form of both malignant tumors. It should be noted, however, that such a statement may not be valid based on the very small series of PNETs studied as compared with the much greater number of documented series of Ewing's sarcomas.[11,13,15,20,21]

Treatment

As a caretaking physician, it is essential to remember some factors about Ewing's sarcoma. Despite the rarity of the lesion, if one encounters a patient aged 5 to 15 years, with pain in an extremity, tenderness and swelling over the site, and imaging changes as described above, the most likely diagnosis is Ewing's sarcoma, particularly if there is no suggestion of osteomyelitis on the basis of laboratory studies.[11,13,16] Once the imaging studies, including plain radiographs, CT, and MRI are obtained, the site should be biopsied. Most surgeons agree that an incisional or even CT-guided core needle biopsy is most appropriate.[41] The incisional biopsy should be performed through a longitudinal incision over a site that shows active disease on imaging studies.[41] Frozen section, permanent sections, and culture should be carefully studied before additional treatment is instituted. If the diagnosis of Ewing's sarcoma is suspected, a bone scan, a CT scan of the chest, and a fluorodeoxyglucose (FDG)-PET scan are essential to determine the presence of metastases or multifocal disease.[13,38-40]

Before the era of chemotherapy, less than 10% of the patients with Ewing's sarcoma survived, despite surgical resection and radiation to the site.[2,10,11,18,42] Recently, with the advent of multimodal therapy including chemotherapy, surgery, and radiation, a much higher percentage of patients survive and often retain reasonable function of the affected part.[8,10,11,13,16,20,21,43-46] If at all possible, surgery should be performed with wide margins to reduce the likelihood of local recurrence.[10,11,16,19,21,35,44,47,48] This is sometimes difficult because of the proximity to vessels and nerves, and occasionally

vascular reconstruction and/or plastic surgical muscle and skin transfers may be necessary.[16,19] Amputation may also be performed and, if the level is midfemoral shaft or lower, function may be quite acceptable to the patient and family.[49] Reconstruction after wide resection may employ metallic devices, often modular systems, or for many lesions, cadaveric allografts.[11,16,19,21,35,50,51] The latter are particularly useful if the resection does not include the adjacent joints or epiphyseal growth plates.[50]

Radiation was introduced early for the treatment of Ewing's sarcoma and was useful in destroying the primary tumor,[10,11,13,52] but the survival rate remained poor until the advent of chemotherapy. The first reports of chemotherapy occurred in the early 1960s; the chosen drug was initially cyclophosphamide.[10,20,53] In 1968, Hustu and associates[54] suggested the combination of cyclophosphamide and vincristine along with radiation. In 1974, Rosen and associates[46] proposed the use of radiation in association with vincristine, actinomycin D, cyclophosphamide, and doxorubicin (VACD), and this became the standard four-agent therapeutic approach. More recently, ifosfamide and etoposide have been added.[10,55-59] Both the radiation and chemotherapy may be given preoperatively, but the doses may differ if they are given postoperatively.[10,43,55,56,60-62]

Metastatic disease is an adverse prognostic sign for survival of patients with Ewing's sarcoma.[10,11,13,20] It must be treated aggressively, including, if necessary, surgical resection of lung lesions, radiation therapy, and chemotherapy.[10,11,13,63] Local recurrences after surgery also decrease survival rates and duration, and often require more extensive chemotherapy and sometimes ablative surgery.[10,47,64-66]

Long-term effects of chemotherapy and radiation are sometimes problems for survivors. Growth disturbances can occur; for females, menstrual abnormalities and infertility can be a problem. Of greater concern is malignant disease related to the treatment.[10,60] These include late-onset leukemias (believed to occur in 1% to 2% of the patients who received chemotherapy) and osteosarcomas at the primary site as a result of radiation.[67] Both are risks, but are infrequent in occurrence and are often treatable by appropriate methods.

Current experimental approaches for treatment of Ewing's sarcomas are related to attempted biologic alterations such as introduction of stem cells or modulation of EWS, both of which may result in inhibition of tumor growth.[10,68,69] Another approach is interference with or silencing of CD99[MIC2], which may induce apoptosis in Ewing's sarcoma cells.[10,70]

Conclusions

Ewing's sarcoma was first described in 1921 and was an enigma then. Here we are, more than 85 years later, and the tumor still remains enigmatic. We have no real evidence for cell origin or for biologic character of the tissue. Although a gene error has been established, there remains no evidence that allows us to label it a genetic disease. It is clearly related to another enigmatic disorder, PNET, but the nature of that relationship remains unclear. Despite all of that, the most remarkable part of this somewhat distressing story is that we have made enormous strides in the management of the patients. What started with a less than 10% survival rate for children and adolescents has now extended to 70% to 80%. Because of advances in surgical technology, most of the patients are restored to reasonable function. Of some interest is the current group of experimental procedures that may lead to biologic treatment protocols in the not-too-distant future. What a joy that will be for the pediatric oncologists and especially their patients and families!

References

1. Ewing J: Diffuse endothelioma of bone. *Proc NY Pathol Soc* 1921;21:17-24.

2. Jaffe HL: *Tumors and Tumorous Conditions of Bones and Joints*. Philadelphia, PA, Lea and Febiger, 1958, pp 350-368.

3. Connor CL: Endothelial myeloma of Ewing: Report of fifty-four cases. *Arch Surg* 1926;12:789-829.

4. Oberling C: Les reticulosarcomes et les retculoendotheliosarcomes de la moelle osseuse (sarcomes d'Ewing). *Bull Assoc Fr Etude Cancer* 1928;17:259-296.

5. Parker F Jr, Jackson H Jr: Primary reticulum cell sarcoma of bone. *Surg Gynecol Obstet* 1939;68:45-53.

6. Colville HC, Willis RA: Neuroblastoma metastases in bone, with a criticism of Ewing's endothelioma. *Am J Pathol* 1933;9:421-430.

7. Willis RA: Metastatic neuroblastoma in bone presenting the Ewing's syndrome, with a discussion of "Ewing's sarcoma." *Am J Pathol* 1940;16:317-332.

8. Bacci G, Ferrari S, Bertoni F: Prognostic factors in nonmetastatic Ewing's sarcoma of bone treated with adjuvant chemotherapy: Analysis of 359 patients at the Istituto Ortopedico Rizzoli. *J Clin Oncol* 2000;18:4-11.

9. Ban J, Siligan C, Kreppel M, Aryee D, Kovar H: EWS-FLI1 in Ewing's sarcoma: Real targets and collateral damage. *Adv Exp Med Biol* 2006;587:41-52.

10. Bernstein M, Kovar H, Paulussen M, et al: Ewing's sarcoma family of tumors: Current management. *Oncologist* 2006;11:503-519.

11. Campanacci M: *Bone and Soft Tissue Tumors*, ed 2. New York, NY, SpringerVerlag, 1999, pp 653-682.

12. Dehner LP: Primitive neuroectodermal tumor and Ewing's sarcoma. *Am J Surg Pathol* 1993;17:1-13.

13. Dorfman HD, Czerniak B: *Bone Tumors*. St. Louis, MO, Mosby, 1998, pp 607-663.

14. Ferrari S, Bertoni F, Mercuri M, et al: Ewing's sarcoma of bone: Relation between clinical characteristics and staging. *Oncol Rep* 2001;8:553-556.

15. Grier HE: The Ewing family of tumors: Ewing's sarcoma and primitive neuroectodermal tumors. *Pediatr Clin North Am* 1997;44:991-1004.

16. Mankin HJ: Ewing sarcoma. *Curr Opin Orthop* 2000;11:479-485.

17. Paulussen M, Ahrens S, Craft AW, et al: Ewing's tumours with primary lung metastases: Survival analysis of 114 (European intergroup) Cooperative Ewing's Sarcoma Studies patients. *J Clin Oncol* 1998;16:3044-3052.

18. Phillips RF, Higinbotham NL: The curability of Ewing's endothelioma of bone in children. *J Pediatr* 1967;70:391-397.

19. Sailer S, Harmon D, Mankin HJ, Truman JT, Suit HD: Ewing's sarcoma: Surgical resection as prognostic factor. *Int J Radiat Oncol Biol Phys* 1988;15:43-52.

20. Schajowicz F: *Tumors and Tumorlike Lesions of Bone and Joints*. New York, NY, Springer Verlag. 1981, pp 243-302.

21. Unni KK: *Dahlin's Bone Tumors*, ed 5. Philadelphia, PA, Lippincott Raven, 1996, pp 249-261.

22. Abudu A, Mangham DC, Reynolds GM, et al: Overexpresssion of p53 protein in primary Ewing's sarcoma of bone: Relationship to tumour stage, response and prognosis. *Br J Cancer* 1999;79:1185-1189.

23. De Alava E, Antonescu CR, Panizo A, et al: Prognostic impact of p53 status in Ewing's sarcoma. *Cancer* 2000;89:783-792.

24. Gu M, Antonescu CR, Guiter G, et al: Cytokeratin immunoreactivity in Ewing's sarcoma: Prevalence in 50 cases confirmed by molecular diagnostic studies. *Am J Surg Pathol* 2000;24:410-416.

25. Huang H-Y, Illei PB, Zhao Z, et al: Ewing sarcomas with p53 mutation or p16/p14 ARF homozygous deletion: A highly lethal subset associated

with poor chemoresponse. *J Clin Oncol* 2005;23:548-558.

26. Folpe AL, Goldblum JR, Rubin BR, et al: Morphologic and immunophenotypic diversity in Ewing family tumors: A study of 66 genetically confirmed cases. *Am J Surg Pathol* 2005;29:1025-1033.

27. Hattinger CM, Potschger U, Tarkkanen M, et al: Prognostic impact of chromosomal aberrations in Ewing tumours. *Br J Cancer* 2002;86:1763-1769.

28. Dc Alava E, Kawai A, Healey JH, et al: EWS-FLI1 fusion transcript structure is an independent determinant of prognosis in Ewing's sarcoma. *J Clin Oncol* 1998;16:1248-1255.

29. Janknecht R: EWS-ETS oncoproteins: The linchpins of Ewings tumors. *Gene* 2005;363:1-14.

30. Llombart-Bosch A, Navarro S: Immunohistochemical detection of EWS and FLI-1 proteins in Ewing's sarcomas and primitive neuroectodermal tumors: Comparative analysis with CD99 (MIC-2) expression. *Appl Immunohistochem Mol Morphol* 2001;9:255-260.

31. Owen LA, Lessnick SL: Identification of target genes in their native cellular context: An analysis of EWS/FLI in Ewing's sarcoma. *Cell Cycle* 2006;5:2049-2053.

32. Kreuter M, Paulussen M, Boeckeler J, et al: Clinical significance of vascular endothelial growth Factor-A expression in Ewing's sarcoma. *Eur J Cancer* 2006;42:1904-1911.

33. Lee TH, Bolatrade MF, Worth LL, et al: Production of VEGF165 by Ewing's sarcoma cells induces vasculogenesis and incorporation of CD34+ stem cells into the expanding tumor vasculature. *Int J Cancer* 2006;119:839-846.

34. Ambros IM, Ambros PF, Strehl S, et al: MIC2 is a specific marker for Ewing's sarcoma and peripheral primitive neuroectodermal tumors. *Cancer* 1991;67:1886-1893.

35. Scully SP, Temple HT, O'Keefe RJ, et al: Role of surgical resection in pelvic Ewing's sarcoma. *J Clin Oncol* 1995;13:2336-2341.

36. Askin FB, Rosai J, Sibley RK, Dehner LP, McAlister WH: Malignant small cell tumor of the thoracopulmonary region in childhood: A distinctive clinicopathologic entity of uncertain histogenesis. *Cancer* 1979;43:2438-2451.

37. Mankin HJ, Fondren G, Hornicek FJ, Gebhardt MD, Rosenberg AE: The use of flow cytometry in assessing malignancy in bone and soft tissue tumors. *Clin Orthop Relat Res* 2002;397:96-105.

38. Frouge C, Vanel D, Coffre C, et al: The role of magnetic resonance imaging in the evaluation of Ewing's sarcoma: A report of 27 cases. *Skeletal Radiol* 1988;17:387-392.

39. Daldrup-Link HE, Franzius C, Link TM, et al: Whole-body MR imaging for detection of bone metastases in children and young adults: Comparison with skeletal scintigraphy and FDG PET. *AJR Am J Roentgenol* 2001;177:229-236.

40. Hawkins DS, Scheutze SM, Butrynski JE, et al: [18 F] Fluorodeoxyglucose positron emission tomography predicts outcome for Ewing sarcoma family of tumors. *J Clin Oncol* 2005;23:8828-8834.

41. Mankin HJ, Mankin CJ, Simon MA: The hazards of biopsy revisited: Members of the Musculoskeletal Tumor Society. *J Bone Joint Surg Am* 1996;78:656-663.

42. Jenkin RD: Ewing's sarcoma: A study of treatment methods. *Clin Radiol* 1966;17:97-106.

43. Bacci G, Forni C, Longhi A, et al: Long-term outcome for patients with non-metastatic Ewing's sarcoma treated with adjuvant and neoadjuvant chemotherapies: 402 patients treated at Rizzoli between 1972 and 1992. *Eur J Cancer* 2004;40:73-83.

44. Bacci G, Longhi A, Briccoll A, et al: The role of surgical margins in treatment of Ewing's sarcoma family tumors: Experience of a single institution with 512 patients treated with adjuvant and neoadjuvant chemotherapy. *Int J Radiat Oncol Biol Phys* 2006;65:766-772.

45. Kolb EA, Kushner BH, Gorlick R, et al: Long-term event-free survival after intensive chemotherapy for Ewing's family of tumors in children and young adults. *J Clin Oncol* 2003;21:3423-3430.

46. Rosen G, Wollner N, Tan C, et al: Proceedings: Disease-free survival in children with Ewing's sarcoma treated with radiation therapy and adjuvant four-drug sequential chemotherapy. *Cancer* 1974;33:384-393.

47. Bacci G, Longhi A, Ferrari S, et al: Pattern of relapse in 290 patients with nonmetastatic Ewing's sarcoma family tumors treated at a single institution with adjuvant and neoadjuvant chemotherapy between 1972 and 1992. *Eur J Surg Oncol* 2006;34:974-979.

48. Jurgens HM, Exner U, Gadner H, et al: Multidisciplinary treatment of primary Ewing's sarcoma of bone: A 6 year experience of a European Cooperative Trial. *Cancer* 1988;61:23-32.

49. Pardasaney PK, Sullivan PE, Portney LG, Mankin HJ: Advantage of limb salvage over amputation for proximal lower extremity tumors. *Clin Orthop Relat Res* 2006;444:201-208.

50. Gebhardt MC, Jaffe K, Mankin HJ: Bone allografts for tumors and other reconstructions in children, in Langlais F, Tomeno B (eds): *Limb Salvage—Major Reconstructions in Oncologic and Nontumoral Conditions*. Berlin, Germany, Springer-Verlag, 1991, pp 561-572.

51. Wafa H, Grimer RJ: Surgical options and outcomes in bone sarcoma. *Expert Rev Anticancer Ther* 2006;6:239-248.

52. Dunst J, Sauer R, Burgers JM, et al: Radiation therapy as local treatment in Ewing's sarcoma: Results of the Cooperative Ewing's Sarcoma studies CESS 81 and CESS 86. *Cancer* 1991;67:2818-2825.

53. Pinkel D: Cyclophosphamide in children with cancer. *Cancer* 1962;15:42-49.

54. Hustu HO, Holton C, James D Jr, Pinkel D: Treatment of Ewing's sarcoma with concurrent radiotherapy and chemotherapy. *J Pediatr* 1968;73:249-251.

55. Bacci G, Mercuri M, Longhi A, et al: Neoadjuvant chemotherapy for Ewing's tumour of bone: Recent experience at the Rizzoli Orthopaedic Institute. *Eur J Cancer* 2002;38:2243-2251.

56. Burgert EO Jr, Nesbit ME, Garnsey LA, et al: Multimodal therapy for the management of nonplevic localized Ewing's sarcoma of bone: Intergroup study IESS-II. *J Clin Oncol* 1990;8:1514-1524.

57. Grier H, Krailo M, Tarbell NJ, et al: Addition of ifosfamide and etoposide to standard chemo-

therapy for Ewing's sarcoma and primitive neuro-ectodermal tumor of bone. *N Engl J Med* 2003;348:694-701.

58. Meyer WH, Kun L, Marina N, et al: Ifosfamide plus etoposide in newly diagnosed Ewing's sarcoma of bone. *J Clin Oncol* 1992;10:1737-1742.

59. Miser JS, Akinsella TJ, Triche TJ, et al: Ifosfamide with mesna uroprotection and etoposide: An effective regimen in the treatment of recurrent sarcoma and other tumors of children and young adults. *J Clin Oncol* 1987;5:1191-1198.

60. Gibbs IC, Tuamokumo N, Yock TI: Role of radiation therapy in pediatric cancer. *Hematol Oncol Clin North Am* 2006;20:455-470.

61. Kushner BH, Meyers PA, Gerald WL et al: Very-high-dose short–term chemotherapy for poor-risk peripheral primitive neuroectodermal tumors, including Ewing's sarcoma in children and young adults. *J Clin Oncol* 1995;13:2796-2804.

62. La TH, Meyers PA, Wexler LH, et al: Radiation therapy for Ewing's sarcoma: Results from Memorial Sloan-Kettering in the modern era. *Int J Radiat Oncol Biol Phys* 2006;64:544-550.

63. McTiernan A, Drier D, Michelagnoli MP, Kilby Am, Whelan JS: High dose chemotherapy with bone marrow or peripheral stem cell rescue is an effective treatment option for patients with relapse or progressive Ewing's sarcoma family of tumours. *Ann Oncol* 2006;17:1301-1305.

64. Barker LM, Pendergrass TW, Sanders JE, Hawkins DS: Survival after recurrence of Ewing's sarcoma family of tumors. *J Clin Oncol* 2005;23:4354-4362.

65. Shankar AG, Ashley S, Craft AW, Pinkerton CR: Outcomes after relapse in an unselected cohort of children and adolescents with Ewing's sarcoma. *Med Pediatr Oncol* 2003;40:141-147.

66. Shankar AG, Pinkerton CR, Atra A: Local therapy and other factors influencing site of relapse in patients with localized Ewing's sarcomas: United Kingdom Children's Cancer Study Group (UKCCSG). *Eur J Cancer* 1999;35:1698-1704.

67. Koshy M, Paulino AC, Mai WY, Teh BS: Radiation-induced osteosarcomas in the pediatric population. *Int J Radiat Oncol Biol Phys* 2005;63:1169-1174.

68. Kotny U: Regulation of apoptosis and proliferation in Ewing's sarcoma: Opportunities for targeted therapy. *Hematol Oncol* 2006;34:14-21.

69. Meyers PA: High-dose therapy with autologous stem cell rescue for pediatric sarcomas. *Curr Opin Oncol* 2004;16:120-125.

70. Scotlandi K: Targeted therapies in Ewing's sarcoma. *Adv Exp Med Biol* 2006;587:13-22.

Chapter 5

Lymphoma and Myeloma of Bone

Lymphoma and myeloma are both malignant neoplasms that can arise from and materially affect the structure of bone. Lymphoma arises principally from lymphocytes in lymphoid tissues, but may also occur in the bone marrow, which is the cause of the bone lesions. Myeloma develops from plasma cells, which are ordinarily located within the marrow cavity. In orthopaedic presentations, the two disorders may closely resemble one another clinically or radiographically. Although the difference is relatively easy to establish with biochemical studies and biopsy, the finding of a single destructive lesion in a long bone, spine, or pelvis may be confusing. One must not only consider lymphoma or myeloma as the source, but metastatic disease to bone or even some primary lesions, all of which may resemble the two lesions that are the subject of this chapter. Although there are several types of lymphoma, the two principal ones to be considered in a primary bone setting are non-Hodgkin's lymphoma and, less commonly, Hodgkin's lymphoma. Myeloma may occur as a solitary lesion in bone but most often occurs in multiple sites with extensive alterations in biochemical data, especially the monoclonal immunoelectrophoretic pattern.

Lymphoma of Bone

Although both Hodgkin's and non-Hodgkin's lymphomas are not really rare disorders, involvement of the bones is unusual and is most often associated with diffuse disease. Either of the diseases occurring primarily in bone is considered to be uncommon, particularly for Hodgkin's disease.[1] Both disorders arise from lymphocytes. Hodgkin's disease was first described by Thomas Hodgkin in 1832,[2] and the disease came to be known by his name as a result of a report by Wilks in 1865.[3] The disorder is of unknown cause but was originally thought to resemble tuberculosis, partly because of the histologic appearance and particularly because of the presence of cells resembling Langhans giant cells.[3] These quite distinctive and diagnostic cells were described near the turn of the century separately by Reed[4] and Sternberg[5] and are eponymically known by their names. The disease is most often a diffuse one, affecting the lymph nodes, liver, spleen, lung, and other organs, and was initially thought to be uniformly fatal.[6,7] Various causes such as Epstein-Barr virus (EBV) infection, genetic errors, and immunologic abnormalities have been proposed, but to date there is no evidence to support any of these explanations and the disease is postulated to be a neoplasm of unknown origin.[7] Primary bone lesions in patients with Hodgkin's disease are considered very rare and most reports are of a small number of patients.[6,8-15] Of some interest is the finding of CD15 and CD30 antigens in the bone lesions on immunohistologic staining, but no evidence has been presented to support a true genetic error or a familial transmission of the disorder.[6] Familial disease occurs in less than 1% of the affected patients, although siblings may have a higher incidence of both Hodgkin's and non-Hodgkin's disease.[6,16,17] EBV has been implicated as a cause of Hodgkin's disease and although the cells may be EBV-positive, the finding has not been considered to be a cause of the disease.[7,17-20] Infections with *Helicobacter pylori* have also been implicated in the genesis of lymphomas, and the incidence of the lymphomatous disease in patients with human immunodeficiency virus (HIV) seems to be increased.[7,17-20]

Non-Hodgkin's lymphoma is a different entity; it was first called reticulum cell sarcoma[21] and subsequently defined as a primary disease of the lymphatic system. Although this disorder is similar in presentation to Hodgkin's disease, it has few of the histologic or clinical features.[17] The disease has multiple forms, including entities such as B-cell lymphoma, T-cell lymphoma, Burkitt's lymphoma, large-cell lym-

Table 1 | Ann Arbor Staging System for Non-Hodgkin's Lymphomas	
I_E	Involvement of a single extranodal site
II_E	Involvement of a single extranodal site with multiple nodal sites on the same side of the diaphragm
III_E	Involvement of single extranodal site with multiple nodal sites on both sides of the diaphragm
IV	Diffuse or disseminated involvement in distant extranodal sites

phoma, and lymphoplasmacytic lymphoma, all of which have similarities in presentation but have different prognoses.[22] Non-Hodgkin's lymphoma located primarily in the bone was first described by Oberling in 1928[23] and subsequently by Parker and Jackson in 1939.[21] Since then, there have been numerous reports of the clinical presentation, histologic pattern, and outcome for patients with this entity.[16,22,24-50] The disease itself is common and the bone tumors, although still unusual, are much more frequently encountered than in patients with Hodgkin's disease.[7] The disease that affects the bone most frequently is diffuse B-cell lymphoma, typically composed of large centroblastic cells with multilobated nuclei.[22] Most such lesions are believed to be immunologically positive for CD3 and some for CD10, which is believed to offer a better prognosis.[17,20,51] Recurrent translocations in large B-cell lymphomas include t(3;14)(q27;32) and several others involving 3q27 have been described. There is still no evidence for a genetic error or familial transmission.[17,52]

Both Hodgkin's and non-Hodgkin's lymphomas are more common in males than females and both occur in the middle years (age 40 to 65).[6,17,21,33,48] There are, however, groups of both types of tumors that occur in children and appear to have a better prognosis.[27,37,53]

The staging system ordinarily used by hematologists and oncologists for non-Hodgkins lymphoma is known as the Ann Arbor Staging System[17,54] (Table 1). It should be evident that those lesions that are confined to a single bone are stage 1_E and those tumors with other sites such as lymph nodes, viscera, or lungs have higher stages.

Clinical Course for Lymphoma of Bone

Imaging studies for lymphomas affecting the bones are fairly straightforward.[25,33,55] Most of the non-Hodgkin's lymphomas are lytic on radiographs and are most often confined

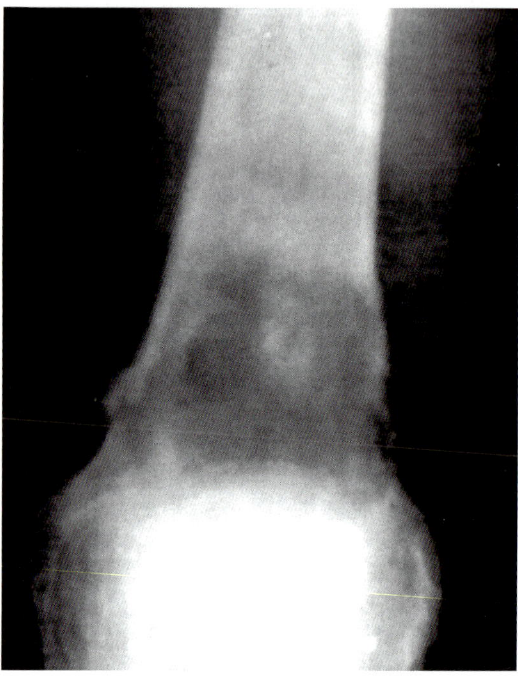

Figure 1
Radiograph of the distal femur in a patient with non-Hodgkin's lymphoma. The lesion is lytic and destructive but does not seem to have a soft-tissue mass.

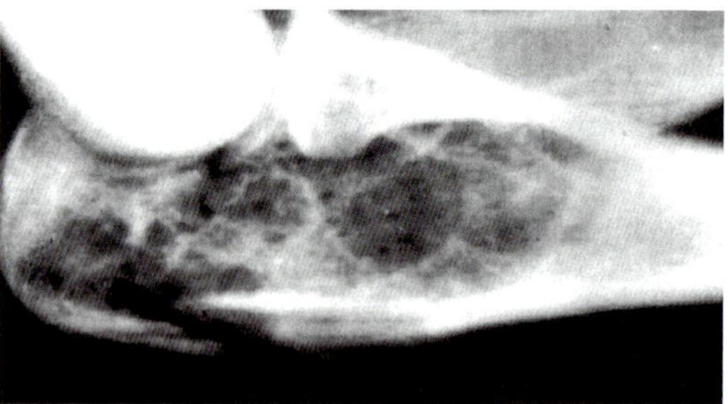

Figure 2
Radiograph of the proximal ulna in a patient with non-Hodgkin's lymphoma. The lesion appears to be irregular in structure and expansile, and has resulted in a fracture.

entirely within the bone[25,33,55] (Figure 1 and Figure 2). Some cases of very severe disease may have soft-tissue extensions, especially if fractures have occurred. In a report from Massachusetts General Hospital (MGH) on 140 cases of lymphoma of bone (130 were

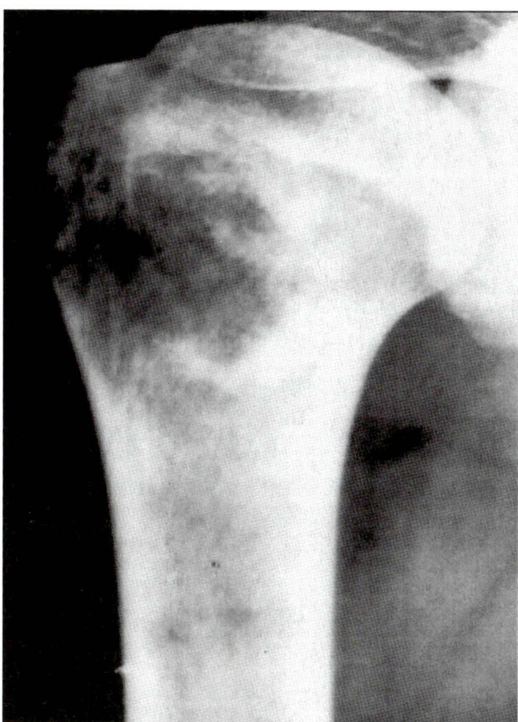

Figure 3

Radiograph of the proximal humerus with some sclerosis of the bone, suggestive of a diagnosis of Hodgkin's lymphoma.

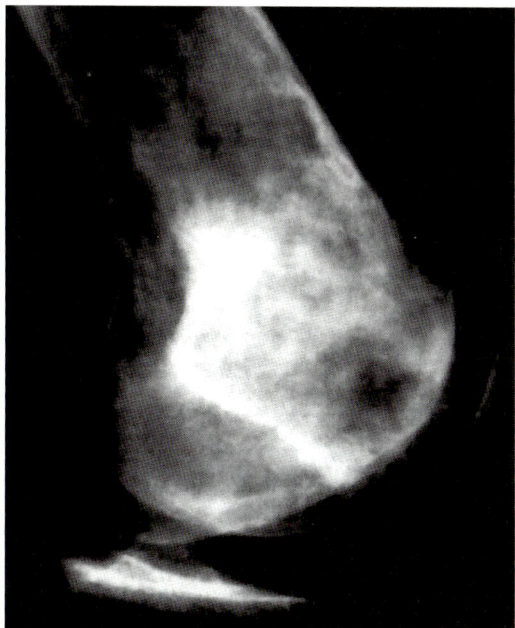

Figure 4

Radiograph of a very productive and destructive lesion of the distal femur, which was diagnosed as Hodgkin's lymphoma.

non-Hodgkin's lymphoma and 10 were Hodgkin's), approximately 35% were in the femur, 20% in the tibia, 20% in the shoulder region, and 20% in the spine or pelvis.[56] Very few lesions were located in acral parts. The non-Hodgkin's lesions were all lytic in appearance, but the Hodgkin's lymphomas of bone were sometimes productive and quite osteosclerotic (Figure 3 and Figure 4). All of the lesions in the MGH and other series were positive on bone scan. CT and MRI are helpful in defining the presence of a pathologic fracture or, in some cases, the presence of a soft-tissue mass surrounding the bone.[7,25,45,55,57] MRI and positron emission tomography (PET) scanning are valuable in defining the presence of lesions outside the bone in lymph nodes, lungs, or viscera.[7,17,25,45,51,55,57]

Histologic examination of the tissues from patients with either form of lymphoma of bone show principally lymphocytes, usually of B-cell type[17,25,33,55,57] (Figure 5). Hodgkin's lymphoma histology is quite distinctive related to the presence of multinucleated Reed-Sternberg cells (Figure 6) and sometimes large numbers of eosinophils.[6,7,11,17,25,55,57]

Laboratory studies are usually of limited value in defining the nature of the bone disease. The erythrocyte sedimentation rate and white count is often increased and occasionally one encounters patients with reduced hemoglobin, but there are no specific diagnostic studies that help with the diagnosis. Alkaline phosphatase may be elevated in patients with extensive bone disease. A biopsy is usually necessary to establish the diagnosis.[17,25,36,55,57]

The clinical course for lymphomas of bone is highly variable. Some of the lesions are small, totally within a bone, and are relatively easy to treat with surgical resection or radiation. Large lesions are more difficult to treat and often require the use of chemotherapy. The principal agents used are mechorethamine, vincristine, procarbazine, and prednisone; cyclophosphamide, doxorubicin, vincristine, and prednisone; or doxorubicin, bleomycin, vinblastine, and dacarbazine—all with or without radiation.[7,17,18,25,28,44,57-60] In some patients with extensive disease and severe marrow disorders, granulocyte colony-stimulating factor or autogenous or allograft stem cells have been used.[17,59] The overall survival rate for primary non-Hodgkin's bone lesions (without extension into lymph nodes or vis-

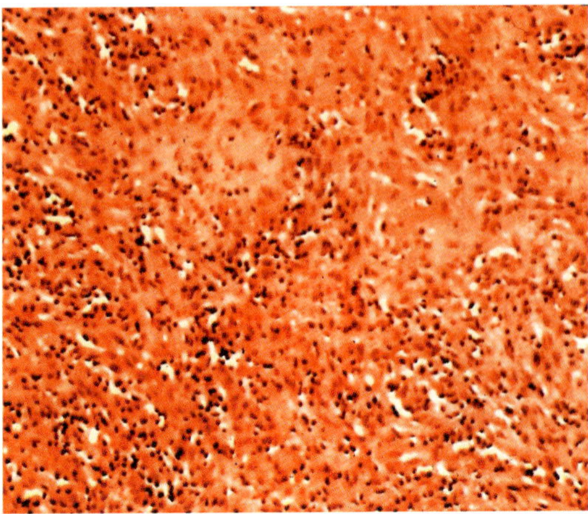

Figure 5

Histology of non-Hodgkin's lymphoma shows multiple round lymphoid B cells with increased density.

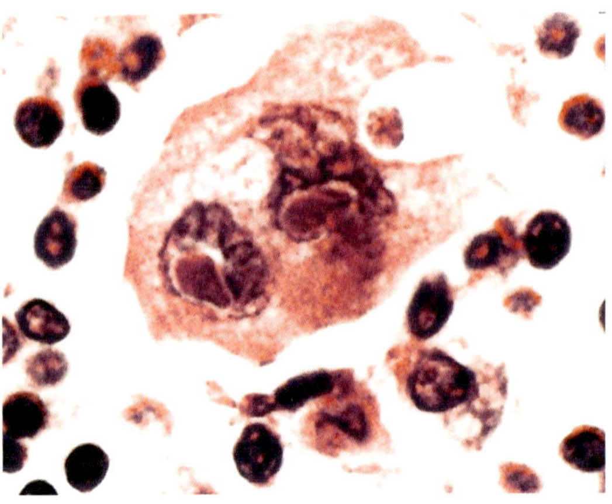

Figure 6

A Reed-Sternberg cell is characteristic of Hodgkin's lymphoma and is a characteristically bilobular giant cell. Eosinophils may also be present.

cera) is approximately 75% in several series, while reports on survival for patients with Hodgkin's lymphoma show a significantly increased death rate, even with extensive treatment.[56]

Myeloma

Myeloma is a common neoplasm principally occurring in the bones of mature adults. It was first described in 1850 by MacIntyre,[61] who reported on a patient with episodes of fatigue and bone pain. MacIntyre called the disorder "mollities and fragilitas ossium." Henry Bence Jones[62] tested urine specimens provided by MacIntyre's patient and described the abnormal light chains, which later became known as Bence-Jones protein. In 1846, Dalrymple[63] described the microscopic features of the disorder. The term multiple myeloma was introduced by Rustizky[64] in 1873, and in 1889 Otto Kahler[65] published an extensive review that resulted in the disease becoming known as Kahler's disease. At the turn of the century, the increased serum proteins and rapid erythrocyte sedimentation rate were identified as characteristic and the origin of the tumor was defined as arising from plasma cells.[66-70] The diagnosis was established by bone marrow aspiration in 1929, and the value of immunoelectrophoresis as a diagnostic instrument was reported in 1937.[68-70]

Disease that appears in a single site with few biochemical findings is known as "solitary plasmacytoma;" however, many of these become multiple over time.[66-69,71,72] In addi-

tion, there are some entities known as monoclonal gammopathies of unknown significance (MGUS), which may or may not be directly related to myeloma.[68-70] Another entity that is often included in descriptions of myeloma is Waldenström's macroglobulinemia, which is a form of the myeloid disease associated with plasma cell abnormalities but principally presenting as a bleeding and visceral disorder.[68-70,73]

Myeloma occurs principally in older individuals with a mean age of 68 years for men and 70 for women.[66-69,72,74,75] Fewer than 2% of the patients are younger than 40 years of age, whereas more than 50% are older than 70.[66-69,72,75] The male-to-female ratio in several series has been estimated as 2:1 or 3:2, and the disease is considerably more frequent in African-Americans than in Caucasians or Asians.[66-69,75] The disease also can occur in some animals, principally mice and dogs.[69]

The pathogenesis of multiple myeloma is obscure. Increased familial incidence is uncommon, although it occasionally is seen, particularly in African-American patients.[66-70,74-76] Endogenous retrovirus infection has been suggested and an initial unsubstantiated report suggested human herpes virus 8 as the cause.[66-69,72] Exposure to chemical and physical agents including benzene, petroleum products, pesticides, and radiation have all been implicated, but none has been clearly established as being causative.[66,69] Cytogenetic abnormalities are present in at least 60% of the cases and these are often complex, with translocations mostly involving chromosome 14q; however, 11q, 4p, and 8q have also been identified.[66-69,77-84] Interleukin 6 has been described as being essential to both the growth and maintenance of myelomatous plasma cells and may lead to the production of receptor activator of nuclear factor κB ligand (RANKL), which is known to increase the number of osteoclasts.[68,69,85,86] The vascular abnormalities may be related to the production of vascular endothelial growth factor (VEGF) by myeloma plasma cells.[68,69,85,87] Despite these findings there is no evidence for a genetic causation and there does not seem to be familial pattern of transmission.

Clinical Presentation of Multiple Myeloma

Myeloma can be limited, asymptomatic, and insidious;[71,88,89] or it can be a very severe, disabling, and life-threatening disorder.[90] In the latter disorder, known as multiple myeloma, production of plasma cells in the bone marrow not only cause weakness of bone structure, pathologic fractures, and spinal cord compression, but in addition may result in leukopenia, anemia, and thrombocytopenia[7,66,68-70,74,75,89-93] (Figure 7). Bone destruction can lead to hypercalcemia, which may severely affect the patients. Aberrant antibody production can lead to impaired immunity and many patients have a high prevalence of infection. The overproduction of antibodies can lead to hyperviscosity, amyloidosis, and renal failure. Immunoelectrophoretic studies show increased amounts of immunoglobulin G (IgG) or IgA, and bone-marrow aspirate is likely to show bone-marrow plasma cells.[66,68,69,80] Bence-Jones protein is often present in the urine.[66,68,69,80] The majority of these patients require extensive treatment but still have a relatively poor survival rate. A system for staging introduced in 1975 by Durie and Salmon[91] establishes the various patterns related to the extent of the disease (Table 2).

In sharp contrast with the above pattern is the picture of solitary plasmacytoma of bone, which occurs principally in the axial skeleton.[66,68,69,71,72,74,88-90,94,95] The bone-marrow studies, bone scans, and PET scanning fail to reveal other lesions and immunoelectrophoretic studies and search for

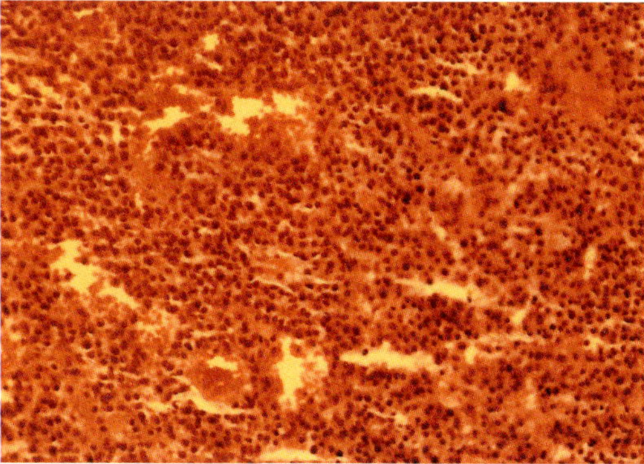

Figure 7

Histology of myeloma shows small round plasma cells, somewhat resembling lymphoid tissue.

Bence-Jones protein usually fail to support the presence of extensive disease. These patients respond well to radiation alone or excision of the local lesion with surgery.[66,68,69,71,72,74,88-90,94-96]

Still another form of the disease that remains a puzzle is MGUS.[7,34,66-69,72,88,89,97,98] These patients are found by chance to have an IgG or IgA paraprotein in the serum but with no other features to suggest myeloma. The affected individuals may include those with Gaucher disease or Hashimoto's disease, as well as other diseases. The bone marrow is normal, with less than 10% plasma cells, and the patients are asymptomatic. They still must be watched and have serial immunoelectrophoretic studies to be certain that the values for the paraproteins do not rise.

Another very rare and quite puzzling entity associated with myeloma is POEMS syndrome, which includes polyneuropathy (P), organomegaly (O), endocrinopathy (E), myeloma (M), and skin changes (S).[69,99] These patients have a very complex presentation consisting of all of the findings indicated in the name of the disease. Fortunately, they seem to respond well to high-dose chemotherapy and stem cell transplant.

Clinical Studies in Patients With Multiple Myeloma

Patients with multiple myeloma often present with bone pain associated with a fracture, most often of one or several vertebrae.[66,69,70,74,75,90,93,100] They may appear chronically ill and many have weight loss, fevers, abdominal distress, and neurologic disturbances. Physical examination shows

Table 2	Durie-Salmon Staging System for Multiple Myeloma		
	Stage I	Stage II	Stage III
Tumor cell mass	Low	Medium	High
Monoclonal IgG	<50	All in between	>70
Monoclonal IgA	<30		>50
Bence-Jones protein	<4		>12
Hemoglobin	<10		<8.5
Lytic lesions	0 or 1		Many
Stage A: Serum creatinine	<175		
Stage B: Serum creatinine	>175		

bone tenderness in multiple sites including the spine, pelvis, ribs, calvarium, and long bones (Figure 8). Laboratory studies show increased amounts of IgG or IgA paraproteins on immunoelectrophoresis, Bence-Jones protein in the urine, and a series of abnormalities in blood studies, including anemia, leukopenia, and thrombocytopenia.[7,66,69,74,75,80,90,100] The erythrocyte sedimentation rate is almost always elevated and the alkaline phosphatase is usually normal or low. Calcium may be greatly elevated. Bone marrow studies are likely to show greater than 10% plasma cells.[7,66,69,74,75,80,90,100]

Radiographic studies are helpful in that they sometimes show diffuse osteopenia in the skeleton and multiple lytic lesions in the spine, pelvis, ribs, and calvarium[66,69,74,75,80,94,100] (Figure 8). Compression fractures of the spine are often present and cause tensive pressure on the spinal cord (Figure 9). The bone scan is not always helpful because 25% of the lesions may be "cold" on standard studies, and PET scanning appears to be much more accurate in defining the extent of the disease.[69,94,100,101] As indicated above, the patients with solitary plasmacytoma of bone may show only one lesion, frequently in a vertebra, and the patients with MGUS may show no abnormalities other than the altered immunoelectrophoretic pattern.[13,66,69,71,74,88,89,94]

Treatment of Multiple Myeloma

There are many forms of treatment of patients with multiple myeloma. Chemotherapy with agents such as vincristine, dexamethasone, bis chloroethylnitrosourea, melphalan, cyclophosphamide, prednisone, and doxorubicin have all been introduced and are often helpful in reducing the pa-

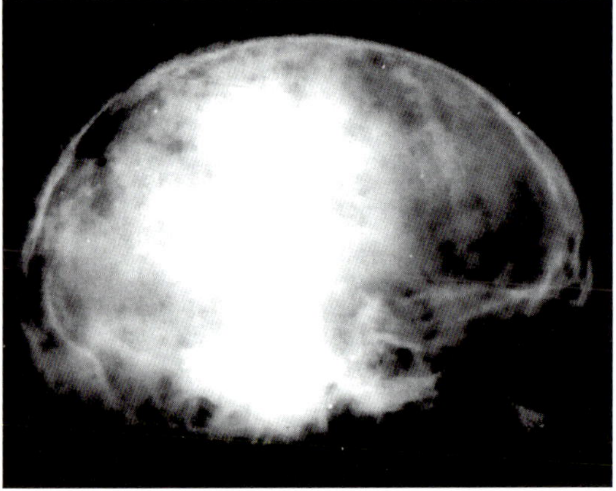

Figure 8
Radiograph of the calvarium showing multiple lytic sites. Serious neurologic problems may develop as a result.

tient's symptomatology and decreasing the extent of the marrow disease.[66,69,82,102-106] A recent addition that seems to be very effective is bortezomib (Velcade).[107] Radiation for local lesions is often successful in reducing pain and preventing further fractures.[66,108,109] Allogeneic marrow transplantation is used for severe cases,[110-116] but in elderly patients the technique has a high risk of complications. Stem cell transfer is safer, particularly for older individuals, but much more difficult to effectively administer.[69,82,116,117] Orthopaedic management for diffuse disease is principally that of treating fractures, spinal collapses with damage to the cord, or destroyed joints.[28,68,69,74,75] Most recently, bisphosphonates, in the form of pamidronate or zoledronate, seem to be helpful in strengthening the bones.[19,118,119] However, a recent concern regarding osteonecrosis of the mandible has reduced some physicians' enthusiasm for this method of therapy.[120] In patients with soli-

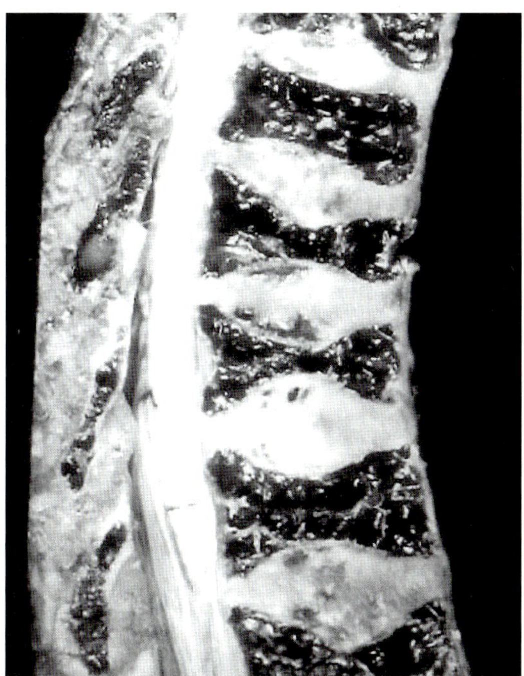

Figure 9

Photograph of an autopsy specimen showing multiple collapsed vertebrae with evidence of spinal cord compression.

tary plasmacytomas, resection or radiation or both have had good success and many patients have become asymptomatic.

Comments and Conclusions

Lymphoma and myeloma are fairly common neoplasms that can severely affect patients and in many cases result in their death. Lymphoma, particularly Hodgkin's, is rarely confined to bone, but non-Hodgkin's disease has a reasonably common presentation as a solitary bone lesion. Myeloma is principally a marrow disease and hence usually severely affects the bones. Both of the lesions have a wide range, however. They can cause solitary lesions, with few additional clinical problems, or extensive disease, with marked bony and visceral changes and great threat to life.

The remarkable feature related to both of these is that despite the fact that both disorders were first identified more than 100 years ago, we still have no real understanding as to the origin of the processes. Genetic abnormalities are present for both lymphoma and myeloma, but no clearly defined familial incidence. There are many identified characteristics and relationships to other disorders but no real knowledge as to causation. Despite that lack of knowledge, physicians have developed protocols to define the diseases, classify and stage them, determine the patient's risks, and treat them—in many cases very effectively. Bone disease for each of these disorders represents threats to structure and function, but with appropriate applications of chemotherapy, radiation, and marrow transplants, as many as 50% to 75% of the patients can continue to maintain a reasonably productive life.

References

1. Blount WP: Hodgkin's disease: An orthopedic problem. *J Bone Joint Surg Am* 1929;11: 761-770.

2. Hodgkin T: On some morbid appearances of the absorbent glands and spleen. *Med Chir Soc Trans* 1832;17:69-97.

3. Wilks S: Cases of enlargement of the lymphatic glands and spleen (or Hodgkin's disease), with remarks. *Guys Hosp Rep* 1865;11:56-67.

4. Reed D: On the pathological changes in Hodgkin's disease with special reference to its relation to tuberculosis. *Johns Hopkins Hosp Rep* 1902;10:133-196.

5. Sternberg C: Uber eine eigenartige unter dem Bilde der pseudoleukamie verlanfende tuberculose des lymphatischen apparatus. *Ztschr Heilk* 1898;19:21-90.

6. Kaplan HS: *Hodgkin's Disease*, ed 2. Cambridge, Harvard University Press, 1980.

7. Mauch P, Armitage JO: Hodgkin's disease, in Bast RC Jr, Kufe DW, Pollock RE, Weichselbaum RR, Holland JF, Frei E (eds): *Cancer Medicine*, ed 5. Hamilton, BC, Decker, 2000, pp 2010-2033.

8. Borg MF, Chowdhury AD, Bhoopal S, Benjamin CS: Bone involvement in Hodgkin's disease. *Australas Radiol* 1993;37:63-66.

9. Chan KW, Rosen G, Miller DR, Tan CT: Hodgkin's disease in adolescents presenting as a primary bone lesion: A report of four cases and review of the literature. *Am J Pediatr Hematol Oncol* 1982;4:11-17.

10. Cowie F, Benghiat A, Holgate C: Primary Hodgkin's disease of bone. *Clin Oncol (R Coll Radiol)* 1991;3:233-235.

11. Fried G, Ben Arieh Y, Haim N, Dale J, Stein M: Primary Hodgkin's disease of bone. *Med Pediatr Oncol* 1995;24:204-207.

12. Gross SB, Robertson WW Jr, Lange BJ, Bunin NJ, Drummond DS: Primary Hodgkin's disease of bone: A report of two cases in adolescents and review of the literature. *Clin Orthop Relat Res* 1992;283:276-280.

13. Moridaira K, Handa H, Murakami H, et al: Primary Hodgkin's disease of the bone presenting with an extradural tumor. *Acta Haematol* 1994;92:148-149.

14. Newcomer LN, Silverstein MB, Cadman EC, Farber LR, Bertino JR, Prosnitz LR: Bone involvement in Hodgkin's disease. *Cancer* 1982;49:338-342.

15. Ozdemirli M, Mankin HJ, Aisenberg AC, Harris NL: Hodgkin's disease presenting as a solitary bone tumor: A report of four cases and review of the literature. *Cancer* 1996;77:79-88.

16. Baar J, Burkes RL, Bell R, Blackstein ME, Fernandes B, Langer F: Primary non-Hodgkin's lymphoma of bone: A clinicopathologic study. *Cancer* 1994;73:1194-1199.

17. Freedman AS, Nadler LM: Non-Hodgkin's lymphoma, in Bast RC Jr, Kufe DW, Pollock RE, Weichselbaum RR, Holland JF, Frei E (eds): *Cancer Medicine*, ed 5. Hamilton, BC, Decker, 2000, pp 2034-2058.

18. Barbieri E, Cammelli S, Mauro F, et al: Primary non-Hodgkin's lymphoma of the bone: Treatment and analysis of prognostic factors for stage I and stage II. *Int J Radiat Oncol Biol Phys* 2004;59:760-764.

19. Berenson JR, Rosen LS, Howell A, et al: Zoledronic acid reduces skeletal-related events in patients with osteolytic metastases. *Cancer* 2001;91:1191-1200.

20. de Leval L, Braaten KM, Ancukiewicz M, et al: Diffuse large B-cell lymphoma of bone: An analysis of differentiation-associated antigens with clinical correlation. *Am J Surg Pathol* 2003;27:1269-1277.

21. Parker F, Jackson H: Primary reticulum cell sarcoma of bone. *Surg Gynecol Obstet* 1939;68:45-53.

22. Pettit CK, Zukerberg LR, Gray MH, et al: Primary lymphoma of bone: A B-cell neoplasm with a high frequency of mutilobated cells. *Am J Surg Pathol* 1990;14:329-334.

23. Oberling C: Les reticulosarcomes et les reticuloendotheliosarcomes de la moelle ossseuse. *Bull Assoc Fr Etud Cancer* 1928;17:259-296.

24. Brousse C, Baumelou E, Morel P: Primary lymphoma of bone: A prospective study of 28 cases. *Joint Bone Spine* 2000;67:446-451.

25. Campanacci M: Primary lymphoma of bone, in Campanacci M (ed): *Bone and Soft Tissue Tumors*, ed 2. New York, NY, Springer Verlag, 1999, pp 559-578.

26. Christie DR, Barton MB, Bryant G, et al: Osteolymphoma (primary bone lymphoma): An Australian review of 70 cases. Australian Radiation Oncology Lymphoma Group (AROLG). *Aust N Z J Med* 1999;29:214-219.

27. Coppes MJ, Patte C, Couanet D, et al: Childhood malignant lymphoma of bone. *Med Pediatr Oncol* 1991;19:22-27.

28. Dürr HR, Müller PE, Hiller E, et al: Malignant lymphoma of bone. *Arch Orthop Trauma Surg* 2002;122:10-16.

29. Falini B, Binazzi R, Pileri S, et al: Large cell lymphoma of bone: A report of three cases of B-cell origin. *Histopathology* 1988;12:177-190.

30. Francis KC, Higinbotham NL, Coley BL: Primary reticulum cell sarcoma of bone: Report of 44 cases. *Surg Gynecol Obstet* 1954;92:142-146.

31. Freeman C, Berg JW, Cutler SJ: Occurrence and prognosis of extranodal lymphomas. *Cancer* 1972;29:252-260.

32. Baar J, Burkes RL, Gospaoradowicz M: Primary non-Hodgkin's lymphoma of bone. *Semin Oncol* 1999;26:270-275.

33. Heyning FH, Hogendoorn PC, Kramer MH, et al: Primary non-Hodgkin's lymphoma of bone: A clincopathological investigation of 60 cases. *Leukemia* 1999;13:2094-2098.

34. Kyle RA, Therneau TM, Rajkumar SV, et al: A long-term study of prognosis in monoclonal gammopathy of undetermined significance. *N Engl J Med* 2002;346:564-569.

35. Lacor P, Cocquyt V, Schots R, Mathijs R, Van Camp B: Malignant lymphoma of the bone. *Acta Clin Belg* 1990;45:386-393.

36. Lin F, Staerkel G, Fanning TV: Cytodiagnosis of primary lymphoma of bone on fine-needle aspiration cytology specimens: Review of 25 cases. *Diagn Cytopathol* 2003;28:205-211.

37. Lones MA, Perkins SL, Sposto R, et al: Non-Hodgkin's lymphoma arising in bone in children and adolescents is associated with an excellent outcome: A Children's Cancer Group report. *J Clin Oncol* 2002;20:2293-2301.

38. Luna-Ortiz K, Cervera-Ceballos E, Doninguez-Malagon H, et al: Primary lymphoma of bone. *Rev Invest Clin* 2003;55:502-506.

39. Marshall DT, Amdur RJ, Scarborough MT, Mendenhall NP, Virkus WW: Stage 1E primary non-Hodgkin's lymphoma of bone. *Clin Orthop Relat Res* 2002;405:216-222.

40. McCormack LJ, Ivins JC, Dahlin DC, Johnson EW Jr: Primary reticulum-cell sarcoma of bone. *Cancer* 1952;5:1182-1192.

41. Misgeld E, Wehmeier A, Krömeke O, Gattermann N: Primary non-Hodgkin's lymphoma of bone: Three cases and a short review of the literature. *Ann Hematol* 2003;82:440-443.

42. Ostrowski ML, Unni KK, Banks PM, et al: Malignant lymphoma of bone. *Cancer* 1986;58:2646-2655.

43. Radaszkiewicz T, Hansmann ML: Primary high-grade malignant lymphoma of bone. *Virchows Arch A Pathol Anat Histopathol* 1988;413:269-274.

44. Rathmell AJ, Gospodarowicz MK, Sutcliffe SB, Clark RM: Localized lymphoma of bone: Prognostic factors and treatment recommendations. The Princess Margaret Hospital Lymphoma Group. *Br J Cancer* 1992;66:603-606.

45. Ruzek KA, Wenger DE: The multiple faces of lymphoma of the musculoskeletal system. *Skeletal Radiol* 2004;33:1-8.

46. Shannon JA, Bell DR, Levi JA, Wheeler HR, Boyle FM: Bone presentation of non-Hodgkin's lymphoma: Experience in the Royal North Shore Hospital, Sydney. Highlighting primary bone lymphoma. *Aust N Z J Med* 1994;24:701-704.

47. Ueda T, Aozasa K, Ohsawa M, et al: Malignant lymphomas of bone in Japan. *Cancer* 1989;64:2387-2392.

48. Unni KK: Malignant lymphoma of bone, in Unni KK (ed): *Dahlin's Bone Tumors*, ed 5. Philadelphia, PA, Lippincott, Raven, 1996, pp 237-248.

49. Valls J, Muscolo D, Schajowicz R: Reticulum cell sarcoma of bone. *J Bone Joint Surg Br* 1952;34:588-598.

50. Yuste AL, Segura A, López-Tendero P, Gironés R, Montalar J, Gómez-Codina J: Primary lymphoma of bone: A clinico-pathological review and analysis of prognostic factors. *Leuk Lymphoma* 2004;45:853-855.

51. Fabiani B, Delmer A, Lepage E, et al: Prognostic

significance and morphologic features of diffuse large B-cell lymphomas expressing CD10. *J Clin Pathol* 2002;55:A14.

52. Alizadeh AA, Eisen MB, Davis RE, et al: Distinct types of diffuse large B-cell lymphoma identified by gene expression profiling. *Nature* 2000;403:503-511.

53. Glotzbecker MP, Kersun LS, Choi JK, Wills BP, Schaffer AA, Dormans JP: Primary non-Hodgkin's lymphoma of bone in children. *J Bone Joint Surg Am* 2006;88:583-594.

54. Harris NL, Jaffe ES, Diebold J, et al: World Health Organization classification of neoplastic diseases of the hematopoietic and lymphoid tissues: Report of the Clinical Advisory Committee meeting-Airlie House, Virginia, November 7, 1997. *J Clin Oncol* 1999;17:3835-3849.

55. Melamed JW, Martinez S, Hoffman CJ: Imaging of primary multifocal osseous lymphoma. *Skeletal Radiol* 1997;26:35-41.

56. Mankin HJ, Hornicek FJ, Harmon DC, Gebhardt MC: Lymphoma of bone: A review of 140 patients. *Therapy* 2006;3:499-508.

57. Clayton F, Butler JJ, Ayala AG, Ro JY, Zornoza J: Non-Hodgkin's lymphoma in bone: Pathologic and radiologic features with clinical correlates. *Cancer* 1987;60:2494-2501.

58. Bacci G, Jaffe N, Emiliani E, et al: Therapy for primary non-Hodgkin's lymphoma of bone and a comparison of results with Ewing's sarcoma: Ten years' experience at the Istituto Orthopedico Rizzoli. *Cancer* 1986;57:1468-1472.

59. Beal K, Allen L, Yahalom J: Primary bone lymphoma: Treatment results and prognostic factors with long-term follow-up of 82 patients. *Cancer* 2006;106:2652-2656.

60. Fidias P, Spiro I, Sobczak M, et al: Long-term results of combined modality therapy in primary bone lymphomas. *Int J Radiat Oncol Biol Phys* 1999;45:1213-1218.

61. MacIntyre W: Case of mollities and fragilitas ossium, accompanied with urine strongly charged with animal matter. *Med Chir Trans Lond* 1850;33:211-232.

62. Bence Jones H: On the new substance occurring in the urine of patient with mollities ossium. *Philo Trans Royal Soc London* 1848;138:55-62.

63. Dalrymple J: On the microscopical character of mollities ossium. *Dublin Q J Med Sci* 1846;2:85-95.

64. Rustizky J: Multiple myeloma. *Dtsch Z Chir* 1873;3:162-172.

65. Kahler O: Zur symptomatologie des multiplen myeloms: Beobachtung von albuminosurie. *Prag Med Wschr* 1889;14:33-35.

66. Anderson K: Plasma cell tumors, in Bast RC Jr, Kufe DW, Pollock RE, Weichselbaum RR, Holland JE, Frei E III (eds): *Cancer Medicine*, ed 5. Hamilton, BC, Decker. 2000, pp 2066-2086.

67. Hussein MA, Oken MM: Multiple myeloma, macroglobulinemia and amyloidosis, in Furie B, Casileth PA, Atkins MB, Mayer RJ (eds): *Clinical Hematology and Oncology: Presentation, Diagnosis and Treatment*. Philadelphia, PA, Churchill Livingstone, 2003, pp 581-600.

68. Munshi NC, Anderson KC: Plasma cell neoplasms, in DeVita VT Jr, Hellman S, Rosenberg SA (eds): *Cancer Principles and Practices of Oncol-ogy*, ed 7. Philadelphia, PA, Lippincott, Williams & Wilkins, 2005, pp 2155-2188.

69. Samson D: Multiple myeloma, in Price P, Sikora K (eds): *Treatment of Cancer*, ed 4. London, Arnold Publishers, 2002, pp 997-1016

70. Schajowicz F: *Tumors and Tumorlike Lesions of Bone and Joints*. New York, NY, Springer-Verlag 1981, pp 281-302.

71. Bataille R: Localized plasmacytomas. *Clin Haematol* 1982;11:113-122.

72. Kyle RA: "Benign" monoclonal gammopathy—after 20-35 years of follow-up. *Mayo Clin Proc* 1993;68:26-36.

73. Waldenström J: Incipient myelomatosis or "essential" hyperglobulinemia with fibrogenopenia: A new syndrome? *Acta Med Scand* 1944;117:217-224.

74. Callander NS, Roodman GD: Myeloma bone disease. *Semin Hematol* 2001;38:276-285.

75. Campanacci M: Multiple myeloma, in Campanacci M (ed): *Bone and Soft Tissue Tumors*, ed 2. New York, NY, Springer Verlag, 1999 pp 581-594.

76. Ogmundsdóttir HM, Haraldsdóttirm V, Jóhannesson GM, et al: Familiality of benign and malignant paraproteinemias: A population-based cancer-registry study of multiple myeloma families. *Haematologica* 2005;90:66-71.

77. Bergsagel PL, Kuehl WM: Chromosome translocations in multiple myeloma. *Oncogene* 2001;20:5611-5622.

78. Epstein J, Xiao HQ, He XY: Markers of multiple hematopoietic cell-lineages in multiple myeloma. *N Engl J Med* 1990;322:664-668.

79. Harada H, Kawano MM, Huang N, et al: Phenotypic difference of normal plasma cells from mature myeloma cells. *Blood* 1993;81:2658-2663.

80. Kyle RA: Diagnostic criteria of multiple myeloma. *Hematol Oncol Clin North Am* 1992;6:347-358.

81. Shaughnessy J, Tian E, Sawyer J, et al: High incidence of chromosome 13 deletion in multiple myeloma detected by mutiprobe intephase FISH. *Blood* 2000;96:1505-1511.

82. Tosi P, Gamberi B, Giuliani N: Biology and treatment of multiple myeloma. *Biol Blood Marrow Transplant* 2006;12:81-86.

83. Van Camp B, Durie BG, Spier C, et al: Plasma cells in multiple myeloma express natural killer cell-associated antigen: CD56 (NKH-1;Leu-19). *Blood* 1990;76:377-382.

84. Zandecki M, Laï JL, Facon T: Multiple myeloma: Almost all patients are cytogenetically abnormal. *Br J Haematol* 1996;94:217-227.

85. Klein B, Zhang XG, Lu ZY, Bataille R: Interleukin-6 in human multiple myeloma. *Blood* 1995;85:863-872.

86. Roux S, Meignin V, Quillard J: RANK (receptor activator of nuclear factor-kappa B) and RANKL expression in multiple myeloma. *Br J Haematol* 2002;117:86-92.

87. Bellamy WT: Expression of vascular endothelial growth factor and its receptors in multiple myeloma and other hematopoietic malignancies. *Semin Oncol* 2001;28:551-559.

88. Alexanian R: Localized and indolent myeloma. *Blood* 1980;56:521-525.

89. Corwin J, Lindberg RD: Solitary plasmacytoma of bone versus extramedullary plasmacytoma and

their relationship to multiple myeloma. *Cancer* 1979;43:1007-1013.

90. Bartl R, Frisch B, Fateh-Moghadam A, Kettner G, Jaeger K, Sommerfeld W: Histologic classification and staging of multiple myeloma: A retrospective and prospective study of 674 cases. *Am J Clin Pathol* 1987;87:342-355.

91. Durie BG, Salmon SE: A clinical staging system for multiple myeloma: Correlation of measured myeloma cell mass with presenting clinical features, response to treatment, and survival. *Cancer* 1975;36:842-854.

92. Kamble R, Rosenzweig T: Diffuse pulmonary parenchymal involvement in multiple myeloma: Antemortem diagnosis. *Int J Hematol* 2006;83:259-261.

93. Matsumoto T, Abe M: Bone destruction in multiple myeloma. *Ann N Y Acad Sci* 2006;1068:319-326.

94. Hess T, Egerer G, Kasper B, Rasul KI, Goldschmidt H, Kauffmann GW: Atypical manifestations of multiple myeloma: Radiological appearance. *Eur J Radiol* 2006;58:280-285.

95. Knobel D, Zouhair A, Tsang RW, et al: Prognostic factors in solitary plasmacytoma of the bone: A multicenter Rare Cancer Network study. *BMC Cancer* 2006;6:118.

96. Dimopoulos MA, Goldstein J, Fuller L, Delasalle K, Alexanian R: Curability of solitary bone plasmacytoma. *J Clin Oncol* 1992;10:587-590.

97. Kuwatsuka Y, Suzuki R, Ichihashi R, Kodera Y: Psuedo-Gaucher cells in light chain plasma cell myeloma. *Am J Hematol* 2006;81:468-469.

98. Martín MG, Romero Colás MS, Dourdil Sahún MV, Olave P, Alba PR, Banzo JB: BaselinTc99-MIBI scanning predicts survival in multiple myeloma and helps to differentiate this disease from monoclonal gammopathy of unknown significance. *Haematologica* 2005;90:1141-1143.

99. Rovira M, Carreras E, Bladé J: Dramatic improvement of POEMS syndrome following autologous haematopoetic cell transplantation. *Br J Haematol* 2001;115:373-375.

100. Healy JC, Armstong P: Radiological features of multiple myeloma, in Malpas JS, Bergsagel DE, Kyle RA, Anderson KC (eds): *Myeloma: Biology and Management*. Oxford, Oxford University Press, 1998, pp 235-265

101. Orchard K, Barrington S, Buscombe J, Hilson A, Prentice HG, Mehta A: Fluoro-deoxyglucose positron emission tomography imaging for the detection of occult disease in multiple myeloma. *Br J Haematol* 2002;117:133-135.

102. Alexanian R, Dimopoulos M: The treatment of multiple myeloma. *N Engl J Med* 1994;330:484-489.

103. Barlogie B, Zangari M, Spencer T, et al: Thalidomide in the management of multiple myeloma. *Semin Hematol* 2001;38:250-259.

104. Garcia-Sanz R: Thalidomide in multiple myeloma. *Expert Opin Pharmacother* 2006;7:195-213.

105. Kumar L, Viram P, Kochupillai V: Recent advances in the management of multiple myeloma. *Natl Med J India* 2006;19:80-89.

106. Tosi P, Zamagni E, Cellini C, et al: First line therapy with thalidomide, dexamethasone and zoledronic acid decrease bone resorption markers in patients with multiple myeloma. *Eur J Haematol* 2006;76:399-404.

107. Goronov SE, Goanova-Marinova VS: Bortezomib (Velcade)—A new therapeutic strategy for patients with refractory multiple myeloma. *Folia Med (Plovdiv)* 2005;47:11-19.

108. Ampil FL, Chin HW: Radiotherapy alone for extradural compression by spinal myeloma. *Radiat Med* 1995;13:129-131.

109. Rowell NP, Tobias JS: The role of radiotherapy in the management of multiple myeloma. *Blood Rev* 1991;5:84-89.

110. Alyea E, Weller E, Schlossman R, et al: T-cell–depleted allogeneic bone marrow transplantation followed by donor lymphocyte infusion in patients with multiple myeloma: Induction of graft-versus-myeloma effect. *Blood* 2001;98:934-939.

111. Bellucci R, Alyea EP, Weller E, et al: Immunologic effects of prophylactic donor lymphocyte infusion after allogeneic marrow transplantation in multiple myeloma. *Blood* 2002;99:4610-4617.

112. Björkstrand BB, Ljungman P, Svensson H, et al: Allogeneic bone marrow transplantation versus autologous stem cell transplantation in multiple myeloma: A retrospective case-matched study from the European Group for Blood and Marrow Transplantation. *Blood* 1996;88:4711-4718.

113. Gahrton G, Svensson H, Cavo M, et al: Progress in allogeneic bone marrow and peripheral blood stem cell transplantation for multiple myeloma: A comparison between transplants performed 1983-93 and 1994-8 at European Group for Blood and Marrow Transplantation centres. *Br J Haematol* 2001;113:209-216.

114. Gerull S, Goerner M, Benner A, et al: Long-term outcome of non-myeloablative allogeneic transplantation in patients with high-risk multiple myeloma. *Bone Marrow Transplant* 2005;36:963-969.

115. Speer SA, Semenza JC, Kurosaki T, Anton-Culver H: Risk factors for acute myeloid leukemia and multiple myeloma: A combination of GIS and case-control studies. *J Environ Health* 2002;64:9-16.

116. Vesole DH, Simic A, Lazarus HM: Controversy in multiple myeloma transplants: Tandem autotransplants and mini-allografts. *Bone Marrow Transplant* 2001;28:725-735.

117. Badros A, Barlogie B, Siegel E, et al: Autologous stem cell transplantation in elderly multiple myeloma patients over the age of 70 years. *Br J Haematol* 2001;114:600-607.

118. Berenson JR, Lichtenstein A, Porter L, et al: Efficacy of pamidronate in reducing skeletal events in patients with advanced multiple myeloma: Myeloma Aredia Study Group. *N Engl J Med* 1996;334:488-493.

119. Jantunen E, Laakso M: Bisphosphonates in multiple myeloma: Current status. Future perspectives. *Br J Haematol* 1996;93:501-506.

120. Dimopoulos MA, Kastritis E, Anagnostopoulos A, et al: Osteonecrosis of the jaw in patients with multiple myeloma treated with bisphosphonates: Evidence of increased risk after treatment with zoledronic acid. *Haematologica* 2006;91:968-971.

Chapter 6

Metastatic Carcinoma to Bone

Bone metastases from primary carcinomas are frequent occurrences and certainly represent a major threat to survival and a source of great concern. The lesions are more common in patients with breast or prostatic carcinomas, occurring in up to 70% of untreated patients with these primary lesions. They are considerably less common but still a major concern for patients with primary cancers of the lung, thyroid, and kidney (approximately 30% of them get bone metastases); even fewer patients have bone metastases with gastrointestinal, uterine, rectum, and bladder primary cancers. Bone metastases from lung, kidney, and prostate carcinomas have a high likelihood of rapid demise, while those patients with breast and thyroid primary tumors can live longer. The problems associated with bone metastases are often significant, with pain, hematologic abnormalities, fractures, deformities, neurovascular problems, and physical disabilities that greatly affect the patient. Until relatively recently, there was little that could be done, particularly for extensive disease, but there are now some approaches that may make life easier for some of the patients and, for a few others, may provide a "cure."

History of Bone Metastatic Disease

Cancer was well recognized by physicians, even in ancient times. Evidence of primary and metastatic carcinomas was found in Egyptian mummies,[1-3] and Hippocrates described the changes seen in some types of cancer in the early days of Grecian medicine.[4,5] Hippocrates and, subsequently, Galen introduced the terms "karkinoi" and "karkinoma" for nodules that arose in a variety of organs.[4-7] Galen decided that the cause of these lesions was "black bile,"[5-7] and it was not until the 16th and 17th centuries that this concept was no longer considered to be a cause. Vesalius advanced the theory that the cancer grew at a primary site and then spread to other foci via lymphatic or vascular pathways.[8] He and others proposed that treatment by excising lymphatic structures, bleeding the patient to reduce the marrow elements, coagulation of the primary tumor, and even excisional surgery or amputation might be of some value.[3,5,8,9] The identification of metastases to bone became apparent after histologic studies of the bony site were found to be identical to the primary site.[10] The key question is why the lesions metastasize to bone. According to a concept originally proposed by Stephen Paget[11] in 1889, the cells find the bone marrow an ideal setting for survival in terms of vascularity, oxygen, nutritional elements, etc; he called it the "seed-and-soil hypothesis." Although initial trials of radiation at the turn of the last century seemed to help,[12] bone metastases became known as evidence of widespread disease and most often represented the end of hope for the patient. Happily, in more recent times it seems possible to moderate the disease and even cure it by appropriate surgery, radiation, and chemotherapy.

Primary Sites and Variation in Metastatic Bone Characteristics

There are five principal sites for primary carcinomas that metastasize to bone.

Breast

Breast cancer is one of the most common causes of metastatic bone disease.[13-19] The osseous lesions are generally located in the pelvis, ribs, spine, proximal humerus, and proximal femur, and only rarely below the knees and elbows.[15,20,21] When lytic, they show considerable cortical expansion and often fracture. About half of these show osteoblastic activity on imaging studies, with considerable amounts of dense bone present at the sites.[15,16,20] The tumors are often associated with lymph node and lung metastases, both of which markedly decrease the potential for survival[13-19] (Figure 1).

Prostate

Prostatic carcinoma is a common cause of metastatic tumors.[15,22-26] Most of these result from involvement of an unusual venous

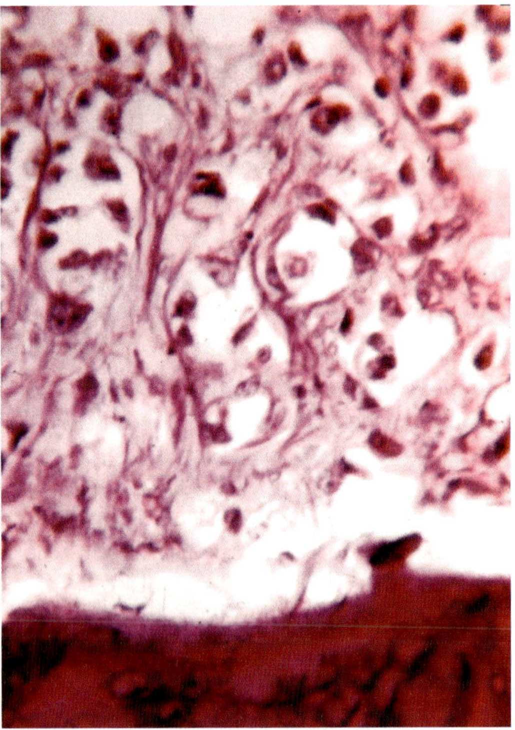

Figure 1
Histologic image of a lesion metastatic to bone from a breast cancer. The cells are small, round, and typical of lesions within the breast.

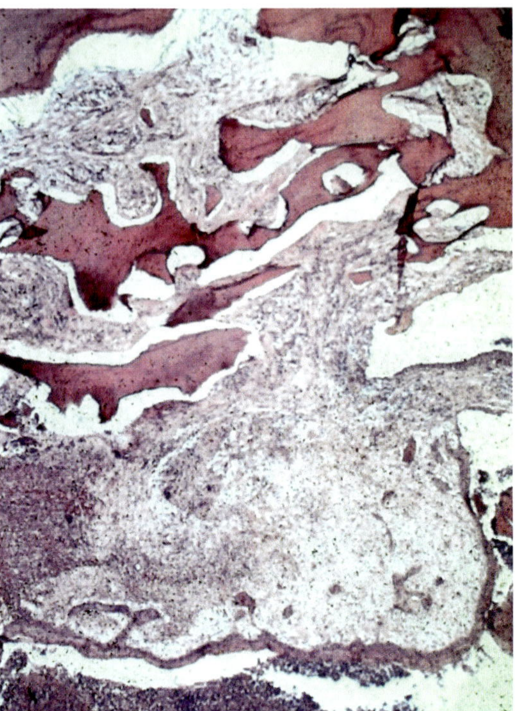

Figure 2
Prostatic cancer metastasis is histologically similar to the prostate primary lesion. Note the presence of bone formation, which occurs in 90% of the lesions.

system known as Batson's plexus.[15,16,20] The plexus has no valvular components and extends from the pelvic region up into the paravertebral and vertebral regions to enter the vena cava. Most of these metastases involve the pelvis, proximal femora, and vertebral segments.[15,16,20,22,23,26] They are almost always very dense on imaging studies and may materially enlarge the bone.[15,16,20,22,23,26] Despite the increase in bone density, fractures are not uncommon.[14,20,21] Pulmonary metastases are less common than lymph nodal extensions from the primary site. Hypercalcemia may develop based on the rapid turnover of affected bones (Figure 2).[15,21,23-26]

Lung

Pulmonary metastases to bone are often extensive and mostly destructive, with little new bone formation (only about 30% show increased density on imaging studies).[20,21,25,27-29] They may occur in any bones, but especially the pelvis, ribs, shoulder, and clavicle.[15,20] The metastatic deposits, unlike those from breast, prostate, or other sites, frequently appear in the hands

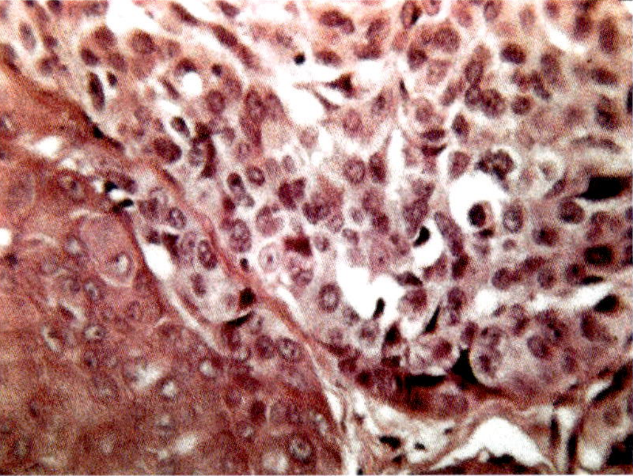

Figure 3
The metastatic lung cancer histologic pattern is very aggressive, with large numbers of atypical cells.

and feet.[15,20,29] The prognosis for patients with lung cancer in whom bone metastases develop is generally very poor, and their death often occurs a short time after discovery of the lesions[15,20,27-29] (Figure 3).

Thyroid

Bone metastases do not regularly develop in patients with carcinoma of the thyroid. When they do occur, they are often in the region around the shoulder, clavicles, or cervical spine, most of which are in close relationship to the vascular and lymphatic sites adjacent to the thyroid gland.[15,20,21,30,31] The lesions are lytic and generally neither aggressive nor destructive. The prognosis is considerably better than for lesions that occur in relation to breast, lung, or prostate primary tumors.[15,20,25]

Kidney

Renal cancers are often very vascular and their osseous metastases often have an enormous blood supply that may result in major bleeding at the time of biopsy or surgical excision.[15,20,25,32,33] The lesions are always destructive and may result in fractures. Unlike some of the other lesions, such as breast or prostate, they may be solitary. Surgical removal of nonpelvic lesions may be curative.

Other Primary Sites

Much less commonly, primary cancers of the uterus, bowel, liver, stomach, or rectum may metastasize to bone.[15,16,20,21,25,34-36] Some of these lesions are very destructive and may principally affect the adjacent vertebral sites, pelvis, and especially the pubic bones. The tumors are much more rarely encountered than the five described above and the prognosis is difficult to predict.

Myeloma and lymphoma within bone are both considered by some to be metastatic tumors. Both of these, however, seem to arise from proliferation of malignant plasma cells or atypical lymphocytes, which are normally present in the marrow.

Pathophysiology

As noted earlier in this chapter, in the past, the only two ways of assessing the origin of an osseous metastasis was to search for a primary lesion and/or to view the histology of the bony lesion.[10,12,16,20] This was not always easily done, as primary tumors may be occult and, before positron emission tomography (PET) scanning,[37] could sometimes not be found even at autopsy. The second issue was that the bone biopsy was sometimes materially altered by fractures or bony repair and as a result was difficult to read.[15,16,20]

First, one must consider how a tumor confined to the prostate, breast, lung, or kidney goes to bone.[15,34,35,38-40] Initially, the tu-mor cells must proliferate and then escape from the primary site by destroying the surrounding membrane, using some form of collagenase. They must then adhere to a vascular wall and cause a defect in the wall of sufficient magnitude to allow the cells to enter, but not great enough to produce extensive local bleeding. Finally, the tumor cells must break free of the vascular membrane and go off into the blood vessel to enter the marrow cavity.[15,34,35,40] These steps require an array of cytokine agents, including laminin, fibronectin, interleukins, some special collagenases, and other metalloproteases.[15,34,35,38,39] Once the cells enter the marrow, they generally activate osteoclastic activity by production of receptor activator of nuclear factor κB ligand (RANKL), osteoprotegerin, vascular endothelial growth factor (VEGF),[41-43] parathyroid hormone-related peptide, and interleukins 1, 6, and 11.[44] They also increase tumor cell DNA synthesis by production of transforming growth factor-beta (TGF-β) or its receptor TGF-β RII,[45-47] prostaglandins, and other stimulants,[15,34,35] including Wnts, an array of genetic materials that regulate cell growth.[48-50]

In addition, these activities vary depending on the type of tumor, the tumor cell survival rates, the response of the marrow elements to the new cells, and the ability of the cells to synthesize osteoblasts in response to the tumor cell cytokine production.[24,34,51,52] Furthermore, some tumor cells, such as those from prostate and breast cancers, actively stimulate osteoblast production, while others, especially lung, thyroid, and kidney tumors, are much more likely to promote marked osteoclast production.[23,26,35,38,48,49]

Given the remarkable number of agents that appear to influence the spread of cancer into bones, several of these may be used as biomarkers for the detection of metastases. These include bone resorption markers (osteoprotegein, RANKL, VEGF, tartrate-resistant acid phosphatase 5b, and parathyroid hormone-related peptide)[41-43,53-56] and bone production markers (calcium receptor, alkaline phosphatase, and bone-specific alkaline phosphatase).[38,56-58] Prostate-specific antigen (PSA)[22] and thyroid studies (thyroid-stimulating hormone and T4 [thyroxine])[59] are also helpful in distinguishing prostate, breast, and thyroid cancers from others.[19,26]

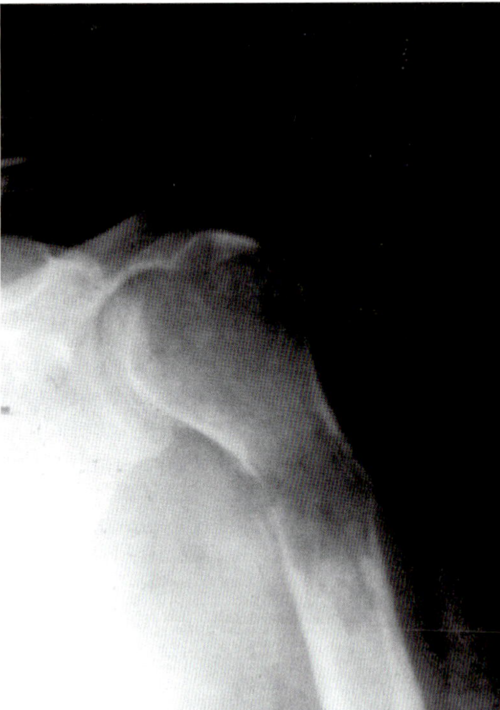

Figure 4
Radiograph of a destructive lesion of the humerus in a patient with breast cancer.

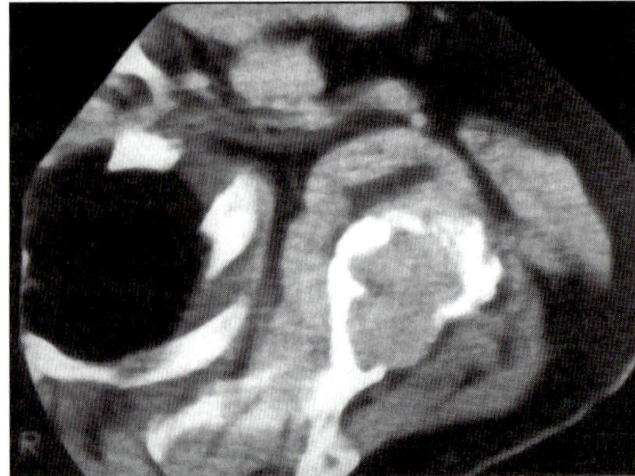

Figure 5
CT scan of the proximal humerus, showing a lytic lesion in a patient with thyroid cancer.

Imaging Studies

The appearance of bone metastases from carcinomatous primary foci may vary enormously based on the type of tumor and its aggressiveness, the size of the lesion, the anatomic site, the patient's age, the degree of osteopenia (particularly in older women), the vascular supply of the bone, and the presence of a pathologic fracture.[13,15,16,18,20,23,26,29,31,59] Lesions of the spine differ from those of the long bones, and those of the pelvis sometimes result in major structural abnormalities and neurovascular compromise.[15,20] The "0-30-60-90-rule" applies to the presence of increased bone density; 0% osteoblastic metastases applies to thyroid and renal primaries, 30% to lung cancers, 60% to breast cancers, and 90% to prostate primary tumors.[17,20,23,27,31,33]

Lytic bone metastases are often expanded on radiographic, CT, or MRI studies and have some structural distortion and thin cortices[15,20] (Figure 4). Pathologic fractures are frequent. The lesions are virtually always very active on both bone scintigraphy and PET scan.[37,59] Renal cell tumors are often highly vascular and surgeons often do angiographic occlusive procedures before

biopsy or surgical resection.[33] Thyroid tumors are usually smaller; located in the clavicles, upper extremities, or cervical spine; and are less destructive[31] (Figure 5). Lesions in the acral parts and even hand or foot bones are usually due to lung cancer and are typically lytic and often quite destructive.[27-29] Most calvarial lesions are also lytic and often multiple. Those located in the spine may be the cause of a collapse of one or several vertebral segments and may show damage to the cord or neural structures on MRI[15,16,60] (Figure 6).

Productive bone metastases are often located proximally in the long bones or in the pelvis and possibly the spinal segments, based largely on the prostatic relationship to Batson's plexus[23,26] (Figure 7).

Treatment

All patients with destructive or productive lesions of the bones must be carefully evaluated. Metastatic cancer in bone is unusual in children; however, in adults, particularly those older than age 45 years, a metastasis is believed to be more than 100 times more frequent than primary lesions.[35] The system for evaluation includes the following:

- A careful history and physical examination. All possible factors (smoking, alcoholism, estrogen or progesterone intake, exposure to radiation or toxic substances, etc) are important parts of the review and should be documented.

- Imaging studies of the lesion. Radiographs, CT, and MRI are useful and helpful in defining the nature of the lesion and especially the likelihood of a pathologic fracture.[15,60]

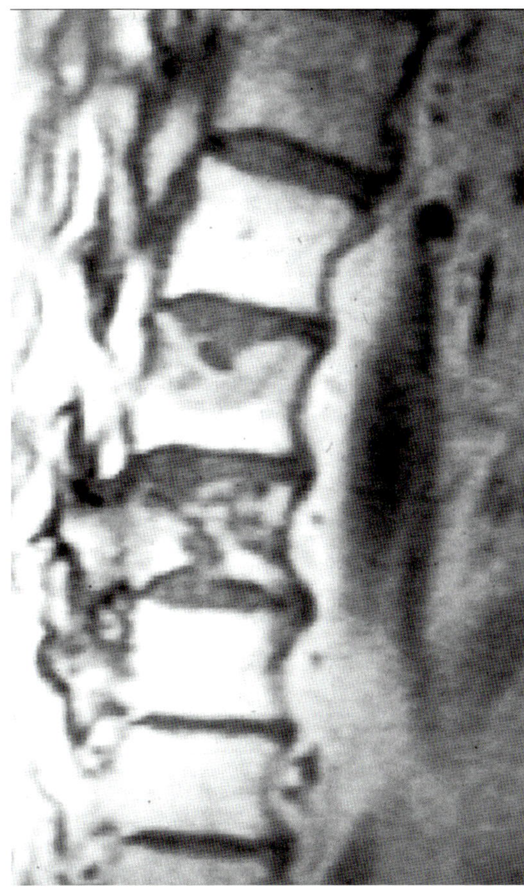

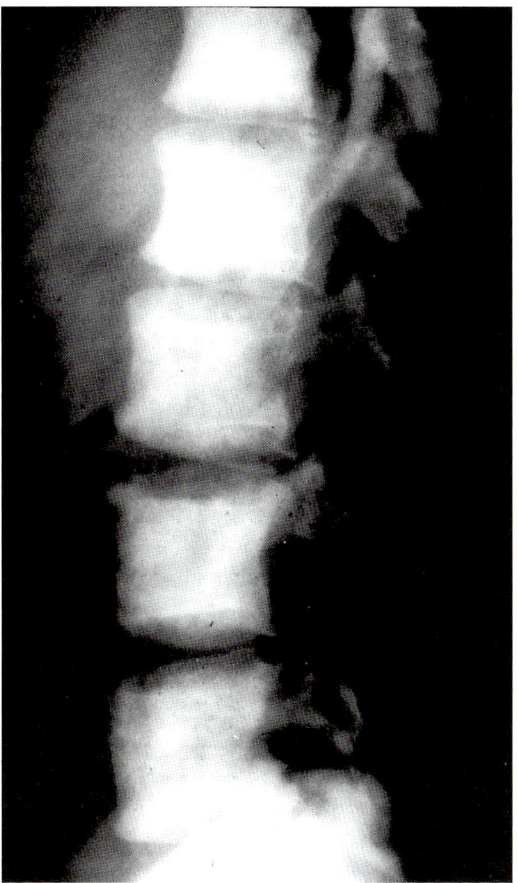

Figure 6
MRI scan of the spine in a patient with carcinoma of the lung, showing destruction of two adjacent vertebrae.

Figure 7
Radiograph of the spine in a patient with metastatic prostate carcinoma, showing marked productive changes in multiple segments.

- Bone scanning. Both standard scintigraphy and PET scans are very helpful, not only in evaluating the lesional site but in identifying other sites of metastases.[37,59] The PET scan may be useful in identifying the primary lesion as well.

- Laboratory studies to rule out such problems as myeloma, lymphoma, leukemia, hyperparathyroidism, osteomalacia, osteopetrosis, etc. Many patients with extensive metastatic disease become dangerously hypercalcemic, and it is essential to repeatedly perform these studies.

- Mammography in female patients; PSA and MRI of the pelvis in males; chest CT scans for all patients; thyroid scans and CT and MRI scans of the abdomen to evaluate liver, kidneys, and uterus; colonoscopy for suspected lesions of the bowel. Studies of lymph node sites to seek sentinel nodes for breast, prostate, or thyroid cancers should also be performed.

- Family history is important, particularly for breast cancer. Possible genetic analysis for breast, lung, or prostatic tumors should be done because all these tumors have recently been described as having some fairly specific markers. The error for breast cancer is believed to be at del(1p),[17,19] for prostate at del(10)(q26),[23,26] and for lung at either del(3)(p14-23) for small cell tumors[28] or at del(9p) for non–small cell lesions.[27] For renal cell tumors, the genetic error is at either del(3)(p25) or t(3,8)(pp21;q24).[33] In addition, markers for these tumors have been at least partially established.[60,61] For breast cancer, these include KI-67, c-ERBB2;[12,17,19] for lung, HER2, MYC, BCL2, CDK4, and HDM2[27-29]; and for prostate, HER-2, CAPB, HSD3B, HPC1, HPC20, and HPCX.[23,26]

Treatment Protocols

- The first issue is a careful definition of the location and degree of malignancy of the primary lesion. This is not always as simple as it seems; at times, the only way the primary lesion can be discovered is at autopsy. A careful history, thorough physical examination, full range of imaging studies (especially PET scanning[37]), and then biopsy studies on the tissue will most often define the primary lesion.[15,20]

- Standard external beam radiation ranging up to or even greater than 60 Gy has often been effective for the treatment of either the primary lesion or the metastatic deposit. Brachytherapy or proton-beam treatment can be used, the latter mentioned particularly for tumors of the vertebrae, calvarium, or sacrum.[62]

- Chemotherapy has varied considerably over the years, with the introduction of several agents for each of the primary diseases and the resultant bone metastases. Tamoxifen, anastrozole, letrozole, exemestane, doxorubicin, cyclophosphamide, docetaxel, paclitaxel, vinorelbine tartrate, and trastuzumab are used for patients with breast cancer.[12,17,19] For those with prostate cancer, calcitriol,[63] estrogens,[64] paclitaxel, vinblastine, etoposide, carboplatin, docetaxel, and mitoxantrone have been used with some success.[23,26] For primary lung cancer with metastases, cisplatin, vindesine, paclitaxel, carboplatin, and vinorelbine have been used, but none very successfully.[27-29] Patients with renal cell carcinoma have been treated with titanocene, pyrazine, treosulfan, irinotecan, capecitabine, suramin, methotrexate, tetrathiomolybdate, and bryostatin.[33] For thyroid carcinoma, radioiodine administration and thyroxine are used to suppress thyroid-stimulating hormone, and the patient may be treated with doxorubicin or doxorubicin plus platinum.[31]

- Use of agents to strengthen the bones. In the last decade, the bisphosphonates and calcitonin have been used to decrease the level of destruction of bone metastases based on the ability of these materials to prevent osteoclastic bone destruction.[35,65-69] Most recently, zoledronate has been extensively used and has markedly improved the quality of the bone and prevented fractures.[59,67-69]

- Surgical procedures on the primary lesion are often indicated, particularly for breast, prostate, renal, or thyroid cancers.[31,70,71] Surgical treatment of bone metastases are often required to deal with fractures, shaft expansion and deformity, joint destruction, or neurovascular compromise, particularly for tumors affecting the calvarium, femurs, vertebrae, or pelvis.[3,20,72] If the metastatic deposit is relatively small and solitary, wide resection is often an appropriate choice and may be successful in leading to long-term survival.[3,72,73] Amputation, once advocated as the treatment of choice, is rarely necessary at present.[20]

Conclusion

In the past, metastatic cancer to bone was considered to be disastrous and a sign of impending bad outcome. Furthermore, it was sometimes difficult to identify the primary tumor, even at autopsy. Patients had fractures, severe bone pain, became hypercalcemic, and had osteoarthritic or neurovascular complications that were sometimes devastating. The survival rate was poor, even for thyroid cancer and some of the less common tumors that were not as aggressive either locally or in bone settings.

The situation has changed considerably. First, if the primary lesion is discovered early, surgical excision, chemotherapy, and radiation may prevent the development of metastases. If the metastasis is discovered after the malignant primary lesion is identified, chemotherapy, radiation, and local treatment to both the primary and the metastatic process has led to a much higher percentage of survival and, even with persistent disease, to a better and sometimes much longer course. We are now able to identify metastatic deposits very early in their course by CT, MRI, scintigraphy, and especially PET scanning that makes local treatment much more effective and possibly curative. Additionally, the use of bisphosphonates has strengthened the bones and prevented fractures.

We still have a way to go, however. With the current knowledge of genetic characteristics of the tumors and more information about the tumor cells' growth and survival characteristics, protocols such as antiangiogenesis factors, gene modifications, agents that induce apoptosis by interference with cytokine production, and drugs that alter cyclooxygenase-2 (COX-2) development may change the future. Furthermore, improved metallic devices and allografts with fewer complications may make it easier to resect and replace a solitary lesion, which may also improve survival. What a joy that would be for the patients, their families, and their orthopaedic surgeons.

References

1. Bryan CP: *The Papyrus Ebers*. Chicago, IL, Ares, 1974.

2. Ebbell B: *The Ebers Papyrus: The Greatest Egyptian Medical Document*. Copenhagen, Denmark, Levin & Munksgaard, 1937.

3. Mankin HJ: History of the treatment of musculoskeletal tumours, in Klenerman L (ed): *The Evolution of Orthopaedic Surgery*. London, Royal Society of Medicine, 2002, pp 191-210.

4. Hippocrates: *The Genuine Works of Hippocrates* (translated from the Greek by Francis Adams). London, Sydenham Society, 1849.

5. Segrist HE: The historical development of the pathology and therapy of cancer, in *On the History of Medicine*. New York, NY, MD Publications, 1960, pp 57-65.

6. Galen C: *De Tumoribus Praeter Naturaum*. [On Abnormal Swellings]. 192 AD.

7. Galen on abnormal swellings. *J Hist Med Allied Sci* 1978;33:531-549.

8. Vesalius A: *De Humani Corporis Fabrica*. Basel, Switzerland, 1543.

9. Abernethy J: *Surgical Observations on Tumors*. London, Longman and Rees, 1804.

10. Beale L: *The Microscope in its Application to Practical Medicine*. London, John Churchill, 1858.

11. Paget S: The distribution of secondary growths in cancer of the breast: 1889. *Cancer Metastasis Rev* 1989;8:98-101.

12. Coley WB: I: Final results in the X-ray treatment of cancer, including sarcoma. *Ann Surg* 1905;42:161-184.

13. Coleman RE, Rubens RD: The clinical course of bone metastases from breast cancer. *Br J Cancer* 1987;55:61-66.

14. Cristofanilli M, Budd GT, Ellis MJ, et al: Circulating tumor cells, disease progression, and survival in metastatic breast cancer. *N Engl J Med* 2004;351:781-791.

15. Dorfman HD, Czerniak B: *Bone Tumors*. St. Louis, MO, Mosby, 1998.

16. Jaffe HL: *Tumors and Tumorous Conditions of Bones and Joints*. Philadelphia, PA, Lea and Febiger, 1958.

17. Margolese RG, Fisher B, Hortobagyi GN, Bloomer WD: Neoplasms of the breast, in Bast RC Jr, Pollock RE, Weichselbaum RR, Holland JF, Frei E III (eds): *Holland and Frei Cancer Medicine*, ed 5. Hamilton, BC, Decker, 2000, pp 1735-1822.

18. Shapiro CL: Metastatic breast cancer, in Furie B, Cassileth PA, Atkins MB, Mayer RJ (eds): *Clinical Hematology and Oncology: Presentation, Diagnosis and Treatment*. Philadelphia, PA, Churchill Livingstone, 2003, pp 750-762.

19. Wood WC, Muss HB, Solin LJ, et al: Cancer of the breast, in DeVita VT Jr, Hellman S, Rosenberg SA (eds): *Cancer Principles and Practice of Oncology*. Philadelphia, PA, Lippincott, Williams & Wilkins, 2005, pp 1453-1462.

20. Campanacci M: *Bone and Soft Tissue Tumors*. New York, NY, Springer, 1999.

21. Coleman RE: Skeletal complications of malignancy. *Cancer* 1997;80:1588-1594.

22. D'Amico AV, Whittington R, Malkowicz SB, et al: Combination of the preoperative PSA level, biopsy gleason score, percentage of positive biopsies, and MRI T-stage to predict early PSA failure in men with clinically localized prostate cancer. *Urology* 2000;55:572-577.

23. Keller ET, Brown J: Prostate cancer bone metastases promote both osteolytic and osteoblastic activity. *J Cell Biochem* 2004;91:718-729.

24. Ko Y-J, Bubley GJ: Prostate cancer, in Furie B, Cassileth PA, Atkins MB, Mayer RJ (eds): *Clinical Hematology and Oncology: Presentation, Diagnosis and Treatment*. Philadelphia, PA, Churchill Livingstone, 2003, pp 859-873.

25. Mundy GR: Metastasis to bone: Causes, consequences and therapeutic opportunities. *Nat Rev Cancer* 2002;2:584-593.

26. Scher HI, Leiger SA, Fuks Z, et al: Cancer of the prostate, in DeVita VT Jr, Hellman S, Rosenberg SA (eds): *Cancer Principles and Practice of Oncology*. Philadelphia, PA, Lippincott, Williams & Wilkins, 2005, pp 1192-1259.

27. Karp DD, Thurer RJ: Non-small cell lung cancer, in Furie B, Cassileth PA, Atkins MB, Mayer RJ (eds): *Clinical Hematology and Oncology: Presentation, Diagnosis and Treatment*. Philadelphia, PA, Churchill Livingstone, 2003, pp 958-982.

28. Merchant JJ, Schiller JH: Small cell lung cancer, in Furie B, Cassileth PA, Atkins MB, Mayer RJ (eds): *Clinical Hematology and Oncology: Presentation, Diagnosis and Treatment*. Philadelphia, PA, Churchill Livingstone, 2003, pp 943-957.

29. Vaporciyan AA, Nesbitt JC, Lee JS, et al: Cancer of the lung, in Bast RC Jr, Pollock RE, Weichselbaum RR, Holland JF, Frei E III (eds): *Holland and Frei Cancer Medicine*, ed 5. Hamilton, BC, Decker, 2000, pp 1227-1292.

30. Carling T, Udelsman R: Thyroid tumors, in DeVita VT Jr, Hellman S, Rosenberg SA (eds): *Cancer Principles and Practice of Oncology*, Philadelphia, PA, Lippincott, Williams & Wilkins, 2005, pp 1502-1520.

31. Do MY, Rhee Y, Kim DJ, et al: Clinical features of bone metastases resulting from thyroid cancer: A review of 28 patients over a 20-year period. *Endocr J* 2005;52:701-707.

32. Donskov F, von der Maase H: Impact of immune parameters on long-term survival in metastatic

renal cell carcinoma. *J Clin Oncol* 2006;24:1997-2005.

33. Richie JR, Kanloff PW, Shapiro CL: Renal cell carcinoma, in Bast RC Jr, Pollock RE, Weichselbaum RR, Holland JF, Frei E III (eds): *Holland and Frei Cancer Medicine*, ed 5. Hamilton, BC, Decker, 2000, pp 1530-1538.

34. Mundy GR: Mechanisms of bone metastases. *Cancer* 1997;80:1546-1556.

35. Roodman GD: Mechanisms of bone metastasis. *N Engl J Med* 2004;350:1655-1664.

36. Selvaggi G, Scagliotti GV: Management of bone metastases in cancer: A review. *Crit Rev Oncol Hematol* 2005;56:365-378.

37. Cook GJ, Fogelman I: The role of positron emission tomography in the management of bone metastases. *Cancer* 2000;88:2927-2933.

38. Boyce BF, Yoneda T, Guise TA: Factors regulating the growth of metastatic cancer in bone. *Endocr Relat Cancer* 1999;6:333-347.

39. Lizardi PM: Molecular methods in oncology, in DeVita VT Jr, Hellman S, Rosenberg SA (eds): *Cancer Principles and Practice of Oncology*. Philadelphia, PA, Lippincott, Williams & Wilkins, 2005, pp 3-7.

40. Phadke PA, Mercer RR, Harms JF, et al: Kinetics of metastatic breast cancer cell trafficking in bone. *Clin Cancer Res* 2006;12:1431-1440.

41. Aldridge SE, Lennard TWJ, Williams JR, Birch MA: Vascular endothelial growth factor acts as an osteolytic factor in breast cancer metastases to bone. *Br J Cancer* 2005;92:1531-1537.

42. Henriksen K, Karsdal M, Delaisse JM, Engsig MT: RANKL and vascular endothelial growth factor (VEGF) induce osteoclast chemotaxis through an ERK1/2 dependent mechanism. *J Biol Chem* 2003;278:48745-48753.

43. Jones DH, Nakashima T, Sanchez OH, et al: Regulation of cancer cell migration and bone metastasis by RANKL. *Nature* 2006;440:692-696.

44. Singh B, Berry JA, Shoher A, Lucci A: COX-2 induces IL-11 production in human breast cancer cells. *J Surg Res* 2006;131:267-275.

45. Barrett JM, Rovedo MA, Tajuddin AM, et al: Prostate cancer cells regulate growth and differentiation of bone marrow endothelial cells through TGFbeta and its receptor TGFbetaRII. *Prostate* 2006;66:632-650.

46. Hiraga T, Myoui A, Choi ME, Yoshikawa H, Yoneda T: Stimulation of cyclooxygenase-2 expression by bone-derived transforming growth factor-beta enhances bone metastases in breast cancer. *Cancer Res* 2006;66:2067-2073.

47. Roberts AB, Wakefield LM: The two faces of transforming growth factor beta in carcinogenesis. *Proc Natl Acad Sci USA* 2003;100:8621-8623.

48. Hall CL, Bafico A, Dai J, Aaronson SA, Keller ET: Prostate cancer cells promote osteoblastic bone metastases through Wnts. *Cancer Res* 2005;65:7554-7560.

49. Hall CL, Kang S, MacDougald OA, Keller ET: Role of Wnts in prostate cancer bone metastases. *J Cell Biochem* 2006;97:661-672.

50. Miller JR: The Wnts. *Genome Biol* 2002;3:REVIEWS 3001.

51. Mastro AM, Gay CV, Welch DR, et al: Breast cancer cells induce osteoblast apoptosis: A possible contributor to bone degradation. *J Cell Biochem* 2004;91:265-276.

52. Mercer RR, Miyasaka C, Mastro AM: Metastatic breast cancer cells suppress osteoblast adhesion and differentiation. *Clin Exp Metastasis* 2004;21:427-435.

53. Chao TY, Yu JC, Ku CH, et al: Tartrate-resistant acid phosphatase 5b as a serum marker for extensive bone metastases in breast cancer patients. *Clin Cancer Res* 2005;11:544-550.

54. Chung YC, Ku CH, Chao TY, Yu JC, Chen MM, Lee SH: Tartrate-resistant acid phosphatase 5b activity is a useful bone marker for monitoring bone metastases in breast cancer patients after treatment. *Cancer Epidemiol Biomarkers Prev* 2006;15:424-428.

55. Janckila AJ, Nakasato YR, Neustadt DH, Yam LT: Disease-specific expression of tartrate-resistant acid phosphatase. *J Bone Miner Res* 2003;18:1916-1919.

56. Lipton A, Costa L, Ali S, Demers L: Use of markers of bone turnover for monitoring bone metastases and the response to therapy. *Semin Oncol* 2001;28:54-59.

57. Coleman RE: The role of bone markers in metastatic bone disease. *Cancer Treat Rev* 2006;32:1-2.

58. Mihai R, Stevens J, McKinney C, Ibrahim NB: Expression of the calcium receptor in human breast cancer—a potential new marker predicting the risk of bone metastases. *Eur J Surg Oncol* 2006;32:511-515.

59. Kücük ON, Gültekin SS, Arias G, Ibi E: Radio-iodine whole-body scans, thyroglobulin levels, 99mTc-MIBI scans and computed tomography: Results in patients with lung metastases from differentiated thyroid cancer. *Nucl Med Commun* 2006;27:261-266.

60. Brose MS, Smyrk T, Weber B, Lynch HT: Genetic predisposition to cancer, in Bast RC Jr, Pollock RE, Weichselbaum RR, Holland JF, Frei E III (eds): *Holland and Frei Cancer Medicine*, ed 5. Hamilton, BC, Decker, 2000, pp 168-184.

61. Calvo JR, Petricoin EFIII, Liotta LA: Genomics and proteomics, in DeVita VT Jr, Hellman S, Rosenberg SA (eds): *Cancer Principles and Practice of Oncology*. Philadelphia, PA, Lippincott, Williams & Wilkins, 2005, pp 51-72.

62. Connell PP, Martel K, Hellman S: Principles of radiation oncology, in DeVita VT Jr, Hellman S, Rosenberg SA (eds): *Cancer Principles and Practice of Oncology*. Philadelphia, PA, Lippincott, Williams & Wilkins, 2005, pp 267-285.

63. Trump DL, Potter DM, Muindi J, Brufsky A, Johnson CS: Phase II trail of high-dose, intermittent calcitriol (1,25 dihydroxyvitamin D3) and dexamethasone in androgen-independent prostate cancer. *Cancer* 2006;106:2136-2142.

64. Cox RL, Crawford ED: Estrogens in the treatment of prostate cancer. *J Urol* 1995;154:1991-1998.

65. Powles T, Paterson A, McCloskey E, et al: Reduction in bone relapse and improved survival with oral clodronate for adjuvant treatment of operable breast cancer [ISRCTN83668026]. *Breast Cancer Res* 2006;8:R13.

66. Russell RG: Bisphosphonates: From bench to bedside. *Ann N Y Acad Sci* 2006;1068:367-401.

67. Saad F: Zoledronic acid: Past, present and future roles in cancer treatment. *Future Oncol* 2005;1:149-159.

68. Santini D, Vincenzi B, Hannon RA, et al: Changes in bone resorption and vascular endothelial growth factor after a single zoledronic acid infusion in cancer patients with bone metastases from solid tumours. *Oncol Rep* 2006;15:1351-1357.

69. Storto G, Klain M, Paone G, et al: Combined therapy of Sr-89 and zoledronic acid in patients with painful bone metastases. *Bone* 2006;39:35-41.

70. Kroepfl D, Loewen H, Roggenbuck U, Musch M, Klevecka V: Disease progression and survival in patients with prostate carcinoma and positive lymph nodes after radical retropubic prostatectomy. *BJU Int* 2006;97:985-991.

71. Rapiti E, Verkooijen HM, Vlastos G, et al: Complete excision of primary breast tumor improves survival of patients with metastatic breast cancer at diagnosis. *J Clin Oncol* 2006;24:2743-2749.

72. Zeegen EN, Aponte-Tinao LA, Hornicek FJ, Gebhardt MC, Mankin HJ: Survivorship analysis of 141 modular metallic endoprostheses at early followup. *Clin Orthop Relat Res* 2004;420:239-250.

73. Mankin HJ: The changes in major limb reconstruction as a result of development of allografts, in Birch EV (ed): *Trends in Bone Cancer Research*. New York, NY, Nova Science Publishers, 2006, pp 65-102.

Chapter 7

Aneurysmal Bone Cyst

Aneurysmal bone cysts are uncommon, enigmatic benign bone tumors that are sometimes difficult to distinguish from other, more aggressive lesions. There are two forms of the entity: a primary tumor, for which recent studies have supported a consistent genetic error; and a secondary tumor that seems to arise in relation to an array of benign and sometimes malignant bone tumors. Aneurysmal bone cysts are usually located eccentrically in the metaphyseal-diaphyseal regions of the long bones or pelvis, occasionally in the spine and facial bones and less commonly in the hands and feet. They appear in late adolescence or young adulthood and are slightly more frequent in women than in men. The principal problem with these benign lesions is the difficulty of distinguishing the primary form from other lesions of bone or, for secondary lesions, identifying the neoplastic tissue of origin. Another problem is defining an effective treatment, as the recurrence rate after local therapy is cited to be as much as 40% in several large series. A major issue is the great concern that some of the tumors defined as aneurysmal bone cysts on the basis of imaging and biopsy may be or may become malignant tumors.

History and Biologic Studies

Aneurysmal bone cyst was first clearly defined and named in 1942 by Henry Jaffe and Louis Lichtenstein[1] and was subsequently further defined by these investigators in several additional studies.[2-5] In his 1958 pathology book, Henry Jaffe stated: "one occasionally encounters a rather arresting benign bone lesion for which the writer has formulated the name *aneurysmal bone cyst* as being descriptive in a general way."[6] The entity became known as Jaffe-Lichtenstein disease,[7] although that term is rarely used today. Before Jaffe and Lichtenstein defined the disorder as an aneurysmal bone cyst, it was called an atypical or subperiosteal giant cell tumor, benign bone aneurysm, hemangiomatous bone cyst, multilocular hematic bone cyst, and even hemangioma of

bone.[8-17] Numerous authors subsequently reported series of cases that defined the anatomic localization, imaging characteristics, clinical presentation, and the problems of management.[6,12,18-30] Several articles further described the possible nature of aneurysmal bone cysts as secondary lesions in association with other types of tumors.[16,19,25,30-33] Surgical approaches were introduced and were most often intralesional, but occasionally marginal excison was proposed, suggesting that it was likely to reduce the high rate of local recurrence.[12,19,20,27-30,34,35] The relationship to other tumors, especially malignant ones, remains an enigma and a concern. Aneurysmal bone cysts may resemble other lesions such as chondroblastoma, giant cell tumor, osteoblastoma, and some forms of osteosarcoma; and if they are secondary lesions, they can arise from them.[4,11,14,19,30-33]

The term aneurysmal bone cyst remains purely descriptive and does not provide any evidence for a causation or for any concept of pathogenesis.[8,27,30,36-38] Trauma, bleeding, and neoplastic processes have been suggested.[4,10,12,13,30,31,33,39-41] In recent years, prodigious efforts by several investigators have defined some specific genetic alterations that strongly suggest a neoplastic origin for the primary lesions. Oliveira and associates[42-44] and others[45,46] have reported that chromosome bands 16q22 and 17p13 are nonrandomly arranged in primary aneurysmal bone cysts. As a result of these studies, aneurysmal bone cysts are defined as genetic disorders or neoplasms driven by upregulation of the USP6 oncogene (ubiquitin specific protease 6). A recurrent t(16;17)(q22;p13) has been identified, but in addition several other chromosomal segments have been defined that serve as translocation partners for each chromosome. Of importance is the evidence that shows that these genetic changes may be absent in those aneurysmal cysts considered to be secondary, which seem to be arising in relation to other types of tumors.[44]

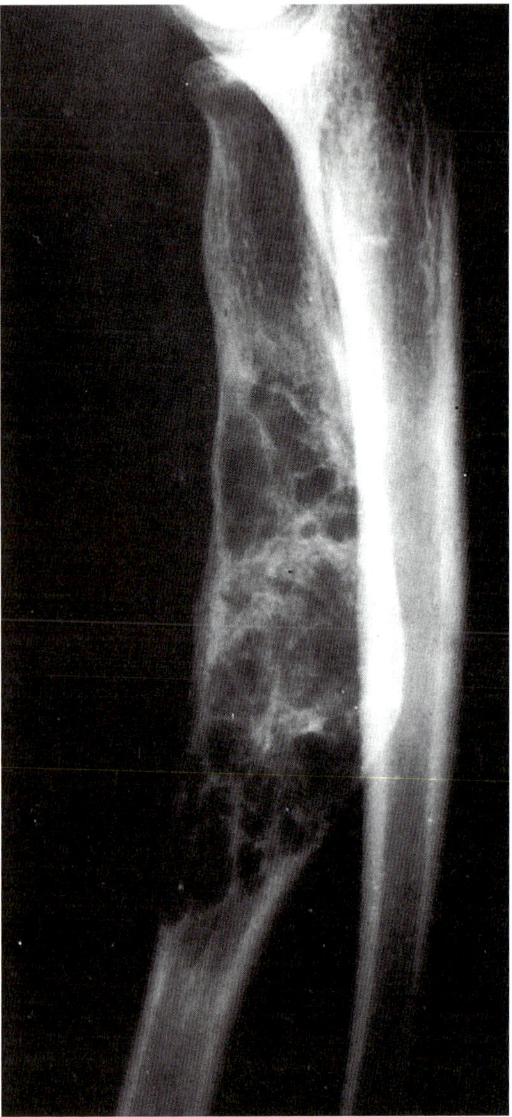

Figure 1
An aneurysmal bone cyst of the proximal radius diaphysis. Note the expansion of the cortex, the modest bowing deformity, and the multiple cyst-like structures.

Gross and Histologic Studies

Perhaps the most difficult issue with regard to the definition of aneurysmal bone cyst is the fact that the cystic, hemorrhagic, and reactive changes seen in the tumor may either focally or extensively resemble the changes seen in giant cell tumors, chondroblastoma, osteoblastoma, hemangioendothelioma, fibrous dysplasia, hyperparathyroidism, or even telangiectatic osteosarcoma.[4,6,8,11,16,30] Furthermore, "secondary" aneurysmal bone cysts may arise in relation to such lesions; this can make it difficult to distinguish the primary tumor as the cause of the le-

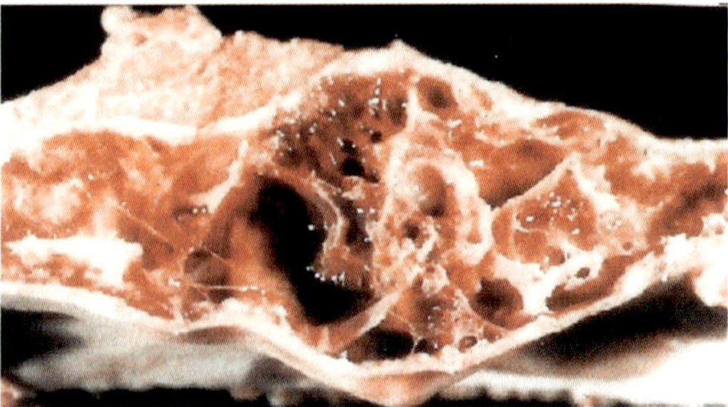

Figure 2
Gross photograph of an aneurysmal bone cyst disclosing the expansion of the bone, thinning of the cortices, and irregular cyst-like structures present within the tumor. These areas are usually filled with bloody fluid.

sion.[8,30,31,33,41] Lesions principally occur in the long bones of the upper and lower extremity, are usually metaphyseal-diaphyseal in location, and are fairly characteristic in gross structure and appearance.[3,6,8,11,16,22,27,36,38,47,48] The tumors are most often eccentrically located, lytic on radiography, thin, and expand the cortex without creating a soft-tissue extension (Figure 1). The periosteum is usually intact but may have a rind of new bone over the site of the lesion. Some of the lesions actually extend into the soft tissues overlying the bone.[8,11,22,49] (Figure 2) The lesions are often bluish. Bleeding occurs when the cyst is opened but it is not pulsatile. The content of the cyst is usually spongy, with multiple irregular cavities filled with blood. The term "aneurysmal" appears to relate to the "blow-out distension," and the word "cyst" reflects the fact that the tumor often presents as a blood-filled cavity.[3,6,8,11,16,22,27,36,38,47,48] The lesional sites are similar for young children but are sometimes more extensive and destructive in appearance.[50-54] Lesions of the spine and pelvis present problems in diagnosis because of their resemblance to other types of destructive tumors and also yield difficulty in planning and executing therapy.[8,11,48,51,55-59] Tumors of the jaw also pose challenges in terms of the difficulty posed by reconstruction.[8,11,20] Tumors located in the foot may affect the calcaneus, talus, distal tibia, or fibula.[8,16,35] Very rarely are they located in multiple sites in the body and discovered either simultaneously or as metachronous tumors.[60]

Histologic examination demonstrates fibrous cells, macrophages, endothelioid cells,

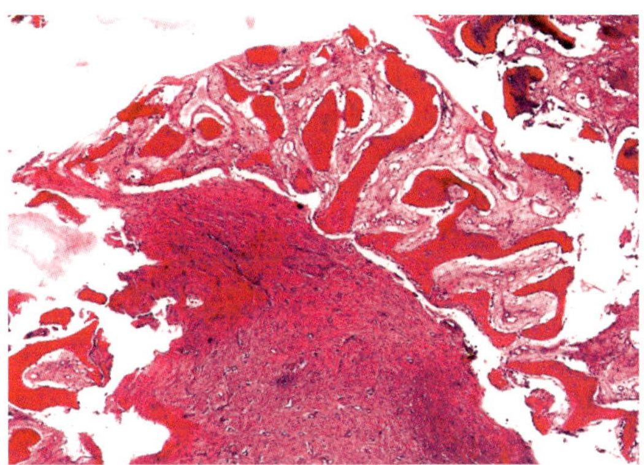

Figure 3
Histologic pattern of an aneurysmal bone cyst. Note the fibrous cells, macrophages, endothelioid cells, and giant cells, along with islands of bone lying in relation to spaces filled with partially clotted blood.

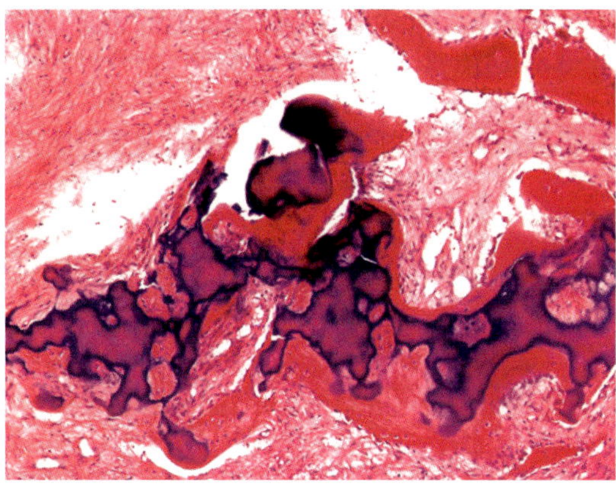

Figure 4
Histology showing that the bone formed is abnormal, with irregular structure and osteoid seams around the sites. Note the fibrous, vascular tissue surrounding the sites of bone formation.

and giant cells, along with islands of bone lying in relation to spaces filled with partially clotted blood.[6,8,11,16,22,27,38,48,61,62] Although there is no specific cell type, according to Mario Campanacci,[8] there are collections of filamentous, bluish, chondro-osteoid calcified matrix known as "blue reticulated chondroid tissue" (Figure 3). If fractures or local recurrences have occurred, nonspecific repair tissue composed of loose collagen fibers, dilated sinusoids, giant cells, and osteoid or chondroid trabeculae may be present.[6,11,22,63,64] (Figure 4) The giant cells are multinucleated and may be associated with mitotic activity, particularly if a fracture has occurred.[8,11,16] Of some concern is the fact that the changes described above are not specific and that within the lesions, one occasionally finds components suggestive of the possibility that the lesion actually results from hemorrhagic or degradative events occurring in patients with other types of tumors.[8,11,30,33]

Clinical Presentation and Imaging Studies

Aneurysmal bone cysts occur most frequently in patients between 10 and 25 years of age, and females are slightly more often affected than males (approximately 54% to 46%).[8,11,16,22,27,36,38,48] No evidence has been presented for a familial genetic origin for the tumors.[8,12,50,63,65] Some patients report the appearance of the lesion in relation to some form of injury, but this may represent a pathologic fracture of a preexisting lesion.[39] The most common anatomic sites are the distal and proximal femur, proximal tibia, proximal humerus, pelvis, spine, and facial bones.[3,6,8,11,16,22,27,36,38,47,48] The forearms, ribs, hands, and feet have fewer tumors than the other sites. The patients often report pain and tenderness at the site and, with large lesions, may display a mass firmly attached to the bone. The tumors grow slowly, although they are subject to fracture and then may enlarge rapidly and show a collection of blood in the subfascial region.[8,11,16,22,33,38,48,49] The fractures are often the cause of severe pain. Nerve injury and pain may result from spinal tumors, and vascular compromise can occur from peripheral or pelvic tumors, particularly with rapid expansion as a result of pathologic fracture.[8,51,56-58]

Radiographic studies show a lytic lesion often eccentrically located in the proximal or distal end of a long bone, with a "blow-out" appearance to the thin cortical shell. In earlier days, angiography was proposed to better define the vascular nature of the lesion but the results were disappointing.[8,66] Lesions are located in the metaphyseal-diaphyseal region and are most often eccentric, which helps to distinguish them from unicameral bone cysts or giant cell tumors, both of which are usually centrally placed.[6,8,11,22,25,27,36,67] Despite the statement that the tumors are aneurysmal and hence "filled with blood," plain radiographs and especially CT and MRI may show an irregular pattern within the tissue consisting of small spots of calcium-containing structures and sometimes a "soap-bubble" appearance.[1,8,11,22,67,68] The periosteum may be thickened and occasionally perforated, particularly if a fracture has occurred. This may result in a soft-tissue mass.[49] Bone scan is almost always positive, and on MRI, the lesions are usually dark on T1 and bright on T2.[8,11,67,68]

Treatment

The most important aspect of initial treatment is to be certain of the diagnosis and the extent of the disease. History of injury and review of complaints suggestive of other types of lesions should be obtained. The lesion itself should be imaged with radiographs, CT, and MRI; a bone scan may be helpful in ruling out lesions at other sites. CT of the chest is sometimes helpful if the lesion is believed to be secondary and there is concern about the nature of the primary tumor. A biopsy, either a CT-guided core biopsy or even an open one, is important and should be carefully evaluated for evidence of other types of lesions.[8,11,22,48]

Most aneurysmal bone cysts are now being treated with thorough curettage with or without sclerotherapy and filling the cavity with allograft bone chips, autogenous bone marrow, bone substitutes, polymethylmethacrylate, or sometimes combinations of these.[26,48,55,59,69-75] Injections of fibrosing agents are sometimes used, but have at times been associated with complications in children and increased rate of recurrence.[76] The surgeon who treats the disease should be aware of the high risk of local recurrence, which ranges up to 40% in the international literature.[8,22,34,48,51,63,72] Patients who are treated surgically should be carefully followed, sometimes for long periods.

Occasionally, for very destructive lesions or those that recur locally, resection and allograft or metallic implant are the best choices.[48] Radiation has now been proposed as either the primary treatment or in association with surgical procedures and appears in several series to be reasonably successful.[8,77,78]

The key problem with any treatment of aneurysmal bone cyst is the appearance of a malignant tumor at the site of the surgery. Several reports have suggested that this may occur; although admittedly rare, it surely represents a serious issue related to this benign entity.[61,79-81]

Conclusions

Aneurysmal bone cysts should be relatively simple tumors to diagnose and treat. They are not very locally aggressive and are located for the most part in anatomic sites that allow intralesional or sometimes marginal surgical procedures. Despite the genetic information that has been recently defined, the tumors are still not clearly defined as either familial lesions or neoplasms, and there is only limited information as to how the genetic data can be used to identify lesions of greater aggressive potential.

There are two major concerns. First is the diagnosis, which may be in error and has not defined an additional underlying bone tumor that may be more aggressive or possibly malignant. The second issue is the high rate of local recurrence, ranging from 10% to 40% in published series, which requires careful observation of the patient for long periods and sometimes more extensive surgery.

References

1. Jaffe HL, Lichtenstein L: Solitary unicameral bone cyst, with emphasis on the roentgen picture, the pathologic appearance and the pathogenesis. *Arch Surg* 1942;44:1004-1025.

2. Jaffe HL: Aneurysmal bone cyst. *Bull Hosp Joint Dis* 1950;11:3-13.

3. Lichtenstein L: Aneurysmal bone cyst: Observations on fifty cases. *J Bone Joint Surg Am* 1957;39:873-882.

4. Lichtenstein L: Aneurysmal bone cyst: A pathological entity commonly mistaken for giant-cell tumor and occasionally for hemangioma and osteogenic sarcoma. *Cancer* 1950;3:279-289.

5. Lichtenstein L: Aneurysmal bone cyst: Further observations. *Cancer* 1953;6:1228-1237.

6. Jaffe HL: *Tumors and Tumorous Conditions of the Bones and Joints*. Philadelphia, PA, Lea and Febiger, 1958.

7. Nasser A: Aneurysmal bone cyst (Jaffe-Lichtenstein Disease). *Rev Paulista Med* 1953;43:49-55.

8. Campanacci M: Aneurysmal bone cyst, in Campanacci M (ed): *Bone and Soft Tissue Tumors*, ed 2. New York, NY, Springer Verlag, 1999, pp 812-840.

9. Coley BL, Miller LB: Atypical giant cell tumor. *AJR Am J Roentgenol* 1942;47:541-548.

10. Cone SM: Ossifying hematoma. *J Bone Joint Surg Am* 1928;10:474-482.

11. Dorfman HD, Czerniak B: Cystic bone tumors, in

Dorfman HD, Czerniak B (eds): *Bone Tumors.* St. Louis, MO, Mosby, 1998, pp 855-912.

12. Donaldson WF Jr : Aneurysmal bone cyst. *J Bone Joint Surg Am* 1962;44:25-40.

13. Hadders HN, Oterdoom HJ: The identification of aneurysmal bone cyst with hemangioma of the skeleton. *J Pathol Bacteriol* 1956;71:193-200.

14. Hodgen JT, Frantz CH: Sub-periosteal giant-cell tumor: Report of a case. *J Bone Joint Surg* 1947;29:781-784.

15. Mider GB, Morton JJ: Pulsating, benign giant cell tumors of bone. *Ann Surg* 1939;109:126-134.

16. Schajowicz F: *Tumors and Tumorlike Lesions of Bone and Joints.* New York, NY, Springer-Verlag, 1981, pp 426-441.

17. Thompson PC: Subperiosteal giant cell tumor: Ossifying subperiosteal hematoma, aneurysmal bone cyst. *J Bone Joint Surg Am* 1954;36:281-291.

18. Barnes R: Aneurysmal bone cyst. *J Bone Joint Surg Br* 1956;38:301-311.

19. Besse BE Jr, Dahlin DC, Ghormley RK, Pugh DG: Aneurysmal bone cysts: Additional considerations. *Clin Orthop* 1956;7:93-102.

20. Bhasker SN, Bernier JL, Godby F: Aneurysmal bone cyst and other giant cell lesions of the jaws: Report of 104 cases. *J Oral Surg Anesth Hosp Dent Serv* 1959;17:30-41.

21. Campanacci M, Capanna R, Picci P: Unicameral and aneurysmal bone cysts. *Clin Orthop Relat Res* 1986;204:25-36.

22. Campanacci M, Cervallati C, Donati U, Bertoni F: Aneurysmal bone cyst (a study of 127 cases, 72 with long term follow up). *Ital J Orthop Traumatol* 1976;2:341-353.

23. Clough JR, Price CH: Aneurysmal bone cyst: Pathogenesis and long term results of treatment. *Clin Orthop Relat Res* 1973;97:52-63.

24. Cruz M, Coley BL: Aneurysmal bone cyst. *Surg Gynecol Obstet* 1956;103:67-77.

25. Dahlin DC, Besse BE Jr, Pugh DG, Ghormley RK: Aneurysmal bone cysts. *Radiology* 1955;64:56-65.

26. Koskinen EV, Visuri TI, Holmström T, Roukkola MA: Aneurysmal bone cyst: Evaluation of resection and of curettage in 20 cases. *Clin Orthop Relat Res* 1976;118:136-146.

27. Ruiter DJ, van Rijssel TG, van der Velde EA: Aneurysmal bone cysts: A clinicopathological study of 105 cases. *Cancer* 1977;39:2231-2239.

28. Taylor FW: Aneurysmal bone cyst: A report of three cases. *J Bone Joint Surg Br* 1956;38:293-300.

29. Tillman BP, Dahlin DC, Lipscomb PR, Stewart JR: Aneurysmal bone cyst: An analysis of ninety-five cases. *Mayo Clin Proc* 1968;43:478-495.

30. Levy WM, Miller AS, Bonakdarpour A, Aegerter E: Aneurysmal bone cyst secondary to other osseous lesions: Report of 57 cases *Am J Clin Pathol* 1975;63:1-8.

31. Bonakdarpour A, Levy WM, Aegerter E: Primary and secondary aneurysmal bone cyst: A radiological study of 75 cases. *Radiology* 1978;126:75-83.

32. Buraczewski J, Dabska M: Pathogenesis of aneurysmal bone cyst: Relationship between aneurysmal bone cyst and fibrous dysplasia of bone. *Cancer* 1971;28:597-604.

33. Martinez V, Sissons HA: Aneurysmal bone cyst: A review of 123 cases including primary lesions and those secondary to other bone pathology. *Cancer* 1988;61:2291-2304.

34. Dormans JP, Hanna BG, Johnston DR, Khurana JS: Surgical treatment and recurrence rate of aneurysmal bone cysts in children. *Clin Orthop Relat Res* 2004;421:205-211.

35. Yu GV, Roth LS, Sellers CS: Aneurysmal bone cyst of the fibula. *J Foot Ankle Surg* 1998;37:426-436.

36. Kransdorf MJ, Sweet DE: Aneurysmal bone cyst: Concept, controversy, clinical presentation, and imaging. *AJR Am J Roentgenol* 1995;164:573-580.

37. Szendroi M, Arató G, Ezzati A, Hüttl K, Szavcsur P: Aneurysmal bone cyst: Its pathogenesis based on angiographic, immunohistochemical and electron microscopic studies. *Pathol Oncol Res* 1998;4:277-281.

38. Vergel De Dios AM, Bond JR, Shives TC, McLeod RA, Unni KK: Aneurysmal bone cyst: A clinicopathological study of 238 cases. *Cancer* 1992;69:2921-2931.

39. Haft GE, Buckwalter JA: Aneurysmal bone cyst following tibial fracture: A case report. *Iowa Orthop J* 2003;23:100-102.

40. Ly JQ, LaGatta LM, Beall DP: Calcaneal chondroblastoma with secondary aneurysmal bone cyst. *AJR Am J Roentgenol* 2004;182:130.

41. Sessions W, Siegel JJ, Thomas J, Pitt M, Said-Al-Naief N, Casillas MA: Chondroblastoma with associated aneurysmal bone cyst of the cuboid. *J Foot Ankle Surg* 2005;44:64-67.

42. Oliveira AM, Hsi BL, Weremowicz S, et al: USP6 (Tre2) fusion oncogenes in aneurysmal bone cyst. *Cancer Res* 2004;64:1920-1923.

43. Oliveira AM, Perez-Atayde AR, Dal Cin P, et al: Aneurysmal bone cyst variant translocations upregulate USP6 transcription by promoter swapping with the ZNF9, COL1A1, TRAP150 and OMD genes. *Oncogene* 2005;24:3419-3426.

44. Oliveira AM, Perez-Atayde AR, Inwards CY, et al: USP6 and CDH11 oncogenes identify the neoplastic cell in primary aneurysmal bone cysts and are absent in so-called secondary aneurysmal bone cysts. *Am J Pathol* 2004;165:1773-1780.

45. Dal Cin PD, Kozakewich HP, Goumnerova L, Mankin HJ, Rosenberg AE, Fletcher JA: Variant translocations involving 16q22 and 17p13 in solid variant and extraosseous forms of aneurysmal bone cyst. *Genes Chromosomes Cancer* 2000;28:233-234.

46. Herens C, Thiry A, Dresse MF, et al: Translocation (16;17)(q22;p13) is a recurrent anomaly of aneurysmal bone cysts. *Cancer Genet Cytogenet* 2001;127:83-84.

47. Leithner A, Windhager R, Lang S, Haas OA, Kainberger F, Kotz R: Aneurysmal bone cyst: A population based epidemiologic study and literature review. *Clin Orthop Relat Res* 1999;363:176-179.

48. Mankin HJ, Hornicek FJ, Ortiz-Cruz E, Villafuerte J, Gebhardt MC: Aneurysmal bone cyst: A review of 150 patients. *J Clin Oncol* 2005;23:6756-6762.

49. Nielsen GP, Fletcher CD, Smith MA, Rybak L, Rosenberg AE: Soft tissue aneurysmal bone cyst: A clinicopathologic study of five cases. *Am J Surg Pathol* 2002;26:64-69.

50. Bollini G, Jouve JL, Cottalorda J, Petit P, Panuel M, Jacquemier M: Aneurysmal bone cyst in chil-

dren: Analysis of twenty-seven patients. *J Pediatr Orthop B* 1998;7:274-285.

51. Cottalorda J, Chotel F, Kohler R, et al: Aneurysmal bone cysts of the pelvis in children: A multicenter study and literature review. *J Pediatr Orthop* 2005;25:471-475.

52. Freiberg AA, Loder RT, Heidelburger KP, Hensinger RN: Aneurysmal bone cysts in young children. *J Pediatr Orthop* 1994;14:86-91.

53. Ozaki T, Hillmann A, Lindner N, Winkelmann W: Aneurysmal bone cysts in children. *J Cancer Res Clin Oncol* 1996;122:767-769.

54. Ramírez AR, Stanton RP: Aneurysmal bone cyst in 29 children. *J Pediatr Orthop* 2002;22:533-539.

55. Garg S, Mehta S, Dormans JP: Modern surgical treatment of primary aneurysmal bone cysts of the spine in children and adolescents. *J Pediatr Orthop* 2005;25:387-392.

56. Giddings CE, Bray D, Stapleton S, Daya H: Aneurysmal bone cyst of the spine. *J Laryngol Otol* 2005;119:495-497.

57. Gupta VK, Gupta SK, Khosla VK, Vashisth RK, Kak VK: Aneurysmal bone cysts of the spine. *Surg Neurol* 1994;42:428-432.

58. Hay MC, Paterson D, Taylor TK: Aneurysmal bone cyst of the spine. *J Bone Joint Surg Br* 1978;60:406-411.

59. Papagelopoulos PJ, Choudhury SN, Frassica FJ, Bond JR, Unni KK, Sim FH: Treatment of aneurysmal bone cysts of the pelvis and sacrum. *J Bone Joint Surg Am* 2001;83:1674-1681.

60. Scheil-Bertram S, Hartwig E, Brüderlein S, et al: Metachronous and multiple aneurysmal bone cysts: A rare variant of primary aneurysmal bone cysts. *Virchows Arch* 2004;444:293-299.

61. Aho HJ, Aho AJ, Einola S: Aneurysmal bone cyst, a study of ultrastructure and malignant transformation. *Virchows Arch A Pathol Anat Histol* 1982;395:169-179.

62. Aho HJ, Aho AJ, Peliniemi LJ, Ekfors TO, Foidart JM: Endothelium in aneurysmal bone cyst. *Histopathology* 1985;9:381-387.

63. Cottalorda J, Kohler R, Chotel F, et al: Recurrence of aneurysmal bone cysts in young children: A multicentre study. *J Pediatr Orthop B* 2005;14:212-218.

64. de Silva MV, Raby N, Reid R: Fibromyxoid areas and immature osteoid are associated with recurrence of primary aneurysmal bone cysts. *Histopathology* 2003;43:180-188.

65. Leithner A, Machacek F, Haas OA, et al: Aneurysmal bone cyst: A hereditary disease? *J Pediatr Orthop B* 2004;13:214-217.

66. Lindbom A, Soderberg G, Spjut HJ, Sunnqvist O: Angiography of aneurysmal bone cyst. *Acta Radiol* 1961;55:12-16.

67. Mahnken AH, Nolte-Ernsting CC, Wildberger JE, et al: Aneurysmal bone cyst: Value of MR imaging and conventional radiography. *Eur Radiol* 2003;13:1118-1124.

68. Sullivan RJ, Meyer JS, Dormans JP, Davidson RS: Diagnosing aneurysmal and unicameral bone cysts with magnetic resonance imaging. *Clin Orthop Relat Res* 1999;366:186-190.

69. Docquier PL, Delloye C: Treatment of aneurysmal bone cysts by introduction of demineralized bone and autogenous bone marrow. *J Bone Joint Surg Am* 2005;87:2253-2258.

70. Dubois J, Chigot V, Grimard G, Isler M, Garel L: Sclerotherapy in aneurysmal bone cysts in children: A review of 17 cases. *Pediatr Radiol* 2003;33:365-372.

71. Hemmadi SS, Cole WG: Treatment of aneurysmal bone cysts with saucerization and bone marrow injection in children. *J Pediatr Orthop* 1999;19:540-542.

72. Marcove RC, Sheth DS, Takemoto S, Healey JH: The treatment of aneurysmal bone cyst. *Clin Orthop Relat Res* 1995;311:157-163.

73. Nonnenmacher J, Bahm J, Laforest P, Kempf I: Aneurysmal cyst of the radius: Resection and free vascularized fibular bone graft. *Microsurgery* 1993;14:280-284.

74. Schreuder HW, Veth RP, Pruszczynski M, Lemmens JA, Koops HS, Molenaar WM: Aneurysmal bone cysts treated by curettage, cryotherapy and bone grafting. *J Bone Joint Surg Br* 1997;79:20-25.

75. Carpenter B, Motley T: Bone matrix therapy for aneurysmal bone cysts. *J Am Podiatr Med Assoc* 2005;95:394-397.

76. Topouchian V, Mazda K, Hamze B, Laredo JD, Penneçot GF: Aneurysmal bone cysts in children: Complications of fibrosing agent injection. *Radiology* 2004;232:522-526.

77. Feigenberg SJ, Marcus RB Jr , Zlotecki RA, Scarborough MT, Berrey BH, Enneking WF: Megavoltage radiotherapy for aneurysmal bone cysts. *Int J Radiat Oncol Biol Phys* 2001;49:1243-1247.

78. Nobler MP, Higinbotham NL, Phillips RF: The cure of aneurysmal bone cyst: Irradiation superior to surgery in an analysis of 33 cases. *Radiology* 1968;90:1185-1192.

79. Brindley GW, Greene JF Jr, Frankel LS: Case reports: Malignant transformation of aneurysmal bone cysts. *Clin Orthop Relat Res* 2005;438:282-287.

80. Hsu CC, Wang JW, Huang CH, Chen WJ: Osteosarcoma at the site of a previously treated aneurysmal bone cyst: A case report. *J Bone Joint Surg Am* 2005;87:395-398.

81. Kyriakos M, Hardy D: Malignant transformation of aneurysmal bone cyst, with an analysis of the literature. *Cancer* 1991;68:1770-1780.

Adamantinoma and Osteofibrous Dysplasia of Long Bones

Adamantinoma and osteofibrous dysplasia of long bones are two uncommon disorders, principally occurring in the tibia, that are disturbingly similar in structure, imaging, biology, and histology. There are, however, differences in terms of patient age, location, effect on the structure of the bone, response to treatment, and even the occurrence of metastasis. Over the years since the first reports, many authors have described various aspects of these lesions; they are sometimes confusing and difficult to further define, partly because of the rarity of the lesions and possibly because of their pattern of unpredictable behavior.

History and Nomenclature

In 1900, Maier[1] described a tumor inside the ulna that he thought might be a form of carcinoma, but it was fibrous in nature and was subsequently defined as a primary bone tumor. In 1913, Fischer[2] described another tumor in the tibia that was similar on imaging and histologic characteristics to Maier's case. Both of these lesions proved to be benign but had histologic similarities to an odontogenic jaw tumor known as ameloblastoma or adamantinoma.[3] Additional cases reported by Ryrie[4] in 1932 and in the early 1940s by Hebbel,[5] Anderson and Saunders,[6] and Dockerty and Meyerding[7] suggested that the tumor was aggressive; all of these authors supported the name adamantinoma. In 1954, however, Baker and associates[8] described three new cases of this rare lesion located in the tibia; in their opinion, the tumors resembled fibrous dysplasia, a concept supported subsequently by Cohen and associates,[9] Weiss and Dorfman,[10] and Campbell and Hawk.[11] In 1954, both Hicks[12] and Lederer and Sinclair[13] expressed the opinion that the tumor was a form of synovial sarcoma. In 3 different decades, Changus and associates,[14] Elliott,[15]

and Llombart-Bosch and Ortuño-Pacheco[16] suggested the likelihood that the lesion was a form of angioblastoma rather than a primary tumor. Rosai and Pinkus[17,18] were impressed by the epithelioid nature of the tissue and expressed the opinion that the tumor arose from epithelial tissue. More recent studies, however, have strongly suggested that the tumor is a specific lesion, which is best described according to Campanacci and associates[19] as an "adamantinoma of the long bones" and may be aggressive, destructive, and even metastasize.[3,19-31] As nearly as can now be defined, the adamantinoma is not related to other neoplasms or metabolic alterations in bone and appears to occur principally in the tibia or occasionally the fibula or ulna in young adults.[3,19,20,26,28,30-32] The only disorder to which this lesion seems to have any form of relationship is the osteofibrous dysplasia of the long bones.

Osteofibrous dysplasia of the long bones is an equally rare tumor, first described in 1966 by Kempson.[33] The lesion was originally known as ossifying fibroma, intracortical fibrous dysplasia, or localized osteitis fibrosa.[20,33-39] It is also principally present in the tibia or, less commonly, the fibula, and occurs in younger patients. In 1976, Campanacci[35] eliminated some of the confusion with other disorders by calling the tumor "osteofibrous dysplasia of long bones." As a result, some authors refer to the disease as Campanacci's disease.[3,32] The origin of the lesion was as mysterious as the adamantinoma and several reviewers suggested that the two disorders were not only similar but were in fact the result of the same process—one less severe, occurring in children and unlikely to metastasize, and the other a more aggressive form in older patients with danger of malignant behavior.[40-44]

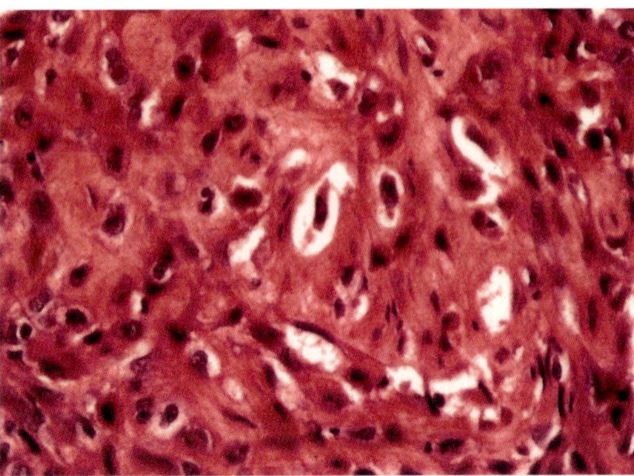

Figure 1
The typical histologic pattern for adamantinoma consists of fascicles of epithelioid or fibroblastic cells arranged in a storiform pattern. The tissue is constructed of collagen fibers that, along with the cellular elements, fill the center of the lesion.

Disease Definition

Adamantinoma of long bones is a very rare condition, accounting for less than 1% of the connective tissue disorders seen annually in the United States.[3,26-29,31,45,46] Most of the lesions occur in the tibia, with rare occurrence in the fibula and even lower incidence in the ulna.[3,20,27,32,46] The patient's age range varies depending on the series reported, but most are young adults (20 to 45 years of age) and most of the tumors occur in the anterior and medial midshaft of the tibia.[3,20,27,31,32] No ethnic frequency differences have been described, but the lesion appears to occur slightly more often in males.[20,26,32] The affected bone is expanded but usually not bowed, and the cortex adjacent to the lesion is often thin but rarely destroyed unless a fracture has occurred.[3,20,22,27,28,32,46] The tumors are epithelial in nature with prominent desmosomes, tubular structures, and squamoid patterns.[3,17,18,32] Biologic studies show that most of the tumors are strongly positive for cytokeratin and vimentin but are negative for actin and S-100 protein.[24,47,48] Cytogenetic studies have shown multiple translocations involving the region 13q14 in the tumor tissue, but very rarely is the same defect found constitutionally in the patient.[3,24,49-53] Fibroblast growth factor-2 and epithelial growth factor are present in many of the tumors.[3,50,54] Despite the suggestions by early investigators, there is no evidence for the presence of classic fibrous dysplasia, fibrosarcoma, angioblastoma, or synovial cell sarcoma in adamantinoma.

Of some importance is the recent suggestion that there are two types of adamantinomas. Those that are "classical" may behave in a very aggressive fashion, and those that are "differentiated" are much more benign and, in fact, resemble and behave very similarly to osteofibrous dysplasia.[3,40-42,55,56] Studies of osteofibrous dysplasia of the long bones show many similarities to those of adamantinoma, but with some distinctive features. The frequency of occurrence is perhaps slightly less than adamantinoma, and the patients are often younger.[20,35,36,40,41,44,56,57] A report by Anderson and associates[58] in 1993 described a lesion in a newborn child. Many of the affected patients are younger than 10 years of age and most have open epiphyseal plates on the tibia or fibula. The lesions are usually located on the anterior face of the tibia, but may be somewhat distal in the bone as compared with adamantinoma. The bone is almost always substantially bowed.[3,20,35,57] Histologically, the lesions show fibrous tissue with small bone trabeculae and the cells may present a classic storiform pattern.[3,20,35,38,39,44] The results of biologic studies are similar to those for adamantinoma, in that most of the osteofibrous dysplasia tumors are cytokeratin- and vimentin-positive but are negative for actin and S-100 protein. The alterations in the genetic structure for the tumors are often quite similar to those for adamantinoma as well.[47,49,59] There are, however, rather distinct trisomies noted on these tumors that are different from the classical adamantinoma but similar to that seen in the differentiated form.[3,55]

Histologic Studies

The characteristic findings in adamantinoma are the presence of fascicles of epithelioid or fibroblastic cells arranged in a storiform pattern[3,18,20,25,26,29,31,32] (Figure 1). The tissue is constructed of collagen fibers that, along with the cellular elements, fill the center of the lesion. In addition, surrounding the centrally placed epithelioid and fibroblastic elements are osteocytes, which are found in irregularly shaped trabeculae of bone with prominent rims of osteoblasts (Figure 2). Occasional giant cells are encountered that may represent osteoclasts. There is a progressive trabeculation from woven to lamel-

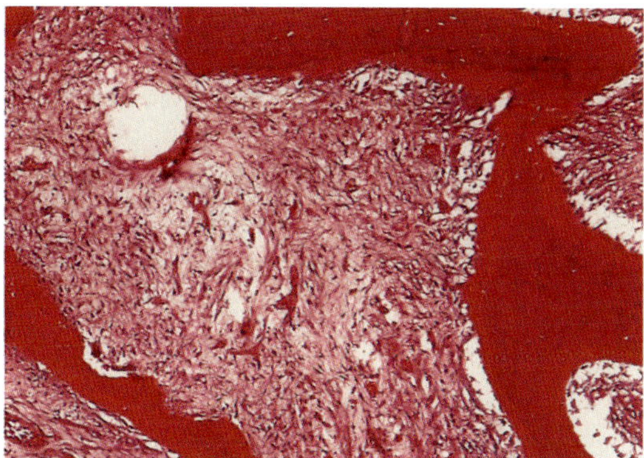

Figure 2

Bone formation occurs and surrounds the fibroblastic cells and vascular channels.

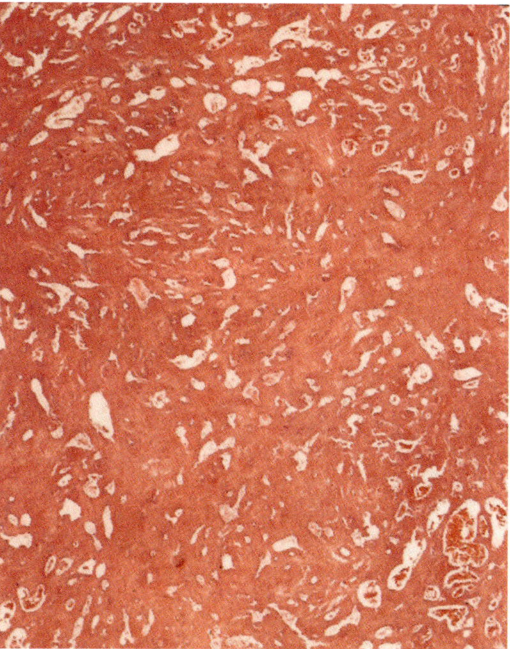

Figure 3

Histologic pattern for osteofibrous dysplasia shows cellular elements but mostly fibrous components, with little to suggest aggressive behavior.

lar bone and increasing numbers of bone trabeculae at the periphery. Vascular channels present in the tissue are sometimes quite large; this has in the past suggested that the lesion is actually a form of angioblastoma.[14-16,25] The overall appearance is of a benign lesion, with few mitotic figures and only occasional cellular atypia.[3,20,26,29,32]

The changes seen in osteofibrous dysplasia are almost identical to those reported for adamantinoma. Loose bundles of collagenous fibrous tissue compose the central portion of the lesions and the storiform pattern of hyalinized collagen bands is characteristic.[3,11,20,32,34,36,37,40,57] Mineralized bone trabeculae form the periphery of the tumor, with increased numbers of osteoblasts that range in appearance from mature woven bone to lamellar bone. There is very limited mitotic activity and only occasional giant cells are seen, mostly at the periphery of the lesion. Histologic experts could find very little difference between differentiated adamantinoma and osteofibrous dysplasia.[3,20,27,32,34,40,43] The classical adamantinoma, however, shows areas with more aggressive-appearing cellular elements and more atypism and mitotic activity[3,40,56] (Figure 3).

Imaging

The two lesions, adamantinoma and osteofibrous dysplasia, are difficult to distinguish on imaging. The tibiae in young patients with osteofibrous dysplasia show normal epiphyseal plates.[3,20,27,40,60] The lesions may be located in the metaphyseal regions rather than the mid- or proximal diaphysis as occurs with adamantinoma.[3,20,27,40] Both lesions are usually located eccentrically, more toward the anterior cortex of the tibia, and are very active on bone scan. Anterior bowing is more frequent with osteofibrous dysplasia than with adamantinoma and can sometimes be deforming (Figure 4). The cortex is markedly expanded in many patients but rarely, even with classical adamantinoma, is there cortical destruction or a soft-tissue mass[3,20,27] (Figure 5).

Synchronous involvement of the tibia and fibula at approximately the same level is more frequent in patients with osteofibrous dysplasia but can occur with either disorder.[3,20,32] The characteristic findings are multiple radiolucencies, sclerotic foci involving the anterior cortex, and associated cortical expansion (Figure 6). MRI shows similar changes for both types of tumors with intermediate signal intensity on T1-weighted images and high signal intensity on T2.[3,20,61-63] CT studies are helpful in defining the cortical thickness and the extent of the eccentric radiolucent component.[3,20]

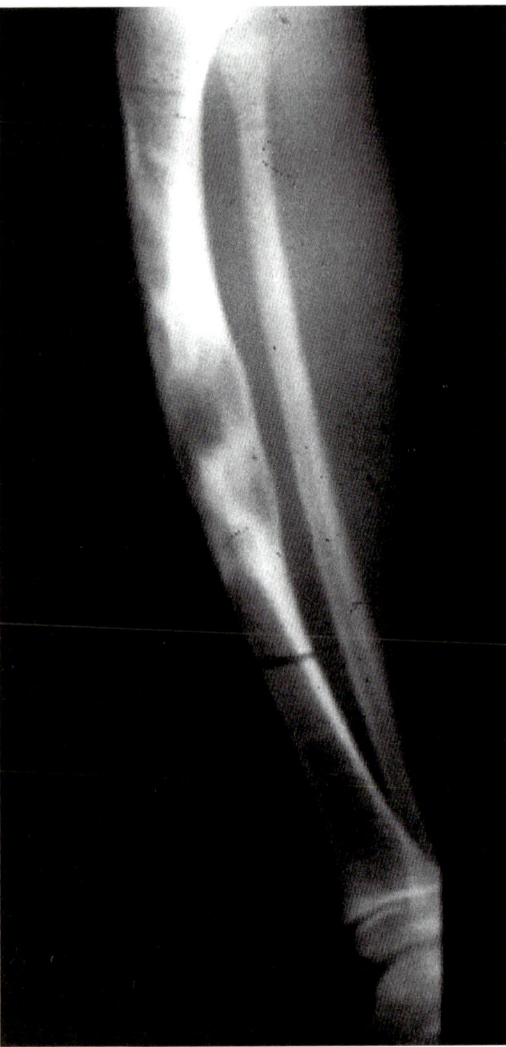

Figure 4
Radiograph of osteofibrous dysplasia of the tibia shows bowing and anterior expansion of the bone but little evidence of active destruction of the cortex.

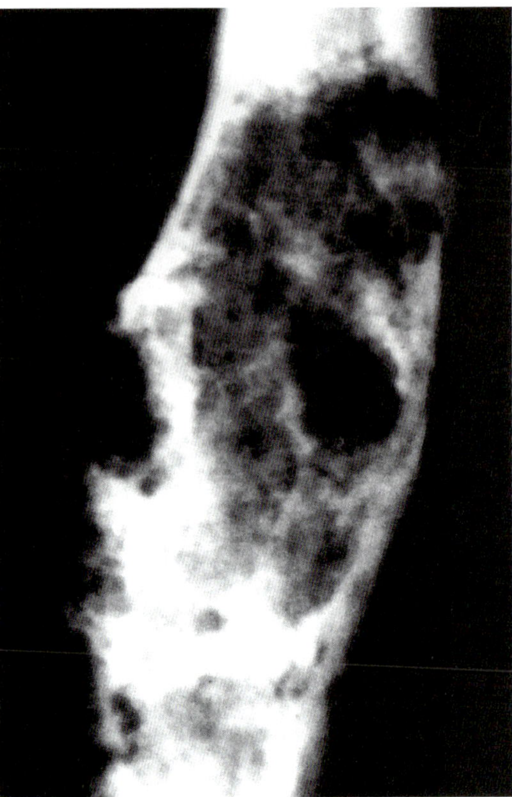

Figure 5
Radiograph of an adamantinoma demonstrates very aggressive changes with cortical expansion, a lytic destructive region anteriorly, and gross deformity of the bone.

Outcome and Treatment

Adamantinoma is considered to be a low-grade malignancy, and metastases occur in approximately 10% to 15% of the patients reported in most current series.[3,19,20,26,27,32,64] Approximately 5% to 10% of the patients die of disease. The problem with metastasis is that the event may not occur until quite late in the course, sometimes as long as 20 years after the primary treatment.[3,10,20,32] In contrast, osteofibrous dysplasia is a benign process that has no potential for metastasis and no resultant fatality. The differentiated adamantinoma that clinically, radiographically, and histologically closely resembles the osteofibrous dysplasia is also believed to be a benign disorder.[3,20,24,40,56] However, all three of these lesions can locally recur after surgical procedures and it is believed that the lesions that do recur have a higher incidence of metastasis.[3,20,32,65]

The treatment of the lesions has been the subject of several studies and remains a controversial issue. The original approach to osteofibrous dysplasia in young children was one of curettage and packing with bone graft or, in some cases, the introduction of a fibular graft.[3,20,32,34,66] The recurrence and fracture rates with this protocol are both high, which can cause problems in management and potentially be disabling. If the lesion is characteristically an osteofibrous dysplasia in a child younger than the age of 8 years, it now seems reasonable to follow the child with serial imaging studies and at the age of 10 years or older, perform a partial or complete resection.[3,41,66]

For adamantinomas, especially lesions designated as classical, wide resection is a reasonable approach. Allograft or autograft

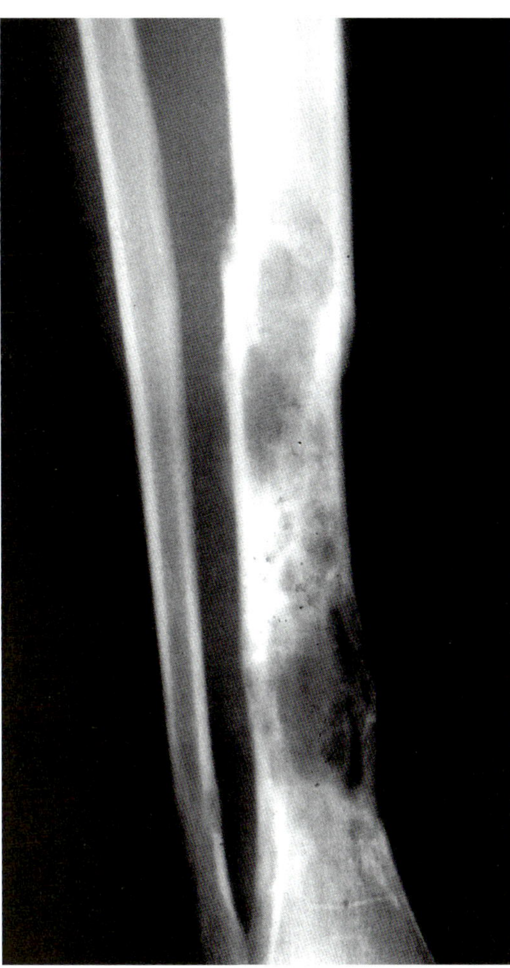

Figure 6
A large, very aggressive adamantinoma of the tibia is seen in this radiograph. The bone is distorted and a fracture has occurred at the proximal junction.

transplants have been used and, although the fracture and nonunion complication rates for both are high, the success rate from a standpoint of no recurrence and prolonged survival is generally excellent.[3,20,26,41,45,67-69] The difficulty is that this may be considered excessive treatment of patients with differentiated adamantinoma or osteofibrous dysplasia.[57,66] The problem lies in attempting to decide on the basis of patient age, clinical history, repeated imaging studies, and histologic studies of biopsy tissue whether extensive surgery is required. This is not a simple issue; until we can define with certainty the potential for malignancy in the lesion by biologic, imaging, or histologic analysis, it remains a major challenge. The rule used by most physicians who care for these patients is that it

is probably better to be a bit more radical in the primary treatment than to subsequently lose a limb or a life.

Comments and Conclusions

The first real concern about these disorders is related to origin. Are they really neoplastic? Do they arise from epithelioid or fibrous tissue? Could they be of vascular origin? Are they somehow related to other fibrous diseases of bone, such as fibrous dysplasia or nonossifying fibroma? Is there some relationship to ameloblastic disease of the jaws? Despite a long history of observation of these tumors by very competent biologists, pathologists, radiologists, and orthopaedists, we still do not have an answer!

A second issue is related to the site of occurrence. More than 80% of the lesions for both disorders are in the tibia—more specifically, in the anterior surface of the tibia. Some additional cases occur in the fibula or the ulna. The principal feature that the tibia and ulna have in common is a segment of the shaft that is free of attached muscular structures. The periosteal sleeve of the bone lies deep to the subcutaneous fibrous layers of the skin. The only other bones that have the same relationship to the skin and soft tissues are the clavicle and a portion of the mandible. These data would possibly suggest that the origin of the tumors is from the subcutaneous fibrous sheath, but that seems unlikely. There is currently no answer to that question.

Adamantinoma and osteofibrous dysplasia of long bones are not simple problems for the patient or treating physician. The two forms of the disease (or indeed the three forms, as it has now been postulated that the differentiated adamantinoma is very similar in character and outcome to osteofibrous dysplasia) are very similar in all aspects of study. Because they look similar on imaging and histologic studies and are not biologically distinct from one another, it is sometimes very difficult to decide which of the three tumors is present in the limb of an individual older than age 15 years. Sometimes, depending on the nature of the lesion, the surgical treatment may be considered excessive or, conversely, inadequate. A number of publications have addressed this issue in an attempt to establish specific protocols for evaluation and design of a treatment protocol. Fortunately, the risk is not great as not only are the tumors rare, but even the classical adamantinoma has a relatively low rate of metastasis. If followed closely over perhaps 10 or more years after surgery, the likelihood of long-term survival is very high.

References:

1. Maier C: Ein primares myelogenes platen epithelcarcinoma der ulna. *Bruns Beitr Klin Chir* 1900;26:553.

2. Fischer B: Über ein primares adamatinom der tibia. *Franfurt Z Pathol* 1913;12:422-441.

3. Dorfman HD, Czerniak B: *Bone Tumors*. St. Louis, MO, Mosby, 1998, pp 481-491, 949-973.

4. Ryrie BJ: Adamantinoma of the tibia: Aetiology and pathogenesis. *BMJ* 1932;2:1000-1003.

5. Hebbel R: Adamantinoma of the tibia. *Surgery* 1940;7:860-868.

6. Anderson CE, Saunders JB de CM: Primary adamantinoma of the ulna. *Surg Gynecol Obstet* 1942;75:351-356.

7. Dockerty MB, Meyerding HW: Adamantinoma of the tibia: Report of two new cases. *JAMA* 1942;119:932-937.

8. Baker PL, Dockerty MB, Coventry MB: Adamantinomas (so called) of the long bones: Review of the literature and report of three new cases. *J Bone Joint Surg Am* 1954;36:704-720.

9. Cohen DM, Dahlin DC, Pugh DG: Fibrous dysplasia associated with adamantinoma of the long bones. *Cancer* 1962;15:515-521.

10. Weiss SW, Dorfman HD: Adamantinoma of long bone: An analysis of nine new cases with emphasis on metastasizing lesions and fibrous dysplasia-like changes. *Hum Pathol* 1977;8:141-153.

11. Campbell CJ, Hawk T: A variant of fibrous dysplasia (osteofibrous dysplasia). *J Bone Joint Surg Am* 1982;64:231-236.

12. Hicks JD: Synovial sarcoma of the tibia. *J Pathol Bacteriol* 1954;67:151-161.

13. Lederer H, Sinclair AJ: Malignant synovioma simulating "adamantinoma of the tibia." *J Pathol Bacteriol* 1954;67:163-168.

14. Changus GW, Speed JS, Stewart FW: Malignant angioblastoma of bone: A reappraisal of adamantinoma of long bone. *Cancer* 1957;10:540-559.

15. Elliott GB: Malignant angioblastoma of long bone, so-called "tibial" adamantinoma. *J Bone Joint Surg Br* 1962;44:25-33.

16. Llombart-Bosch A, Ortuño-Pacheco G: Ultrastructural findings supporting the angioblastic nature of the so-called adamantinoma of the tibia. *Histopathology* 1978;2:189-200.

17. Rosai J: Adamantinoma of the tibia: Electron microscopic evidence of its epithelial origin. *Am J Clin Pathol* 1969;51:786-792.

18. Rosai J, Pinkus GS: Immunohistochemical demonstration of epithelial differentiation in adamantinoma of the tibia. *Am J Surg Pathol* 1982;6:427-434.

19. Campanacci M, Giunti A, Bertoni F, Laus M, Gitelis S: Adamantinoma of the long bones: The experience at the Istituto Ortopedico Rizzoli. *Am J Surg Pathol* 1981;5:533-542.

20. Campanacci M: *Bone and Soft Tissue Tumors*, ed 2. New York, NY, Springer Verlag, 1999, pp 707-732.

21. Cohn BT, Brahms MA, Froimson AI: Metastasis of adamantinoma sixteen years after knee disarticulation: Report of a case. *J Bone Joint Surg Am* 1986;68:772-776.

22. Dameron TB Jr: Adamantinoma of the appendicular skeleton. *Johns Hopkins Med J* 1979;145:107-111.

23. Donner R, Dikland R: Adamantinoma of the tibia: A long-standing case with unusual histologic features. *J Bone Joint Surg Br* 1966;48:138-144.

24. Hazelbag HM, Taminiau AH, Fleuren GJ, Hagendoorn PC: Adamantinoma of long bones: A clinicopathological study of thirty-two patients with emphasis on histological subtype, precursor lesion, and biologic behavior. *J Bone Joint Surg Am* 1994;76:1482-1499.

25. Huvos AG, Marcove RC: Adamantinoma of long bones: A clinicopathological study of fourteen cases with vascular origin suggested. *J Bone Joint Surg Am* 1975;57:148-154.

26. Keeney GL, Unni KK, Beabout JW, Pritchard DJ: Adamantinoma of long bones: A clinicopathologic study of 85 cases. *Cancer* 1989;64:730-737.

27. Mirra JM: *Bone Tumors: Clinical, Radiologic, and Pathologic Correlations*. Philadelphia, PA, Lea and Febiger, 1989, pp 1204-1231.

28. Moon NF, Mori H: Adamantinoma of the appendicular skeleton: Updated. *Clin Orthop Relat Res* 1986;204:215-237.

29. Pieterse AS, Smith PS, McClure J: Adamantinoma of long bones: Clinical, pathological and ultrastructural features. *J Clin Pathol* 1982;35:780-786.

30. Unni KK, Dahlin DC, Beabout JW, Ivins JC: Adamantinoma of long bones. *Cancer* 1974;34:1796-1805.

31. Zehr RJ, Recht MP, Bauer TW: Adamantinoma. *Skeletal Radiol* 1995;24:553-555.

32. Schajowicz F: *Tumors and Tumorlike Lesions of Bone and Joints*. New York, NY, Springer Verlag, 1981, pp 383-398

33. Kempson RL: Ossifying fibroma of the long bones: A light and electron microscopic study. *Arch Pathol* 1966;82:218-233.

34. Alguacil-Garcia A, Alonso A, Pettigrew NM: Osteofibrous dysplasia (ossifying fibroma) of the tibia and fibula and adamantinoma: A case report. *Am J Clin Pathol* 1984;82:470-474.

35. Campanacci M: Osteofibrous dysplasia of long bones: A new clinical entity. *Ital J Orthop Traumatol* 1976;2:221-237.

36. Campanacci M, Laus M: Osteofibrous dysplasia of the tibia and fibula. *J Bone Joint Surg Am* 1981;63:367-375.

37. Goergen TG, Dickman PS, Resnick D, Saltzstein SL, O'Dell CW, Akeson WH: Long bone ossifying fibromas. *Cancer* 1977;39:2067-2072.

38. Markel SF: Ossifying fibroma of long bone: Its distinction from fibrous dysplasia and its associa-

tion with adamantnoma of long bone. *Am J Clin Pathol* 1978;69:91-97.

39. Schoenecker PL, Swanson K, Sheridan JJ: Ossifying fibroma of the tibia: Report of a new case and review of the literature. *J Bone Joint Surg Am* 1981;63:483-488.

40. Ishida T, Iijima T, Kikuchi F, et al: A clinicopathological and immunohistochemical study of osteofibrous dysplasia, differentiated adamantinoma, and adamantinoma of long bones. *Skeletal Radiol* 1992;21:493-502.

41. Springfield DS, Rosenberg AE, Mankin HJ, Mindell ER: Relationship between osteofibrous dysplasia and adamantinoma. *Clin Orthop Relat Res* 1994;309:234-244.

42. Sweet DE, Vinh TN, Devaney K: Cortical osteofibrous dysplasia of long bone and its relationship to adamantinoma: A clinicopathologic study of 30 cases. *Am J Surg Pathol* 1992;16:282-290.

43. Ueda Y, Blasius S, Edel G, Wuisman P, Böcker W, Roessner A: Osteofibrous dysplasia of long bones: A reactive process to adamantinoma tissue. *J Cancer Res Clin Oncol* 1992;118:152-156.

44. Wang JW, Shih CH, Chen WJ: Osteofibrous dysplasia (ossifying fibroma of long bones): A report of four cases and review of the literature. *Clin Orthop Relat Res* 1992;278:235-243.

45. Qureshi AA, Shott S, Mallin BA, Gitelis S: Current trends in the management of adamantinoma of long bones: An international study. *J Bone Joint Surg Am* 2000;82:1122-1131.

46. Unni KK: *Dahlin's Bone Tumors: General Aspects and Data on 11,087 Cases*, ed 5. Philadelphia, PA, Lippincott Raven, 1996.

47. Benassi MS, Campanacci L, Gamberi G, et al: Cytokeratin expression and distribution in adamantinoma of long bones and osteofibrous dysplasia of tibia and fibula: An immunohistochemical study correlated to histogenesis. *Histopathology* 1994;25:71-76.

48. Bovée JV, van den Broek LJ, de Boer WI, Hagendoorn PC: Expression of growth factors and their receptors in adamantinoma of long bones and the implication for its histogenesis. *J Pathol* 1998;184:24-30.

49. Bridge JA, Dembinski A, DeBoer J, Travis J, Neff JR: Clonal chromosomal abnormalities in osteofibrous dysplasia: Implications for histopathogenesis and its relationship with adamantinoma. *Cancer* 1994;73:1746-1752.

50. Maki M, Saitoh K, Kaneko Y, Fukayama M, Morohoshi T: Expression of cytokeratin 1, 5, 14, 19 and transforming growth factors-beta 1, beta 2, beta 3 in osteofibrous dysplasia and adamantinoma: A possible association of transforming growth factor-beta with basal cell phenotype promotion. *Pathol Int* 2000;50:801-807.

51. Mandahl N, Heim S, Rydholm A, Willén H, Mitelman F: Structural chromosome aberrations in an adamantinoma. *Cancer Genet Cytogenet* 1989;42:187-190.

52. Perez-Atayde AR, Kozakewich HP, Vawter GF: Adamantinoma of the tibia: An ultrastructural and immunohistochemical study. *Cancer* 1985;55:1015-1023.

53. Sozzi G, Miozzo M, Di Palma S, et al: Involvement of the region 13q14 in a patient with ada-

mantinoma of the long bones. *Hum Genet* 1990;85:513-515.

54. Maki M, Athanasou N: Osteofibrous dysplasia and adamantinoma: Correlation of proto-oncogene product and matrix protein expression. *Hum Pathol* 2004;35:69-74.

55. Czerniak B, Rojas-Corona RR, Dorfman HD: Morphologic diversity of long bone adamantinoma: The concept of differentiated (regressing) adamantinoma and its relationship to osteofibrous dysplasia. *Cancer* 1989;64:2319-2334.

56. Kahn LB: Adamantinoma, osteofibrous dysplasia and differentiated adamantinoma. *Skeletal Radiol* 2003;32:245-258.

57. Park YK, Unni KK, McLeod RA, Pritchard DJ: Osteofibrous dysplasia: Clinicopathologic study of 80 cases. *Hum Pathol* 1993;24:1339-1347.

58. Anderson MJ, Townsend DR, Johnston JO, Bohay DR: Osteofibrous dysplasia in the newborn: Report of a case. *J Bone Joint Surg Am* 1993;75:265-267.

59. Hazelbag HM, Wessels JW, Mollevangers P, van den Berg E, Molenaar WM, Hogendoorn PC: Cytogenetic analysis of adamantinoma of long bones: Further indications for a common histogenesis with osteofibrous dysplasia. *Cancer Genet Cytogenet* 1997;97:5-11.

60. Garces P, Romano CC, Vellet AD, Alakija P, Schachar NS: Adamantinoma of the tibia: Plain film, computed tomography and magnetic resonance imaging appearance. *Can Assoc Radiol J* 1994;45:314-317.

61. Judmaier W, Perr S, Krejzi T, Dessl A, Kühberger R: MR findings in tibial adamantinoma: A case report. *Acta Radiol* 1998;39:276-278.

62. Torriani M, Dertkigil SS, Etchebehere M, Amstalden EM: Magnetic resonance imaging of tibial classic adamantinoma at 2 tesla. *J Comput Assist Tomogr* 2002;26:855-859.

63. Van der Woude HJ, Hazelbag HM, Bloem JL, Taminiau AH, Hogendoorn PC: MRI of adamantinoma of long bones in correlation with histopathology. *AJR Am J Roentgenol* 2004;183:1737-1744.

64. Naji AF, Murphy JA, Stasney RJ, Neville WE, Chrenka P: So-called adamantinoma of long bones. *J Bone Joint Surg Am* 1964;46:151-158.

65. Lokich J: Metastatic adamantinoma of bone to lung: A case report of the natural history and the use of chemotherapy and radiation therapy. *Am J Clin Oncol* 1994;17:157-159.

66. Lee RS, Weitzel S, Eastwood DM, et al: Osteofibrous dysplasia of the tibia: Is there a need for a radical surgical approach? *J Bone Joint Surg Br* 2006;88:658-664.

67. Gebhardt MC, Lord FC, Rosenberg AE, Mankin HJ: The treatment of adamantinoma of the tibia by wide resection and allograft bone transplantation. *J Bone Joint Surg Am* 1987;69:1177-1188.

68. Ortiz-Cruz E, Gebhardt MC, Jennings LC, Springfield DS, Mankin HJ: The results of transplantation of intercalary allografts after resection of tumors: A long-term follow up study. *J Bone Joint Surg Am* 1997;79:97-106.

69. Papagelopoulos PJ, Savvidou OD, Mavrogenis AF, et al: Lateral malleolus en bloc resection and ankle reconstruction for malignant tumors. *Clin Orthop Relat Res* 2005;437:209-218.

Chapter 9

Hemangiomas of Bone, Joint, and Soft Tissue

One of the most common soft-tissue lesions, particularly in children, is the hemangioma. The lesion is benign and limited in extent and effect on the patient. Problems often disappear spontaneously. If this were to be the only lesion included in this discussion, the chapter would be short indeed. However, one of the difficulties with defining the entity is the remarkable number of disorders to which the name "hemangioma" can be applied. These include benign vascular tumor, senile hemangioma, cherry hemangioma, strawberry hemangioma, capillary hemangioma, cavernous hemangioma, intramuscular hemangioma, intraosseous hemangioma, arteriovenous hemangioma, and blue rubber bleb nevus syndrome. There are also several more extensive disorders, some of which are genetic and have hemangiomatous vascular abnormalities as one of their presenting features—Klippel-Trénaunay-Weber syndrome, Osler-Weber-Rendu disease, Kasabach-Merritt syndrome, Gorham disappearing bone disease, and Maffucci syndrome. Some of these rare disorders are very aggressive and destructive and resemble malignant tumors, including angiosarcoma, in many ways.

Histologic and Genetic Characteristics

The most common forms of histologic characteristics are seen in the capillary hemangiomas, located in the skin or subcutaneous tissues.[1-9] They are composed of nodules of small capillary-size vessels that are each subserved by a "feeder vessel," also known as a lobular pattern.[1-3,7,9] A second form is known as cavernous hemangioma; these lesions are far less common and occur in older individuals.[1-3,9] They are larger and less circumscribed and more frequently located in muscle, bone, and viscera.[9,10] The blood vessels are widely dilated; in most cases, cavernous hemangiomas are associated with venous structures and are much more symptomatic and destructive.[1,9,10]

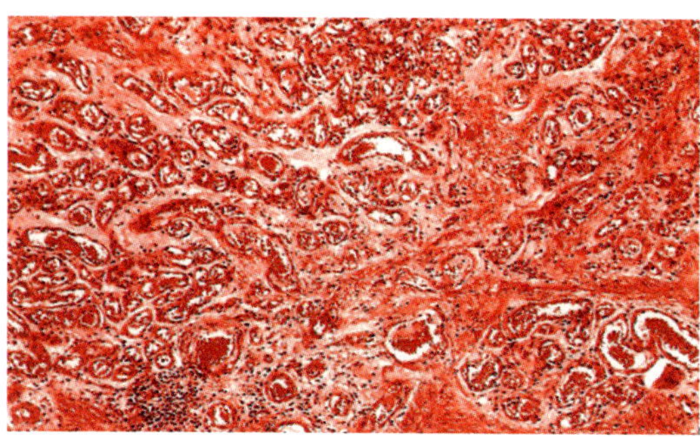

Figure 1

Histologic pattern for a hemangioma of bone. Note the enormous number of small vessels that contain blood elements and the fibrous and sometimes osseous or cartilaginous components surrounding them.

Although most of the vascular tumors are not genetic or familial, some hemangiomatous cases have been linked to chromosome 5, with characteristic presence of fibroblast growth factor and platelet-derived growth factor.[9,11,12] With advancing growth, collagenase IV is frequently identified. Furthermore, a recent study has described increased circulating endothelial progenitor cells AC133, CD34, and VEGFR2/KDR in children with congenital capillary hemangiomas.[13]

Histologically, all forms of the lesion arise from angioblasts, which subsequently differentiate to form flattened, mature endothelial cells.[1-4,6,7,9,14] The cells create atypical vascular systems that show thickening of walls, dilatation of vessels, and hyperplasia by some mitotic activity (Figure 1). Mast cells are often present.[15] Histology is fairly typical, but electron microscopy is sometimes helpful in defining the vascular nature of the tumors.[7,9] Solid nests of endothelium are frequently encircled by cuffs of pericytes. Calcification can occur and consists of tiny crystals embedded in organizing thrombi and in the collagen wall of the blood vessels.[1,9] Infarction of the vessels may occur.

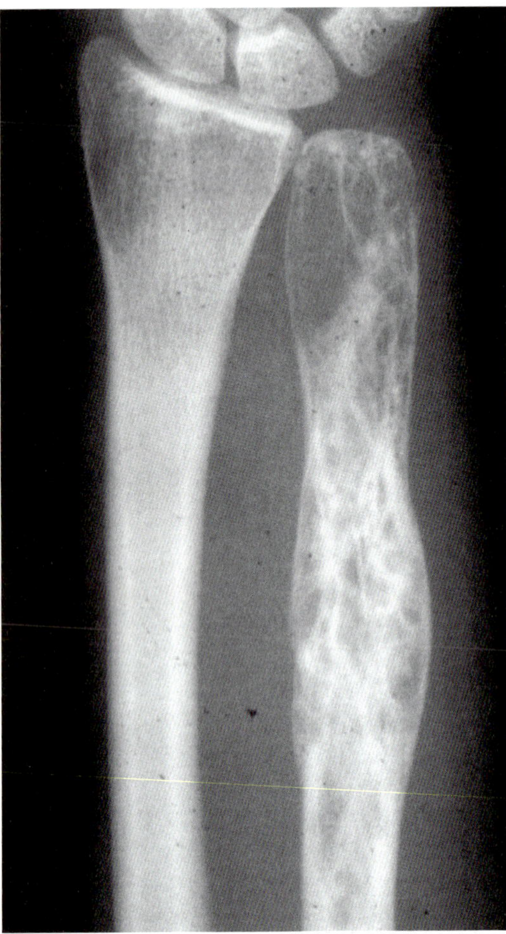

Figure 2

A hemangioma of bone in the ulna. Note the expansion and thinning of the cortex and the irregular bony elements within the medullary cavity. The bone is deformed and led to a limitation of arm movement.

Clinical Forms

The most common form of hemangioma is described as the *senile* or *cherry hemangioma*. These are small, benign, asymptomatic, self-limited red-purple papules that appear in the skin of elderly patients.[2,3,5,6,9] A second common disorder is the *"strawberry nevus,"* which is seen in approximately 0.5% of infants.[9,16] About one fifth of the cases are multiple and most appear on the head and neck. The lesions may resemble "birthmarks" but produce a strawberry color when the infant cries. Most of the lesions spontaneously regress over a period of a few years and appear as a gray, somewhat wrinkled spot at the location.[9,16]

Hemangiomas of deep soft tissue may be much larger and more difficult to treat. They are frequently cavernous in structure and

may cause bleeding and significant pain and disability.[9,10,17,18] A distinctive form of multiple cavernous hemangiomata delineated by Bean[19] in 1958 is known as *blue rubber bleb nevus syndrome* (BRBNS) or Bean syndrome. The lesions are cutaneous, blue, and look and feel like rubber nipples. Many patients with BRNBS also have gastrointestinal hemangiomas of a similar type.[20,21]

Hemangiomas of joint tissue appear to arise from synovium.[22-24] They are sometimes associated with fat cells and may be a component of lipoma arborescens (Hoffa's disease). They may produce articular hemorrhages and joint disorders. Small *intramuscular hemangiomas* are often unnoticed, but the larger ones occur in young people and most occur before 30 years of age. They may become large and deforming, and hemorrhaging can sometimes cause severe muscular abnormalities.[9,17,18,25]

Hemangiomas of bone occur more commonly in females than males, and the peak age incidence is the fifth decade.[9,14,26-33] Although they are not believed to be familial, suggestive case reports describe some hemangiomas as multiple.[9,30,34-36] Vertebral hemangiomas are the most common form; the lesions are most often solitary but may expand the bone posteriorly to cause cord compression.[9,17,27,37,38] Calvarial hemangiomas are common and are centered in a diploic space in the frontal and parietal regions.[9,39,40] They can be expansile and produce palpable lumps in the skull. The mandible is occasionally involved and may cause considerable abnormality in dentition.[9,41] Long-bone hemangiomas are less common, but are almost always cavernous in nature; they can be quite large and cause bony deformity[9,26-29,31-33] (Figure 2). The tumors have a predilection for the metaphyseal or diaphyseal sites, but can involve the epiphysis and may on rare occasions extend across joints. The bones are expanded as a rule and may show calcification in the vascular tissue within the bone.[1,9,14,31,32] Occasionally, one may see a surface-based osseous hemangioma, which can be symptomatic and present a confusing radiographic image.[9,42,43]

Still another rare entity that can be very disabling is known as *diffuse angiomatosis*. The disorder occurs during childhood and is clinically often very extensive and symptomatic.[2,5,9,26,29,39,44,45] The lesions appear during the child's intrauterine life and grow proportionally with the fetus. Thus within the first decade of life, the tumors can cause massive enlargement of a limb or abdomen.[5,6,9,23] When the lesions are capillary, they may be smaller and less disabling; when the lesions are cavernous, however, the child may have an enormous enlargement of a limb and be quite disabled.[2,9]

Kasabach-Merritt syndrome was first described in an article in the *American Journal of Diseases of Children* in 1940.[46] The patient was a male infant with a discolored, indurated lesion of the thigh that rapidly grew and involved the entire extremity, scrotum, abdomen, and thorax. The patient was also noted to have a severe thrombocytopenia.[46] It is believed that the vascular lesion present in the soft tissues causes intravascular coagulation and platelet trapping. Several publications have subsequently expanded the description.[2,3,47-49] The disorder is uncommon, more frequent in males, and can be lethal (with an estimated mortality rate of 25%). Histologically, the lesions show a Kaposiform hemangioendothelioma with many spindle cells, rounded endothelial cells, and pericytes.[9] The appearance has sometimes been described as a tufted angioma.[9] The disorder is of unknown cause and is not considered to be hereditary.

Osler-Weber-Rendu disease was first described in 1896 by Rendu[50] and then in 1904 by Weber.[51] Both described children with peculiar skin changes thought to be telangiectasia. It was Sir William Osler,[52] however, who defined the hereditary nature of the disease and the clinical features of vascular anomalies consisting of dilated capillaries and small veins that caused discoloration and bruising of the skin and mucous membranes. The disorder is autosomal dominant and is characterized by the development of numerous small red papules on the face, lips, and tongue, as well as similar findings in the gastrointestinal tract.[9,53] As the patient ages, the lesions have been described as having the features of a "vascular spider."[9,53] Patients have repeated episodes of bleeding that may be life-threatening.

Klippel-Trénaunay-Weber syndrome was first described in 1900 by Klippel and Trénaunay[54] and then several years later by Weber.[55] This rare condition consists of the triad of cutaneous hemangiomas, bone and soft-tissue hypertrophy, and varicose veins.[9,48,54] The disorder does not appear to be hereditary, and males and females are equally affected. The capillary hemangiomas are large and infiltrative and may expand sufficiently to cause gigantism involving an entire extremity. Venous varicosities are characteristically present in the affected part of the body; these may occlude and cause swelling or bleed if damaged.[1-3,9,47,48]

Gorham disease, also known as "disappearing bone disease," was first described in 1838 by Jackson,[56] but then in considerable detail in 1955 by Lemuel Gorham and Arthur Purdy Stout.[57] It is an extremely rare disorder characterized by the progressive dissolution of a bone, associated with abnormal vascular swelling described as angiomatosis.[1,5,9,14,44,57,58] The disorder often extends to adjacent bones. The disease is of unknown cause, occurs in all age groups (but mostly in patients younger than 30 years of age), and affects males more frequently than females. The bones most frequently affected are in the hand, arm, shoulder, ribs, pelvis, femur, and jaw. Cases affecting the skull and spine have also been reported. Histologically, the findings are those of a markedly vascular and destructive angiomatosis of the medullary cavity, which extends to the cortex and sometimes completely destroys the bone.[1,14,27,57,58] Fractures are common. The disorder extends from one bone to an adjacent one so that the lesion of the humerus extends to the scapula, which then further extends to the clavicle, and so forth.

Maffucci syndrome, first described in 1881 by Angelo Maffucci,[59] is a nonhereditary, rare, mesodermal dysplastic disorder with the principal lesions being enchondromas of the bones.[1,14] The disease has a mild male predilection and principally affects the long bones (especially the pelvis, femur, and humerus), but also the hands and feet.[1,14] Malignancy in the chondral tissue occurs in approximately 50% of the patients, which is much more frequent than in Ollier's disease.[1,14] Patients with Maffucci syndrome are also noted to have small, soft-tissue cavernous hemangiomas that are highly vascular, can break through the skin, and even occasionally become malignant.[1,60] The lesions are sometimes painful. Patients with Maffucci syndrome occasionally have gastrointestinal involvement.[61]

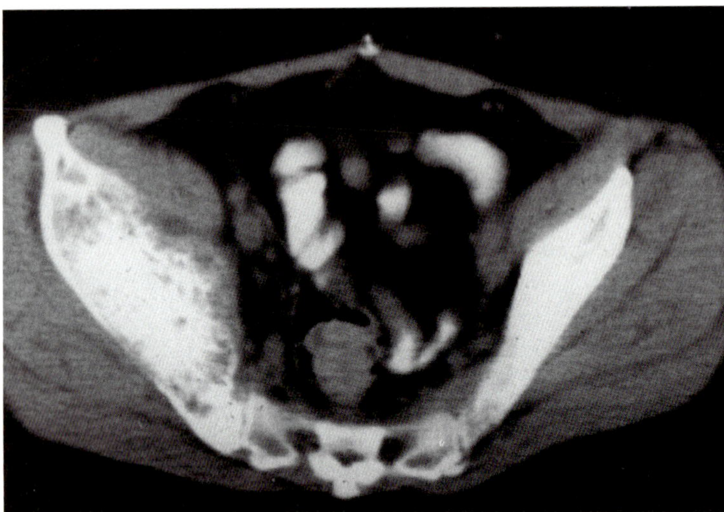

Figure 3
MRI scan of the pelvis showing an enormous lesion of the ilium with a soft-tissue component and gross distortion of the bony structure.

Imaging and Diagnosis

Imaging of hemangiomatous lesions has been the subject of multiple studies. Standard radiographs disclose the lesions as soft-tissue shadows, although they are isodense with muscle; hence small lesions, adjacent lesions, or those within muscle may be difficult to identify.[1,7,9,34,62] When adjacent to bone, they may cause periosteal ossification, but usually just as a thin shell. Calcification and phleboliths may be seen occasionally in hemangiomas studied with plain radiographs.[1,9]

MRI is currently the technique of choice to identify the lesions and to distinguish them from other tumors.[1,9,63-66] Hemangiomas show an increased signal on both T1 and T2 but some sites have areas of signal void.[63,66] The void areas correspond to the presence of dense fibrous tissue, thrombi, phleboliths, or areas of high vascular flow rate. The serpentine pattern of vascular structures may be present and is strongly supportive of the diagnosis of a hemangioma. Increased gadolinium enhancement is characteristic of these lesions and may be very helpful in distinguishing hemangiomas from other soft-tissue lesions.[9,10,65,66] In the past, angiography was performed and was helpful in disclosing increased presence of the dye within the lesion, but could not be considered diagnostic for hemangiomas because many other aggressive tumors had a similar pattern. Recently, ultrasound technology and positron emission tomography

have been introduced to aid in distinguishing the lesions from other types of tumors.[67,68]

Synovial hemangiomas may be seen best using MRI, which shows an intra-articular pedunculated or diffuse mass with increased signals on T1 and T2.[9,23] Erosion of bones, particularly of the knee or hip joint, may be seen as well, either with plain radiography or MRI.[23]

Osseous hemangiomas may have different imaging characteristics, depending on the location of the lesion.[1,9,14,33-35] In the calvarium or pelvis, the lesions are characterized by what is described as a "honeycomb" appearance[9,35,39,69] (Figure 3). The cortex is often thin and expanded; fine radiating striations may be present, creating a "sunburst" appearance. The appearance of vertebral hemangiomas on plain radiographs is virtually diagnostic. The image consists of parallel vertical trabeculae referred to as a "jailhouse appearance."[38] The cortex is rarely thinned or expanded. In the long bones, the appearance is less specific but the bones are irregularly lytic on radiographs, with sometimes expanded and thinned cortices. The medullary region may show a coarse, bubbly appearance.[1,14,34,41] CT scans of the lesions, particularly those in the pelvis, sometimes show a pattern described as "filigree lace."[1,37,38,64,69] MRI shows the classic pattern of T1 and T2 enhancement and the presence of vascular structures.[38,64]

Bones from patients with Gorham disease show marked medullary and cortical destruction with ultimate dissolution and frequently involvement of the adjacent bone.[58] Lesions seen in patients with Kasabach-Merritt syndrome or Klippel-Trénaunay-Weber syndrome are often of enormous size and have soft-tissue abnormalities. The lesions may show the characteristic appearance of cavernous hemangiomas.[5,9,34,35,63]

The principal problem related to benign hemangiomatous lesions is distinguishing them from malignant tumors.[18,45,70] The small lesions of the skin and subjacent soft tissues are not difficult to assess and follow, but lesions that are deeper—especially those in the muscles—can be very puzzling in terms of diagnosis. Hemangiomatous tumors may appear quite similar to a vast array of benign (especially soft-tissue) sarcomas on physical examination and even on imaging studies. Angiosarcomas of various presentations may be the most confusing as they have similar MRI features to those of benign hemangiomatous lesions.[18,45] Patients with Kasabach-Merritt syndrome, Osler-Weber-Rendu disease, and Klippel-Trénaunay-Weber syndrome are less of a problem in diagnosis, based on the other physical and laboratory findings that support the systemic illness and make the possibility of overlooking a malignant tumor of soft tissue less likely. A biopsy is often necessary to be certain of the nature of the lesion, but it should also be noted that the vascular components of the tumors may be difficult to identify or separate from other types of neoplasms. Furthermore, open and even needle biopsies may result in excessive bleeding, particularly for patients with platelet disorders.

Treatment

It should be quite evident that the majority of hemangiomatous lesions need no treatment other than periodic observation.[2,3,16] Cherry lesions in the elderly and strawberry lesions in children are usually asymptomatic and need only be occasionally observed.[2,3,16] Similarly, small asymptomatic subcutaneous or even muscular lesions should be assessed clinically to be certain that they appear benign on imaging, but usually need no further treatment.[9,10,17] Laser treatment has been introduced for small lesions, particularly in the face and neck of children.[2,9,16] Similarly, asymptomatic hemangiomas of the vertebral segments and many small lesions of bone often do not require any treatment other than periodic observation.[1,14,31,33,41]

The concern lies with large lesions in soft tissue, bone, or joint that are painful and continue to enlarge.[22-24] These frequently require some form of biopsy, followed by embolization, if sufficiently vascular, or even radiation or surgical excision if neces

sary.[1,2,9,14,32,71,72] Pneumatic compression has been helpful for patients with Kasabach-Merritt syndrome.[69] Radiation may also be helpful, particularly for the lesions of Gorham disease and some of the very destructive lesions of Kasabach-Merritt or Klippel-Trénaunay-Weber syndromes.[71] Diffuse angiogenesis, which causes major alterations in limb structure, often requires radiation and some forms of surgery as well.

Some chemotherapeutic agents have been introduced in an attempt to decrease the rapidity of development and the possible impairment as a result of large, destructive, painful lesions. These include corticosteroids, interferon-2α, theophylline, vincristine, cyclophosphamide, and other agents that help stop bone destruction and vascular alterations that can lead to excessive bleeding, decrease in the number of red and white cells, and thrombocytopenia.[6,9,73]

Conclusions

Musculoskeletal hemangiomatous lesions remain mysterious entities with a vast array of presentations, ranging from small cherry lesions to extensive vascular lesions with resultant severe damage to the involved site and sometimes marked loss of blood components. The diagnosis can be difficult in view of the infrequency with which the lesions appear and the variability of their presentation. Imaging studies are helpful, and biopsy may provide an accurate diagnosis for large or aggressive lesions. Treatment of many of the lesions is simply periodic observation; but for the more aggressive, deforming, or painful lesions, there does not appear to be much that can be done other than surgery or radiation. The key problem that faces the physician who treats patients with these lesions is that they must be carefully distinguished from angiosarcomas and other forms of connective-tissue cancer that have similar presentations. That, along with maintaining reasonable function for the affected part, represents the challenge.

References

1. Campanacci M: *Bone and Soft Tissue Tumors*, ed 2. New York, NY, Springer Verlag, 1999, pp 599-618.

2. Coffin CM, Dehner LP: Vascular tumors in children and adolescents: A clinicopathologic study of 228 tumors in 222 patients. *Pathol Annu* 1993;28:97-120.

3. Esterly NB: Cutaneous hemangiomas, vascular stains and malformations, and associated syndromes. *Curr Probl Pediatr* 1996;26:3-39.

4. Geschickter CF, Keasbey LE: Tumors of blood vessels. *Am J Cancer* 1935;23:568-591.

5. Paley D, Evans DC: Angiomatous involvement of an extremity: A spectrum of syndromes. *Clin Orthop Relat Res* 1986;206 :215-218.

6. Rao VK, Weiss SW: Angiomatosis of soft tissue: An analysis of the histologic features and clinical outcome in 51 cases. *Am J Surg Pathol* 1992;16:764-771.

7. Stout AP, Lattes R: *Tumors of the Soft Tissues*. Washington, DC, Armed Forces Institute of Pathology, 1967, pp 67-73.

8. Tan ST, Velickovic M, Ruger BM, Davis PF: Cellular and extracellular markers of hemangioma. *Plast Reconstr Surg* 2000;106:529-538.

9. Weiss SW, Goldblum JR: *Enzinger and Weiss's Soft Tissue Tumors*, ed 4. St. Louis, MO, Mosby, 2001, pp 837-915.

10. Wild AT, Raab P, Krauspe R: Hemangioma of skeletal muscle. *Arch Orthop Trauma Surg* 2000;120:139-143.

11. Blei F, Walter J, Orlow SJ, Marchuk DA: Familial segregation of hemangiomas and vascular malformations as an autosomal dominant trait. *Arch Dermatol* 1998;134:718-722.

12. Chang J, Most D, Bresnick S, et al: Proliferative hemangiomas: Analysis of cytokine gene expression and angiogenesis. *Plast Reconstr Surg* 1999;103:1-10.

13. Kleinman ME, Tepper OM, Capla JM: Increased circulating AC133+ CD34+ endothelial progenitor cells in children with hemangiomas. *Lymphat Res Biol* 2003;1:301-307.

14. Dorfman HD, Czerniak B: *Bone Tumors*. St. Louis, MO, Mosby, 1998, pp 729-761.

15. Glowacki J, Mulliken JB: Mast cells in hemangiomas and vascular malformations. *Pediatrics* 1982;70:48-51.

16. Tompkins VN, Walsh TS Jr : Some observations on the strawberry nevus of infancy. *Cancer* 1956;9:869-904.

17. Beham A, Fletcher CD: Intramuscular angioma: A clinicopathological analysis of 74 cases. *Histopathology* 1991;18:53-59.

18. Meis-Kindblom JM, Kindblom LG: Angiosarcoma of soft tissue: A study of 80 cases. *Am J Surg Pathol* 1998;22:683-697.

19. Bean WB: Blue rubber bleb nevi of the skin and gastrointestinal tract, in Bean WB (ed): *Vascular Spiders and Related Lesions of the Skin*. Springfield, IL, Charles C. Thomas, 1958, pp 17-185.

20. Fishman SJ, Smithers CJ, Folkman J, et al: Blue rubber bleb nevus syndrome: Surgical eradication of gastrointestinal bleeding. *Ann Surg* 2005;241:523-528.

21. Walshe MM, Evans CD, Warin RP: Blue rubber bleb naevus. *Br Med J* 1966;2:931-932.

22. Eichhorn JH, Rosenberg AE: Intravascular papillary endothelial hyperplasia involving the synovium. *Arch Pathol Lab Med* 1988;112:647-650.

23. Greenspan A, Azouz EM, Matthews J II, Décarie JC: Synovial hemangioma: Imaging features in eight histologically proven cases, review of the literature, and differential diagnosis. *Skeletal Radiol* 1995;24:583-590.

24. Price NJ, Cundy PJ: Synovial hemangioma of the knee. *J Pediatr Orthop* 1997;17:74-77.

25. Cohen AJ, Youkey JR, Clagett GP, Huggins M, Nadalo L, d'Avis JC: Intramuscular hemangioma. *JAMA* 1983;249:2680-2682.

26. Boyle WJ: Cystic angiomatosis of bone: A report of three cases and review of the literature. *J Bone Joint Surg Br* 1972;54:626-636.

27. Dorfman HD, Steiner GC, Jaffe HL: Vascular tumors of bone. *Hum Pathol* 1971;2:349-376.

28. Goidanich IF, Campanacci M: Vascular hamartoma and infantile angioectatic osteohyperplasia of the extremities. *J Bone Joint Surg Am* 1962;44:815-842.

29. Gutierrez RM, Spjut HJ: Skeletal angiomatosis: Report of three cases and review of the literature. *Clin Orthop Relat Res* 1972;85:82-97.

30. Karlin CA, Brower AC: Multiple primary hemangiomas of bone. *AJR Am J Roentgenol* 1977;129:162-164.

31. Kenan S, Abdelwahab IF, Klein MJ, Lewis MM: Hemangiomas of the long tubular bone. *Clin Orthop Relat Res* 1992;280:256-260.

32. Unni KK, Ivins JC, Beabout JW, Dahlin DC: Hemangioma, hemangiopericytoma and hemangioendothelioma (angiosarcoma) of bone. *Cancer* 1971;27:1403-1414.

33. Wenger DE, Wold LE: Benign vascular lesions of bone: Radiologic and pathologic features. *Skeletal Radiol* 2000;29:63-74.

34. Crone MD, Wallace RG: The radiographic features of familial expansile osteolysis. *Skeletal Radiol* 1990;19:245-250.

35. Lomasney LM, Martinez S, Demos TC, Harrelson JM: Multifocal vascular lesions of bone: Imaging characteristics. *Skeletal Radiol* 1996;25:255-261.

36. Reid AB, Reid IL, Johnson G, Hamonic M, Major P: Familial diffuse cystic angiomatosis of bone. *Clin Orthop Relat Res* 1989;238:211-218.

37. Ghormley RK, Adson AW: Hemangioma of vertebrae. *J Bone Joint Surg Am* 1941;23:887-895.

38. Laredo JD, Rezine D, Bard M, Merland JJ: Vertebral hemangiomas: Radiologic interpretation. *Radiology* 1986;161:183-189.

39. Abdullah DC, Hallisey MJ, Muraki AS, Schellinger DR: Diffuse calvarial hemangiomatosis associated with hereditary hemorrhagic telangiectasia. *AJNR Am J Neuroradiol* 1989;10:S59.

40. Khanam H, Lipper MH, Wolf CL, Lopes MB: Calvarial hemangiomas: Report of two cases and review of the literature. *Surg Neurol* 2001;55:63-67.

41. Devaney K, Vinh TN, Sweet DE: Skeletal-extraskeletal angiomatosis: A clinicopathological study of fourteen patients and nosologic considerations. *J Bone Joint Surg Am* 1994;76:878-891.

42. Devaney K, Vinh TN, Sweet DE: Surface-based hemangiomas of bone: A review of 11 cases.

Clin Orthop Relat Res 1994;300:233-240.

43. Ly JQ, Sanders TG, Mulloy JP: Osseous changes adjacent to soft-tissue hemangiomas of the extremities: Correlation with lesion size and proximity to bone. *AJR Am J Roentgenol* 2003;180:1695-1700.

44. Cannon SR: Massive osteolysis: A review of seven cases. *J Bone Joint Surg Br* 1986;68:24-28.

45. Ishida T, Dorfman HD, Steiner GC, Norman A: Cystic angiomatosis of bone with sclerotic changes mimicking osteoblastic metastases. *Skeletal Radiol* 1994;23:247-252.

46. Kasabach HH, Merritt KK: Capillary hemangioma with extensive purpura: Report of a case. *Am J Dis Child* 1940;59:1063-1070.

47. Aylett SE, Williams AF, Bevan DH, Holmes SJ: The Kasabach-Merritt syndrome: Treatment with intermittent pneumatic compression. *Arch Dis Child* 1990;65:790-791.

48. Mueller-Lessmann V, Behrendt A, Wetzel WE, Petersen K, Anders D: Orofacial findings in Klippel-Trénaunay syndrome. *Int J Paediatr Dent* 2001;11:225-229.

49. Wananukul S, Nuchprayoon I, Seksarn P: Treatment of Kasabach-Merritt syndrome: A stepwise regimen of prednisolone, dipyridamole, and interferon. *Int J Dermatol* 2003;42:741-748.

50. Rendu M: Epistaxis repetees chez un sujet porteur de petits angiomes cutanes et muqueux. *Bull Mem Soc Med Hop Paris* 1896;13:731-733.

51. Weber FP: A note on cutaneous telangiectasias and their aetiology: Comparison with the aetiology of haemorrhoids and ordinary varicose veins. *Edinburgh Med J* 1904:346-349.

52. Osler W: On multiple hereditary telangiectasias with recurring hemorrhages. *QJ Med* 1907;1:53-58.

53. Calvo-Alén J, Loza E, Alonso JL, Rodríguez-Valverde V: Pseudohaemarthrosis: A new manifestion of Osler-Rendu-Weber disease. *Ann Rheum Dis* 1992;51:1021.

54. Klippel M, Trénaunay P: Du naevus variqueux osteohypertrophique. *Arch Gen Med (Paris)* 1900;3:641-672.

55. Weber FP: Angioma: Formation in connection with hypertrophy of limbs and hemihypertrophy. *Br J Dermatol* 1907;19:231-235.

56. Jackson JBS: A boneless arm. *Boston Med Surg J* 1838;18:368-369.

57. Gorham LW, Stout AP: Massive osteolysis (acute spontaneous absorption of bone, phantom bone, disappearing bone): Its relation to hemangiomatosis. *J Bone Joint Surg Am* 1955;37:985-1004.

58. Möller G, Priemel M, Amling M, Werner M, Kuhlmey AS, Delling G: The Gorham-Stout syndrome (Gorham's massive osteolysis): A report of six cases with histopathological findings. *J Bone Joint Surg Br* 1999;81:501-506.

59. Maffucci A: Di un caso di enchondroma ed angioma multiplo: Contribuzione alla genesi embrionale dei tumori. *Mov Med Chir* 1881;3:399-412.

60. Davidson TI, Kissin MW, Bradish CF, Westbury G: Angiosarcoma arising in a patient with Maffucci syndrome. *Eur J Surg Oncol* 1985;11:381-384.

61. Shepherd V, Godbolt A, Casey T: Maffucci's syndrome with extensive gastrointestinal involvement. *Australas J Dermatol* 2005;46:33-37.

62. Sherman RS, Wilner D: The roentgen diagnosis of hemangioma of bone. *Am J Roentgenol Ther Nucl Med* 1961;86:1146-1159.

63. Buetow PC, Kransdorf MJ, Moser RP Jr, Jelinek JS, Berrey BH: Radiologic appearance of intramuscular hemangioma with emphasis on MR imaging. *AJR Am J Roentgenol* 1990;154:563-567.

64. Hawnaur JM, Whitehouse RW, Jenkins JP, Isherwood I: Musculoskeletal haemangionas: Comparison of MRI with CT. *Skeletal Radiol* 1990;19:251-258.

65. Rak KM, Yakes WF, Ray RL, et al: MR imaging of symptomatic peripheral vascular malformations. *AJR Am J Roentgenol* 1992;159:107-112.

66. Vilanova JC, Barceló J, Villalón M: MR and MR angiography characterization of soft tissue vascular malformations. *Curr Probl Diagn Radiol* 2004;33:161-170.

67. Hatayama K, Watanabe H, Ahmed AR, et al: Evaluation of hemangioma by positron emission tomography: Role in a multimodality approach. *J Comput Assist Tomogr* 2003;27:70-77.

68. Paltiel HJ, Burrows PE, Kozakewich HP, Zurakowski D, Mulliken JB: Soft tissue vascular anomalies: Utility of US for diagnosis. *Radiology* 2000;214:747-754.

69. Bandiera S, Gasbarrini A, De Iure F, Cappuccio M, Picci P, Boriani S: Symptomatic vertebral hemangioma: The treatment of 23 cases and a review of the literature. *Chir Organi Mov* 2002;87:1-15.

70. O'Connell JX, Kattapuram SV, Mankin HJ, Bhan AK, Rosenberg AE: Epithelioid hemangioma of bone: A tumor often mistaken for low-grade angiosarcoma or malignant hemangioendothelioma. *Am J Surg Pathol* 1993;17:610-617.

71. Bremnes RM, Hauge HN, Sagsveen R: Radiotherapy in the treatment of symptomatic vertebral hemangiomas: Technical case report. *Neurosurgery* 1996;39:1054-1058.

72. Tang P, Hornicek FJ, Gebhardt MC, Cates J, Mankin HJ: Surgical treatment of hemangiomas of soft tissue. *Clin Orthop Relat Res* 2002;399:205-210.

73. Akyüz C, Emir S, Büyükpamukçu M, et al: Successful treatment with interferon alfa in infiltrating angiolipoma: A case presenting with Kasabach-Merritt syndrome. *Arch Dis Child* 2003;88:67-68.

Chapter 10

Osteoid Osteoma and Osteoblastoma

Since the discovery of osteoid osteoma by Henry Jaffe[1] in 1935 and the subsequent separate reports on osteoblastoma by Henry Jaffe[2] and Louis Lichtenstein[3] in 1956, these two clinical entities have been described as closely related (doubtful), benign (although not always), and virtually identical in structure (probably not quite true). Osteoid osteoma, osteoblastoma, and osteosarcoma have been described as the only three bone-forming neoplasms, which is also not true because the statement ignores osteoma, ossifying fibroma, and fibrous dysplasia. Furthermore, despite having similar histologic structure, the clinical presentations for the osteoid osteoma and osteoblastoma are quite dissimilar and the imaging characteristics are distinctly different, and both are quite different from the standard osteosarcoma. The purpose of this chapter, then, is to describe these two somewhat mysterious entities and to try to more clearly define their distinctive clinical presentations, outcome, and, based on these data, the best form of treatment.

History and Biology

A signal article written by Henry Jaffe and Leo Mayer in 1932[4] first identified the two benign osteoblastic tumors. Both osteoid osteoma and osteoblastoma were included in their description, but because Jaffe's 1935 article defined the specific nature and characteristics of osteoid osteoma, he was responsible for providing the lesion with that name.[1] In 1956, Henry Jaffe[2] and Louis Lichtenstein[3] independently described the larger, somewhat more aggressive entity and named it a benign osteoblastoma. Over the next 2 decades, the entities were the subject of many descriptive articles.[5-16] It soon became apparent that there was yet another tumor, similar in structure to the benign form of osteoblastoma, which was histologically and clinically more malignant; this became known as the aggressive osteoblastoma.[13,17-25] Although the aggressive lesions grew more rapidly and were more locally destructive, metastasis was rare; indeed, when it did occur, the primary lesion was thought to be a low-grade osteosarcoma.[18-20,22,24-28] Although there have been many studies of patients with both forms of tumors over the years, no genetic abnormalities have been described for either entity.[17,18] In recent studies, the osteoid osteoma has been thought to contain large amounts of prostaglandin E_2 and prostacyclin.[18,29-32] The urinary excretion rate of 2,3-dinor-6-keto-$PGF_{1\alpha}$, the major metabolite of prostacycline, has been discovered to be increased in patients with osteoid osteoma; the values decline with removal of the tumor.[29,30] These changes have not been observed in osteoblastoma.

Gross Structural Characteristics

The osteoid osteoma is quite distinctive in gross structure. The lesion is virtually always small by definition and is less than 2 cm in its widest diameter.[6,17,18,24,33-36] The central area known as the "nidus" has virtually no bone and consists of tumor tissue, while the structure of the external bone surrounding the nidus is usually quite dense[17,18,24,36] (Figure 1). Occasionally the central lytic area has a zone of slightly increased bone density[18] so that the rounded osteoma lesion resembles a "rondelle," similar to the appearance of the symbol on the wings of British war planes (Figure 2). Rarely, more than one osteoid osteoma will appear in a single patient.[37,38]

The osteoblastoma is almost always considerably larger and is described as never being less than 4 cm in its largest diameter.[8,10,13,17,18,21,33,34,39,40] The lesions are more irregular in contour and the nidus is much larger and more irregular in structure. The bone surrounding it varies considerably from very dense osseous tissue to lytic areas with sometimes very thin and expanded cortices[17,18,24,40] (Figure 3). The structure is sometimes lace-like in character, and aneu-

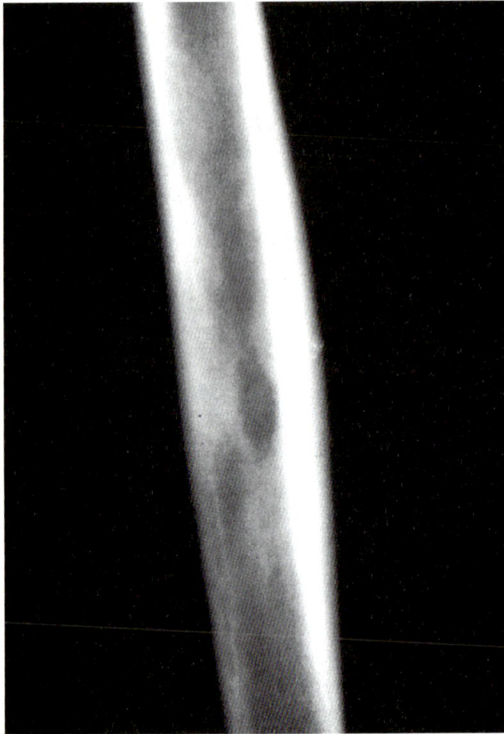

Figure 1
Radiograph of an osteoid osteoma of the humeral shaft. The lesion is small and lytic and there is a surrounding increase in bone density.

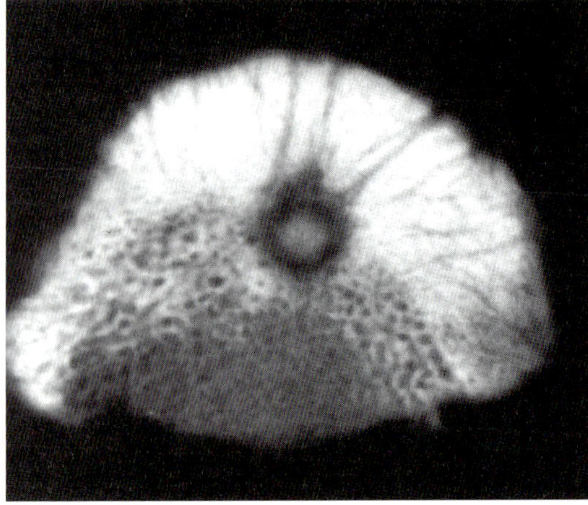

Figure 2
Radiograph of a resected osteoid osteoma specimen. Note the central nidus and the surrounding dense bone.

rysmal bone cysts are known to occur quite frequently in osteoblastoma but not ordinarily in osteoid osteomas.[21,24,29,40,41]

Histologic Characteristics

As indicated in the introduction to this chapter, one of the reasons for the confusion in nomenclature over the years since the two diseases were first discovered has been the remarkably similar histologic pattern.[8,17,18,24] In the osteoid osteoma, the histologic picture represents a process of bone remodeling with active osteoblastic activity producing osteoid and small, coarse-fibered irregular immature bone (Figure 4). Simultaneous osteoclastic bone resorption is occurring that results in a clearer area, known as the nidus, which is almost never greater than 1 cm in size.[8,18,24,34,35,39] Surrounding the nidus is a region of very active bone formation producing new osseous tissue, which is almost always dense on histologic study and positive on bone scan. In some cases, the bone formation is slightly more active in the central area of the nidus, producing a small region that is more dense than the major part of the nidus.[18,24]

The microscopic features of benign osteoblastoma are similar to those of osteoid osteoma but the lesions are generally much larger, usually more than 4 cm.[17,18,33,40] The nidus tissue consists of an interlacing network of tiny bone trabeculae, evenly distributed in a fibrous stroma with prominent vasculature. The osteoblasts and osteoclasts are present in large numbers. Mitotic activ-

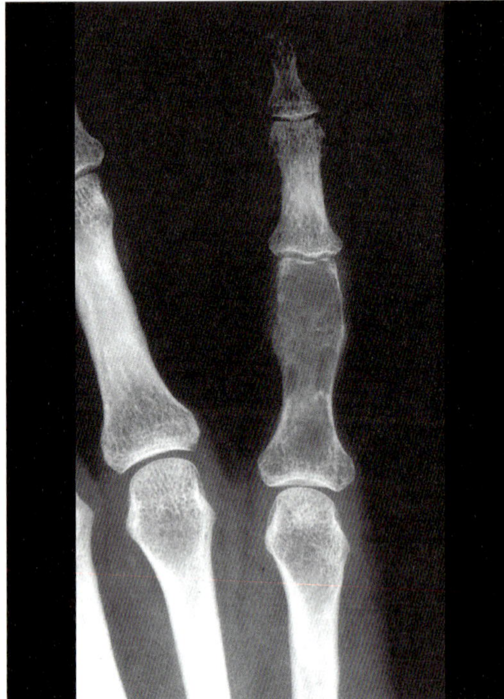

Figure 3
An osteoblastoma of the proximal phalanx of a digit showing a lytic area and modest bone expansion surrounding it.

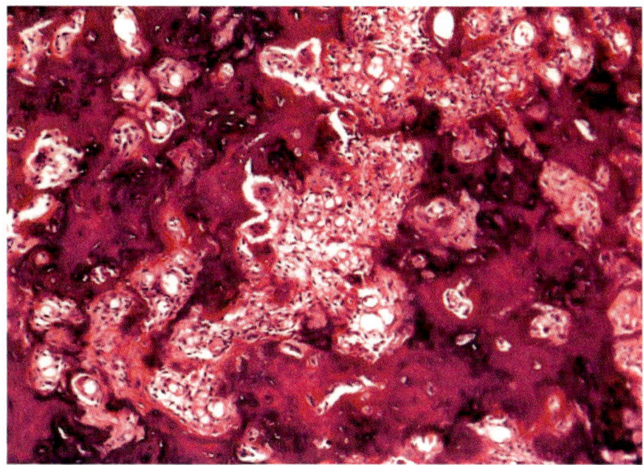

Figure 4
Histologic pattern for osteoid osteoma shows the central region of osteofibrous elements and a surrounding zone of dense bone. Note the presence of both osteoblasts and osteoclasts.

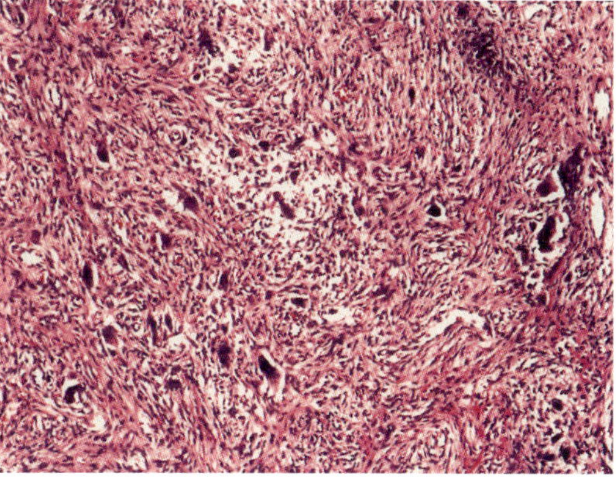

Figure 5
Histology for a low-grade osteoblastoma, showing a very active cellular structure with fibroblasts, some cellular atypism, and the presence of osteoclastic elements.

ity may be seen in the osteoblasts as well as the stromal cells, and bone formation is irregular[24,29,34,40] (Figure 5). The aggressive osteoblastomas have similar histologic findings, but in addition there are some cells known as epithelioid osteoblasts that rim the bony trabeculae and are more aggressive in appearance than the cells seen in osteoid osteoma or in benign osteoblastoma.[13,17-19,40] Despite these differences, the surrounding dense bony shell is similar to that seen in the other two lesions. The osteoid osteoma and both forms of osteoblastoma are different from the osteosarcoma, which presents with a high mitotic rate, cellular atypism, permeative growth into adjacent tissue, and presence of neoplastic cartilage.[17-19,24,34] In addition, the bony shell surrounding the lesion in patients with even the aggressive form of osteoblastoma does not support the diagnosis of osteosarcoma.

Clinical Presentation

Osteoid osteoma is a common tumor; estimates have suggested that it accounts for more than 10% of all bone neoplasms seen in the United States.[18] The most common skeletal sites are the femur and tibia, but the lesion may be present in the posterior elements of the spine,[42-45] upper extremity,[46-48] pelvis,[49-51] sacrum,[52] ribs,[53] and the hands and feet.[54-56] Tumors of the spine may result in scoliosis and occasionally nerve compression syndromes.[42,43,45] In the foot, the talus and calcaneus are commonly affected.[11,18,24] Most of the lesions are cortical

in location, although cancellous lesions may occur as well as tumors in the epiphyseal and subchondral regions, which can affect the joint and sometimes lead to osteoarthritis.[57-60] The average age of patients is in the 20s, with a range from approximately 5 to 50 years. Males are twice as often affected as females.[17,24,30] The striking feature related to this disorder is the pain pattern that exists for most of the patients with the tumors.[17,24,29,61,62] The pain is more frequent at night, associated with tenderness, and relieved by non-steroidal anti-inflammatory drugs (NSAIDs).[18,62] The finding of cyclooxygenase (COX)-1 and COX-2 in the nidus of the tumors supports the sensitivity of the pain to NSAIDs.[63] A 1970 study by Schulman and Dorfman[61] suggested that the cause of the pain was related to their finding of nerves within the tumor, but it seems equally likely that it is associated with the presence of prostaglandin E_2 and prostacyclin.[29-32] The tumors are not malignant, do not grow, and sometimes spontaneously disappear, especially in young children. Rarely, they are multiple in location.[38]

Osteoblastomas are much less common, accounting for approximately 1% of all primary tumors of bone.[17,18,24] Like the osteoid osteomas, they occur twice as frequently in males as in females, and the mean age for patients is approximately 20 years.[18,21,24,26,40] Approximately 40% of osteoblastomas occur in the spine, most often in the posterior elements, and can cause painful scoliosis.[21,24,40,42,43,45,52,64] The pain associated with osteoblastoma is less intense than in patients with osteoid osteoma and not worse at night.[18] If the lesion is superficial, it may cause localized swelling and tenderness.[17,18,24,65] Osteoblastomas may affect the maxilla and mandible, and even the calvarium.[9,24,40,66-69] The aggressive osteoblastoma is larger, has a more destructive effect on the surrounding bone, and is more painful.[18,23,24]

Imaging Studies

Osteoid osteomas located in the proximal femur or the femoral or tibial shafts all have a highly characteristic appearance on radiographs. The lesions are cortical or adjacent to the cortex, symmetric, and consist of a 1- to 2-cm central nidus surrounded by dense bone.[6,35,36,70] Occasionally there is an area of increased density within the nidus, which provides the rondelle appearance.[18,24] The lesions are virtually always very active on bone scan.[18,54,70] CT is sometimes more effective for definition, particularly when the lesions are located in the spine or in the epiphyseometaphyseal regions of the bone.[6,18,34,35,44,45,70,71] MRI may be difficult to interpret and is often not as useful as CT.[18,72]

The osteoblastoma is much more difficult to identify. The lesions are larger and less rounded and sometimes quite irregular in outline on radiography.[21,43,49,67,71] The bone around the margins is less dense, and if the lesion is near the cortex it may be thin and expanded.[17,18,40,73] The lesions of the spine and sacrum are more difficult and can best be seen on CT and sometimes MRI.[17,18,42,43,64,71] The lesions are often hypointense on T1 and may show structural distortion.[18,44,72]

The principal problem with osteoblastomas is distinguishing the aggressive lesions from osteosarcomas.[17-19,22,23,25-28,34] The aggressive lesions may have significant cortical thinning and erosion, and even occasionally relatively small soft-tissue extensions outside the bone.[18,23] Lesions of the spine can be very disruptive to normal structure.[18,21,40,43,64,71,74]

Treatment

With either of these lesions, it is essential to be as certain of the diagnosis as possible. Imaging studies are useful in this regard.

As far as the osteoid osteoma is concerned, there are some other possibilities, including osteomyelitis (specifically the sclerosing osteomyelitis of Garré), small ganglion cyst, and nonossifying fibroma.[14,18,33,34,36,47,54,58,70] For osteoblastoma, the differential diagnoses include osteomyelitis, aneurysmal bone cyst, giant cell tumor of bone, Hodgkin's lymphoma, low-grade osteosarcoma, or even metastatic bone disease.[3,17-19,26,34,40,65] Bone scan, CT, and MRI studies are useful for these lesions as well. A biopsy is particularly useful for osteoblastoma and is usually less necessary for osteoid osteoma.

Some patients with osteoid osteoma do not require treatment.[18,24,34,42] After several years, particularly with use of NSAIDs, the pain and in fact the lesion may disappear. However, most patients require some treatment, and in prior years the lesions were treated by surgical excision.[17,18,24,49,54,57,58] With the exception of the tumors in the spinal elements, these procedures were relatively simple and usually successful. In recent years, many patients with osteoid osteoma have been treated by percutaneous radiofrequency ablation, which appears to be successful with only a few complications reported.[47,75-79]

The management of osteoblastoma is a bit more complicated, particularly because the recurrence rate after curettage and packing with bone graft or cement is relatively high. Recurrences after surgery may suggest the possibility of a diagnosis of osteosarcoma and may require wide excision as the treatment of choice.[18,19,40,52,64,66,71,74,75] Radiation has been recommended for some of these lesions as well, particularly after recurrence.[18,80]

Conclusions

Osteoid osteoma and osteoblastoma are really quite different lesions that have some remarkably similar features. The age and gender distribution is identical and the histologic features are very similar. The benign nature for even the aggressive osteoblastoma is characteristic for both. However, osteoid osteoma is very small and does not enlarge or commonly recur. The pain pattern is highly characteristic, and the findings of prostaglandin E_2 and prostacyclin are quite distinctive from osteoblastoma. Furthermore osteoblastoma can be aggressive and behave in a sufficiently malignant fashion so as to be called a low-grade osteosarcoma. The recurrence rate is high, and the difficulties of treating lesions of the spine make this disorder much more complicated. So are osteoid osteoma and osteoblastoma "brothers"—one small and very benign, and the other larger and sometimes aggressive? They are certainly not "twins" in terms of size, structure, and outcome, but with respect to their histologic nature, they may be of similar "familial" origin. One thing that appears to be true is that the brothers, such as they are, may occasionally be confused with one another but are not directly related to their "malignant cousin," the osteosarcoma.

References

1. Jaffe HL: "Osteoid osteoma": A benign osteoblastic tumor composed of osteoid and atypical bone. *Arch Surg* 1935;31:709-728.

2. Jaffe HL: Benign osteoblastoma. *Bull Hosp Joint Dis* 1956;17:141-151.

3. Lichtenstein L: Benign osteoblastoma: A category of osteoid- and bone-forming tumor other than the classical osteoid osteoma, which may be mistaken for giant-cell tumor or osteogenic sarcoma. *Cancer* 1956;9:1044-1052.

4. Jaffe HL, Mayer L: An osteoblastic-osteoid tissue-forming tumor of a metacarpal bone. *Arch Surg* 1932;24:550-564.

5. Dahlin DC, Johnson EW Jr: Giant osteoid osteoma. *J Bone Joint Surg Am* 1954;36:559-572.

6. Freiberger RH, Lotman BS, Helpern M, Thompson TC: Osteoid osteoma: A report of 80 cases. *Am J Roentgenol Radium Ther Nucl Med* 1959;82:194-205.

7. Jaffe HL, Lichtenstein L: Osteoid-osteoma: Further experience with this benign tumor of bone with special reference to cases showing the lesion in relation to shaft cortices and commonly misclassified as instances of sclerosing nonsuppurative osteomyelitis of cortical bone abscess. *J Bone Joint Surg Am* 1940;22:645-682.

8. Jaffe HL: *Tumors and Tumorous Conditions of Bones and Joints*. Philadelphia, Lea and Febiger, 1958, pp 92-116.

9. Kent JN, Castro HF, Girotti WR: Benign osteoblastoma of the maxilla: Case report and review of the literature. *Oral Surg Oral Med Oral Pathol* 1969;27:209-219.

10. Lichtenstein L, Sawyer WF: Benign osteoblastoma: Further observations and report of twenty additional cases. *J Bone Joint Surg Am* 1964;46:755-765.

11. Marsh BW, Bonfiglio M, Brady LP, Enneking WF: Benign osteoblastoma: Range of manifestations. *J Bone Joint Surg Am* 1975;57:1-9.

12. Mayer L: Malignant degeneration of so-called benign osteoblastoma. *Bull Hosp Joint Dis* 1967;28:4-13.

13. McLeod RA, Dahlin DC, Beabout JW: The spectrum of osteoblastoma. *AJR Am J Roentgenol* 1976;126:321-335.

14. Norman A, Dorfman HD: Osteoid osteoma inducing pronounced overgrowth and deformity of bone. *Clin Orthop Relat Res* 1975;110:233-238.

15. Ponseti I, Barta CK: Osteoid osteoma. *J Bone Joint Surg Am* 1947;29:767-776.

16. Tonai M, Campbell CJ, Ahn GH, Schiller AL, Mankin HJ: Osteoblastoma: Classification and report of 16 patients. *Clin Orthop Relat Res* 1982;167:222-235.

17. Campanacci M: *Bone and Soft Tissue Tumors*, ed 2. New York, NY, Springer Verlag, 1999, pp 391-433.

18. Dorfman HD, Czerniak B: *Bone Tumors*. St Louis, MO, Mosby, 1998, pp 85-128.

19. Dorfman HD, Weiss SW: Borderline osteoblastic tumors: Problems in the differential diagnosis of aggressive osteoblastoma and low-grade osteosarcoma. *Semin Diagn Pathol* 1984;1:215-234.

20. Kenan S, Floman Y, Robin GC, Laufer A: Aggressive osteoblastoma: A case report and review of the literature. *Clin Orthop Relat Res* 1985;195:294-298.

21. Kroon HM, Schurmans J: Osteoblastoma: Clinical and radiological findings in 98 new cases. *Radiology* 1990;175:783-790.

22. Merryweather R, Middelmiss JH, Sanerkin NG: Malignant transformation of osteoblastoma. *J Bone Joint Surg Br* 1980;62:381-384.

23. Revell PA, Scholtz CI: Aggressive osteoblastoma. *J Pathol* 1979;127:195-198.

24. Schajowicz F: *Tumors and Tumorlike Lesions of Bone and Joints*. New York, NY, Springer Verlag, 1981, pp 25-64.

25. Schajowicz F, Lemos C: Malignant osteoblastoma. *J Bone Joint Surg Br* 1976;58:202-211.

26. Bertoni F, Unni KK, McLeod RA, Dahlin DC: Osteosarcoma resembling osteoblastoma. *Cancer* 1985;55:416-426.

27. Bonar F, McCarthy S, Stalley P, et al: Epiphyseal osteoblastoma-like osteosarcoma. *Skeletal Radiol* 2004;33:46-50.

28. Hermann G, Klein MJ, Springfield D, Abdelwahab IF: Osteoblastoma like osteosarcoma. *Clin Radiol* 2004;59:105-108.

29. Ciabattoni G, Tamburrelli F, Greco F: Increased prostacyline biosynthesis in patients with osteoid osteoma. *Eicosanoids* 1991;4:165-167.

30. Greco F, Tamburrelli F, Ciabattoni G: Prostaglandins in osteoid osteoma. *Int Orthop* 1991;15:35-37.

31. Wold LE, Pritchard DJ, Bergen J, Wilson DM: Prostaglandin synthesis by osteoid osteoma and osteoblastoma. *Mod Pathol* 1988;1:129-131.

32. Yamamura S, Sato K, Sugiura H, et al: Prostaglandin levels of primary bone tumor tissues correlate with peritumoral edema demonstrated by magnet resonance imaging. *Cancer* 1997;79:255-261.

33. Frassica FJ, Waltrip RL, Sponseller PD, Ma LD, McCarthy EF Jr: Clinicopathologic features and treatment of osteoid osteoma and osteoblas-

toma in children and adolescents. *Orthop Clin North Am* 1996;27:559-574.

34. Greenspan A: Benign bone-forming lesions: Osteoma, osteoid osteoma and osteoblastoma: Clinical, imaging, pathologic and differential considerations. *Skeletal Radiol* 1993;22:485-500.

35. Klein MH, Shankman S: Osteoid osteoma: Radiologic and pathologic correlation. *Skeletal Radiol* 1992;21:23-31.

36. Sim FH, Dahlin CD, Beabout JW: Osteoidosteoma: Diagnostic problems. *J Bone Joint Surg Am* 1975;57:154-159.

37. Matera D, Campanacci DA, Caldora P, Mazza E, Capanna R: Osteoid osteoma of the femur with a double nidus: A case report. *Chir Organi Mov* 2005;90:75-79.

38. Zmurko MG, Mott MP, Lucas DR, Hamre MR, Miller PR: Multicentric osteoid osteoma. *Orthopedics* 2004;27:1294-1296.

39. Gitelis S, Schajowicz F: Osteoid osteoma and osteoblastoma. *Orthop Clin North Am* 1989;20:313-325.

40. Lucas DR, Unni K, McLeod RA, O'Connor MI, Sim FH: Osteoblastoma: Clinicopathologic study of 306 cases. *Hum Pathol* 1994;25:117-134.

41. Wang YC, Huang JS, Wu CJ, et al: A huge osteoblastoma with aneurysmal bone cyst of the skull base. *Clin Imaging* 2001;25:247-250.

42. Azouz EM, Kozlowski K, Marton D, et al: Osteoid osteoma and osteoblastoma of the spine in children: Report of 22 cases with brief literature review. *Pediatr Radiol* 1986;16:25-31.

43. Bruneau M, Cornelius JF, George B: Osteoid osteomas and osteoblastomas of the occipitocervical junction. *Spine* 2005;30:E567-E571.

44. Harish S, Saifuddin A: Imaging features of spinal osteoid osteoma with emphasis on MRI findings. *Eur Radiol* 2005;15:2396-2403.

45. Ozaki T, Liljenqvist U, Hillmann A: Osteoid osteoma and osteoblastoma of the spine: Experiences with 22 patients. *Clin Orthop Relat Res* 2002;397:394-402.

46. Ruggieri P, Biagini R, Ferraro A: Osteoid osteoma of the elbow: A study of twelve cases. *Ital J Orthop Traumatol* 1989;15:154-163.

47. Soong M, Jupiter J, Rosenthal D: Radiofrequency ablation of osteoid osteoma of the upper extremity. *J Hand Surg [Am]* 2006;31:279-283.

48. Themistocleous GS, Chloros GD, Benetos IS, et al: Osteoid osteoma of the upper extremity: A diagnostic challenge. *Chir Main* 2006;25:69-76.

49. Bettelli G, Capanna R, van Horn JR, et al: Osteoid osteoma and osteoblastoma of the pelvis. *Clin Orthop Relat Res* 1989;247:261-271.

50. Gille P, Gross P, Brax P, et al: Osteoid osteoma of the acetabulum: Two cases. *J Pediatr Orthop* 1990;10:416-418.

51. Weits T, van der Werf GJ: Subperiosteal osteoid osteoma of the right acetabulum. *JBR-BTR* 2006;89:162-163.

52. Biagini R, Orsini U, Demitri S, et al: Osteoid osteoma and osteoblastoma of the sacrum. *Orthopedics* 2001;24:1061-1064.

53. McGuire MH, Mankin HJ: Osteoid osteoma: An unusual presentation as a rib lesion. *Orthopaedics* 1984;7:305-307

54. Burger IM, McCarthy EF: Phalangeal osteoid osteomas of the hand: A diagnostic problem. *Clin Orthop Relat Res* 2004;427:198-203.

55. Laffosse JM, Trcoire JL, Catagrel A, Wagner A, Puget J: Osteoid osteoma of the carpal bones: Two case reports. *Joint Bone Spine* 2006;73:560-563.

56. Lee GK, Kang IW, Lee ES, et al: Osteoid osteoma of the tarsal cuboid mimicking osteomyelitis. *AJR Am J Roentgenol* 2004;183:341-342.

57. Banerjee D, Eriksson K, Morris H: Arthroscopically treated intraarticular osteoid osteoma of the ankle: A report of three cases. *Acta Orthop* 2005;76:721-724.

58. Bauer TW, Zehr JR, Belhobek GH, Marks KE: Juxta-articular osteoid osteoma. *Am J Surg Pathol* 1991;15:381-387.

59. Kattapuram SV, Kushner DC, Phillips WC, Rosenthal DI: Osteoid osteoma: An unusual cause of articular pain. *Radiology* 1983;147:383-387.

60. Koos Z, Than P: Rare localization of osteoid osteoma in the patella. *Pediatr Radiol* 2005;35:929-930.

61. Schulman L, Dorfman HD: Nerve fibers in osteoid osteoma. *J Bone Joint Surg Am* 1970;52:1351-1356.

62. Sherman MS, McFarland G: Mechanism of pain in osteoid osteomas. *South Med J* 1965;58:163-166.

63. Mungo DV, Zhang X, O'Keefe RJ, et al: COX-1 and COX-2 expression in osteoid osteomas. *J Orthop Res* 2002;20:159-162.

64. Nemoto O, Moser RP Jr, Van Dam E, Aoki J, Gilkey FW: Osteoblastoma of the spine: A review of 75 cases. *Spine* 1990;15:1272-1280.

65. Van Giffen N, De Smet L: Osteoblastoma of the proximal ulna, an unusual cause of ulnar wrist pain: A case report. *Acta Orthop Belg* 2005;71:736-739.

66. Capodiferro S, Maiorano E, Giardina C, et al: Osteoblastoma of the mandible: Clinicopathologic study of four cases and a literature review. *Head Neck* 2005;27:616-621.

67. Jones AC, Prihoda TJ, Kacher JE, Odingo NA, Freedman PD: Osteoblastoma of the maxilla and mandible: A report of 24 cases, review of the literature, and discussion of its relationship to osteoid osteoma of the jaws. *Oral Surg Oral Med Oral Pathol Oral Radiol Endod* 2006;102:639-650.

68. Moon KS, Jung S, Lee JH, et al: Benign osteoblastoma of the occipital bone: Case report and literature review. *Neuropathology* 2006;26:141-146.

69. William RN, Boop WC Jr: Benign osteoblastoma of the skull: Case report. *J Neurosurg* 1974;41:769-772.

70. Bilchik T, Hayman S, Siegel A, Alavi A: Osteoid osteoma: The role of radionuclide bone imaging, conventional radiography and computed tomography in its management. *J Nucl Med* 1992;33:269-271.

71. Boriani S, Capanna R, Donati D, et al: Osteoblastoma of the spine. *Clin Orthop Relat Res* 1992;278:37-45.

72. Hosalkar HS, Garg S, Moroz L, Pollack A, Dormans JP: The diagnostic accuracy of MRI versus CT imaging for osteoid osteoma in children. *Clin Orthop Relat Res* 2005;433:171-177.

73. Nakatani T, Yamamoto T, Akisue T, et al: Periosteal osteoblastoma of the distal femur. *Skeletal Radiol* 2004;33:107-111.

74. Bruneau M, Polivka M, Cornelius JF, George B: Progression of an osteoid osteoma to an osteoblastoma: Case report. *J Neurosurg Spine* 2005;3:238-241.

75. Finstein JL, Hosalkar HS, Ogilvie CM, Lackman RD: Case reports: An unusual complication of radiofrequency ablation treatment of osteoid osteoma. *Clin Orthop Relat Res* 2006;448:248-251.

76. Rosenthal DI, Alexander A, Rosenberg AE, Springfield D: Ablation of osteoid osteoma with percutaneously placed electrode: A new procedure. *Radiology* 1992;183:29-33.

77. Rosenthal DI, Hornicek FJ, Toriani M, Gebhardt MC, Mankin HJ: Osteoid osteoma: Percutaneous treatment with radiofrequency energy. *Radiology* 2003;229:171-175.

78. Rosenthal DI: Radiofrequency treatment. *Orthop Clin North Am* 2006;37:475-484.

79. Simon CJ, Dupuy DE: Percutaneous minimally invasive therapies in the treatment of bone tumors: Thermal ablation. *Semin Musculoskelet Radiol* 2006;10:137-144.

80. Rajkumar A, Basu R, Datta NR, Dhingra S, Gupta RK: Radiation therapy for sacral osteoblastoma. *Clin Oncol (R Coll Radiol)* 2003;15:85-86.

Chapter 11

Benign Tumors of Cartilage

Benign tumors that contain cartilage are relatively common and affect many people of all ages. Although there are some rare tumors such as chondroblastoma, chondromyxoid fibroma, juxtacortical chondroma, and synovial chondromatosis, the most frequently encountered are the enchondroma and the osteocartilaginous exostosis, followed by hereditary multiple osteocartilaginous exostoses, and the two forms of enchondromatosis—Ollier's disease and Maffucci's syndrome. All of these tumors are defined as benign, but some have the potential for local destruction of bone, recurrence after surgical excision, and even true malignancy with metastasis and death. Of almost equal concern is the fact that the lesions may behave in an aggressive fashion and histologically resemble chondrosarcoma, so that they are sometimes overtreated. This chapter will define and review information about the most common of the tumors, the solitary and multiple osteocartilaginous exostoses and enchondromas.

Exostotic Lesions
Nomenclature and History
Benign exostotic cartilage tumors have been described as osteochondromatosis, exostosis multiplex cartilaginea, osteogenic multiple exostosis, chondral osteogenic dysplasia, chondral osteoma, dyschondroplasia, exostotic dysplasia, diaphyseal aclasis, osteocartilaginous exostoses, osteochondrodystrophy, or hereditary multiple osteocartilaginous exostoses.[1-13]

Although Boyer[14] provided a brief description of the multiple form of the exostotic disease in 1814, it was Sir Astley Cooper[15] who first described the disorder in some detail, in a chapter in his book published in 1818. Friedrich von Recklinghausen[16] described a case in 1866, and Gibney[17] described four cases in 1876, introducing the name hereditary multiple exostosis for the multisite form of the disease. Bessel-Hagen[18] described the relationship of the osteocartilaginous masses to the structure of bone in 1891 and proposed that the

disease arose from an abnormality in epiphyseal cartilage. This view was contested in 1895 by Rudolf Virchow,[19] who related the exostotic lesions to the cartilaginous joint structure. Although Louis Ollier later described enchondromatosis, his interest in cartilage-containing tumors was first noted in an article published in 1898 on exostotic lesions.[10] In an article in the *Journal of the American Medical Association* in 1915, Ehrenfried[4] clearly described the entity and declared it to be hereditary. In 1919, Sir Arthur Keith[20] proposed that the origin of the lesion is a defect in the periosteal ring on the growth plate and named the disease diaphyseal aclasis. In his 1930 article in the *Annals of Surgery*, Rixford[21] defined the nature of the multiple osteocartilaginous tumors and described their common anatomic sites. Several other investigators attempted to relate the disorder to abnormalities of the bone or epiphyseal plate, including Jansen,[22] Hume,[23] and Geschickter and Copeland.[7] Henry Jaffe,[8] Harsha,[24] Fairbank,[5] and Langenskiöld[25] proposed several possible methods of development for the exostotic cartilage lesions, an issue that, despite fairly extensive research in both humans and animals,[26,27] remains somewhat mysterious to this day.

Solitary Osteocartilaginous Exostosis
Incidence, Age, and Sex Distribution
The solitary form of osteocartilaginous exostosis is believed to be the most common benign bone lesion, accounting for 10% to 15% of all primary skeletal tumors.[1,3,11,13,27-30] The lesion is usually discovered in childhood or adolescence as a mass physically evident in the region adjacent to a joint, or identified as an incidental finding during radiographic evaluation.[1,3,9,11,31] Most authors believe that the lesions are more frequent in males than in females.[1,3,11,13,31] The masses are located in the metaphyseal regions of the distal femur or proximal tibia (together accounting for approximately half of the solitary lesions), proximal humerus, distal

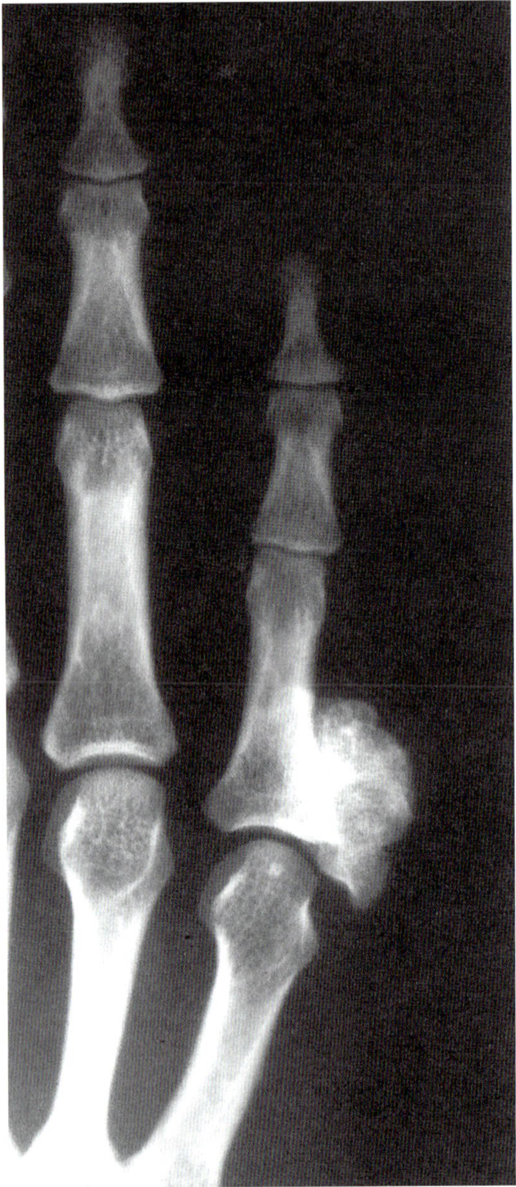

Figure 1

A solitary osteocartilaginous exostosis arising from the fifth digit of the hand.

radius, distal tibia, and both ends of the fibula.[1,3,13] In this regard, they seem to obey Phemister's law, which suggests that tumors and infection occur in the fastest growing end of the longest bone in the body and go downhill from there. Tumors in the pelvis, scapula, spine, skull, and digits are less common.[1,3,13]

Pathogenesis

As indicated in the discussion regarding history of these lesions, the pathologic causes of both the solitary and multiple forms have been and continue to be somewhat mysteri-ous. The lesion occurs near the epiphyseal growth plate and is, at least in part, cartilag-inous; thus it is believed to arise from some form of error in growth plate structure that allows cartilage cells to escape and develop their own bone growth system adjacent to the cortex.[1,3,9,24,28,32] The fact that the le-sions share a cortex, rather than developing adjacent to one, supports this concept. The bone that is produced by the cartilaginous "cap" is normal in structure, but clearly has no real relationship to the normal functional bone site, nor does it obey Wolff's law.[1,3] One possible explanation is the develop-ment of an anomalous metaphyseal-diaphyseal blood vessel, which then contin-ues to grow cartilage and bone.[1,3,13,29,31]

Clinical Findings

The solitary lesions themselves are almost al-ways asymptomatic unless fracture has oc-curred.[1,3] The complaints expressed by pa-tients with the lesions are more related to limitation of movement, pressure on adja-cent structures, bursa formation, nerve compression (usually of the popliteal, me-dian, or ulnar nerve), or vascular com-pression with pseudoaneurysm forma-tion.[1,3,13,33-36] Enlarging lesions of the spine may cause neural abnormalities or even paralysis,[37-39] and those arising from the fa-cial or skull bones ("ivory exostoses") can cause deformities of the face or cranial nerve injuries.[7] Lesions of the digits, espe-cially the great toe ("subungual exostosis"), may erode the skin and present as ulcerous lesions overlying the tumorous bone and cartilage.[3,40]

Imaging and Histology

Imaging studies of osteocartilaginous exos-toses demonstrate that the bone formed is normal in appearance and the cortical struc-ture arises from the underlying normal bone[1,3,9,13,24,28,31] (Figure 1). The cortex is "shared" with the normal bone and may ac-tually produce some deformation in the structure of the bone. The cartilage cap is sometimes quite large, particularly in young patients, as seen in gross specimens or CT or MRI studies. With advancing age, the carti-lage may show calcification and irregular os-sification of the underlying bone[1,3,31] (Fig-ure 2).

The histologic appearance of the cartilage cap shows an abnormal structural configura-

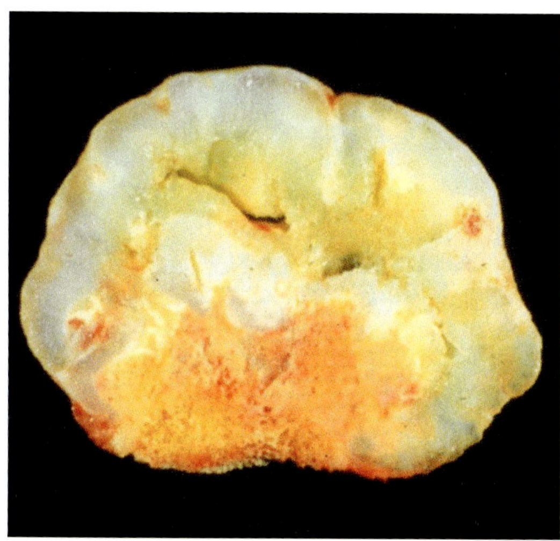

Figure 2
Cut section of an osteocartilaginous mass, disclosing the underlying bone and the cartilage cap, which is similar in structure to the epiphyseal plate.

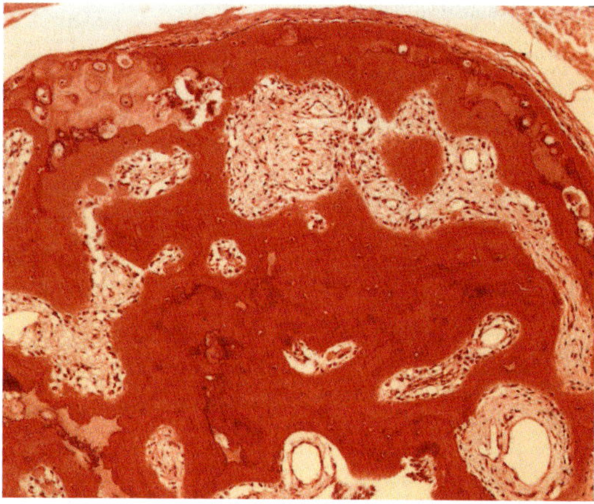

Figure 3
Histology of an osteocartilaginous exostosis, showing the cartilage adjacent to the bone. The cartilage appears benign and the bony segments are well structured.

tion similar to that seen in the epiphyseal plate in young children.[1,3] The chondrocytes are not arranged in an orderly linear fashion, however, and show some atypism and occasionally double nuclei. The bone structure is characteristically woven bone initially. This converts to mature medullary bone, but with distorted and atypical structure (Figure 3). As indicated in the imaging studies, the surrounding bone is cortical and joins to the cortex of the bone of origin.[1,3,13,31] With advancing age, the cartilage matures and calcifies, often with focal collections of heavily calcified cartilage resembling "popcorn balls."[1] Of interest is the occasional finding of an osteocartilaginous exostosis at the site of radiation, particularly in a child.[41]

Chondrosarcoma has been reported to arise in solitary lesions, but the frequency is very low (probably less than 1% to 2%).[1,3,9,13,42-46] The tumors are relatively benign; metastases or patient death are very unusual, except for those tumors that arise in relation to lesions of the pelvis.

Hereditary Multiple Osteocartilaginous Exostoses (HMOCE)

Incidence, Age, and Sex Distribution
By standards of other genetic bone disorders, HMOCE are quite common and believed to occur in approximately 1 in 20,000 children.[3,11-13,28,29,31] The disease appears to result from an autosomal dominant genetic disorder with frequent mutations.[3,47,48] HMOCE occur with equal frequency in males and females, and only one parent with the disease is required for the disorder to appear in progeny.[3,27,47] HMOCE appear to occur with greater frequency in Caucasians and some western hemisphere Indian tribes.[1,3,11,29] The disease is sometimes subtle; although present in children at birth, it usually does not become evident until after age 2 years. Approximately 80% of patients have quite evident disease by 10 years of age, but some are never aware of the disorder until it is accidentally discovered in a routine radiology study.[1,3,11] The anatomic distribution of the lesions includes the same sites as described for the solitary lesions. Because the lesions are located in multiple sites, they sometimes produce significant deformity and even disability related to limited use of the extremities or facial, cranial, or spinal nerve or vessel impingement. Short stature, limb-length discrepancies, valgus deformities of the knees and ankles, pelvic girdle asymmetry, bowing of the radius, ulnar deviation of the wrist, and subluxation of the radial head are common occurrences in children with extensive disease.[1,3,8,9,11,13,24,29,31-35,37,38,40,49-51] The hand is involved in more than 30% of patients and, although not symptomatic, may limit the patient's capacity to write or use a computer.[3,40]

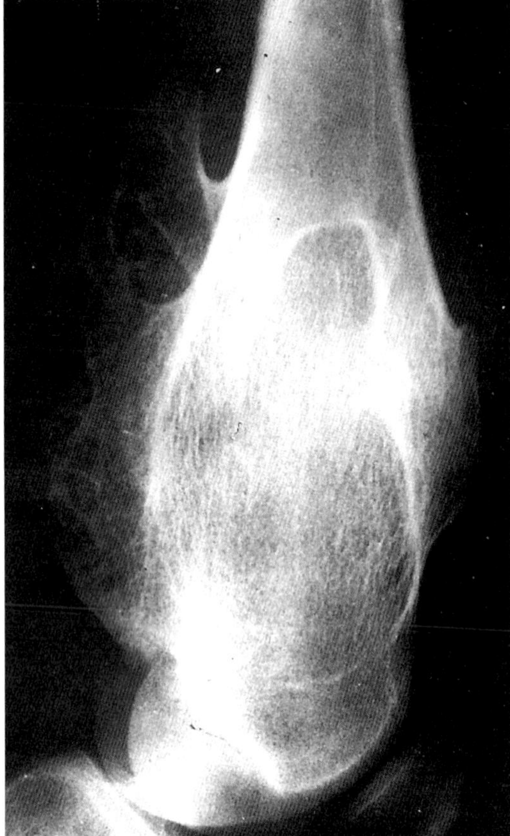

Figure 4
HMOCE arising from the distal femur and distorting the shape of the bone.

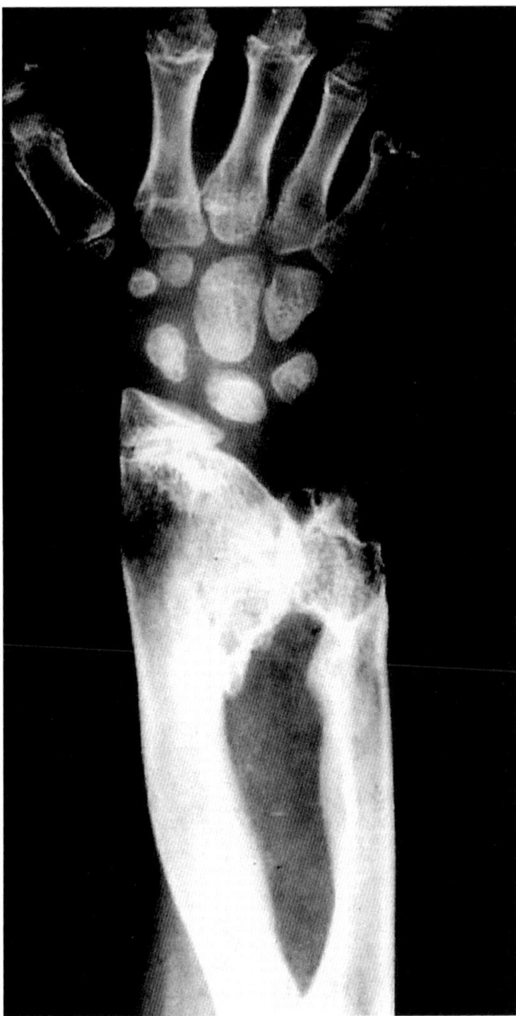

Figure 5
Marked disorganization of the distal radius and ulna in a patient with HMOCE.

Pathogenesis

HMOCE are clearly a genetic disorder, which appears to be associated with mutations in three separate genes called EXT genes.[3,47,48,52,53] Changes in EXT1 and EXT2 genes are most frequent. The EXT1 loci have recently been mapped in chromosomal regions 8q23-q24; EXT2 is on 11p11-p12; and EXT3, which has not been fully characterized and is infrequently noted, is on chromosome arm 19.[52-55] As reported in 2004 by Porter and associates,[45] patients with an EXT1 error appear to have more extensive disease and a higher risk for chondrosarcoma and breast cancer. The EXT genes are also known as tumor suppressors, and some of the EXT-like genes may play a role in the development of breast tumors and other forms of cancer. HMOCE have also been associated with several other disorders, such as the Langer-Giedion, trichorhinophalangeal and DEFECT 11 syndromes, all three of which have additional genetic errors along with EXT gene deletion from the 11p11-p12 chromosome.[3,29,53] Of some concern is the number of patients with the disorder who are relatively asymptomatic and have no knowledge of the presence of the disease. This makes them highly likely to transmit the disorder to their progeny.

Imaging and histologic characteristics for the individual lesions in HMOCE do not differ from the solitary osteochondroma described above. There are, however, considerably greater deformities noted in various body parts but especially the forearms, hands, elbows, knee regions, fibulae, and ankles[1,3,8,9,13,29,33-35,37,38,40,49-51,56,57] (Figures 4 and 5). Several of the features that are virtually diagnostic for HMOCE include enlargement and "sausage shape" of both pu-

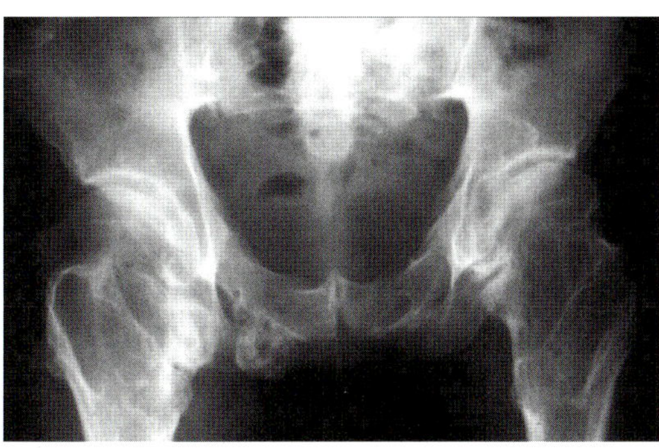

Figure 6
Changes in the pelvic structure and the proximal femora in a patient with HMOCE.

bic rami and oblique tibiotalar joints [1,3](Figure 6).

Malignant degeneration is much more frequent in HMOCE than in the solitary form of the disease and can occur in 5% or more of the patients. Usually this occurs in adults; is more frequent in proximally placed lesions; and is associated with an increase in the size of the mass, increased pain, and limitation.[1,3,9,42-44,58-60] Cartilage caps of large size in adults should be viewed with some suspicion and followed closely,[1,3,9] and one should be concerned if a lesion recurs after surgery.[61] The outcome for patients with exostotic chondrosarcoma is considerably better than that for patients with enostotic lesions.

Enostotic Lesions
Nomenclature and History
Solitary enchondromas and multiple enchondromas (such as occur in patients with Ollier's disease or Maffucci's syndrome) have over the years been labeled with many different terms. These include achondromatosis, chondrodysplasia, chondrodystrophy, dyschondroplasia, multiple enchondromatosis, hemichondrodystrophy, internal chondromatosis, enchondromatosis with hemangiomatosis, and Kast's disease.[1,3,6,7,62-70]

Solitary enchondromas were not recognized early in the history of medicine based on the fact that most of these lesions appear in adults and rarely caused symptoms or deformity. In the days before imaging, only fractures or the occasional case of chondrosarcoma called the attention of the physician to the bony lesion. Jones[71] reported removing a scapula for an enchondroma in 1868, and in 1925 LeConte and associates[72] re-

ported a case of an enchondroma of the femur that recurred and ultimately became a chondrosarcoma. Emanuel Freund[73] described cartilaginous tumors of the skeleton in 1936, and in 1947 Coley and Santoro[2] listed the characteristics of benign solitary intraosseous lesions and indicated that treatment was rarely required. In their 1936 book, Geschickter and Copeland[7] described primary solitary cartilaginous lesions, and Jaffe,[9] in his textbook on bone and joint tumors published in 1958, defined the radiographic, gross, and histologic characteristics of solitary benign enchondromas of bone.

The multiple tumors have a much earlier historical background based on the grossly abnormal bones that cause the patient's deformities and disabilities. The first description of multiple chondromatous lesions along with hemangiomatous tumors was in 1881 by Angelo Maffucci,[74] an Italian pathologist. Alfred Kast and Friedrich von Recklinghausen[67] clearly described a patient with multiple enchondromas but no vascular abnormalities in 1889; shortly thereafter, in 1900, Louis Ollier published his remarkable description of that entity.[75,76] The disease was originally known as Kast syndrome and then as Kast-Ollier's disease, but then became Ollier's disease.[65] Subsequent references to these entities include that of Jemma in 1929,[77] Fairbank in 1948,[65] and Strang and Rannie in 1950,[69] all of whom defined the multiple nature of the cartilaginous lesions and their appearance on radiographs. In 1965, Cowan[78] described malignant change in the lesions, particularly those in the pelvis and proximal femur. In 1976, Schnall and Genuth[79] described patients with Maffucci's syndrome who had multiple endocrine abnormalities. Numerous other investigators reported on this syndrome that, although rare, may be very damaging. The most remarkable publication on Maffucci's syndrome is that of Lewis and Ketcham[80] in *The Journal of Bone and Joint Surgery* in 1973; this article not only provided data on a patient with severe changes, but listed 87 references to various aspects of the disease. Contributory comments on the presentation, radiographic appearance, complications, and chondrosarcoma development in patients with Maffucci's syndrome were introduced by early reports by Carleton and associates in 1942,[64] Umansky in 1946,[70] Coppens in

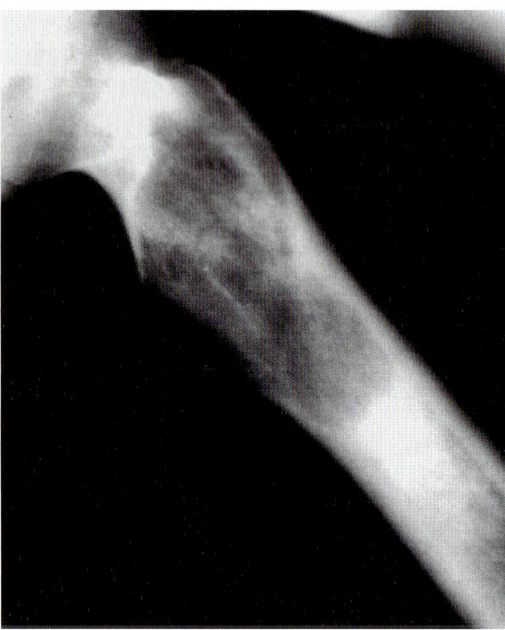

Figure 7
An enchondroma of the proximal femur. The lesion is solitary but has expanded the bone.

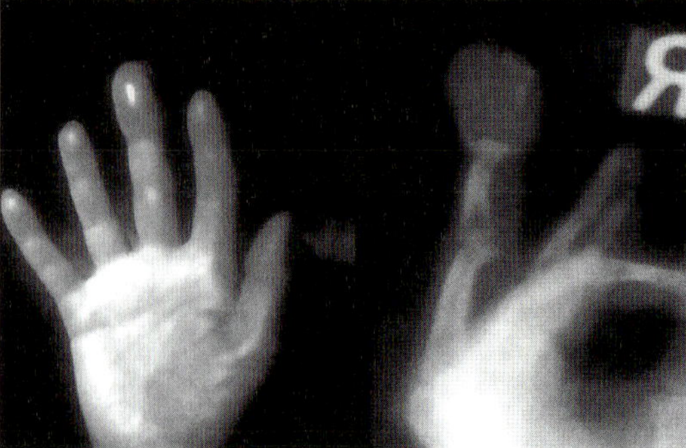

Figure 8
A solitary enchondroma of the terminal phalanx of the finger as seen clinically (left) and on a radiograph.

1947,[81] Langenskiöld in 1947,[68] Zellweger and Uhlinger in 1948,[82] Bean in 1958,[62] and Anderson in 1965.[83]

Solitary Enchondroma of Bone
Incidence, Age, and Sex Distribution
Solitary enchondromas are common disorders, occurring as frequently as in 2% of the population and accounting for up to 20% of all bone tumors. The lesions are equally present in males and females, and they generally are not discovered before the late teens or early adulthood.[1-3,9,28] Some patients are never aware of the presence of the tumor until late in life, when discovered as an incidental finding on radiographs. Painless swelling is the most common presentation, particularly for lesions of the hand or, less frequently, the foot; the hand and foot together account for more than 30% of the lesions.[84,85] The lesions are most often metaphyseal in location, but can be located in the diaphysis or even the epiphysis in young children.[1,3,9,28]

Pathogenesis
Enchondromas occur in bones; they arise from cartilage and presumably represent an error in the normal chondromatous development of mature medullary and cortical bone that occurs in the growing fetus or in in-

fancy.[1,3] The nature of the error is not clear, as there is very limited evidence to support the possibility that this disease is genetically related to multiple enchondromatous disorders such as Ollier's disease or Maffucci's syndrome. All histologic evidence strongly suggests that the origin of the disorder is related to a chondromatous focus inside the bone that does not undergo endochondral ossification, possibly as a result of injury in utero.[28]

Clinical Findings
Aside from the hands and feet, the lesions of the long bones are mostly in the femur (approximately 17% of the total) and humerus (7%), and less commonly in the pelvis, ribs, scapulae, and vertebrae.[1,3,28] Craniofacial bones are usually spared. Patients with a solitary enchondroma are most often asymptomatic and only note the abnormality when a fracture occurs or when palpation of a digit, the femur, or the humerus discloses a painless enlargement of the bone (Figure 7). Occasionally, with very large lesions that have undergone alterations in structure, a limb may be slightly deformed or vary in appearance from the opposite side.[1,3,28]

Radiographic findings usually show a symmetric mild expansion of the bone, with slight to moderate internal scalloping of the cortex[1,3,9,13,85] (Figure 8). With larger lesions, particularly those in the femur or humerus, calcification or ossification may be present in the central cartilaginous portion. Calcification is irregular, punctate, or stippled, and has been described as appearing like popcorn balls.[3] These sites may be

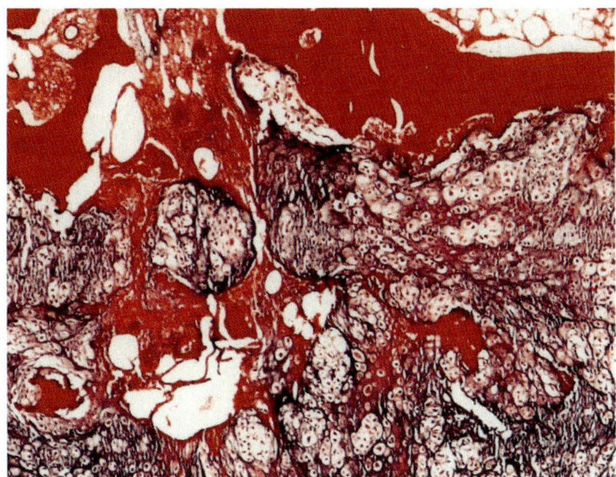

Figure 9

Histologic study of a solitary enchondroma, showing the presence of modestly atypical cartilage and adjacent bone production.

more easily detected with CT. MRI usually shows the lesion to have a low intensity signal on T1 and a high intensity on T2.[1,3] Bone scan is sometimes negative but more often, for those lesions with calcification or ossification, the scan is active.[86]

Histologically, enchondromas are composed of collections of immature cartilage separated by thin fibrous septae[1,3,9] (Figure 9). Cellularity is low and the lesions appear quite bland in character, with little evidence of DNA synthesis or cells with double nuclei. The cells themselves are small and the nuclei dark on hematoxylin and eosin stains. Fine or coarse calcification and sometimes ossification may be present. Myxoid change may be noted in lesions located in the hands and feet. The flow cytometric pattern is almost always diploid and the lesions are often positive for S100 protein and vimentin.[3]

Treatment of Enchondromas

Enchondromas that are small and asymptomatic and not in a site where a fracture could be a problem can be observed at regular intervals to see if changes occur or pain develops.[1,3,9] Lesions of the hand or foot bones need not be treated unless they enlarge or cause pain. One of the key issues in lesions of the proximal femur, proximal humerus, or pelvis is the possibility that the diagnosis is a low-grade or myxoid chondrosarcoma and that observing it may allow it to grow or even metastasize.[87] If the lesion is painful or enlarges, the most appropriate treatment is open biopsy, examination of the tissue on frozen section, and, if it is convinc-

ingly benign, curettage of the lesion and filling of the space with bone chips or methylmethacrylate.[1,3] Sometimes it may be necessary to use hardware to reduce the risk of fracture. If the frozen section is not diagnostic, permanent sections may be more accurate; the wound should be closed, and then further surgery performed when the diagnosis is established. Resection may be indicated for lesions that too closely resemble chondrosarcoma. Local recurrences are relatively frequent if the lesion is not completely removed and may be a source of concern regarding the possibility of development of a chondrosarcoma.[72,87,88]

Multiple Enchondromatosis of Bone (Ollier's Disease and Maffucci's Syndrome)
Incidence, Age, and Sex Distribution

Ollier's disease and Maffucci's syndrome are uncommon, with an estimated frequency of less than 1 in 100,000 live births—yet they remain a major problem for the patients, their families, and their physicians. Both disorders affect males and females equally and have no really clearly defined system of familial transmission.[1,3,9,80,83,89] The diseases may appear at birth or by 2 or 3 years of age and show gradual increases in the extent of the lesions and the other findings, some of which (particularly for Maffucci's syndrome) can be very deforming and even life-threatening.[3,80]

Pathogenesis

Parathyroid hormone–related protein (PTHrP) and Indian hedgehog, acting on the receptors PTHR1 and PTCH1 (patched 1), exert a signaling relay that is critical for the regulation of endochondral ossification.[90-92] A mutant PTHR1 has been identified as occurring in several patients with Ollier's disease, and it has been proposed that this is the genetic cause of the disorder.[93,94] Concern exists chiefly because there have been very limited findings to support a possible gene error or familial transmission, and evaluating the families of affected patients has failed to show a clearly defined autosomal recessive or dominant pattern.[95]

Clinical Findings

Patients with Ollier's disease or Maffucci's syndrome have multiple sites of enchondro-

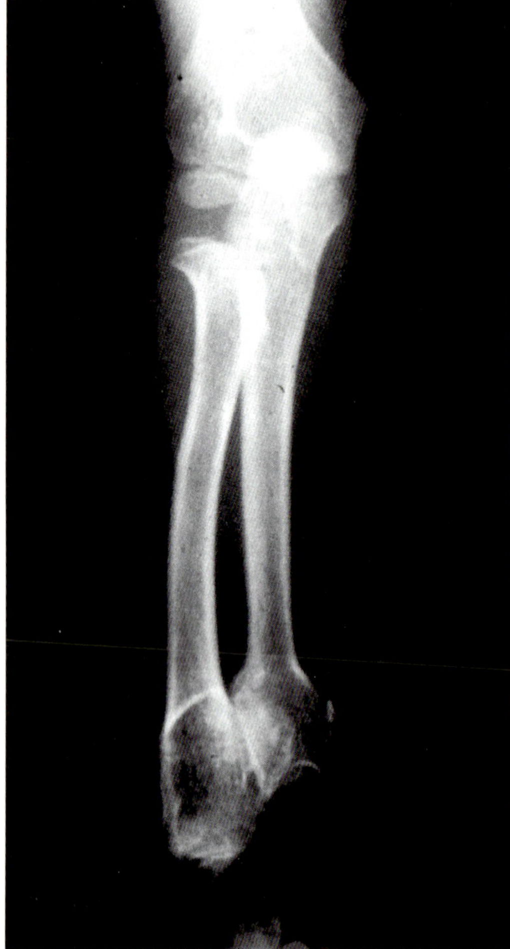

Figure 10

Ollier's disease affecting the radius and ulna and producing marked structural alteration.

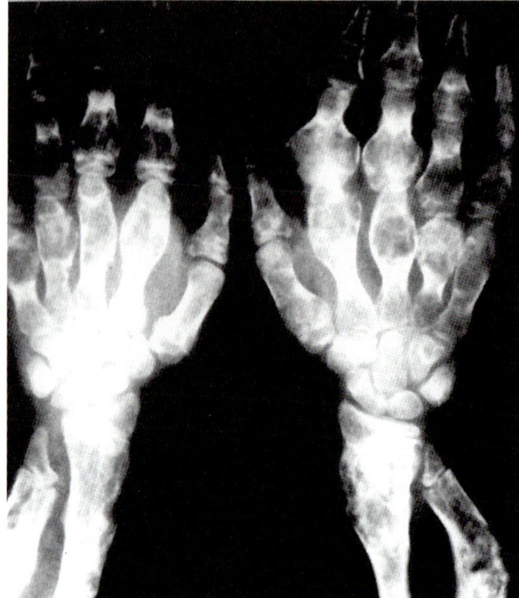

Figure 11

Ollier's disease producing very marked alteration in structure of the hands and considerably limiting the patient's function.

mas in their limbs, which cause sometimes significant deformities.[1,3,83,89,96] The lesions sometimes occur in one extremity, or even on one side of the body, which may cause deformity and shortening (Figure 10). The limbs occasionally show bowing or knock knees, and the hands and feet are distorted in shape (Figure 11). Of greater concern is the frequency of the disease in relation to the hip or knee, which may result in microfractures and lead to osteoarthritic changes. Deformity of the pelvis is frequent and occasional partial dislocation of the hip is encountered. The skull, facial bones, and spine are rarely involved but when they are, they may become very deformed.[97,98]

Maffucci's syndrome has another extraordinary feature related to vascular malformations, which can occur and sometimes dominate the presentation. The vascular lesions are usually soft-tissue hemangiomas that typically occur in the skin but may be present in the viscera, pharynx, or even lungs (Figure 12). The types of lesions that may occur in extraosseous sites include spindle-cell hemangioendotheliomas, arteriovenous aneurysms, endocrine adenomas, vascular fistulae, lymphangiomas, and even angiosarcoma and gastrointestinal adenocarcinoma.[1,3,62,64,79,80,99,100]

Imaging and Histology

Imaging and histology are similar to that reported for enchondromas, with several notable exceptions. The lesions are usually larger and much more damaging to the cortex, which may appear frayed and markedly thinned on imaging.[1,3,70,83,96] The result is frequent microfractures, with changes in the bone alignment and sometimes significant decrease in the length of the bone. Calcification and ossification in the central portion of the lesion is frequently present and the pattern of popcorn balls is quite characteristic.[1,3,96] Pelvic structural abnormalities are often the rule and may result in abnormalities of the hip joint.[96] CT and MRI results are similar to those reported for solitary enchondromas, but the lesions are far less subtle and fewer are in the hands or feet. The bone scan is virtually always positive, particularly over the large lesions.[86]

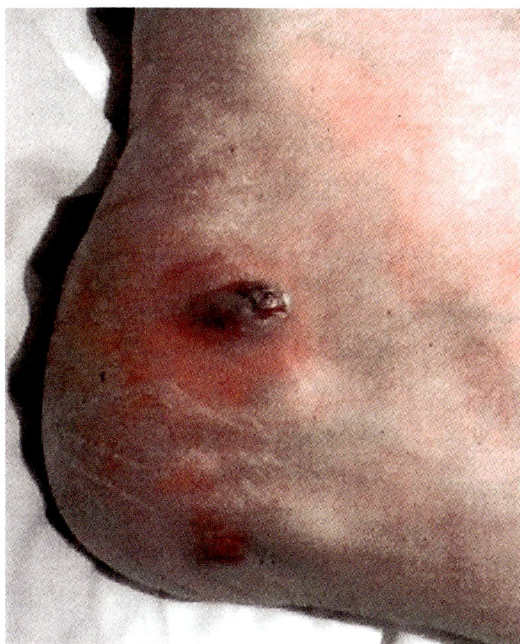

Figure 12
Typical vascular lesion in the foot of a patient with Maffucci's syndrome.

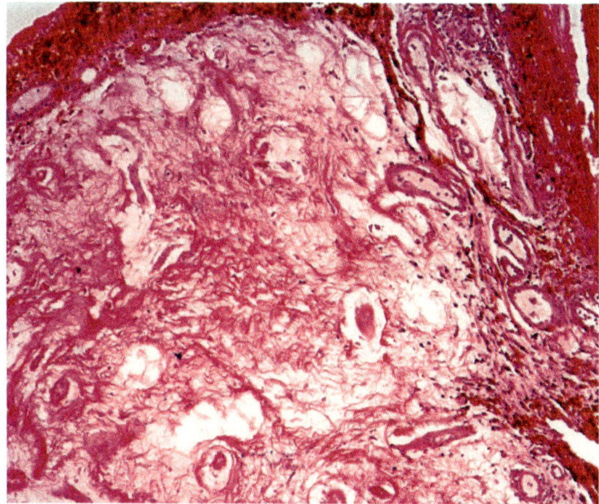

Figure 13
Histology for Ollier's and Maffucci's syndromes, showing markedly distorted cartilage with bone segments. A number of atypical cells and some multinuclear cells are present.

Histologically, the lesions are clearly cartilaginous but there are more cells and they are larger and show much more atypism than enchondromas (Figure 13). Double nuclei and occasional mitotic figures are seen.[1,3,28,96] The calcification and ossification is sometimes dominant and other types of cells may be present, particularly vascular components in patients with Maffucci's syndrome. Many of the features of the cartilage lesions seem identical to grade 1 chondrosarcoma.[9,47,72,87,101,102]

Risk of Chondrosarcoma and Other Tumors

Patients with Ollier's disease, and especially those with Maffucci's syndrome, have a much higher risk of chondrosarcoma than any other benign cartilage lesions, including hereditary multiple osteocartilaginous enchondromas.[9,47,72,87,96,101-103] The statistics for Ollier's disease suggest that the likelihood is ≥20% and, for Maffucci's syndrome, closer to ≥50%.[1,3,30,43,63,78,87,101] Patients with Maffucci's syndrome also have a high incidence of bowel and ovarian cancer, and it is estimated that with the frequency of chondrosarcoma, vascular tumors, and adenocarcinoma of the bowel, the patients have a low survival rate.[3,62,87,98,99,102-106] Fortunately, the chondrosarcomas that develop in patients with both entities are relatively low grade and, if resected, have a low rate of recurrence or metastasis. It is possible for chondrosarcomas to develop at different sites at intervals after the initial tumor is treated.

Treatment of Patients With Ollier's Disease and Maffucci's Syndrome

Unfortunately, there are no effective treatments of patients with these two entities. They must be carefully watched for evidence of increased size or pain at a site; biopsies and, if necessary, resective surgery should be performed.[1,3,9,102,106] Local recurrence of the tumor after surgery can be a major problem and suggests the possibility of chondrosarcoma; this may require more extensive and sometimes disabling surgery.[13,70,72] If a genetic error were identified, it might be possible to alter it by appropriate treatment or the use of marrow transplant or stem cell therapy, but currently there is no evidence that those protocols would be successful. The vascular hemangiomatous lesions in patients with Maffucci's syndrome should be watched closely as well; although they are unlikely to become malignant, they may produce problems, particularly when located in the foot.[3,62,79,100] Patients with Maffucci's syndrome should be evaluated regularly for colon problems by colonoscopy or imaging studies.[105]

Conclusions

Benign cartilage tumors have a broad series of presentations ranging from a solitary osteocartilaginous exostosis, which is essentially of no problem or risk to the patient, to Maffucci's syndrome, for which the likelihood of some form of cancer developing can be as high as 90%. The tumors all have distinctive and readily identifiable appearances on imaging studies. The ecchondrotic lesions lie outside the bone but share a cortex and may be calcified, while the enchondrotic lesions lie inside the bone and not only produce scalloping of the cortex, but irregularity of structure along with calcification. Although there are many problems for these patients, two are critical. The first is the likelihood that in some of them, particularly those with extensive disease, a chondrosarcoma may develop. Fortunately, most of the chondrosarcomas that occur are low grade; although the death rate is not insignificant, it is less than for patients with osteosarcoma or Ewing's tumor. The second problem is that it is sometimes very difficult with any of the entities to determine if a lesion that is large, painful, recurrent after surgery, or very active on bone scan is not a chondrosarcoma. Biopsies are not always easy to perform and are sometimes difficult to read with accuracy; the concern is the possibility of either undertreatment of malignant tumors or overtreatment of benign ones. Genetic or biologic markers for chondrosarcoma would be enormously helpful to these patients, their families, and physicians, and thus research must continue to address this issue.

References

1. Campanacci M: *Bone and Soft Tissue Tumors*, ed 2. New York, NY, Springer Verlag, 1999, pp 179-196, 213-228, 235-246.

2. Coley BL, Santoro AJ: Benign central cartilaginous tumors of bone. *Surgery* 1947;22:411-423.

3. Dorfman HD, Czerniak B: *Bone Tumors*. St Louis, MO, Mosby, 1997, pp 253-352.

4. Ehrenfried A: Multiple cartilaginous exostoses—hereditary deforming chondrodysplasia: A brief report on a little known disease. *JAMA* 1915;64:1642-1646.

5. Fairbank HA: Diaphyseal aclasis: Synonyms. Multiple exotoses, hereditary deforming chondrodysplasia. *J Bone Joint Surg Am* 1949;31:105-113.

6. Gabos PG, Bowen JR: Epiphyseal-metaphyseal enchondromatosis: A new clinical entity. *J Bone Joint Surg Am* 1998;80:782-792.

7. Geschickter CF, Copeland MM: *Tumors of Bone (Including the Jaws and Joints)*, ed 2. New York, NY, American Journal of Cancer, 1936, pp 11-70.

8. Jaffe HL: Hereditary multiple exostosis. *Arch Pathol* 1943;36:335-357.

9. Jaffe HL: Solitary and multiple osteocartilaginous exostosis: Solitary enchondroma and multiple enchondromatosis, in *Tumors and Tumorous Conditions of the Bones and Joints*. Philadelphia, PA, Lea and Febiger, 1958, pp 143-168.

10. Ollier M: Exostoses osteogeniques multiples. *Lyon Med* 1898;88:484-486.

11. Peterson HA: Multiple hereditary osteochondromata. *Clin Orthop Relat Res* 1989;239:222-230.

12. Solomon L: Hereditary multiple exostosis. *Am J Hum Genet* 1964;16:351-363.

13. Unni KK: Cartilaginous lesions of bone. *J Orthop Sci* 2001;6:457-472.

14. Boyer A: *Traité des Maladies Chirurgicales et des Operations qui leur Conviennent*. Paris, France, Migneret, 1814, p 594.

15. Cooper A: Exostosis, in Cooper A, Travers B (eds): *Surgical Essays*, ed 3. London, Cox and Son, 1818, pp 169-226.

16. Von Recklinghausen F: Ein fall von multiplen exostosen. *Arch Pathol Anat Phys* 1866;35:203-207.

17. Gibney VP: Hereditary multiple exostosis: Four cases with remarks. *Am J Med Sci* 1876;72:73-80.

18. Bessel-Hagen F: Uber knochen und gelenkanomalien insbesondere bei partiellem riesenwuchs und bei multiplen cartilaginären exostosen. *Arch Klin Chir* 1891;41:420-466.

19. Virchow R: Exostosen und hyperostosen von extremittäten-knochen des menschen im hiblick auf den pithecanthropus. *Z Ethnol* 1895;27:787-793.

20. Keith A: Studies on the anatomical changes which accompany certain growth-disorders of the human body: I. The nature of the structural alterations in the disorder known as multiple exostoses. *J Anat* 1920;54:101-115.

21. Rixford E: Osteochondromatosis. *Ann Surg* 1930;92:673-680.

22. Jansen M: Dissociation of bone growth (exostoses and enchondromata) or Ollier's dyschondroplasia and associated phenomena, in: *The Robert Jones Birthday Volume*. London, England, Oxford University Press, 1928, pp 43-72.

23. Hume JB: The causation of multiple exostoses. *Brit J Surg* 1929-30;17:236-241.

24. Harsha WN: The natural history of osteocartilaginous exostoses (ostechondroma). *Am Surg* 1954;20:65-72.

25. Langenskiöld A: The development of multiple cartilaginous exostoses. *Acta Orthop Scand* 1967;38:259-266.

26. Banks WC, Bridges CH: Multiple osteocartilaginous exostoses in a dog. *J Am Vet Med Assoc* 1956;129:131-135.

27. Gardner EJ, Shupe JL, Leone NC, Olson AE: Hereditary multiple exostosis: A comparative

genetic study in man and horses. *J Hered* 1975;66:318-326.

28. Milgram JW: The origins of osteochondromas and enchondromas: A histopathologic study. *Clin Orthop Relat Res* 1983;174:264-284.

29. Pierz KA, Stieber JR, Kusumi K, Dormans JP: Hereditary multiple exostoses: One center's experience and review of etiology. *Clin Orthop Relat Res* 2002;401:49-59.

30. Tamimi HK, Bolen JW: Enchondromatosis (Ollier's disease) and ovarian juvenile granulosa cell tumor. *Cancer* 1984;53:1605-1608.

31. Shapiro F, Simon S, Glimcher MJ: Hereditary multiple exostoses: Anthropometric, roentgenographic, and clinical aspects. *J Bone Joint Surg Am* 1979;61:815-824.

32. Mermer MJ, Gupta MC, Salamon PB, Benson DR: Thoracic vertebral body exostosis as a cause of myelopathy in a patient with hereditary multiple exostoses. *J Spinal Disord Tech* 2002;15:144-148.

33. Borges AM, Huvos AG, Smith J: Bursa formation and synovial chondrometaplasia associated with osteochondromas. *Am J Clin Pathol* 1981;75:648-653.

34. Cardelia JM, Dormans JP, Drummond DS, Davidson RS, Duhaime C, Sutton L: Proximal fibular osteochondroma with associated peroneal nerve palsy: A review of six cases. *J Pediatr Orthop* 1995;15:574-577.

35. Griffiths HJ, Thompson RC Jr, Galloway HR, Everson LI, Suh JS: Bursitis in association with solitary osteochondromas presenting as mass lesions. *Skeletal Radiol* 1991;20:513-516.

36. Vallance R, Hamblen DL, Kelly IG: Vascular complications of osteochondroma. *Clin Radiol* 1985;36:639-642.

37. Albrecht S, Crutchfield JS, SeGall GK: On spinal osteochondromas. *J Neurosurg* 1992;77:247-252.

38. Román G: Hereditary multiple exostoses: A rare cause of spinal cord compression. *Spine* 1978;3:230-233.

39. Shapiro SA, Javid T, Putty T: Osteochondroma with cervical cord compression in hereditary multiple exostoses. *Spine* 1990;15:600-602.

40. Cates HE, Burgess RC: Incidence of brachydactyly and hand exostosis in hereditary multiple exostosis. *J Hand Surg Am* 1991;16:127-132.

41. Pogrund H, Yosipovitch Z: Osteochondroma following irradiation: Case report and review of the literature. *Isr J Med Sci* 1976;12:154-157.

42. Ahmed AR, Tan TS, Unni KK, Collins MS, Wenger DE, Sim FH: Secondary chondrosarcoma in osteochondroma: Report of 107 patients. *Clin Orthop Relat Res* 2003;411:193-206.

43. Coley BL, Higinbotham NL: Secondary chondrosarcoma. *Ann Surg* 1954;139:547-559.

44. Garrison RC, Unni KK, McLeod RA, Pritchard DJ, Dahlin DC: Chondrosarcoma arising in osteochondroma. *Cancer* 1982;49:1890-1897.

45. Porter DE, Lonie L, Fraser M, et al: Severity of disease and risk of malignant change in hereditary multiple exostoses: A genotype-phenotype study. *J Bone Joint Surg Br* 2004;86:1041-1046.

46. Schweitzer G, Pirie D: Osteosarcoma arising in a solitary osteochondroma. *S Afr Med J* 1971;45:810-811.

47. Buddingh EP, Naumann S, Nelson M, Neffa JR, Birch N, Bridge JA: Cytogenetic findings in benign cartilaginous neoplasms. *Cancer Genet Cytogenet* 2003;141:164-168.

48. Sandberg AA, Bridge JA: Updates on the cytogenetics and molecular genetics of bone and soft tissue tumors: Chondrosarcoma and other cartilaginous neoplasms. *Cancer Genet Cytogenet* 2003;143:1-31.

49. Bloch AM, Nevo Y, Ben-Sira L, Harel S, Shahar E: Winging of the scapula in a child with hereditary multiple exostoses. *Pediatr Neurol* 2002;26:74-76.

50. Parsons TA: The snapping scapula and subscapular exostoses. *J Bone Joint Surg Br* 1973;55:345-349.

51. Solomon L: Carpal and tarsal exostosis in hereditary multiple exostoses. *Clin Radiol* 1967;18:412-416.

52. Ahn J, Lüdecke HJ, Lindow S, et al: Cloning of the putative tumor suppressor gene for hereditary multiple exostoses (EXT1). *Nat Genet* 1995;11:137-143.

53. Wuyts W, Van Hul W: Molecular basis of multiple exostoses: Mutations in the EXT1 and EXT2 genes. *Hum Mutat* 2000;15:220-227.

54. Le Merrer M, Legeai-Mallet L, Jeannin PM: A gene for hereditary multiple exostoses maps to chromosome 19p. *Hum Mol Genet* 1994;3:717-722.

55. Ligon AH, Potocki L, Shaffer LG, Stickens D, Evans GA: Gene for multiple exostoses (EXT2) maps to 11(p11.2p12) and is deleted in patients with a contiguous gene syndrome. *Am J Med Genet* 1998;75:538-540.

56. Porter DE, Benson MK, Hosney GA: The hip in hereditary multiple exostoses. *J Bone Joint Surg Br* 2001;83:988-995.

57. Solomon L: Bone growth in diaphyseal aclasis. *J Bone Joint Surg Br* 1961;43:700-716.

58. Bennett GE, Berkheimer GA: Malignant degeneration in a case of multiple benign exostoses: With a brief review of the literature. *Surgery* 1941;10:781-792.

59. Creyssel J, Peycelon R: Osteogenic multiple exostosis terminated by malignant development of chondroma. *Lyon Chir* 1930;27:733-749.

60. Solomon L: Chondrosarcoma in hereditary multiple exostosis. *S Afr Med J* 1974;48:671-676.

61. Morton KS: On the question of recurrence of osteochondroma. *J Bone Joint Surg Br* 1964;46:723-725.

62. Bean WB: Dyschondroplasia and hemangiomata (Maffucci Syndrome): II. *AMA Arch Intern Med* 1958;102:544-550.

63. Bükte Y, Necmioglu S, Nazaroglu H, Kilinc N, Yilmaz F: A case of multiple chondrosarcomas secondary to severe multiple symmetrical enchondromatosis (Ollier's disease) at an early age. *Clin Radiol* 2005;60:1306-1310.

64. Carleton A, Elkington JS, Greenfield JG, Robb-Smith AHT: Maffucci's syndrome (dyschondroplasia with hemangiomata). *Q J Med* 1942;11:203-208.

65. Fairbank HA: Dyschondroplasia: Synonyms, Ollier's disease, multiple enchondroma. *J Bone Joint Surg Am* 1948;30:689-704.

66. Hunter D, Wiles P: Dyschondroplasia (Ollier's

disease) with report of a case. *Brit J Surg* 1935;22:507-519.

67. Kast A, von Recklinghausen FD: Ein fall von enchondrom mit ungewöhnlicher multiplikation. *Virchows Arch* 1889;118:1-18.

68. Langenskiöld A: Ollier's disease and its relation to other forms of chondrodysplasia. *Acta Orthop Scand* 1947;17:93-133.

69. Strang C, Rannie I: Dyschondroplasia with haemangiomata (Maffucci syndrome). *J Bone Joint Surg Br* 1950;32:376-383.

70. Umansky AL: Dyschondroplasia with hemangiomata (Maffucci's syndrome). *Bull Hosp Joint Dis* 1946;7:59-68.

71. Jones S: Excision of the scapula for enchondroma. *Lancet* 1868;2:665-667.

72. LeConte RG, Lee WE, Belk WP: Enchondroma of the femur with repeated recurrences and ultimate death: Report of a case. *Arch Surg* 1925;11:93-99.

73. Freund E: Unusual cartilaginous tumor formation of the skeleton. *Arch Surg* 1936;33:1054-1077.

74. Maffucci A: Di un caso di encondroma ed angioma multiplex: Contribuzione alla genesi embrionale dei tumori. *Mov Med Chir Nap* 1881;3:399-412,565-575.

75. Ollier M: Dyschondroplasie. *Lyon Med* 1900;93:23-25.

76. Ollier M: De la dyschondroplasie. *Bull Soc Chir Lyon* 1900;3:22-27.

77. Jemma G: Multiple chondromas of bone. *Riforma Med* 1929;45:1445-1449.

78. Cowan WK: Malignant change and multiple metastases in Ollier's disease. *J Clin Pathol* 1965;18:650-653.

79. Schnall AM, Genuth SM: Multiple endocrine adenomas in a patient with the Maffucci syndrome . *Am J Med* 1976;61:952-956.

80. Lewis RJ, Ketcham AS: Maffucci's syndrome: Functional and neoplastic significance. Case report and reviews of the literature. *J Bone Joint Surg Am* 1973;55:1465-1479.

81. Coppens A: Un cas de syndrome de Maffucci. *Acta Orthop Belg* 1947;13:11-13.

82. Zellweger H, Uhlinger E: Ein fall von halbseitiger knochenchondromatose (Ollier) mit nevus icthyosisformis. *Helvetica Paediatr Acta* 1948;3:153-163.

83. Anderson IF: Maffucci's syndrome: Report of a case and review of the literature. *S Afr Med J* 1965;39:1066-1070.

84. Noble J, Lamb DW: Enchondromata of the bones of the hand: A review of 40 cases. *Hand* 1974;6:275-284.

85. Takigawa K: Chondroma of the bones of the hand: A review of 110 cases. *J Bone Joint Surg Am* 1971;53:1591-1600.

86. Grüning T, Franke WG: Bone scan appearances in a case of Ollier's disease. *Clin Nucl Med* 1999;24:886-887.

87. Flemming DJ, Murphey MD: Enchondroma and chondrosarcoma. *Semin Musculoskelet Radiol* 2000;4:59-71.

88. Mirra JM, Gold R, Downs J, Eckardt JJ: A new histologic approach to the differentiation of enchondroma and chondrosarcoma of bone: A clinicopathologic analysis of 51 cases. *Clin Orthop Relat Res* 1985;201:214-237.

89. Shapiro F: Ollier's disease: An assessment of angular deformity, shortening, and pathological fracture in twenty-one patients. *J Bone Joint Surg Am* 1982;64:95-103.

90. Pateder DB, Gish MW, O'Keefe RJ, Hicks DG, Teot LA, Rosier RN: Parathyroid hormone-related peptide expression in cartilaginous tumors. *Clin Orthop Relat Res* 2002;403 :198-204.

91. Robinson D, Tieder M, Halperin N, Burshtein D, Nevo Z: Maffucci's syndrome—the result of neural abnormalities? Evidence of mitogenic neurotransmitters present in enchondromas and soft tissue hemangiomas. *Cancer* 1994;74:949-957.

92. Rozeman LB, Hameetman L, Cleton-Jansen AM, Taminiau AH, Hogendoorn PC, Bovée JV: Absence of IHH and retention of PTHrP signaling in enchondromas and central chondrosarcomas. *J Pathol* 2005;205:476-482.

93. Hopyan S, Gokgoz N, Poon R, et al: A mutant PTH/PTHrP type I receptor in enchondromatosis. *Nat Genet* 2002;30:306-310.

94. Rozeman LB, Hameetman L, van Wezel T, et al: cDNA expression profiling of chondrosarcomas: Ollier disease resembles solitary tumors and alteration in genes coding for components of energy metabolism occurs with increasing grade. *J Pathol* 2005;207:61-71.

95. Rozeman LB, Sangiorgi L, Briaire-de Bruijn IH, et al: Enchondromatosis (Ollier disease, Maffucci syndrome) is not caused by the PTHR1 mutation p.R150C. *Hum Mutat* 2004;24:466-473.

96. Heckman JA: Ollier's disease. *AMA Arch Surg* 1951;63:861-865.

97. Balcer LJ, Galetta SL, Cornblath WT, Liu GT: Neuro-ophthalmologic manifestations of Maffucci's syndrome and Ollier's disease. *J Neuroophthalmol* 1999;19:62-66.

98. Noël G, Feuvret L, Calugaru V, et al: Chondrosarcomas of the base of the skull in Ollier's disease or Maffucci's syndrome: Three cases and review of the literature. *Acta Oncol* 2004;43:705-710.

99. Davidson TI, Kissin MW, Bradish CF, Westbury G: Angiosarcoma arising in a patient with Maffucci syndrome. *Eur J Surg Oncol* 1985;11:381-384.

100. Yáñez S, Va-Bernal JF, Mira C, Echevarría MA, González-Vela MC, Arce F: Spindle cell hangioendotheliomas associated with multiple skeletal enchondromas: A variant of Maffucci's syndrome. *Gen Diagn Pathol* 1998;143:331-335.

101. Bovée JV, van Roggen JF, Cleton-Jansen AM, Taminiau AH, van der Woude HJ, Hogendoorn PC: Malignant progression in multiple enchondromatosis (Ollier's disease): An autopsy-based molecular genetic study. *Hum Pathol* 2000;31:1299-1303.

102. Schwartz HS, Zimmerman NB, Simon MA, Wroble RR, Millar EA, Bonfiglio M: The malignant potential of enchondromatosis. *J Bone Joint Surg Am* 1987;69:269-274.

103. Banna M, Parwani GS: Multiple sarcomas in Maffucci's syndrome. *Br J Radiol* 1969;42:304-307.

104. Liu J, Hudkins PG, Swee RG, Unni KK: Bone sarcomas associated with Ollier's disease. *Cancer* 1987;59:1376-1385.

105. Shepherd V, Godbolt A, Casey T: Maffucci's syndrome with extensive gastrointestinal involvement. *Australas J Dermatol* 2005;46:33-37.

106. Sun TC, Swee RG, Shives TC, Unni KK: Chondrosarcoma in Maffucci's syndrome. *J Bone Joint Surg Am* 1985;67:1214-1219.

Chapter 12

Unicameral (Solitary) Bone Cyst

Unicameral bone cyst or, as it is otherwise known, either solitary or simple bone cyst is a common skeletal disorder of unknown cause. It has been variously defined as infectious, vascular, traumatic, genetic, or related to the epiphysis, but most agree that the lesion is nonneoplastic. The lesions appear principally in children between 5 and 15 years of age and are more frequently present in males than females. The principal site is the proximal humerus and less commonly the proximal femur, but the lesions can also occur, although less frequently, in the pelvis, spine, talus, facial bones, or calcaneus. The tumors of the proximal humerus tend to disappear over time, while those of other parts may remain problems for years. Local recurrence after treatment is common but the ultimate fate for the child, particularly for humeral lesions, is usually full recovery and return to normal function.

History and Etiology

The first identifiable report on a unicameral bone cyst was that of Rudolf Virchow in 1876.[1] Virchow described a lesion occurring in the proximal humerus of a young child and causing a fracture. In his opinion, the specimen obtained supported the concept that the lesion arose from degeneration of an existing tumor. An 1891 article by Friedrich Von Recklinghausen[2] describing benign bone tumors advanced the concept that the cystic lesions were similar to others that occur in relation to fibrous, neurologic, and vascular lesions. In 1904, Johann Mönckeberg[3] suggested that the lesion was a result of a healing process of an enchondroma. This concept was supported by von Mikulicz[4] in his 1905 article, and subsequently in Geschickter and Copeland's[5] textbook, and in articles by Freund and Meffert[6] and Konjetzny.[7] All these presentations suggested that the parent lesion was either a giant cell tumor or another benign fibrous lesion. This view was supported in the 1960s by Broder,[8] Maeda,[9] and Aegerter and Kirkpatrick.[10] In 1910, Joseph Bloodgood[11] advanced the theory that the tumors were the result of a low-grade infection; this principle was supported by Phemister and Gordon[12] in an article published in 1926 and by Santos[13] in a 1930 report. In their seminal article published in 1942, Henry Jaffe and Louis Lichtenstein[14] expressed the opinion that the lesion was not an infection but represented a dysplastic process resulting from mechanical trauma to the epiphyseal plate, which causes defective endochondral bone formation. In 1919, Pommer[15] considered a hematoma as a possible cause. In 1960, Jonathan Cohen[16] tried to further assess vascular abnormality as a cause and stated that the cyst was the result of a "transient circulatory compromise attributed to a developmental anomaly in the veins of the affected bone." According to his theory, this intraosseous hemorrhage in time becomes a transudate as the erythrocytes disappear.[17] Based on his studies, Cohen voiced the opinion that the fluid within the cyst did not have chemical characteristics of blood, serum, or synovial fluid and more importantly that it was "isolated" from other body fluids.[18] In 1973, Charles Neer and associates[19] supported this concept and defined it as a blockage of the sinusoidal vessels and accumulation of interstitial fluid and resultant cyst formation. They also discovered that the alkaline phosphatase concentration in the fluid was very high, strongly suggesting a repair process. The view was further supported by the studies of Gebhart in 1996.[20] Chigira and associates[21] showed the internal pressure within the cysts to be higher than normal bone marrow. Mirra and associates[22] reported a close association of the cellular material to both fibrous and macrophage types of synovial cells, suggesting that the lesions could possibly be synovial cysts. In 1989, Shindell and associates[23] reported increased prostaglandin E2 levels, and Gerasimov and associates[24] subsequently showed increased lysosomal enzyme activ-

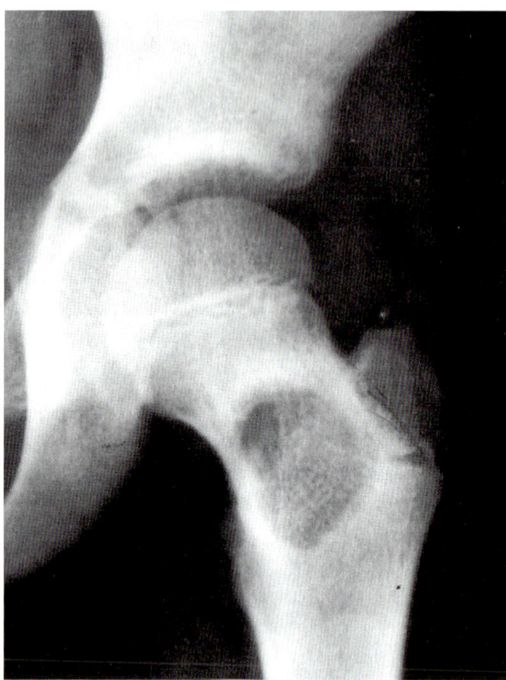

Figure 1

Radiograph of a unicameral bone cyst of the proximal femur. The cortices are thin but the bone is not distorted. The lesion is at the metaphyseal-diaphyseal junction.

ity. Komiya and associates[25] measured oxygen activity in cysts and compared it with other body fluids. They discovered that superoxide dismutase was 15-fold higher than in serum, suggesting that hyperoxygenation may play a role in cyst formation. Vayego and associates[26,27] reported genetic abnormalities in chromosomes 4, 6, 8, 12, and 21 with amino substitutions (arginine for tryptophan and argenine for serine) as well as TP53 mutations. A translocation (16: 20)(p11.2;q13) was reported for a single case by Richkind and associates[28] in 2002. Despite all of that information, there is still no clear definition of the cause of unicameral bone cyst. The best definition of the problem is in the final sentence of the 1926 article by the orthopaedic "giant," Dallas B. Phemister.[12] He and his coauthor Gordon wrote, "Thus far, the various etiologic theories have been of little practical value in our understanding and treatment of solitary cyst."

Clinical Presentation

Unicameral bone cysts are common and cited to be approximately 3% of all bone tumors.[14,29-38] The lesions may in fact occur much more frequently but may not be recognized because they are usually asymptomatic unless fractures occur. Most lesions occur in children between 5 and 15 years of age,[10,30-32,35,36,38-40] but may have been present earlier and not discovered.[41] The fact that they are not seen much later than 15 years of age strongly supports the Jaffe and Lichtenstein concept that the lesions spontaneously resolve after puberty.[14] The disorder is approximately twice as common in males as in females, and most of the lesions are located in the proximal humerus (50% to 60%) or in the proximal femur (20% to 30%).[10,30-32,35,36,38-40] Those that are located in other sites may have less typical behavior patterns, especially those occurring in the pelvis, vertebrae, calcaneus, talus, jaw bones, or patella.[5,30,35,38,42-48]

As indicated above, most of the lesions are asymptomatic until a fracture occurs or until they are seen on a radiograph by chance.[30,31,33,35,40,46,48-51] Because radiographs of the chest usually also show the proximal humerus, in the early part of the 20th century, many of the lesions were discovered when children were required to obtain chest radiographs regularly to diagnose tuberculosis. One of the ways that it was decided that the lesions spontaneously resolved was related to the fact that adults who had chest radiographs for the same reason were rarely, if ever, found to have a humeral cyst. Because the bone is considerably thinned, fractures occur quite frequently and are usually the presenting complaint for most unicameral bone cysts, especially those of the humerus or femur.[30,31,33,35,40,46,48-51]

Unicameral bone cysts of the proximal humerus or proximal femur are centrally placed in the bone and usually appear in the metaphysis or even the diaphysis, but almost always distant from the epiphyseal region[10,14,30,32,38] (Figure 1). The lesions almost never extend more widely than the width of the epiphyseal plate, which helps distinguish them from other lytic lesions such as the aneurysmal bone cyst, the giant cell tumor, or the osteosarcoma.[30,31,38] (Figure 2) With time, the cysts move away from the proximal portions of the bone and become more distal, indicating that the epiphyseal growth pushes the metaphysis away from the cyst, rather than

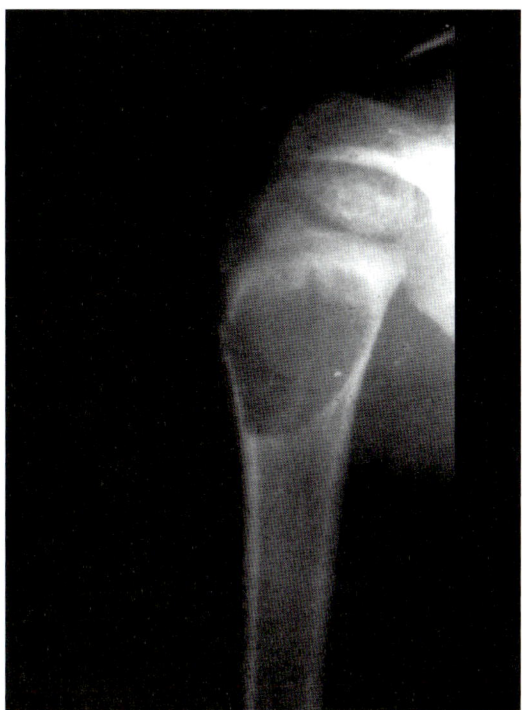

Figure 2
Typical unicameral bone cyst of the proximal humerus in a child. The bone is not expanded but the cortices are thinned.

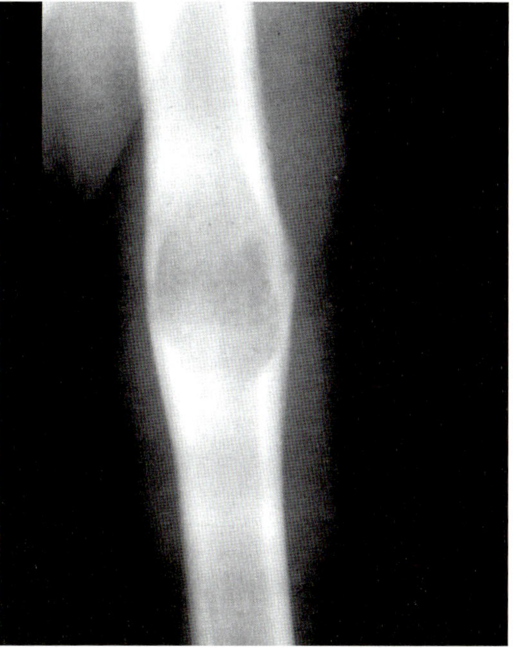

Figure 3
Several years after the original radiograph seen in Figure 1, another image shows that the lesion has extended down the shaft and is beginning to heal.

the cyst itself moving distally in the bone (Figure 3). Spontaneous healing of fractures is certainly possible, although it occurs less frequently than anticipated.[14,30-33,35,36,38-40,50] In most cases, fractures must be treated to achieve restoration of bone structure.

Unicameral cysts are believed to be solitary, although there was a report of 2 sites with the same tumor.[52] Several reports have described a chondrosarcoma and a Ewing tumor arising at the site of a histologically proven unicameral bone cyst.[53-55] It should also be noted that pelvic unicameral cysts are often much more difficult to treat and have a high recurrence rate.[30,31,38,40,48] They do not seem to disappear spontaneously. This is also true for lesions of the calcaneus, mandible, or maxilla, which may be present for years with little structural change but with sometimes continued pain or limitation of motion.[5,10,29-31,38,43] Late recurrences of cysts have been recorded,[56,57] and occasional reports of epiphyseal injury and altered growth have also appeared.[58-60]

Histologic Appearance

Histologic studies have over the years demonstrated a series of characteristic changes.[10,14,18,22,29-31,36,38] The cyst is filled with fluid, which as noted above does not resemble synovial fluid, serum, or blood elements. The bone shows marked cortical thinning, with immature periosteal bone surrounding the remaining cortex and the fluid sac. The cyst membrane consists of loose vascular connective tissue showing fibroblasts, monocytes, giant cells, and cholesterol clefts (Figure 4). The vascular blood supply for the cortical bone is rich in dilated and hyperemic capillaries and venous vessels.

Imaging Studies

Lesions located in the typical sites, specifically the proximal humerus or proximal femur, are centrally located and do not invade or damage the metaphyseal-epiphyseal region.[14,32,35,61,62] There have been several reports of damage of the epiphysis by cysts, but these are presumed to result from fractures.[58-60] The cortices are usually very thin and sometimes appear fragmented.[30,33,38] A characteristic sign that is believed to be diagnostic is the presence of a

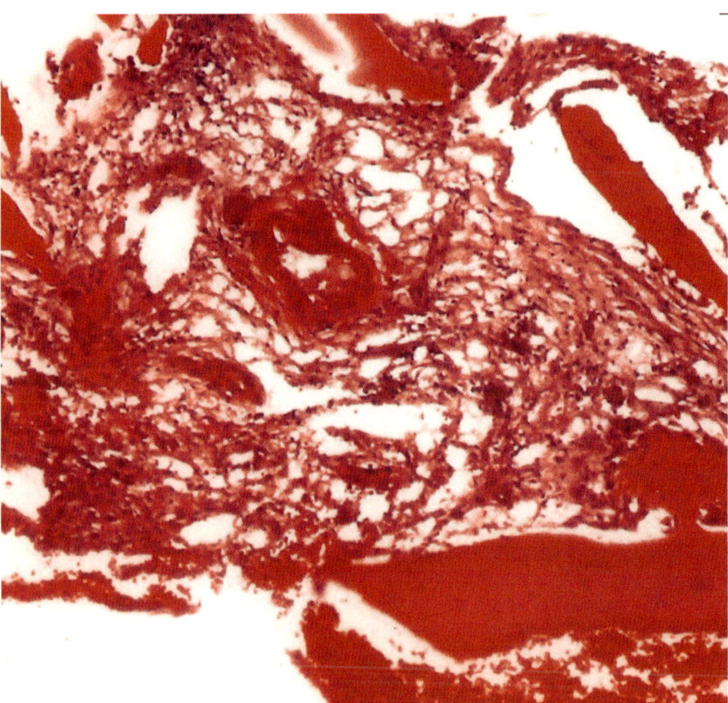

Figure 4

Histologic picture of a unicameral bone cyst showing the fibrous tissue in the central portion of the lesion surrounding fluid-filled spaces. Bone formation is present but very limited in extent. The cells are benign in appearance.

small segment of bone floating at the bottom of the cyst, known as the "fallen fragment sign."[63-65] This is found in approximately 20% of the lesions of the humerus or femur. MRI studies will often show heterogenous fluid signals, suggesting internal fractures that have altered the structure of the cyst.[66,67] Routine radiographs, CT, and MRI scans may be very useful in helping to distinguish the unicameral cyst from other lesions, including aneurysmal bone cyst, fibrous dysplasia, enchondroma, brown tumor of hyperparathyroidism, Langerhans cell histiocytosis, giant cell tumor, nonossifying fibroma, osteosarcoma, or Ewing's tumor.[30,38,68]

Treatment

Surgical treatment of unicameral bone cysts was the earliest technique suggested. In 1962, Fahey and O'Brien[69] introduced a technique for subtotal resection and iliac crest autografting. Neer and associates.[19,40] then reviewed their series of cases and es-

tablished a system to define and establish success based principally on the absence of recurrence. In 1977, McKay and Nason[70] also reported successful resections but without bone grafting, and subsequently allograft implants either as gross segments or as chips were used and were also thought to have reasonable success.[21,36,50,69,71-73]

Percutaneous techniques for treatment were introduced in 1982 by Scaglietti and associates.[74] He and his colleagues were first to introduce steroids through a needle injection, which appeared to have reasonable success. Unfortunately, in some series, this required repeat procedures for as many as 70% of patients.[71,75-77] In the past decade, steroids have been less frequently used and demineralized bone matrix and other bone substitutes have been introduced with seemingly good success.[78-81] Most recently, autogenous bone marrow transplants injected through a needle appear to be very helpful and thus far have a high level of success.[76,81-83] Intramedullary nails have been introduced, particularly for lesions of the calcaneus and especially the proximal femur, to avoid possible shepherd's-crook deformities.[84,85]

Conclusions

Unicameral bone cyst is a common lesion mostly affecting the proximal humerus or femur of young males. The cause is not clear and it is likely that the lesion spontaneously disappears if fractures do not occur. With a true fracture or an impending one, the treatment of choice today appears to be introduction of various materials including bone marrow or bone substitutes through a percutaneous administrative system. The rate of success is relatively high and patients are restored reasonably quickly to an active life.

One major issue remains, however—the determination of the nature of the entity and its causation. Despite efforts by many scientific and numerous clinical approaches, the cause of unicameral bone cyst appears to resist identification at this time. Fortunately, the natural history of the lesion and the current treatment systems allow good restoration of the patient with minimal risk of complications. Nevertheless, it would still be nice to know what these lesions are and how they occur.

References

1. Virchow R: Uber die bildung von knochenzysten. *Monats Akad Wissensch Berlin Phys Math Klasse* 1876;2:369-381.

2. Von Recklinghausen F: Die fibrose oder deformierende ostitis, die osteomalacie und die osteoplatische carzinose, in Reimer G (ed): *Festschrift fur Rudolph Virchow.* Berlin, Germany, Georg Reimer Verlag, 1891, pp 1-89.

3. Mönckeberg J: Uber cystenbildung bei ostitis fibrosa. *Ver Ges Dtsch Naturforsch* 1904;7:232-241.

4. von Mikulicz J: Uber cystische Degeneration der Knochen. *Ver Ges Dtsch Naturforsch* 1905;76:107.

5. Geschickter CF, Copeland MM: *Tumors of Bone (Including the Jaws and Joints).* New York, NY, *American Journal of Cancer*, 1936, pp 267-288.

6. Freund E, Meffert CB: On different forms of non generalized fibrous osteodystrophy, localized, diffuse monostotic, unilateral and monostotic. *Surg Gynec Obstet* 1936;62:541-563.

7. Konjetzny GE: Die sogennante "Lokalisierte Ostitis Fibrosa". *Arch F Clin Chir* 1922;121:567-634.

8. Broder HM: Possible precursor of unicameral bone cysts. *J Bone Joint Surg Am* 1968;50:503-507.

9. Maeda F: Studies on the solitary bone cyst with special reference to its pathogenesis. *Nippon Seikeigeka Gakkai Zasshi* 1963;37:529-547.

10. Aegerter E, Kirkpatrick JA Jr: *Orthopaedic Diseases: Physiology, Pathology, Radiology*, 3rd ed. Philadelphia, PA, WB Saunders Co, 1968, pp 491-500.

11. Bloodgood JC: Benign bone cysts, ostitis fibrosa, giant cell sarcoma and bone aneurysm of long pipe bones: A clinical and pathological study with the conclusion that conservative treatment is justifiable. *Ann Surg* 1910;52:145-185.

12. Phemister DB, Gordon JE: Etiology of solitary bone cyst. *JAMA* 1926;87:1429-1433.

13. Santos JV: Bacteriology of apparently normal bones: Further corroborative evidence of the inflammatory nature of some cases of solitary bone cyst. *J Bone Joint Surg Am* 1930;12:150-155.

14. Jaffe HL, Lichtenstein L: Solitary unicameral bone cyst. *Arch Surg* 1942;44:1004-1025.

15. Pommer G: Zur kentniss der progressiven Haematom und Phlegmasienveranderungen der Rohrenknochen. *Arch Orthop Chir* 1919;17:17-69.

16. Cohen J: Simple bone cyst: Study of cyst fluid in six cases with a theory of pathogenesis. *J Bone Joint Surg Am* 1960;42:609-616.

17. Cohen J: Etiology of simple bone cysts. *J Bone Joint Surg Am* 1970;52:1493-1497.

18. Cohen J: Unicameral bone cysts: A current synthesis of reported cases. *Orthop Clin North Am* 1977;8:715-736.

19. Neer CS, Francis KC, Johnston D, Kiernan HA Jr: Current concepts in the treatment of unicameral bone cyst. *Clin Orthop Relat Res* 1973;97:40-51.

20. Gebhart M, Blaimont P: Contribution to the vascular origin of the unicameral bone cyst. *Acta Orthop Belg* 1996;62:137-143.

21. Chigira M, Machara S, Arita S, et al: The aetiology and treatment of simple bone cysts. *J Bone Joint Surg Br* 1983;65:633-637.

22. Mirra JM, Bernard GW, Bullough PG, Johnston W, Mink G: Cementum-like bone production in solitary bone cysts (so called cementoma of long bones): Report of three cases. Electron microscopic observations supporting a synovial origin to the simple bone cyst. *Clin Orthop Relat Res* 1978;135:295-307.

23. Shindell R, Huurman WW, Lippeillo L, Connolly JF: Prostaglandin levels in unicameral bone cysts treated by intralesional steroid injections. *J Pediatr Orthop* 1989;9:516-519.

24. Gerasimov AM, Toporova SM, Furthseva LN, et al: The role of lysosomes in the pathogenesis of unicameral bone cysts. *Clin Orthop Relat Res* 1991;266:53-63.

25. Komiya S, Tsuzuki K, Mangham DC, Sugiyama M, Inoue A: Oxygen scavengers in simple bone cysts. *Clin Orthop Relat Res* 1994;308:199-206.

26. Vayego SA, DeConti OJ, Varella-Garcia M: Complex cytogenetic rearrangement in a case of unicameral bone cyst. *Cancer Genet Cytogenet* 1996;86:46-49.

27. Vayego-Lourenco SA: TP53 mutations in a recurrent unicameral bone cyst. *Cancer Genet Cytogenet* 2001;124:175-176.

28. Richkind KE, Mortimer E, Mowery-Rushton P, Fraire A: Translocation (16:20)(p11.2;q13), sole cytogenetic abnormality in a unicameral bone cyst. *Cancer Genet Cytogenet* 2002;137:153-155.

29. Boseker EH, Bickel WH, Dahlin DC: A clinicopathologic study of simple unicameral bone cysts. *Surg Gynecol Obstet* 1968;127:550-560.

30. Campanacci M: *Bone and Soft Tissue Tumors*, ed 2. New York, NY, Springer Verlag, 1999, pp 791-812.

31. Campanacci M, Capanna R, Picci P: Unicameral and aneurysmal bone cysts. *Clin Orthop Relat Res* 1986;204:25-36.

32. Garceau GJ, Gregory CF: Solitary unicameral bone cyst. *J Bone Joint Surg Am* 1954;36:267-280.

33. Graham JJ: Solitary unicameral bone cyst: A follow-up study of thirty-one cases with proven pathological diagnoses. *Bull Hosp Joint Dis* 1952;13:106-130.

34. Hecht AC, Gebhardt MC: Diagnosis and treatment of unicameral and aneurysmal bone cysts in children. *Curr Opin Pediatr* 1998;10:87-94.

35. James AG, Coley BL, Higinbotham NL: Solitary (unicameral) bone cyst. *Arch Surg* 1948;57:137-147.

36. Lokiec F, Wientroub S: Simple bone cyst: Etiology, classification, pathology and treatment modalities. *J Pediatr Orthop B* 1998;7:262-273.

37. Norman A, Schiffman M: Simple bone cysts: Factors of age dependency. *Radiology* 1977;124:779-782.

38. Schajowicz F: *Tumors and Tumorlike Lesions of Bones and Joints*. New York, NY, Springer Verlag, 1981, pp 417-424.

39. Beller ML: Solitary bone cyst in the humeral midshaft at age five years. *Bull Hosp Joint Dis* 1952;13:212-216.

40. Neer CS, Francis KC, Marcove RC, Terz J, Carbonara PN: Treatment of unicameral bone cyst: A follow-up study of one hundred seventy-five cases. *J Bone Joint Surg Am* 1966;48:731-745.

41. Brunschwig A: Solitary bone cysts of long duration. *J Bone Joint Surg Am* 1930;12:141-149.

42. Chaudhary D, Bhatia N, Ahmed A, et al: Unicam-

eral bone cyst of the patella. *Orthopedics* 2000;23:1285-1286.

43. Glaser DL, Dormans JP, Stanton RP, Davidson RS: Surgical management of calcaneal unicameral bone cysts. *Clin Orthop Relat Res* 1999;360:231-237.

44. Huch K, Werner M, Puhl W, Delling G: Calcaneal cyst: A classical simple bone cyst? *Z Orthop Ihre Grenzgeb* 2004;142:625-630.

45. Ogata T, Masuda Y, Hino M, et al: A simple bone cyst located in the pedicle of the lumbar vertebra. *J Spinal Disord Tech* 2004;17:339-342.

46. Snell BE, Adesina A, Wolfla CE: Unicameral bone cyst of a cervical vertebra body and lateral mass with associated pathological fracture in a child: Case report and review of the literature. *J Neurosurg* 2001;95(2 Suppl):243-245.

47. Tsirikos AI, Bowen JR: Unicameral bone cyst in the spinous process of a thoracic vertebra. *J Spinal Disord Tech* 2002;15:440-443.

48. Tynan JR, Schachar NS, Marshall GB, Gray R: Pathologic fracture through a unicameral bone cyst of the pelvis: CT guided percutaneous curettage, biopsy and bone matrix injection. *J Vasc Interv Radiol* 2005;16:293-296.

49. Caviglia H, Garrido CP, Palazzi FF, Meana NV: Pediatric fractures of the humerus. *Clin Orthop Relat Res* 2005;432:49-56.

50. Gartland JJ, Cole FL: Modern concepts in the treatment of unicameral bone cysts of the proximal humerus. *Orthop Clin North Am* 1975;6:487-498.

51. Ortiz EJ, Isler MH, Navia JE, Canosa R: Pathologic fractures in children. *Clin Orthop Relat Res* 2005;432:116-126.

52. Keret D, Kumar SJ: Unicameral bone cysts in the humerus and femur in the same child. *J Pediatr Orthop* 1987;7:712-715.

53. Grabias S, Mankin HJ: Chondrosarcoma arising in histological proved unicameral bone cyst: A case report. *J Bone Joint Surg Am* 1974;56:1501-1509.

54. Johnson LC, Vetter H, Putschar WG: Sarcomas arising in bone cysts. *Virchows Arch Pathol Anat Physiol Klin Med* 1962;335:428-451.

55. Steinberg GG: Ewing's sarcoma arising in a unicameral bone cyst. *J Pediatr Orthop* 1985;5:97-100.

56. Bowen RE, Morrissy RT: Recurrence of a unicameral bone cyst in the proximal part of the fibula after en bloc resection: A case report. *J Bone Joint Surg Am* 2004;86:154-158.

57. Tyler W, Frassica FJ, McCarthy EF: Recurrence of a unicameral bone cyst after nineteen years. *Orthopedics* 2002;25:435-436.

58. Haims AH, Desai P, Present D, Beltran J: Epiphyseal extension of a unicameral bone cyst. *Skeletal Radiol* 1997;26:51-54.

59. Stanton RP, Abdel-Mota'al MM: Growth arrest resulting from unicameral bone cyst. *J Pediatr Orthop* 1998;18:198-201.

60. Violas P, Salmeron F, Chapuis M, et al: Simple bone cysts of the proximal humerus complicated with growth arrest. *Acta Orthop Belg* 2004;70:166-170.

61. Copleman B, Vidoli HF, Crimmings FJ: Solitary cyst in a calcaneus. *Radiology* 1946;47:142-148.

62. Lodwick GS: Juvenile unicameral bone cyst: A roentgen reappraisal. *Am J Roentgenol Radium Ther Nucl Med* 1958;80:495-504.

63. McGlynn FJ, Mickelson MR, El-Khoury GY: The fallen fragment sign in unicameral bone cyst. *Clin Orthop Relat Res* 1981;156:157-159.

64. Reynolds J: The "fallen fragment sign" in the diagnosis of unicameral bone cysts. *Radiology* 1969;92:949-953.

65. Struhl S, Edelson C, Pritzker H, Seimon LP, Dorfman HD: Solitary (unicameral) bone cyst: The fallen fragment sign revisited. *Skeletal Radiol* 1989;18:261-265.

66. Margau R, Babyn P, Cole W, Smith C, Lee F: MR imaging of simple bone cysts in children: Not so simple. *Pediatr Radiol* 2000;30:551-557.

67. Maas EJ, Craig JG, Swisher PK, Amin MB, Marcus N: Fluid-fluid levels in a simple bone cyst on magnetic resonance imaging. *Australas Radiol* 1998;42:267-270.

68. Sullivan RJ, Meyer JS, Dormans JP, Davidson RS: Diagnosing aneurysmal and unicameral bone cyst with magnetic resonance imaging. *Clin Orthop Relat Res* 1999;366:186-190.

69. Fahey JJ, O'Brien ET: Subtotal resection and grafting in selected cases of solitary unicameral bone cysts. *J Bone Joint Surg Am* 1973;55:59-68.

70. McKay DW, Nason SS: Treatment of unicameral bone cysts by subtotal resection without grafts. *J Bone Joint Surg Am* 1977;59:515-519.

71. Campanacci M, De Sessa L, Bellando Randone P: Bone cyst: Review of 275 cases. Results of the surgical treatment and early results of closed treatment with methylprednisolone acetate. *Chir Organi Mov* 1976;62:471-482.

72. Komiya S, Minamitani K, Sasaguri Y, et al: Simple bone cyst: Treatment by trepanation and studies on bone resorptive factors in cyst fluid with a theory of its pathogenesis. *Clin Orthop Relat Res* 1993;287:204-211.

73. Spence KF, Sell KW, Brown RH: Solitary bone cyst: Treatment with freeze-dried cancellous bone allograft: A study of one hundred seventy-seven cases. *J Bone Joint Surg Am* 1969;51:87-96.

74. Scaglietti O, Marchetti PG, Bartolozzi P: Final results obtained in the treatment of bone cysts with methylprednisolone acetate (depo-medrol) and a discussion of results achieved in other bone lesions. *Clin Orthop Relat Res* 1982;165:33-42.

75. Capanna R, Dal Monte A, Gitelis S, Campanacci M: The natural history of unicameral bone cyst after steroid injection. *Clin Orthop Relat Res* 1982;166:204-211.

76. Chang CH, Stanton RP, Glutting J: Unicameral bone cysts treated by injection of bone marrow or methylprednisolone. *J Bone Joint Surg Br* 2002;84:407-412.

77. De Palma L, Santucci A: Treatment of bone cysts with methylprednisolone acetate: A 9 to 11 year follow-up. *Int Orthop* 1987;11:23-28.

78. Altermatt S, Schwobel M, Pochon JP: Operative treatment of solitary bone cysts with tricalcium phosphate ceramic: A 1 to 7 year follow-up. *Eur J Pediatr Surg* 1992;2:180-182.

79. Killian JT, Wilkinson L, White S, Brassard M: Treatment of unicameral bone cyst with demineralized bone matrix. *J Pediatr Orthop* 1998;18:621-624.

80. Mirzayan R, Panossian V, Avedian R, Forrester DM, Menendez LR: The use of calcium sulfate in the treatment of benign bone lesions: A preliminary report. *J Bone Joint Surg Am* 2001;83:355-358.

81. Rougraff BT, Kling TJ: Treatment of active unicameral bone cysts with percutaneous injection of demineralized bone matrix and autogenous bone marrow. *J Bone Joint Surg Am* 2002;84:921-929.

82. Docquier PL, Delloye C: Treatment of simple bone cysts with aspiration and a single bone marrow injection. *J Pediatr Orthop* 2003;23:766-773.

83. Kose N, Gokturk E, Turgut A, Gunal I, Seber S: Percutaneous autologous bone marrow grafting for simple bone cysts. *Bull Hosp Joint Dis* 1999;58:105-110.

84. Abdel-Wanis ME, Tsuchiya H, Uehara K, Tomita K: Minimal curettage, multiple drilling and continuous decompression through a cannulated screw for treatment of calcaneal simple bone cysts in children. *J Pediatr Orthop* 2002;22:540-543.

85. Roposch A, Saraph V, Linhard WE: Flexible intramedullary nailing for the treatment of unicameral bone cysts in long bones. *J Bone Joint Surg Am* 2000;82:1447-1453.

Chapter 13

Charcot Arthropathy

Charcot arthropathy, otherwise known as neuropathic arthropathy, has many origins and presentations. The primary entity, as reported by Jean-Martin Charcot[1] in 1868, was probably due to tabes dorsalis in patients with tertiary syphilis; however, in more recent years, this has become much less likely as a cause. Now, diabetes mellitus, spinal injury, syringomyelia, congenital insensitivity to pain, Charcot-Marie-Tooth disease, hemophilia, and neurofibromatosis are more common as the pathologic cause. The anatomic sites of the disorder range from shoulder to spine, hip, knee, and now most commonly the foot. The processes usually result in structural deformities, functional deficits, and sometimes significant skin and soft-tissue disorders. The treatment is complex; not only are there many failures, but complications are common and sometimes devastating.

Nomenclature and History

Synonyms include Charcot arthropathy, Charcot arthrosis, arthropathia neurotica, arthropathia tabica, neurotrophic joint, neuropathic joint disease, tabetic osteoarthropathy, neuroarthropathy, neuropathic osteoarthropathy, and hypertrophic neuropathic osteoarthropathy.

Historically, the original description was reported to be that of Jean-Martin Charcot[1] in 1868, but it is now recognized that an earlier presentation describing the syndrome was that of William Musgrave in 1703.[2] The initial reports related the disease to a form of tertiary syphilis known as tabes dorsalis. Professor Charcot (1825-1893) was a very productive and knowledgeable French neurologist who not only described the neuropathic joint, but also multiple sclerosis, Charcot-Marie-Tooth disease, Parkinson's disease, Gilles de la Tourette syndrome, aspects of gout, and several other disorders.[3,4] Subsequent reports on the relation of the bone structural alteration in patients with tertiary syphilis included those by Taylor[5] in 1913, Eloesser[6] in 1917, Potts[7] in 1927, Arthur Steindler[8] in 1931, J. Albert Key[9] in

1932, and Pomeranz and Rothberg[10] in 1941. Delano[11] and Storey[12] further defined the pathogenesis of Charcot arthropathy in patients with tertiary syphilis, relating it to demyelinization of the spinal posterior columns and damage to the dorsal roots and dorsal root ganglions. In his 1972 textbook, Henry Jaffe[13] provided information about Charcot disease in association with not only tabetic changes in syphilis, but other disorders as well.

The correlation of tabes dorsalis and Charcot arthropathy with impairment of motor control was reported in 1853 by Romberg,[14] although he did not relate the condition directly to syphilis.

In 1886, Professor Charcot and Pierre Marie[15] and, independently, Howard Tooth[16] reported on a form of hereditary sensory neuropathy characterized by muscle atrophy, arthropathic changes, and deformity now known as Charcot-Marie-Tooth disease. In 1893, Joseph Déjérine and Jules Sottas[17] described a slowly progressive hereditary form of hypertrophic neuritis characterized by numbness, paresthesias, bone abnormalities, and pain in the extremities associated with ocular complications. In 1922, Eric Hicks[18] described a patient with a sensory defect in whom a perforating ulcer of the foot developed. In the next two decades, Dearborn[19] and Nelaton[20] described newborn children with almost total analgesia and joint abnormalities. Thévenard[21] also described a child with sensory loss and self-mutilation, and in 1949, Riley and associates[22] described a series of Ashkenazi Jewish children with severe insensitivity to pain resulting in major skeletal defects (a disease that is now known as Riley-Day syndrome). Subsequent reports by Silverman and Gilden[23] in 1959, Abell and Hayes[24] in 1964, Mooney and Mankin[25] in 1966, and MacEwen and Floyd[26] in 1970 described orthopaedic findings in patients with extensive insensitivity to pain disorders.

In the 1950s, Cotler and DePalma[27] related Charcot-type joint abnormalities in patients with hemophilia, and Floyd and associates[28] further described the neuropathic joint in these patients. Rodnan and associates[29] defined the entity of neuropathic joint disease related to genetic errors, and in 1975, Nellhaus[30] reviewed the changes in the bones of seriously neurologically impaired children. In 1976, Peitzman and associates[31] described the changes in joints in patients with amyloid neuropathy. That same year, Hensinger and MacEwen[32] published a key description of the clinical entity of Charcot arthropathy and its relationship to diabetes and several other disorders. These data, as well as several subsequent studies, defined the role of diabetes in the pathogenesis of the Charcot changes and established it as the current leading cause of Charcot arthropathy, particularly of the foot and ankle.

Physiologic Changes in Bone Affected by Charcot Arthropathy

Several features have been implicated in the development of Charcot arthropathy regardless of site or causation. First and foremost is the reduction in deep sensation and proprioception following demyelinization of the spinal posterior columns and damage to the dorsal roots and dorsal root ganglions, which allows the affected bone to undergo injury and microfracture or even macrofracture without the patient having enough pain to recognize the process.[33-36] Another postulate is that some form of vascular disturbance occurs at the site; this may consist of either hyper- or hypovascularity.[34,37-41] The former results in hyperemia, such as is seen in hemophilia, and the latter may occur as a result of diminished blood flow in diabetes.[40,41] Another clinical feature is the impaired sensory status related to the Romberg sign, which may result in microfractures not easily recognized by the patient's impaired sensory capacity.[42]

There are several disorders that have a genetic origin; these include the congenital insensitivities to pain and Charcot-Marie-Tooth disease, which may create additional problems in terms of anatomic structure for bones and joints that render them more susceptible to abnormal stress.[16,25,30,35,36,43-59] Excessive osteoclastic resorbtion of bone has been implicated, especially in some genetic diseases and diabetes, and there has

recently been a suggestion that the presence of osteoporosis may increase the degree of bony damage.[55,60-63]

The genetic errors for some of these disorders seem to affect the neurotrophins, and modification of these may cause sensory, autonomic, and motor alterations.[43,50,57-59,64] The altered materials include serine palmitoyltransferase, small GTPase late endosomal protein, inhibitor of kappa light polypeptide gene enhancer in B cells, tyrosine kinase A receptor, and nerve growth factor β. All of these gene errors have an effect on nerves, chiefly to reduce the sensory capacity and in some cases diminish autonomic function, motor strength, and ocular or auditory function.[43,50,58,59,64,65]

Congenital insensitivity to pain occurs as either an autosomal dominant or X-linked form. The chromosome site is 17p11.2-12 and the gene error is PMP22 (peripheral myelin protein 22). Additional forms of this disorder are linked to 1q22, Xq13-q22, or 17p11-12 and the gene errors may also include connexin 32 or ERG-2 (early growth response 2).[36,49,50,66,67] Another form of the disorder has chromosome sites at 1p35-p36, 3q13-q22, 19q 13.3, 7p14, or 8p21.[49,50,58,66] The gene errors include kinesis family myelin protein, lamin AC, or neurofilament light chain. Many of these patients present with optic atrophy as a major problem. Laryngeal muscle weakness and diaphragmatic paralysis are commonly present.[31,58,59]

Clinical Presentation

Charcot arthropathy was originally described as an entity arising in patients with tabes dorsalis and tertiary syphilis, but this cause is now rarely encountered[29,68,69] (Figure 1). The disorder may be related to many other conditions, shown below.

- *Diabetes mellitus*. Diabetes is the most common form of Charcot arthropathy today, principally occurring in the foot or ankle and associated with a diminution in deep pain sensation and sometimes reduced vascular supply. Most of the patients are elderly and have had type II diabetes for a long time. Skin lesions and areflexia are common[38,62,63,70-76] (Figure 2).
- *Spinal trauma*. Lumbar or cervical spine injury affecting the sensory components of the spinal roots can cause the disorder in the upper or lower extremity.[77-82]
- *Congenital insensitivity to pain*. Several disor-

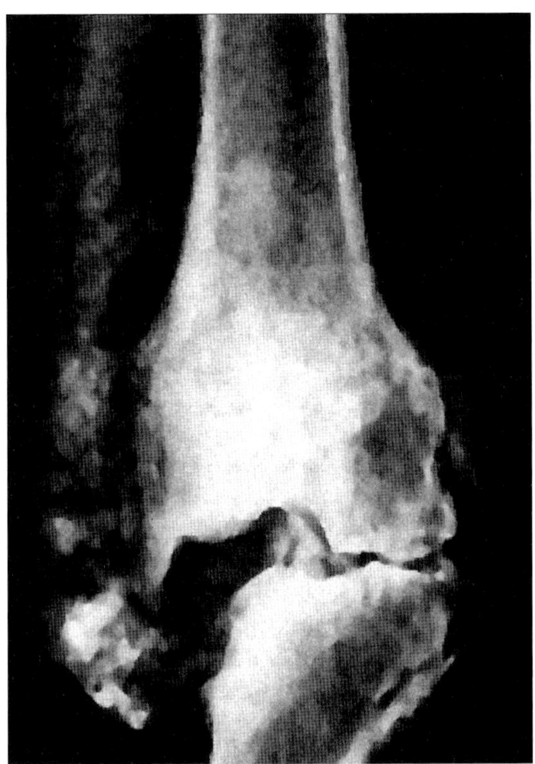
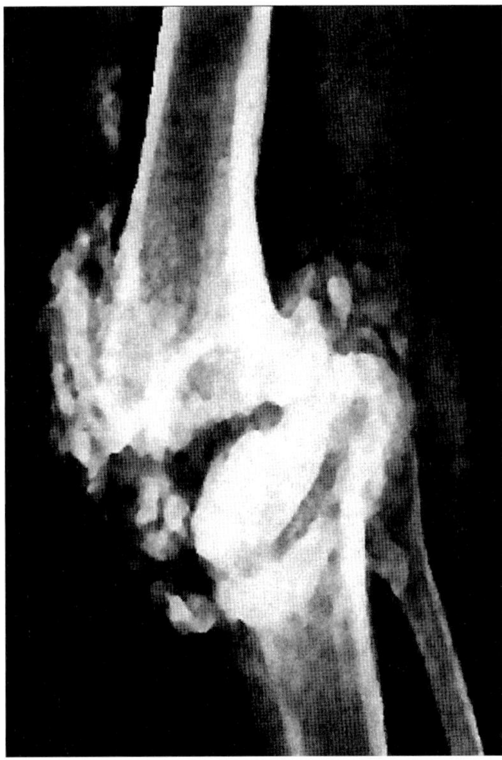

Figure 1

Very severe destructive changes in both knees were once common occurrences in patients with syphilis and tabes dorsalis. The changes are remarkable in their extent, and clearly the patient was disabled by the disorder.

ders associated with reduced deep pain sensation may result in Charcot arthropathy. The condition is rare except for Riley-Day syndrome, which occurs with greater frequency as a genetic error in Ashkenazi Jewish people. Many of these patients present with optic atrophy as a major problem. Laryngeal muscle weakness and diaphragmatic paralysis are commonly present as well.[22,24,35,36,44,47,51,56,57,59,83]

- *Syringomyelia*. This chronic disease, also known as Morvan syndrome, is characterized by cavities in the spinal cord, usually in the cervical region and extending into the medulla or inferiorly into the thoracic or lumbar region. The entity is most common in the neck and produces finger deformities; dissociation anesthesia; areflexia; and humeral, clavicular, or scapular Charcot arthropathy[84-88] (Figure 3).

- *Amyloidosis*. This genetic disorder is characterized by paresthesia and hypesthesia of the limbs and is associated with visual disturbances and skin disorders. The entity may result in either upper or lower extremity Charcot arthropathy related to sensory deficits in spinal canal and nerve roots.[31]

- *Charcot-Marie-Tooth disease*. Charcot-Marie-Tooth disease is a hereditary entity that begins with atrophy of the peroneal musculature and

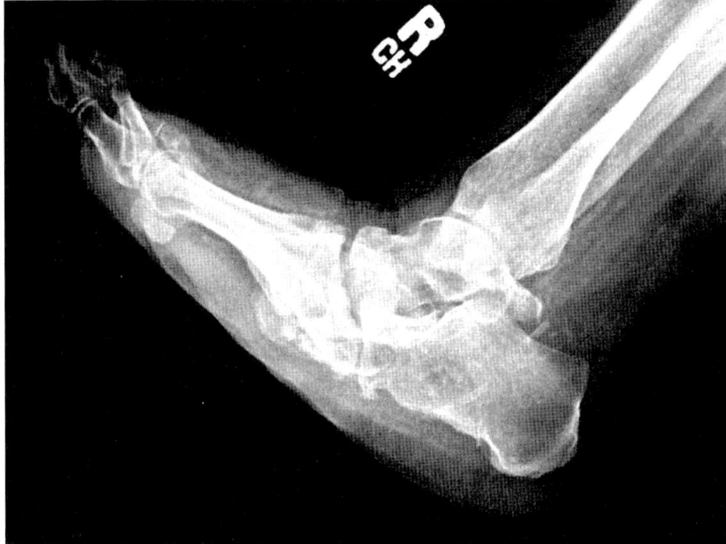

Figure 2

Changes in the foot of a 68-year-old woman with severe diabetes. Note the irregularity of bone structure and several microfractures.

then extends into the lower and upper limb. It is characterized by motor and sensory neuropathy, which can cause upper or lower extremity Charcot arthropathy. It is characterized by generalized weakness and sensory loss, and often

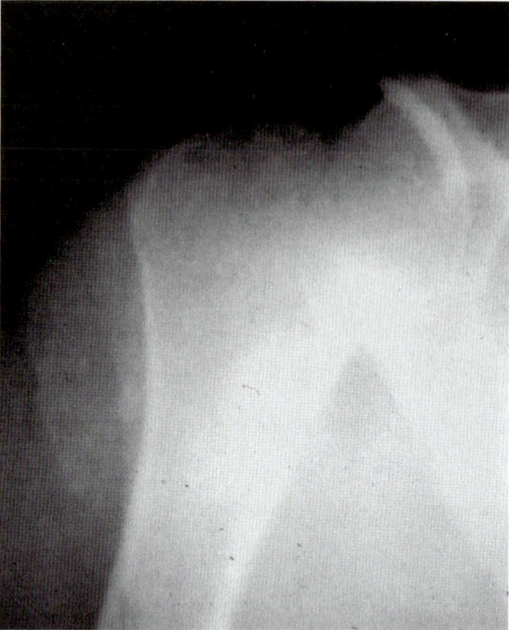

Figure 3
Classic Charcot arthropathy with destruction of the proximal humerus and glenoid sometimes occurs in patients with syringomyelia.

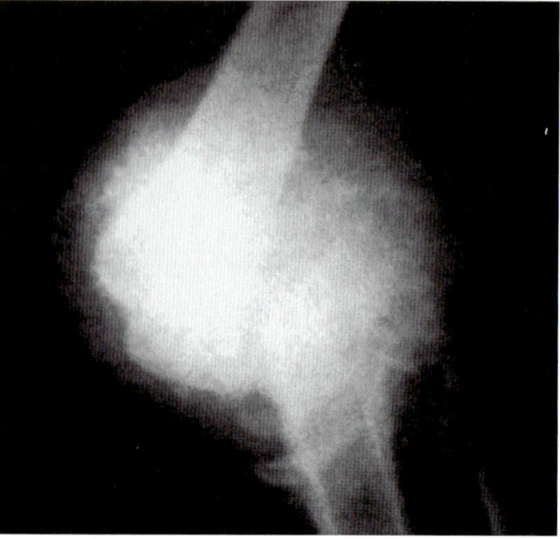

Figure 4
Severe changes may occur in patients with hemophilia and are characterized by marked production of bone.

optic atrophy and severe spinal deformity and pain.[43,48,49,52,57]

- *Multiple sclerosis and other neuropathic disorders*. These entities can cause structural damage as a result of motor and sensory changes in the extremities and may lead to Charcot changes.[5,19,25,74,89-92]
- *Leprosy affecting the spine*. Leprosy may result in damage to the deep sensory system and cause Charcot arthropathy.[93]
- *Hemophilia*. Excessive bleeding into the soft tissue adjacent to a bony site may injure nerves and also produce direct damage to the joint[37,40,41,94] (Figure 4).
- *Neurofibromatosis*. Various neurofibromatous tumors have been implicated in the causation of Charcot arthropathy, principally around the hip, knee, and elbow.[95-97]

Less common causes include pernicious anemia, spina bifida, myelomeningocele, rheumatoid arthritis, scleroderma, Raynaud's disease, Ehlers-Danlos syndrome, and congenital vascular disease. These, as well as the 10 causes listed above, produce a "diagnostic dilemma."[75]

In general, Charcot changes that occur with these disorders are characterized by excessive joint effusion, micro- and macrofractures, fragmentation of bone, subluxation, and soft-tissue swelling.[34,52-55,62,70,78,89,91] Sensation at the site is usually impaired, and reflexes are typically diminished or absent. Cartilage structure is often severely damaged and there is almost always wide structural joint displacement with movement, most often without pain. The skin may show small areas of redness, and in some cases there are defects in the skin with infected sites and drainage.

When the lesion is in the knee, the patient has difficulty walking and sometimes standing erect. When it is located in the shoulder, there is profound limitation of movement. With diabetic lesions in the foot, patients have considerable difficulty putting on shoes and gait can be markedly disturbed, sometimes with severe pain in the distal or proximal sites. Skin defects are common.

Radiographic studies are difficult to interpret. Usually CT or MRI will not only show the bone destruction, but the soft-tissue masses in and around the joint. Cartilage damage and small segments of dead bone within the tissue are common[11,39,55,60,63,71,80] (Figure 5). Positron emission tomographic scanning may be helpful in assessing the presence of multiple sites and the extent of the lesional area.[98]

The critical issue is differentiation from several other joint abnormalities, such as osteonecrosis, osteoarthritis, osteomyelitis, osteopetrosis, gouty arthritis, and even alkaptonuric ochronosis. In addition, however, it is sometimes difficult to determine the cause of the Charcot presentation. Lesions about the foot and ankle should be considered to be caused by diabetes,[38,62,63,70,72,74] while those of the shoulder or upper extremity may result from syringomyelia, Charcot-Marie-Tooth disease, congenital insensitivity to pain, or spinal trauma.[24,33,36,45,47-49,52,54,77,84,88,91,92] Those around the spine, hip, or knee may result from syphilis, spinal disease, congenital insensitivity to pain, or hemophilia.[65,68,69,81] A careful physical examination, family history, evaluation of sensory and motor status, bone scan, MRI, and laboratory studies may be necessary to identify the structure and the causation of the Charcot arthropathy in many cases.

Treatment

Currently the most frequently encountered location is the ankle or foot in patients with diabetes. Corticosteroids and bisphosphonates have been introduced but may be dangerous to the patient's general condition, particularly if diabetes is the cause.[62,71,99-101] If the lesion is small and limited in extent in terms of joint, soft-tissue, and skin damage, then bracing, use of boot-type shoes, or even external fixation may be successful in controlling the problems and allowing the patient to walk and carry on reasonably normal activities.[102] Surgical approaches, including arthrodesis or arthroplasty, are sometimes successful but are fraught with risk of infection or local recurrence problems.[74,103-105] Sometimes, for such entities as congenital insensitivity to pain, syringomyelia, or spinal deformity, eliminating the vertebral lesion and inserting rods to achieve an arthrodesis may be successful.[70,79,83]

Discussion

If this chapter had been written before 1940, it would have simply defined Charcot arthropathy as a consequence of tertiary syphilis and tabes dorsalis. The latter disorder results from a demyelinization of the spinal posterior columns and damage to the dorsal roots and dorsal root ganglions. Patients become unsteady with the eyes closed (Romberg sign) and sometimes injure insensate and hypovascularized joints. This is the original Charcot arthropathy, an entity that, happily, is rarely seen in the United States today.

Instead, the chapter deals with at least 10 other disorders associated with damage to

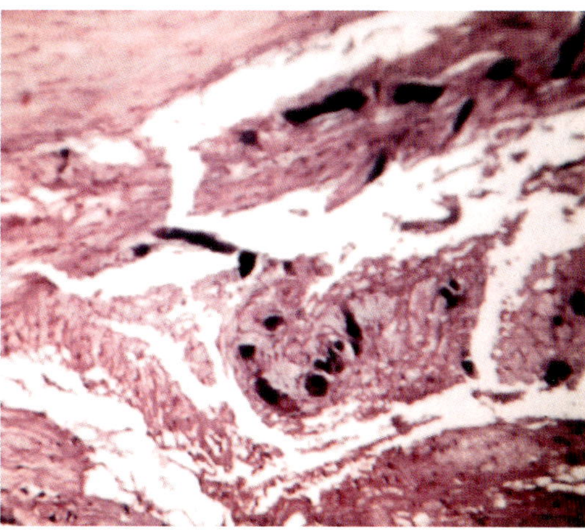

Figure 5

Histologic changes seen in tissue from the joints of patients with Charcot arthropathy. The major tissues are fibrous and monocytic, but frequently there are small segments of dead bone within the tissue.

the posterior columns and altered vascularity; the main one today is clearly diabetes mellitus. This disease is now most often "under control," so that patients live longer, undergoing more trauma to their limbs, which can result in enlarged Charcot joints at the ankle and foot, that may be relatively asymptomatic. The other disorders that cause the Charcot arthropathy are quite uncommon as compared with diabetes, but include not only some spinal disorders, vascular diseases, and spinal and neural abnormalities, but a group of genetic diseases including Riley-Day syndrome, congenital indifference to pain, and Charcot-Marie-Tooth disease.

The problem with these entities today is that it is not always easy to define the nondiabetic causes of Charcot arthropathy, and, furthermore, treatment is almost always a problem in terms of the limited degree of success and the frequency of complications. Similarly, the treatments of diabetic Charcot disorders around the ankle and foot are not always successful and in some cases worsen the patient's disability. Although we have come a long way since Jean-Martin Charcot first described the disorder in 1868, we still cannot provide much help to the unfortunate patients with the disorders. Perhaps in the next 100 years, we will solve the problem!

References

1. Charcot JM: Sur quelques arthropathies qui paraissent dependre d'une lesion du cerveau ou de la moelle epiniere. *Arch Physiol Norm Pathol* 1868;1:161-178.

2. Kelly M: De Arthritide Symptomatica of William Musgrave (1657-1721): His description of neuropathic arthritis. *Bull Hist Med* 1963;37:372-377.

3. Lellouch A: Charcot, discoverer of diseases. *Rev Neurol (Paris)* 1994;150:506-510.

4. Teive HA, Munhoz RP, Barbosa ER: Little-known scientific contributions of J-M Charcot. *Clinics* 2007;62:211-214.

5. Taylor HL: Charcot joints as initial or early symptom in tabes dorsalis. *JAMA* 1913;61:1784-1788.

6. Eloesser L: On the nature of neuropathic affections of the joints. *Ann Surg* 1917;66:201-207.

7. Potts WJ: The pathology of Charcot joints. *Ann Surg* 1927;86:596-606.

8. Steindler A: The tabetic arthropathies. *J Am Med Assoc* 1931;96:250-256.

9. Key JA: Clinical observations of tabetic arthropathies (Charcot's joints). *Amer J Syph* 1932;16:429-446.

10. Pomeranz MM, Rothberg AS: A review of 58 cases of tabetic arthropathy. *Am J Syph Gonorrhea Vener Dis* 1941;25:103-119.

11. Delano PJ: The pathogenesis of Charcot's joint. *AJR Am J Roentgenol* 1946;56:189-200.

12. Storey G: Charcot joints. *Br J Vener Dis* 1964;40:109-117.

13. Jaffe HL: Syphilis of bones and joints, in *Metabolic, Degenerative and Inflammatory Diseases of Bones and Joints*. Philadelphia, PA, Lea and Febiger, 1972, pp 907-952.

14. Romberg MH: *A Manual of the Nervous Diseases of Man*. Sieveking EH, editor and translator. London, England, Sydenham Society, 1853, pp 226-227, 395-401.

15. Charcot JM, Marie P: Sur une forme particulière d'atrophie musculaire progressive souvent familial débutant par les pieds et les jambes et atteignant plus tard les mains. *Rev Med (Paris)* 1886;6:97-138.

16. Tooth HH: *The Peroneal Type of Progressive Muscular Atrophy*. London, England, HK Lewis Co, 1886.

17. Déjérine JJ, Sottas J: Sur la névrite interstitielle hypertrophique et progressive de l'enfance; affection souvent familiale et a debut infantile caracterisee par une atrophie musculaire des extremites, avec troubles marques de la sensibiliste et ataxia des mouvements et relevant d'une névrite interstielle hypertrophique a marche ascendante avec lesions medullaires consecutives. *C R Soc Biol (Paris)* 1893;45:63-82.

18. Hicks EP: Hereditary perforating ulcer of the foot. *Lancet* 1922;1:319-322.

19. Dearborn GV: A case of congenital pure analgesia. *J Nerv Ment Dis* 1932;75:612-615.

20. Nelaton M: Affection singuliere des os du pied. *Gaz Hop Civ et Milit (Paris)* 1942;4:13-20.

21. Thévenard A: L'acropathie ulc éro-mutilante familiale. *Rev Neurol* 1942;74:193-212.

22. Riley CM, Day RL, Greeley DM, Langford WS: Central autonomic dysfunction with defective lacrimation: Report of five cases. *Pediatrics* 1949;3:468-478.

23. Silverman FN, Gilden JJ: Congenital indifference to pain: A neurologic syndrome with bizarre skeletal lesions. *Radiology* 1959;72:176-190.

24. Abell JM Jr , Hayes JT: Charcot knee due to congenital insensitivity to pain. *J Bone Joint Surg Am* 1964;46:1287-1291.

25. Mooney V, Mankin HJ: A case of congenital insensitivity to pain with neuropathic arthropathy. *Arthritis Rheum* 1966;9:820-829.

26. MacEwen GD, Floyd GC: Congenital insensitivity to pain and its orthopedic manifestations. *Clin Orthop Relat Res* 1970;68:100-107.

27. Cotler JM, DePalma AF: Hemophilic arthropathy. *Clin Orthop* 1956;8:163-190.

28. Floyd W, Lovell W, King RE: The neuropathic joint. *South Med J* 1959;52:563-569.

29. Rodnan GP, MacLachlan MJ, Brower TD: Neuropathic joint disease. *Bull Rheum Dis* 1959;9:183-184.

30. Nellhaus G: Neurogenic arthropathies (Charcot's joints) in children. *Clin Pediatr (Phila)* 1975;14:647-653.

31. Peitzman SJ, Miller JL, Ortega L, Schumacher HR, Fernandez PC, et al: Charcot arthropathy secondary to amyloid neuropathy. *JAMA* 1976;235:1345-1347.

32. Hensinger RN, MacEwen GD: Spinal deformity associated with heritable neurological conditions: Spinal muscular atrophy, Friedreich's ataxia, familial dysautonomaia, and Charcot-Marie-Tooth disease. *J Bone Joint Surg Am* 1976;58:13-24.

33. Alpert SW, Koval KJ, Zuckerman JD: Neuropathic arthropathy: Review of current knowledge. *J Am Acad Orthop Surg* 1996;4:100-108.

34. Brower AC, Allman RM: Pathogenesis of the neuropathic joint: Neurotraumatic versus neurovascular. *Radiology* 1981;139:349-354.

35. Guidera KJ, Multhopp H, Ganey T, Ogden JA: Orthopaedic manifestations in congenitally insensate patients. *J Pediatr Orthop* 1990;10:514-521.

36. Houlden H, Blake J, Reilly MM: Hereditary sensory neuropathies. *Curr Opin Neurol* 2004;17:569-577.

37. Gamble JG, Bella J, Rinsky LA, Glader B: Arthropathy of the ankle in hemophilia. *J Bone Joint Surg Br* 1991;73:1008-1015.

38. Jeffcoate WJ: Abnormalities of vasomotor regulation in the pathogenesis of the acute Charcot foot of diabetes mellitus. *Int J Low Extrem Wounds* 2005;4:133-137.

39. Pettersson H, Ahlberg A, Nilsson IM: A radiological classification of hemophilic arthropathy. *Clin Orthop Relat Res* 1980;149:153-159.

40. Raffini L, Manno C: Modern management of haemophilic arthropathy. *Br J Haematol* 2007;136:777-787.

41. Ribbans WJ, Phillips AM: Hemophilic ankle arthropathy. *Clin Orthop Relat Res* 1996;328:39-45.

42. Lanska DJ, Goetz CG: Romberg's sign: Development, adoption, and adaptation in the 19th century. *Neurology* 2000;55:1201-1206.

43. Anand N, Levine DB, Burke S, Bansal M: Neuropathic spinal arthropathy in Charcot-Marie-Tooth

disease: A case report. *J Bone Joint Surg Am* 1997;79:1235-1239.

44. Auer-Grumbach M, De Jonghe P, Vorhoeven K, et al: Autosomal dominant inherited neuropathies with prominent sensory loss and mutilations: A review. *Arch Neurol* 2003;60:329-334.

45. Axelrod FB: Familial dysautonomia. *Muscle Nerve* 2004;29:352-363.

46. Bar-On E, Floman Y, Sagiv S, Katz K, Pollak RD, Maayan C: Orthopaedic manifestations of familial dysautonomia: A review of one hundred and thirty-six cases. *J Bone Joint Surg Am* 2000;82:1563-1570.

47. Bar-On E, Weigl D, Parvari R, Katz K, Weitz R, Steinberg T: Congenital insensitivity to pain: Orthopaedic manifestations. *J Bone Joint Surg Br* 2002;84:252-257.

48. Bertorini T, Narayanaswami P, Rashed H: Charcot-Marie-Tooth disease (hereditary motor sensory neuropathies) and hereditary sensory and autonomic neuropathies. *Neurologist* 2004;10:327-337.

49. Bertorini T, Narayanaswami P, Rashed H: Charcot-Marie-Tooth disease (hereditary motor sensory neuropathies) and hereditary sensory and autonomic neuropathies. *Neurologist* 2004;10:327-337.

50. Chance PF: Genetic evaluation of inherited motor/sensory neuropathy. *Suppl Clin Neurophysiol* 2004;57:228-242.

51. Craigen MA, Clarke NM: Familial congenital pseudoarthrosis of the ulna. *J Hand Surg Br* 1995;20:331-332.

52. Daher YH, Lonstein JE, Winder RB, Bradford DS: Spinal deformities in patients with Charcot-Marie-Tooth disease: A review of 12 patients. *Clin Orthop Relat Res* 1986;202:219-222.

53. Greider TD: Orthopedic aspects of congenital insensitivity to pain. *Clin Orthop Relat Res* 1983;172:177-185.

54. Gwathmey FW, House JH: Clinical manifestations of congenital insensitivity of the hand and classification of syndromes. *J Hand Surg Am* 1984;9:863-869.

55. Jones EA, Manaster BJ, May DA, Disler DG: Neuropathic osteoarthropathy: Diagnostic dilemmas and differential diagnosis. *Radiographics* 2000;20:S279-S293.

56. Karmani S, Shedden R, De Sousa C: Orthopaedic manifestations of congenital insensitivity to pain. *J R Soc Med* 2001;94:139-140.

57. Laura M, Reilly MM: Hereditary neuropathies. *Adv Clin Neurosci Rehabil* 2007;7:22-25.

58. Sly ME, Lupski JR, Chance PF, et al: Hereditary motor and sensory neuropathies: An overview of clinical, genetic electrophysiologic and pathologic features, in Dyck PJ, Thomas PK (eds): *Peripheral Neuropathy*, ed 4. Philadelphia, PA, Saunders, 2005, pp 1623-1658.

59. Verpoorten N, De Jonghe F, Timmerman V: Disease mechanisms in hereditary sensory and autonomic neuropathies. *Neurobiol Dis* 2006;21:247-255.

60. Allman RM, Brower AC, Kotlyarov EB: Neuropathic bone and joint disease. *Radiol Clin North Am* 1988;26:1373-1381.

61. Baumhauer JF, O'Keefe RJ, Schon LC, Pinzur MS: Cytokine-induced osteoclastic bone resorption in charcot arthropathy: An immunohistochemical study. *Foot Ankle Int* 2006;27:797-800.

62. Frykberg RG, Kozak GP: The diabetic Charcot foot, in Kozak GP, Campbell DR, Frykberg RG, Havershaw GM (eds): *Management of Diabetic Foot Problems*, ed 2. Philadelphia, PA, Saunders 1995, pp 88-97.

63. Klenerman L: The Charcot joint in diabetes. *Diabet Med* 1996;13:S52-S54.

64. Bibel M, Barde YA: Neurotrophins: Ky regulators of cell fate and cell shape in the vertebrate nervous system. *Genes Dev* 2000;14:2919-2937.

65. Nagasako EM, Oaklander AL, Dworkin RH: Congenital insensitivity to pain: An update. *Pain* 2003;101:213-219.

66. Bergoffen J, Trofatter J, Pericak-Vance MA, Haines JL, Chance PF, Fischbeck KH: Linkage location of X-linked Charcot-Marie-Tooth disease. *Am J Hum Genet* 1993;52:312-318.

67. Minde J, Toolanen G, Andersson T, et al: Familial insensitivity to pain (HSAN V) and a mutation in the NGFB gene: A neurophysiological and pathological study. *Muscle Nerve* 2004;30:752-760.

68. Mankin HJ: Syphilis and its effect on bones and joints, in *Pathophysiology of Orthopaedic Diseases*. Rosemont, IL, American Academy of Orthopaedic Surgeons, 2006, pp 15-22.

69. Scheck DN, Hook EW III: Neurosyphilis. *Infec Dis Clin North Am* 1994;8:769-795.

70. Jeffcoate W, Lima J, Nobrega L: The Charcot foot. *Diabet Med* 2000;17:253-258.

71. Koop I, Loreck D, Krause A: Diabetic neuropathic arthropathy. *Arthritis Rheum* 1999;42:806.

72. Lee L, Blume PA, Sumpio B: Charcot joint disease in diabetes mellitus. *Ann Vasc Surg* 2003;17:571-580.

73. Pinzur MS: Benchmark analysis of diabetic patients with neuropathic (Charcot) foot deformity. *Foot Ankle Int* 1999;20:564-567.

74. Schon LC, Easley ME, Weinfeld SB: Charcot neuroarthropathy of the foot and ankle. *Clin Orthop Relat Res* 1998;349:116-131.

75. Sommer TC, Lee TH: Charcot foot: The diagnostic dilemma. *Am Fam Physician* 2001;64:1591-1598.

76. Veves A, Akbari CM, Primavera J, et al: Endothelial dysfunction and the expression of endothelial nitric oxide synthetase in diabetic neuropathy, vascular disease, and foot ulceration. *Diabetes* 1998;47:457-463.

77. Campbell CC, Koris MJ: Etiologies of shoulder pain in cervical spinal cord injury. *Clin Orthop Relat Res* 1996;322:140-145.

78. Culling J, Gibberd FB: Charcot's disease of the spine. *Proc R Soc Med* 1974;67:1026-1027.

79. Harrison MJ, Sacher M, Rosenblum BR, Rothman AS: Spinal Charcot arthropathy. *Neurosurgery* 1991;28:273-277.

80. Kapila A, Lines M: Neuropathic spinal arthopathy: CT and MR findings. *J Comput Assist Tomogr* 1987;11:736-739.

81. Nagarkatti DG, Banta JV, Thomson JD: Charcot arthropathy in spina bifida. *J Pediatr Orthop* 2000;20:82-87.

82. Standaert C, Cardenas DD, Anderson P: Charcot spine as a late complication of traumatic spinal

cord injury. *Arch Phys Med Rehabil* 1997;78:221-225.

83. Tsirikos AI, Haddo O, Noordeen HH: Spinal manifestations in a patient with congenital insensitivity to pain. *J Spinal Disord Tech* 2004;17:326-330.

84. Brodbelt AR, Stoodley MA: Post-traumatic syringomyelia: A review. *J Clin Neurosci* 2003;10:401-408.

85. Browne RF, Murphy SM, Torreggiani WC, Munk PL: Musculoskeletal case 29: Neuropathic shoulder secondary to syringomyelia. *Can J Surg* 2003;46:309-310.

86. Jones J, Wolf S: Neuropathic shoulder arthropathy (Charcot joint) associated with syringomyelia. *Neurology* 1998;50:825-827.

87. Klekamp J: The pathophysiology of syringomyelia: Historical overview and current concept. *Acta Neurochir (Wien)* 2002;144:649-664.

88. Nozawa S, Miyamoto K, Nishimoto H, Sakaguchi Y, Hosoe H, Shimizu K: Charcot joint in the elbow associated with syringomyelia. *Orthopedics* 2003;26:731-732.

89. Citron ND, Paterson FW, Jackson AM: Neuropathic osteonecrosis of the lateral femoral condyle in childhood: A report of four cases. *J Bone Joint Surg Br* 1986;68:96-99.

90. Cullen AB, Ofluoglu O, Donthineni R: Neuropathic arthropathy of the shoulder (Charcot shoulder). *MedGenMed* 2005;7:29.

91. Deirmengian CA, Lee SG, Jupiter JB: Neuropathic arthropathy of the elbow: A report of five cases. *J Bone Joint Surg Am* 2001;83:839-844.

92. Kwon YW, Morrey BF: Neuropathic elbow arthropathy: A review of six cases. *J Shoulder Elbow Surg* 2006;15:378-382.

93. Horibe S, Tada K, Nagano J: Neuroarthropathy of the foot in leprosy. *J Bone Joint Surg Br* 1988;70:481-485.

94. Gilbert MS, Radomisli TE: Therapeutic options in the management of hemophilic synovitis. *Clin Orthop Relat Res* 1997;343:88-92.

95. Joseph KN, Bowen JR, MacEwen GD: Unusual orthopaedic manifestations of neurofibromatosis. *Clin Orthop Relat Res* 1992;278:17-28.

96. Lachiewicz PF, Salvati EA, Hely D, Ghelman B: Pathological dislocation of the hip in neurofibromatosis: A case report. *J Bone Joint Surg Am* 1983;65:414-415.

97. Lokiec F, Arbel R, Isakov J, Wientroub S: Neuropathic arthropathy of the knee associated with an intra-articular neurofibroma in a child. *J Bone Joint Surg Br* 1998;80:468-470.

98. Alnfisi N, Yun M, Alavi A: F-18 FDG positron emission tomography to differentiate diabetic osteoarthropathy from septic arthritis. *Clin Nucl Med* 2001;26:638-639.

99. Guis S, Pellissier JF, Arniaud D, et al: Healing of Charcot's joint by pamidronate infusion. *J Rheumatol* 1999;26:1843-1845.

100. Pinzur MS, Shields N, Trepman E, Dawson P, Evans A: Current practice patterns in the treatment of Charcot foot. *Foot Ankle Int* 2000;21:916-920.

101. Selby PL, Young MJ, Boulton AJ: Bisphosphonates: A new treatment for diabetic Charcot neuroarthropathy? *Diabet Med* 1994;11:28-31.

102. Herbst SA: External fixation of Charcot arthropathy. *Foot Ankle Clin* 2004;9:595-609.

103. Kim YH, Kim JS, Oh SW: Total knee arthroplasty in neuropathic arthropathy. *J Bone Joint Surg Br* 2002;84:216-219.

104. Pinzur MS, Sostak J: Surgical stabilization of non-plantigrade Charcot arthropathy of the midfoot. *Am J Orthop* 2007;36:361-365.

105. Simon SR, Tejwani SG, Wilson DL, Santner TJ, Denniston NL: Arthrodesis as an early alternative to nonoperative management of Charcot arthropathy of the diabetic foot. *J Bone Joint Surg Am* 2000;82:939-950.

Chapter 14

Lipomas: Benign Tumors of Fat

Benign tumors of fat, known as lipomas, are the most common form of soft-tissue tumors. These lesions have as their characteristic cell of origin the adipose cell, known as the lipocyte, which has a differentiated spherical or polygonal structure with most of the cytoplasm displaced by lipid droplets. The fat may be white or, much less commonly, brown; in either case, the material fills the cell. The most common entity in the family of lipomatous tumors is the standard lipoma. However, on review of the literature, it is apparent that many other forms of benign lipomatous tumors exist. These include angiolipoma, myolipoma, chondroid lipoma, spindle-cell lipoma, intraosseous lipoma, and lipoblastoma. In addition, there are four other rare lipomatous tumors that have unusual presentations—lipoma arborescens in the knee joint (Hoffa's disease), "horse collar" lipomatosis (Madelung's disease), adiposis dolorosa (Dercum's disease, known as painful fat), and tumors containing brown fat (hibernoma). Although all these lipomatous lesions are benign, they may cause considerable problems in terms of pressure on viscera, nerves, or vascular structures, along with deformity and disability of body parts, fractures of affected bones, and chronic pain. Another major issue is distinguishing benign lipomatous tumors from liposarcomatous ones, particularly the low-grade malignant lesions.

Pathophysiology and Histology

The majority of the lipomatous lesions arise from and resemble lipocytes, the cells of soft-tissue origin that contain white fat.[1-6] These tissues were first identified and described in 1901 by Shaw.[7] Histologically, the lipocyte cell is large, the cytoplasm is replaced by a single large droplet of fat, and the nucleus is small and often eccentrically located.[4-6] Variations in appearance may occur related to the type of tumor[1-6,8] (Figure 1). Angiolipomas have small vascular structures surrounding the lipocytes, myolipomas are surrounded by small smooth muscle structures, chondroid lipomas include

areas of the tissue that appear to arise from immature cartilage, spindle-cell lipomas are surrounded by irregular bundles of collagen, intraosseous lipomas lie either within the bones or subperiosteally, and lipoblastomas consist of multiple lipocytes in several sites and appear more aggressive in structure. The cells that form hibernomas are similar in structure but the cells contain brown fat.[4,6,9,10] The cells in patients with Hoffa's, Madelung's, or Dercum's diseases are rarely different from those seen in simple lipomas. Lipoblastomas and brown fat tumors appear to arise from lipoblasts, the type of cell that serves as the origin of the malignant liposarcomas.[2,4-6]

Except for lipoblastomas, which may occur in young or even newborn children,[4,5,11-14] lipomas are rare in the first 2 decades of life; most become apparent in patients between age 40 and 60 years.[2,4-6,8] Most gender studies suggest that the lesions are more frequently seen in males than females.[2,4-6] There is no variation in presentation among patients of different ethnic origins with the exception of Madelung's disease, which seems to be more common in people from Mediterranean countries, especially Italy.[4,15]

In terms of genetics, the CHOP gene appears to be involved in adipocytic differentiation.[1,4,6,16] Adiposites and both benign and malignant fatty tumors stain positively for vimentin and less consistently for S100 protein.[6] An antibody to the adipocyte lipid-binding protein p422 has been found to stain lipoblasts, liposarcomas, and brown fat cells and hence, at least in theory, may help to distinguish benign from malignant tumors.[4,6] Cytogenetic abnormalities have been found in 50% to 60% of lipomas. The major subgroups of genetic aberrations identified include 12q13-15, 6p21-23, and deletions from q13.[4,6,16-21]

Of considerable interest is the observation initially made during the Holocaust that patients with lipomas who lost as much as 100 pounds of weight lost their body fat but their lipomas were unchanged. These data

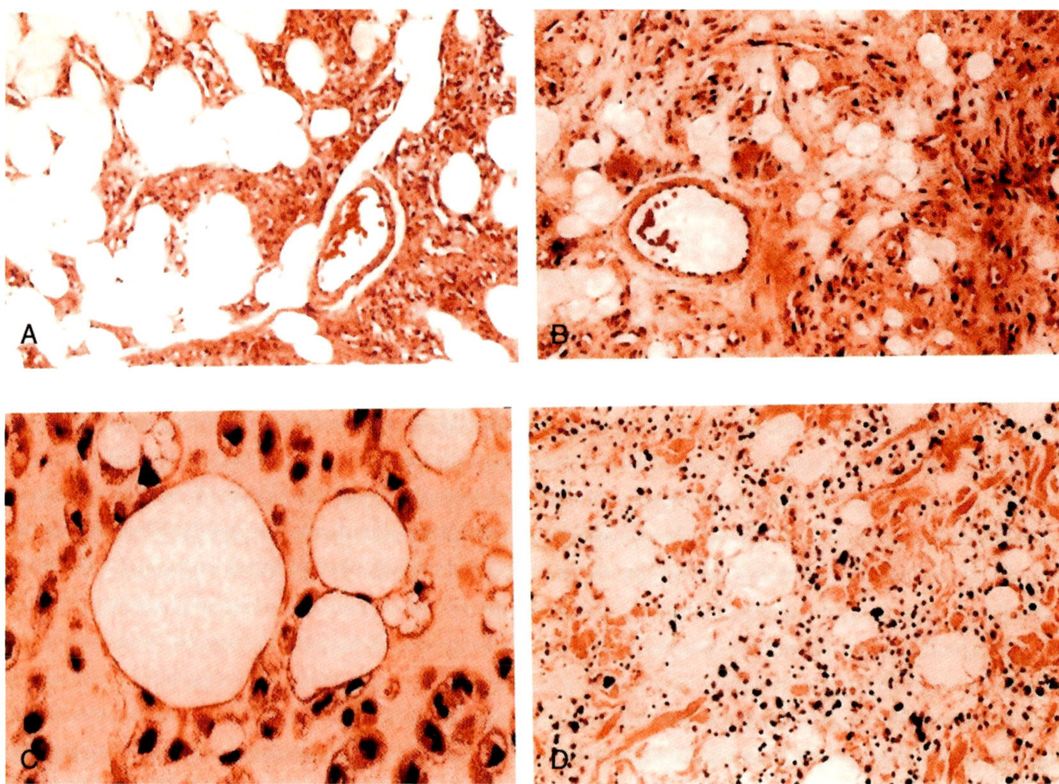

Figure 1
Histologic patterns for lipomatous tumors. **A,** Spindle-cell lipomas are surrounded by irregular bundles of collagen. **B,** Angiolipomas have small vascular structures surrounding the lipocytes. **C,** Chondroid lipomas include areas of the tissue that appear to arise from immature cartilage. **D,** Lipoblastic lesions have collections of fat outside the cells.

suggest that lipomas do not metabolically communicate with body fat.[4,6]

Clinical Presentations of Benign Lipomatous Tissues

Lipoma

Lipomas are the commonest form of soft-tissue neoplasm, estimated at more than 2 cases per 100 population.[2-6,22] They can either be superficial or deep. The *superficial tumors* are subcutaneous; small (usually < 5 cm); and tend to affect the upper back, neck, proximal extremities (especially the shoulder), and abdomen. They commonly occur in the fifth through seventh decades of life and have no ethnic or gender specificity.[2-6,22] The *deep tumors* are often intramuscular and are sometimes called "infiltrating lipomas" (Figure 2). They most frequently occur in patients 30 to 60 years of age and more frequently in males. They most commonly occur in the lower extremity, trunk, and shoulder and are larger than the superficial tumors, ranging up to 20 cm in size[2-6,22] (Figure 3). Both the superficial

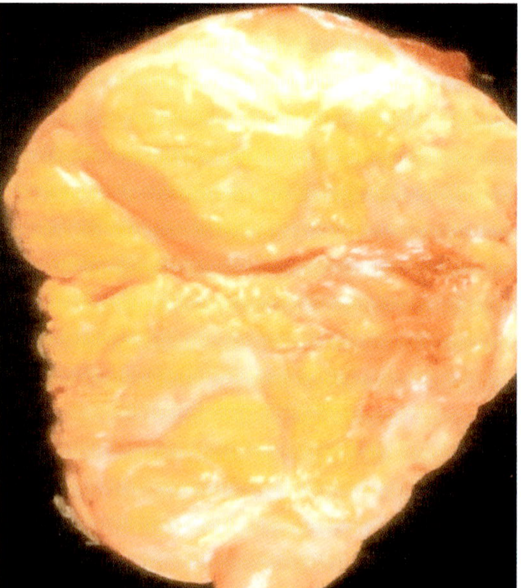

Figure 2
Gross photograph of a lipoma at the time of surgical resection. The tissue is obviously yellow fat.

and the deep lesions may enlarge slowly and, unless the deep lesions cause pressure

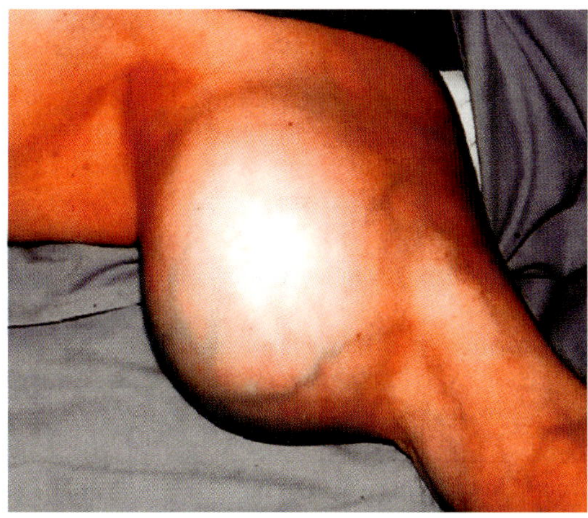

Figure 3
Appearance of a patient's knee with a collection of lipomatous mass in the deep muscular structures. Although it seemed reasonable that this might be a liposarcoma, the lesion was benign.

on nerves or vascular structures, both are relatively asymptomatic.[1,3,4,6,22,23] Both forms of lipomas may be multiple in about 5% to 15% of patients and are thought to occur more frequently in obese patients or diabetic patients[4,6] (Figure 4). Multiple forms of superficial and/or deep lipomas may be a component of some genetic diseases, including such disorders as Bannayan-Zonana syndrome, Cowden disease, Fröhlich syndrome, and Proteus syndrome.[4] In terms of genetics, the major subgroups have been identified as including 12q13-15, 6p21-23, and deletions from q13; these are present in approximately 80% of patients, especially those with familial disease.[1,4,6,16,19,24-26] A recently described entity, consisting of plantar lipomatosis in children with unusual facies and developmental delay, is known as the Pierpont syndrome.[27,28] In 1952, Sternberg[29] reported on a liposarcoma arising in a benign lipoma; however the key problem is distinguishing benign lipomas from low-grade liposarcomas. This difficulty in differentiating them may have been the explanation.[2,5,16,19,22,25,30-37]

Angiolipoma

The tumor known as angiolipoma was first described in 1960 by Howard and Helwig.[38] It is a benign lesion that appears to affect males more frequently than females, and most patients first notice their lesions in the second or third decade of life.[4-6,39,40] Angio-

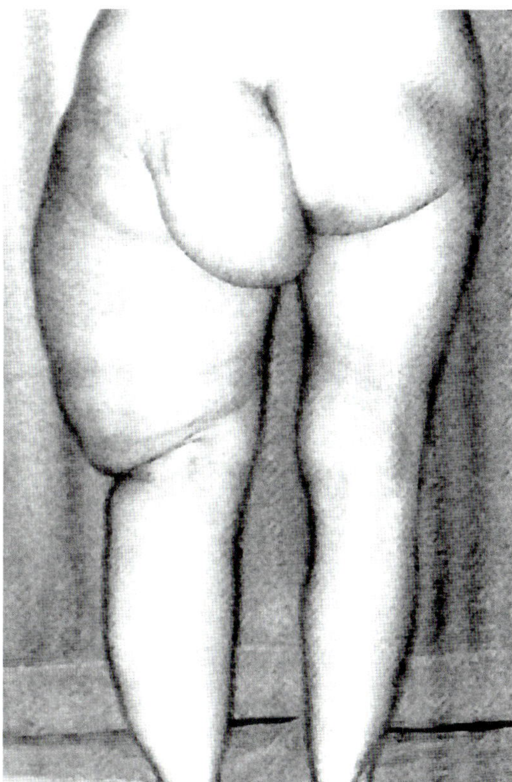

Figure 4
Photograph of a patient with collections of adipose tissue in the entire posterior aspect of the lower extremity. The diagnosis was believed to be Dercum's disease.

lipomatous tumors are quite common in dogs and less common in cats.[41] The lesions occur most frequently in the forearm, the trunk, or the upper arm in humans, and more than 70% of patients are found to have multiple lesions.[2,4,6,39] The tumors are smaller than lipomas (most are < 2 cm) but are painful on palpation. Histologically, the lesions are quite distinct in that the fat cells are surrounded by vascular channels, often containing thrombi.[2,6,39] Mast cells not ordinarily seen in standard lipomas are often present.[4] Genetic abnormalities have been reported for these lesions, which differ somewhat from those for lipomas, but the tumors are believed to be completely benign.[4,6,26,39,42] Surgical excision is ordinarily curative, but several recent reports describe spinal lesions that have resulted in a myelopathy.[40,43,44]

Myolipoma

These adipose tumors, originally described in 1993 by Meis and Enzinger,[34] are very unusual. They appear to consist of adipose cells surrounded by smooth muscle fibers.[2,4-6,34] They affect adults most frequently in the fifth to sixth decade of life and are considerably more frequent in females than in males. The lesions are most commonly located in the abdominal cavity, retroperitoneum, and inguinal areas and much less frequently in the subcutaneous tissues of the trunk or extremities.[45] Unlike some of the other adipose tumors, the myolipomas are almost always large, with a median size of 17 cm, and can be found up to 25 cm in size.[4,5,34] Histologically, muscle usually exceeds the fat in the tumors (2:1) and is regularly interspersed, producing a sieve-like appearance. Coarse calcification may be present in the lesions.[4-6,46] The muscle components are strongly positive for actin and desmin, but no genetic abnormality has been consistently identified.[2,6,16,46] The tumors have no record of malignant degeneration potential and do not ordinarily recur after excisional surgery.

Chondroid Lipoma

This rare tumor was first identified in 1986 by Chan and associates,[47] who suggested that it was a malignant lesion. The tumor was subsequently further evaluated by Meis and Enzinger[34] and named a benign chondroid lipoma. The masses are slow-growing and painless and are usually located in the proximal extremities and limb girdles but occasionally in the trunk, head and neck, or hands.[2,48,49] The tumors are small, with a mean size of 4 cm; occur in the fourth or fifth decade of life; and are much more frequent in women. The tumors are encapsulated and consist of nests and cords of lipocytes and lipoblasts in a mixed body of prominent myxoid and hyalinized chondroid matrix.[49] As indicated by Chan's study and others, the tumors may resemble or be classified as myxoid chondrosarcoma and as a result be overtreated. Cytogenetic aberrations with t(11;16)(q13:p12-13) translocations have been reported.[1,19,26,49,50] Once again, despite the tumors' appearance and resemblance to malignant lesions, the tumors do not metastasize and usually do not recur after simple resection.[34]

Spindle-Cell Lipoma and Pleomorphic Lipoma

Although there are some differences between spindle-cell and pleomorphic lipoma, they are thought to very closely resemble one another and probably have the same origin. Spindle-cell lipoma was originally described in 1975 by Enzinger and Harvey,[51] and pleomorphic lipoma in 1981 by Shmookler and Enzinger.[35] Both of these lesions commonly affect patients between 45 and 65 years of age and approximately 90% of the patients are males.[4-6,51] Both lesions commonly affect the subcutaneous tissues of the posterior neck, shoulder, and back, but may also occur in the oral cavity, larynx, breast, bronchus, or extremities.[4,6,52] Deep lesions are uncommon and are rarely multiple, although a recent study by Fanburg-Smith and associates[53] reported on 18 patients, all of whom had multiple lesions, and 7 of these proved to be familial. The lesions are ordinarily asymptomatic and subcutaneous in location, with most of them less than 5 cm in size. Pathologic examination shows fat cells surrounded by parallel bundles of bland spindle cells and rope-like collagen bundles. Mast cells, lymphocytes, myxoid tissue, and valvular elements are often present.[2,54] In the pleomorphic variant, multinucleated giant cells with radially arranged nuclei are often present. The cytogenetic character of both of these lesions shows a partial loss of chromosomes 13 or 16.[3,4,6,16,20,25,26] Although these tumors resemble sclerosing liposarcomas, they remain benign, do not metastasize, and rarely display a local recurrence after surgical resection.[6,37]

Lipoblastoma

This disorder is also rarely encountered. In 1926, Jaffe[32] introduced the term lipoblastoma to describe an atypical lipomatous tissue of the groin. In 1958, Vellios and associates[14] introduced the term lipoblastomatosis and Chung and Enzinger[11] subsequently described the lesions as benign lipoblastoma or benign lipoblastomatosis to emphasize the nonmalignant nature of the disorder. Lipoblastomas are benign tumors of white fat that occur in infancy or early childhood.[4,6,10,13,55] Males are much more frequently affected than females.[4,6] The lesions principally occur in the superficial or subcutaneous soft tissue of the extremities, while the trunk, neck, and retroperitoneum are less commonly affected.[12,13,55] Children may be ill with respiratory symptoms, fever, and intermittent airway obstructions depending on the number and site of the lesions.[4,12,55,56] Histologic studies show the lipoblastoma is often encapsulated, while tumors in patients with lipoblastomatosis lack a capsule and tend to be infiltrative.[4,6,12,56] Most of the lesions have a plexiform vascular network. The cytogenetic abnormalities include deletions and rearrangements in 8q11-13.[1,6,18,24] Surgical treatment is only successful if the resection margins are wide. The recurrence rate is high, particularly for patients with lipoblastomatosis.[6,12,13,55]

Hibernoma

Hibernomas are rare tumors that contain brown fat (Figure 5). Merkel is credited with first describing the lesion in 1906, naming it pseudolipoma,[4] but in 1914, Gery[57] introduced the term hibernoma, because the brown fat resembled that seen in hibernating animals. In 1923, Rasmussen[58] pointed out that brown fat also occurs in animals that do not hibernate, including humans, in whom the material has been identified in the periscapular region, neck, axilla, shoulder, thorax, retroperitoneum, and less commonly, the thigh. Hibernomas are slowly growing and painless.[4,6,9,10,59] They are generally located in the subcutaneous tissue and are warm to touch, related to hypervascularity.[4] They appear to be more frequent in patients in the third or fourth decade of life, and both males and females seem to be equally affected.[9,10,59] The pathology is quite distinctive. The lesions measure 5 to 10 cm and are well demarcated, encapsulated, soft, and rubbery. Unlike lipomas, which are quite white, these lesions are brown or brownish-yellow. Histologically, they appear lobulated and contain multivacuolar adipocytes and brown cells with a granular eosinophilic cytoplasm.[4-6,9,10,59] They may display myxoid or spindle-cell characteristics. Cytogenetic abnormalities have been identified as occurring in the long arm of chromosome 11 (11q13-21) and 10(10q22).[4,60] Tumors are usually S100 positive and CD34 negative.[6] There are no reports of local recurrences or metastases from lesions clearly identified as hibernomas, but they do bear a close resemblance to well-differentiated liposarcomas, and it is important to be certain on the basis of imaging studies and histology that they are truly hibernomas.[2,4,59]

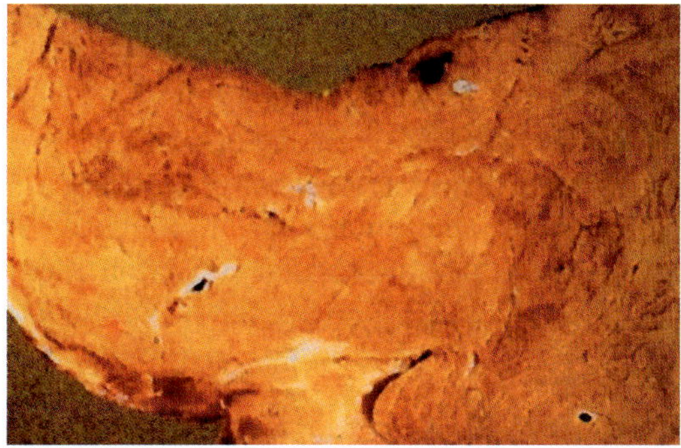

Figure 5
Gross photograph of a rare tumor known as a hibernoma. Note the brownish coloration.

Intraosseous and Subperiosteal Lipomas

Bones of adults ordinarily contain fat in the form of lipocytes but, although uncommon, lipomas of neoplastic origin may occur within or on the surface of bones.[61] The entity is a true tumor, not a response to another type of lesion, and should not be confused with other benign lesions such as aneurysmal bone cyst, unicameral bone cyst, giant cell tumor, enchondroma, or others that have similar appearances on standard radiographic imaging.[61] Patients may be almost any age (they range in the literature from 5 to 85 years of age).[61-64] Males are slightly more commonly affected. Pain is common at the site, possibly related to small pathologic fractures, arthritic changes in an adjacent joint, or ischemic alterations in the bone. The lesions may appear almost anywhere in the skeleton, but the most common sites are the proximal femur, ilium, tibia, fibula, and especially the calcaneus.[61,64-68] The lesions are almost always intramedullary but occasionally cause cortical erosion.[4,61,62,66] Grossly, the lesions show white fat within the medullary cavity, with thinning of the cortex and sometimes small pathologic fractures.[4,61] James Milgram[61] performed a definitive review in 1988 and classified the lesions based on their structure. Lesions with only fat are called Milgram stage 1, while some of the lesions have areas of fat necrosis (Milgram stage 2), which sometimes leads to cystic areas and irregular calcification within the tumor (Milgram stage 3). These changes make the imaging and pathologic diagnosis more difficult as the tumors may resemble other lesions.[4,6,61] Histologic studies show the lipocytes with altered trabecular architecture, fibrous areas, osteonecrotic foci, and sometimes irregular tiny islands of calcification.[4,61,62,66] The cortices are thinned from the inside for the intraosseous lesion and from the outside for the subperiosteal lesion. One of the key diagnostic methods is special imaging studies that can often identify the fat, the necrosis, the calcific material, and the alteration in bone contour.[61,62,64,65] The periosteal lipoma was first described in 1836 by Seering[69] and subsequently better defined in 1888 by Power.[70] The most common sites of origin of these very uncommon lesions are the proximal femur and the radius, but they have also been found in the tibia, humerus, scapula, clavicle, ribs, pelvis, skull, and bones of the hands and feet.[4,47,71,72] Patients range in age from 40 to 60 years and usually present with a slowly growing tender mass that is fixed to the underlying bone. Sciatic, femoral, and radial nerve problems are commonly seen in these patients.[4,47,71,72] The tumors are clearly lipomatous on histologic examination, but they are closely attached to the underlying bone and show cartilaginous, osteoid, or fibrous membranes, which help the tumors to adhere to the bone. Recent genetic studies have demonstrated a 3;12 translocation for these lesions, which is similar to that found in some lipomas.[1,4,16,17,20]

Madelung's Disease

Madelung's disease, otherwise known as the "horse collar syndrome," was first reported in 1846 by Benjamin Brodie,[73] but Otto Madelung[74] extensively described a series of patients in 1888. Launois and Bensaude[75] reported 65 cases in 1889, and the disorder is sometimes known by their names as well. The disorder appears to be more frequent in individuals from the Mediterranean area, especially Italy, and occurs much more frequently in middle-aged males.[4,15,76] Familial disorders can occur, and it has been suggested that the lesions are transmitted as autosomal dominant. The genetic error for some cases appears to consist of a mutation in MERRF (A85446).[77,78] Alcoholism has been reported as a characteristic of the disease, as have gout, hyperlipidemia, and diabetes.[79] The disease consists of a painless progressive deposition of fat in the region of the neck, upper trunk, arms, and cheeks that ultimately produces an enormous and deforming increase in the size of the neck known as "lipoma annulare colli."[4,15,76] The fatty masses are not only subcutaneous, but intramuscular as well, markedly impairing cervical function. Patients have difficulty moving their head and neck and frequently have speaking, hearing, and respiratory difficulties.[17,76] If the lesions enter the chest, cardiac and pulmonary difficulties can be life-threatening.[4,6,17,76] Ultimately, both sensory and motor deficits may develop, and malignant tumors have been reported to occur in these patients.[80] Similar changes in the face, scalp, shoulders, and chest wall have been reported in small numbers of patients; all of these are markedly deforming.[4,6]

Adiposis Dolorosa (Dercum's Disease)

This rare disorder was first described in 1892 by Francis Dercum.[81] The disease consists of a collection of small subcutaneous lipomas in multiple sites that are associated with pain and sometimes marked tenderness, a feature that makes this syndrome different from all other lipomatous disorders, almost all of which are painless.[2,4,6,82-84] The disease occurs principally in obese postmenopausal women and is thought to be autosomal dominant.[85] The major genetic finding in some of the patients is the presence of MERRF, harboring the 8344t mutation.[24,78] Patients with Dercum's disease often have lipid and endocrine diseases, but in addition appear to have psychiatric problems, consisting of emotional instability, sleep disturbances, epilepsy, depression, and dementia.[2,4,6,82-84]

Lipoma Arborescens (Hoffa's Disease)

This is an unusual disorder first described in 1904 by Albert Hoffa.[86] The disease consists of collections of lipomatous fat with inflammatory cells located within a joint—most commonly the knee, but occasionally in other sites, including tendon sheaths.[87-89] The tumors appear in the subsynovial connective tissue and can grow slowly, but are sufficiently extensive so as to produce joint problems including osteoarthritic disorders.[62,87,90] Patients vary considerably in age, and males appear to be affected more frequently than females. The diagnosis is often made by MRI studies of knees for assessment of internal derangements.[91] The lesions of tendon sheaths may grow sufficiently to result in nerve compression or injury.

Imaging Studies

Two of the major issues with lipomatous tumors are distinguishing the tumor from other soft-tissue or even bone neoplasms and the need to be certain that the lesion is not a liposarcoma. These are not easy tasks. In the past, with just careful historical analysis, physical examination, and plain radiographs, it was not simple to do; sometimes errors occurred, that complicated the patient's status and were life-threatening. In recent years, imaging technology has made great strides, and it is now possible using an array of techniques to be fairly secure in the diagnosis and prediction of outcome for lipomatous lesions. Ultrasound studies of a lipoma show that it classically displays a hyperechoic mass.[4,6] The tumor is usually homogeneous, and capsular tissue and fibrous sections of the tumor may be identified but also depend on the nature of the lesion, which can be confusing. CT and MRI have been shown to be of greater diagnostic value[4,6,10,33,37,48,64,72,87,91-93] (Figure 6). CT is useful in assessing the extent of the lesion, the proximity to other structures, and to some extent the homogeneity or heterogeneity of the lesion. MRI will show a characteristic pattern that is, for standard lipomas, essentially identical to subcutaneous fat on both T1 and T2 images.[31,33,93] The capsular tissues are better seen on CT for many lesions, but MRI is very useful for intramuscular and deeply placed lesions. Fat-suppressed T2 and short tau inversion recovery (STIR) sequences are useful in distinguishing benign from malignant tumors and are of particular value for chondroid tumors.[30] Despite the value of MRI with standard superficial lipomas, there are still some problems with distinguishing chondroid lipoma, hibernoma, intraosseous lipoma, and myxoid lipoma from low-grade liposarcoma and other types of soft-tissue or bone lesions. Recently, positron emission tomography (PET) has been very useful in defining the character of the lesion, the extent of the tumor, and also its absence from adjacent lymph nodes. A recent study from Japan describes the use of PDG PET scanning as being of great value in defining the nature of hibernomas and distinguishing them from

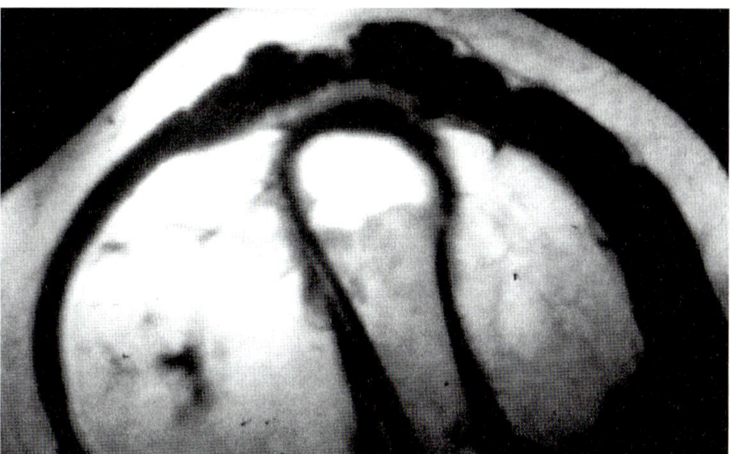

Figure 6

MRI scan of a massive lipoma located in the proximal arm. Fat is bright white on both T1 and T2 images.

liposarcoma.[35,94] In addition, the use of CT-guided needle biopsies of the lesion may be helpful in terms of studying sections that may appear abnormal or possibly liposarcomatous.

Treatment

Small benign asymptomatic solitary lipomas in older individuals should be evaluated by imaging studies but need not be treated except by repeated studies at regular intervals.[4,6] Larger lesions in younger individuals can usually be excised marginally or sometimes widely without difficulty, and generally the recurrence rates for lipomas, lipoblastoma, chondroid lipomas, myxoid lipomas, hibernomas, adiposis dolorosa, and lipoma arborescens are very low.[95] The surgical problems that arise are with attempting resection of Madelung's disease, lipoblastomatosis, and extensive disease in multiple sites. Deep-seated lesions are the most difficult, and at times genetic studies including real-time assessment of MDM2 and CDK4 are useful in distinguishing the tissue obtained from more aggressive tumors.[1,4,6,17,19,92] Liposuction techniques have been helpful with some of the lipomatous lesions.[96] Intraosseous and parosteal lesions sometimes require excision or curettage and packing with bone graft or cement.[61,62] Some patients with extensive disease have been treated with corticosteroids in the past with limited success.[4] Recently interferon alpha-2b has been used with somewhat greater success.[97] Lidocaine injections for patients with Dercum's disease have helped the pain.[98] Patients with Dercum's should also have psychiatric help.

Conclusions and Comments

In earlier times in orthopaedic and surgical oncologic programs, patients with either superficial or deeply placed lipomas were all that were diagnosed and treated. We now face not only these relatively simple disorders, but a host of others that are sometimes difficult to identify and, even more importantly, are hard to distinguish from malignant tumors. Fortunately, these troublesome entities are rare, but they still can cause major difficulties for patients. Lipomatosis in children and chondroid or spindle-cell lipomas in adults, as well as intraosseous lipomas, Dercum's disease, and the disabilities caused by Madelung's disease, represent sometimes very severe problems for patients and their physicians. Because the diseases are so rare, they are not very extensively studied, but it is possible that some forms of chemotherapeutic or genetic treatment should be sought.

References

1. Fletcher CD, Akerman M, Dal Cin P, et al: Correlation between clinicopathological features and karyotype in lipomatous tumors: A report of 178 cases from the Chromosomes and Morphology (CHAMP) Collaborative Study Group. *Am J Pathol* 1996;148:623-630.

2. Kempson R, Fletcher C, Evans H, et al: Lipomatous tumors, in Rosai J, Bethesda MD (eds): *Tumors of the Soft Tissues*, ed 3. Armed Forces Institute of Pathology, 2001, pp 187-238.

3. Miettinen M: Benign fatty tumors, in *Diagnostic Soft Tissue Pathology*. New York, NY, Churchill Livingstone, 2003, pp 207-225.

4. Murphey MD, Carroll JF, Flemming DJ, Pope TL, Gannon FH, Kransdorf MJ: From the archives of the AFIP: Benign musculoskeletal lipomatous lesions. *Radiographics* 2004;24:1433-1466.

5. Weiss SW: Lipomatous tumors. *Monogr Pathol* 1996;38:207-239.

6. Weiss SW, Goldblum JR: Benign lipomatous tumors, in Weiss SW, Goldblum JR (eds): *Enzinger and Weiss's Soft Tissue Tumors*, ed 4. St. Louis, MO, Mosby, 2001, pp 571-640.

7. Shaw HB: A contribution to the study of the morphology of adipose tissue. *J Anat Physiol* 1901;36:1-13.

8. Kransdorf MJ: Benign soft-tissue tumors in a large referral population: Distribution of specific diagnoses by age, sex, and location. *AJR Am J Roentgenol* 1995;164:395-402.

9. Alvine G, Rosenthal H, Murphey M, Huntrakoon M: Hibernoma. *Skeletal Radiol* 1996;25:493-496.

10. Furlong MA, Fanburg-Smith JC, Miettinen M: The morphologic spectrum of hibernoma: A clinicopathologic study of 170 cases. *Am J Surg Pathol* 2001;25:809-814.

11. Chung EB, Enzinger FM: Benign lipoblastomatosis: An analysis of 35 cases. *Cancer* 1973;32:482-492.

12. Collins MH, Chatten J: Lipoblastoma/lipoblastomatosis: A clinicopathologic study of 25 tumors. *Am J Surg Pathol* 1997;21:1131-1137.

13. Jimenez JF: Lipoblastoma in infancy and childhood. *J Surg Oncol* 1986;32:238-244.

14. Vellios F, Baez J, Shumacker HB: Lipoblastomatosis: A tumor of fetal fat different from hibernoma. Report of a case, with observations on the embryogenesis of human adipose tissues. *Am J Pathol* 1958;34:1149-1159.

15. Payne CE: Hereditary Madelung's disease. *J R Soc Med* 2000;93:194-195.

16. Mandahl N, Höglund M, Mertens F, et al: Cytogenetic aberrations in 188 benign and borderline adipose tissue tumors. *Genes Chromosomes Cancer* 1994;9:207-215.

17. Bassett MD, Schuetze SM, Disteche C, et al: Deep-seated, well differentiated lipomatous tumors of the chest wall and extremities: The role of cytogenetics in classification and prognostication. *Cancer* 2005;103:409-416.

18. Brandal P, Bjerkehagen B, Heim S: Rearrangement of chromosomal region 8q11-13 in lipomatous tumours: Correlation with lipoblastoma morphology. *J Pathol* 2006;208:388-394.

19. Dahlén A, Debiec-Rychter M, Pedeutour F, et al: Clustering of deletions on chromosome 13 in benign and low-malignant lipomatous tumors. *Int J Cancer* 2003;103:616-623.

20. Rubin BP, Fletcher CD: The cytogenetics of lipomatous tumours. *Histopathology* 1997;30:507-511.

21. Sandberg AA: Updates on the cytogenetics and molecular genetics of bone and soft tissue tumors: Lipoma. *Cancer Genet Cytogenet* 2004;150:93-115.

22. Rydholm A, Berg NO: Size, site and clinical incidence of lipoma: Factors in the differential diagnosis of lipoma and sarcoma. *Acta Orthop Scand* 1983;54:929-934.

23. Silverman TA, Enzinger FM: Fibrolipomatous hamartoma of nerve: A clinicopathologic analysis of 26 cases. *Am J Surg Pathol* 1985;9:7-14.

24. Gámez J, Playán A, Andreu AL, et al: Familial multiple symmetric lipomatosis associated with the A8344G mutation of mitochondrial DNA. *Neurology* 1998;51:258-260.

25. Skubitz KM, Cheng EY, Clohisy DR, Thompson RC, Skubitz AP: Differential gene expression in liposarcoma, lipoma, and adipose tissue. *Cancer Invest* 2005;23:105-118.

26. Willén H, Akerman M, Dal Cin P, et al: Comparison of chromosomal patterns with clinical features in 165 lipomas: A report of the CHAMP study group. *Cancer Genet Cytogenet* 1998;102:46-49.

27. Oudesluijs GG, Hordijk R, Boon M, Sijens PE, Hennekam RC: Plantar lipomatosis, unusual facies, and developmental delay: Confirmation of the Pierpont syndrome. *Am J Med Genet A* 2005;137:77-80.

28. Pierpont ME, Stewart FJ, Gorlin RJ: Plantar lipomatosis, unusual facial phenotype and developmental delay: A new MCA/MR syndrome. *Am J Med Genet* 1998;75:18-21.

29. Sternberg SS: Liposarcoma arising within a subcutaneous lipoma. *Cancer* 1952;5:975-978.

30. Galant J, Martí-Bonmatí L, Sáez F, Soler R, Alacá-Santaella R, Navarro M: The value of fat-supressed T2 or STIR sequences in distinguishing lipoma from well-differentiated liposarcoma. *Eur Radiol* 2003;13:337-343.

31. Gaskin CM, Helms CA: Lipomas, lipoma variants, and well-differentiated liposarcomas (atypical lipomas): Results of MRI evaluations of 126 consecutive fatty masses. *AJR Am J Roentgenol* 2004;182:733-739.

32. Jaffe RH: Recurrent lipomatous tumors of the groin: Liposarcoma and lipoma psuedomyxomatodes. *AMA Arch Pathol* 1926;1:381-387.

33. Kransdorf MJ, Bancroft LW, Peterson JJ, Murphey MD, Foster WC, Temple HT: Imaging of fatty tumors: Distinction of lipoma and well-differentiated liposarcoma. *Radiology* 2002;224:99-104.

34. Meis JM, Enzinger FM: Chondroid lipoma: A unique tumor simulating liposarcoma and myxoid chondrosarcoma. *Am J Surg Pathol* 1993;17:1103-1112.

35. Shmookler BM, Enzinger FM: Pleomorphic lipoma: A benign tumor simulating liposarcoma. A clinicopathologic analysis of 48 cases. *Cancer* 1981;47:126-133.

36. Suzuki R, Watanabe H, Yanagawa T, et al: PET evaluation of fatty tumors in the extremity: Possibility of using the standardized uptake value (SUV) to differentiate benign tumors from liposarcoma. *Ann Nucl Med* 2005;19:661-670.

37. Yang YJ, Damron TA, Cohen H, Hojnowski L: Distinction of well-differentiated liposarcoma from lipoma in two patients with multiple well-differentiated fatty masses. *Skeletal Radiol* 2001;30:584-589.

38. Howard WR, Helwig EB: Angiolipoma. *Arch Dermatol* 1960;82:924-931.

39. Dixon AY, McGregor DH, Lee SH: Angiolipomas: An ultrastructural and clinicopathological study. *Hum Pathol* 1981;12:739-747.

40. Lin JJ, Lin F: Two entities in angiolipoma: A study of 459 cases of lipoma with review of the literature on infiltrating angiolipoma. *Cancer* 1974;34:720-727.

41. Liggett AD, Frazier KS, Styer EL: Angiolipomatous tumors in dogs and a cat. *Vet Pathol* 2002;39:286-289.

42. Sciot R, Akerman M, Dal Cin P, et al: Cytogenetic analysis of subcutaneous angiolipoma: Further evidence supporting its difference from ordinary pure lipomas. A report of the CHAMP Study Group *Am J Surg Pathol* 1997;21:441-444.

43. Kuroda S, Abe H, Akino M, Iwasaki Y, Nagashima K: Infiltrating spinal angiolipoma causing myelopathy: Case report. *Neurosurgery* 1990;27:315-318.

44. Rabin D, Hon BA, Pelz DM, Ang LC, Lee DH, Duggal N: Infiltrating spinal angiolipoma: A case report and review of the literature. *J Spinal Disord Tech* 2004;17:456-461.

45. Tardío JC, Martín-Fragueiro LM: Angiomyxolipoma (vascular myxolipoma) of subcutaneous tissue. *Am J Dermatopathol* 2004;26:222-224.

46. Meis JM, Enzinger FM: Myolipoma of soft tissue. *Am J Surg Pathol* 1991;15:121-125.

47. Chan JK, Lee KC, Saw D: Extraskeletal chondroma with lipoblast-like cells. *Hum Pathol* 1986;17:1285-1287.

48. Green RA, Cannon SR, Flanagan AM: Chondroid lipoma: Correlation of imaging findings and histopathology of an unusual benign lesion. *Skeletal Radiol* 2004;33:670-673.

49. Thomson TA, Horsman D, Bainbridge TC: Cytogenetics and cytologic features of chondroid lipoma of soft tissue. *Mod Pathol* 1999;12:88-91.

50. Ballaux F, Debiec-Rychter M, De Wever I, Sciot R: Chondroid lipoma is characterized by t(11;16)(q13;p12-13). *Virchows Arch* 2004;444:208-210.

51. Enzinger FM, Harvey DA: Spindle cell lipoma. *Cancer* 1975;36:1852-1859.

52. French CA, Mentzel T, Kutzner H, Fletcher CD: Intradermal spindle cell/pleomorphic lipoma: A distinct subset. *Am J Dermatopathol* 2000;22:496-502.

53. Fanburg-Smith JC, Devaney KO, Miettinen M, Weiss SW: Multiple spindle cell lipomas: A report of 7 familial and 11 nonfamilial cases. *Am J Surg Pathol* 1998;22:40-48.

54. Hawley IC, Krausz T, Evans DJ, Fletcher CD: Spindle cell lipoma: A pseudoangiomatous variant. *Histopathology* 1994;24:565-569.

55. Keskin D, Ezirmik N, Celik H: Familial multiple lipomatosis. *Isr Med Assoc J* 2002;4:1121-1123.

56. Kratz C, Lenard HG, Ruzicka T, Gärtner J: Multiple symmetric lipomatosis: An unusual cause of childhood obesity and mental retardation. *Eur J Paediatr Neurol* 2000;4:63-67.

57. Gery L: Discussions. *Bull Mem Soc Anat (Paris)* 1914;89:111-112.

58. Rasmussen AT: The so-called hibernating gland. *J Morphol* 1923;38:147-205.

59. Lewandowski PJ, Weiner SD: Hibernoma of the medial thigh: Case report and literature review. *Clin Orthop Relat Res* 1996;330:198-201.

60. Mertens F, Rydholm A, Brosjö O, Willén H, Mitelman F, Mandahl N: Hibernomas are characterized by rearrangements of chromosome bands 11q13-21. *Int J Cancer* 1994;58:503-505.

61. Milgram JW: Intraosseous lipomas: A clinicopathologic study of 66 cases. *Clin Orthop Relat Res* 1988;231:277-302.

62. Campbell RS, Grainger AJ, Mangham DC, Beggs I, Teh J, Davies AM: Intraosseous lipoma: Report of 35 new cases and a review of the literature. *Skeletal Radiol* 2003;32:209-222.

63. Chow LT, Lee KC: Intraosseous lipoma: A clinicopathologic study of nine cases. *Am J Surg Pathol* 1992;16:401-410.

64. Hatori M, Hosaka M, Ehara S, Kokubun S: Imaging features of intraosseous lipomas of the calcaneus. *Arch Orthop Trauma Surg* 2001;121:429-432.

65. Hirata M, Kusuzaki K, Hirasawa Y: Eleven cases of intraosseous lipoma of the calcaneus. *Anticancer Res* 2001;21:4099-4103.

66. Leeson MC, Kay D, Smith BS: Intraosseous lipoma. *Clin Orthop Relat Res* 1983;181:186-190.

67. Ragsdale BD, Sweet DE: Intraosseous lipoma. *Am J Surg Pathol* 1993;17:209-211.

68. Weinfeld GD, Yu GV, Good JJ: Intraosseous lipoma of the calcaneus: A review and report of four cases. *J Foot Ankle Surg* 2002;41:398-411.

69. Seering G: Geschichte eines sehr grossen steatoms im hinterhaupte eines 2 und ½ jahrigen kindes. *Mag Ges Heil* 1836:511-514.

70. Power DA: Parosteal lipoma, or congenital fatty tumour, connected with periosteum of femur. *Trans Pathol Soc London* 1888;39:270-272.

71. Henrique A: A high radial neuropathy by parosteal lipoma compression. *J Shoulder Elbow Surg* 2002;11:386-388.

72. Murphey MD, Johnson DL, Bhatia PS: Parosteal lipoma: MR imaging characteristics. *AJR Am J Roentgenol* 1994;162:105-110.

73. Brodie BC: *Lectures Illustrative of Various Subjects in Pathology and Surgery*. London, England, Longman, 1846, pp 275-276.

74. Madelung O: Uber den Fetthals (diffuses lipoma des Halses). *Arch Klin Chir* 1888;37:106-130.

75. Launois P, Bensaude R: De l'adenolipomatose symmetrique. *Soc Med Hosp Paris Bull Mem* 1889;15:298-318.

76. Colella G, Giudice A, Moscariello A: A case of Madelung's disease. *J Oral Maxillofac Surg* 2005;63:1044-1047.

77. Chong P, Vucic S, Hedley-Whyte ET, Dreyer M, Cros D: Multiple symmetric lipomatosis (Madelung's disease) caused by the MERRF (A8344G) mutation: A report of two cases and review of the literature. *J Clin Neuromuscul Dis* 2003;5:1-7.

78. Silvestri G, Ciafaloni E, Santorelli FM, et al: Clinical features associated with the A—> G transition at nucleotide 8344 of mtDNA ("MERRF mutation"). *Neurology* 1993;43:1200-1206.

79. Morelli F, De Benedetto A, Toto P, Tulli A, Feliciani C: Alcoholism is a trigger of multiple symmetric lipomatosis? *J Eur Acad Dermatol Venereol* 2003;17:367-369.

80. Chan ES, Ahuja AT, King AD, Lau WY: Head and neck cancers associated with Madelung's disease. *Ann Surg Oncol* 1999;6:395-397.

81. Dercum F: Three cases of a hitherto unclassified affection resembling in its grosser aspects obesity, but associated with special nervous symptoms: Adiposis dolorosa. *Am J Med Sci* 1892;104:521-535.

82. Amine B, Leguilchard F, Benhamou CL: Dercum's disease (adiposis dolorosa): A new case-report. *Joint Bone Spine* 2004;71:147-149.

83. Bonatus TJ, Alexander AH: Dercum's disease (adiposis dolorosa): A case report and review of the literature. *Clin Orthop Relat Res* 1986;205:251-253.

84. Wortham NC, Tomlinson IP: Dercum's disease. *Skinmed* 2005;4:157-162.

85. Campen R, Mankin H, Louis DN, Hirano M, Maccollin M: Familial occurrence of adiposis dolorosa. *J Am Acad Dermatol* 2001;44:132-136.

86. Hoffa A: Influence of adipose tissue with regard to the pathology of the knee joint. *JAMA* 1904;43:795-796.

87. Doyle AJ, Miller MV, French JG: Lipoma arborescens in the bicipital bursa of the elbow: MRI findings in two cases. *Skeletal Radiol* 2002;31:656-660.

88. Hallel T, Lew S, Bansal M: Villous lipomatous proliferation of the synovial membrane (lipoma arborescens). *J Bone Joint Surg Am* 1988;70:264-270.

89. Kim RS, Song JS, Park SW, et al: Lipoma arborescens of the knee. *Arthroscopy* 2004;20:e95-e99.

90. Hubscher O, Costanza E, Elsner B: Chronic monoarthritis due to lipoma arborescens. *J Rheumatol* 1990;17:861-862.

91. Vilanova JC, Barceló J, Villalón M, Aldomà J, Delgado E, Zapater I: MR imaging of lipoma arborescens and the associated lesions. *Skeletal Radiol* 2003;32:504-509.

92. Einarsdóttir H, Skoog L, Söderlund V, Bauer HC: Accuracy of cytology for diagnosis of lipomatous tumors: Comparison with magnetic resonance and computed tomography findings in 175 cases. *Acta Radiol* 2004;45:840-846.

93. Logan PM, Janzen DL, O'Connell JX, Munk PL, Connell DG: Chondroid lipoma: MRI appearances with clinical and histologic correlation. *Skeletal Radiol* 1996;25:592-595.

94. Tsuchiya T, Osanai T, Ishikawa A, Kato N, Watanabe Y, Ogino T: Hibernomas show intense accumulation of FDG positron emission tomography. *J Comput Assist Tomogr* 2006;30:333-336.

95. Rozental TD, Khoury LD, Donthineni-Rao R, Lackman RD: Atypical lipomatous masses of the extremities: Outcome of surgical treatment. *Clin Orthop Relat Res* 2002;398:203-211.

96. Al-basti HA, El-Khatib HA: The use of suction-assisted surgical extraction of moderate and large lipomas: Long-term follow-up. *Aesthetic Plast Surg* 2002;26:114-117.

97. Gonciarz Z, Mazur W, Hartleb J, et al: Interferon alfa-2b induced long-term relief of pain in two patients with adiposis dolorosa and chronic hepatitis C. *J Hepatol* 1997;27:1141.

98. Juhlin L: Long-standing pain relief of adiposis dolorosa (Dercum's disease) after intravenous infusion of lidocaine. *J Am Acad Dermatol* 1986;15:383-385.

Chapter 15

Achondroplasia

Achondroplasia is a frequently encountered form of dwarfism—probably the commonest form in the world. It is well known in the animal kingdom, and it is believed that dachshund and Pekinese dogs, Dexter cattle, and some rabbit species offer examples of the same disease.

Patients with achondroplasia have short stature, rhizomelic limb shortening, frontal bossing, midface hypoplasia, lumbar lordosis, elbow limitation, and trident hand deformities. The disorder is transmitted as an autosomal dominant genetic error with frequent mutations; thus it is frequent in siblings and believed to occur in the United States at a rate of 1 in every 8,000 to 10,000 births. Although the disease markedly affects epiphyseal growth, the other features, including abnormalities in the cranium, spinal deformities, sleep problems, and obesity, are the principal medical issues for affected patients. Intelligence is generally normal and basic physical capacities are only infrequently impaired. Psychological and sociologic issues are sometimes a major problem in affected individuals who, because of their appearance, find it difficult to enjoy some of life's important functions and social activities.

Nomenclature and History

Many diseases are associated with short stature, including achondrogenesis, camptomelic dwarfism, diastrophic dwarfism, Kniest dwarfism, metatropic dwarfism, thanatophoric dwarfism, hypochondroplasia, and others,[1-3] but none of these is as frequent or as well defined as achondroplasia. Achondroplasia itself has many synonyms, including Kaufmann syndrome, Parrot syndrome, Parrot-Kaufmann syndrome, chondrodysplasia foetalis, chondrodystrophic dwarfism, chondrogenesis imperfecta, fetal achondroplasia, and osteochondrodystrophia foetalis.[1-6]

Persons of short stature are known as "dwarfs," a term of Saxon origin (dwerg, dweorg), but Aristotle introduced the term "pygmy" because the short people were thought to be descendents of Pygmaeus, the son of Dorus (the term pygmy now only applies to some African tribes and is not used for patients with achondroplasia). Ancient Egyptians documented the presence of dwarfs in almost every facet of life.[7] Dwarfs were employed in all capacities; several were important contributors to their governments, including Seneb, Khnumhotpe, and Djeder. There were two dwarf gods in Egypt: Ptah, who was committed and involved in regeneration; and Bes, who was a protector of women, children, and sexuality.[7] In ancient Rome, all emperors had dwarfs as colleagues and associates. Augustus had Conopas and Andromeda, both of whom were supportive and essential to his governmental activities. In ancient Norse culture, Brok and Sindre were described as creating magical objects for the gods. Other famous dwarfs included Attila the Hun; Procopius (a famous historian); Gregory of Tours; King Charles III of Naples; Archbishop Godeau of Grasse; Richard Gibson, a well-known English painter; and Joseph Boruwlaski, a Polish scholar of the 18th century. In more recent times, they include Charles Stratton, the famous circus performer known as General Tom Thumb; Michael Dunn, an actor in "Wild, Wild West"; Verne Troyer, who played the role of "Mini-Me" in the Austin Power movies' and Tom Shakespeare, a current British writer of considerable renown.[1-7]

The first clinical description of the syndrome of achondroplasia was by the Frenchman Parrot[8] in 1878; in 1892, another report was published in Germany by Kaufmann.[9] Both of them described children who were born with large heads and facial deformities and proximally short (rhizomelic) extremities. The children had difficulty in the infant years but when they reached 2 or 3 years of age they seemed to do well and had no intellectual impairment.[1,3,9,10] Subsequent reports by many authors defined limb abnormalities, problems with breathing, abnormal appearance of the hands, spinal deformities, and disabilities.[1,2,4,5,11-18] It was

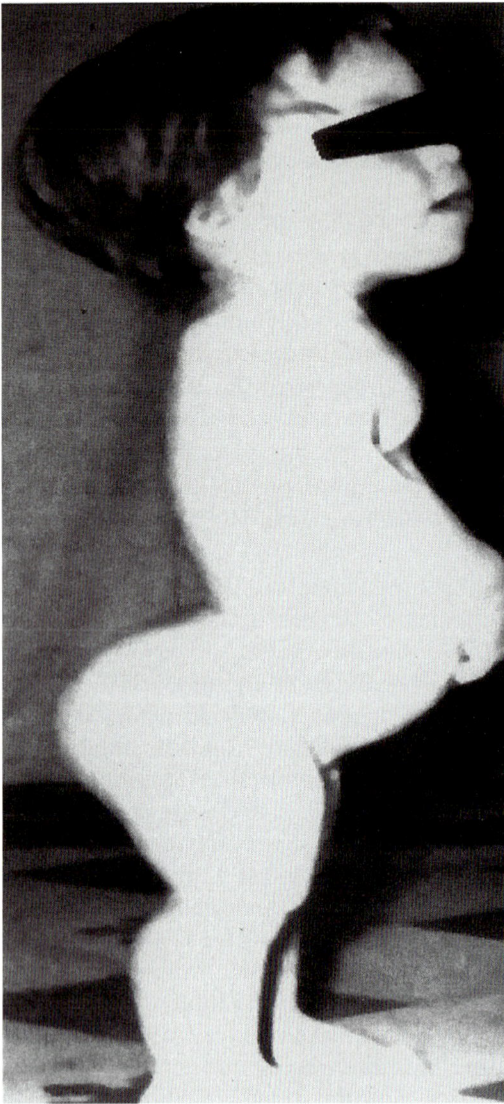

Figure 1
Skeletal structure of a patient with achondroplasia. Note the short and somewhat wider bones, the bowing deformities, and changes in the calvarium.

Ponseti and associates[19,20] who established the biologic changes and histologic abnormalities in the epiphyseal cartilage, which appear to be the cause of the problem; shortly thereafter, several investigators defined the autosomal dominance of the genetic transmission of the disease.[1,3,18-20]

Genetic Causation

Recent studies of the gene structure in patients with achondroplasia strongly support the concept that the error lies with a mutation in the fibroblast growth factor receptor 3 (FGFR3).[21-26] FGFR3 is a membrane-spanning tyrosine kinase receptor with three domains that exert a negative control on growth of connective tissue components. If this material is activated by introducing a substitution, the result is a slowing and alteration in normal epiphyseal and bone growth. In 98% of patients with achondroplasia, the mutation that acts in the system is a G380R substitution resulting from a G to R (glycine to arginine) point mutation at nucleotide 1138. This action enhances the FGFR3 negative function, which interferes with epiphyseal cartilage growth and function. The result is the often markedly altered body structure of the child with achondroplasia. In another 2% of patients, the G380R substitution results from a G to C (glycine to cysteine) point mutation, but there does not appear to be a significant difference in the clinical outcome for the two errors.[21-26] It should be noted that there is another entity known as pseudoachondroplasia, with similar genetic errors but with less severe changes in the bones and cartilage.[1,3,4,27,28]

Pathologic Findings

The genetic error described above results in an altered structure for cartilage, which in the infant and child is responsible for endochondral ossification and especially epiphyseal growth and development.[1-3,19,20,29-31] In patients with achondroplasia, epiphyseal growth is retarded, which results in short and moderately deformed bones (Figure 1). Failure to normally ossify the epiphysis results in an increase in the width of the distal and proximal portions of the long bones and also structural changes to the hands and feet (Figure 2 and 3). In the skull, because the base is developed from cartilage, that portion is smaller than normal and markedly limits the size of the sphenoid and a portion of the occipital bone, which surrounds the foramen magnum.[1-3,19,30] The remainder of the bone is not preformed out of cartilage and hence enlarges even more than normally to cover the underlying neural components. All of these changes result in short stature, rhizomelic shortening and wide epiphyses of the long bones, frontal bossing, midface hypoplasia, narrowing of the foramen magnum, spinal stenosis, diminished size of the innominate bone, thickening of the ribs, lumbar lordosis, thoracic kyphosis, elbow limitation, and trident hand

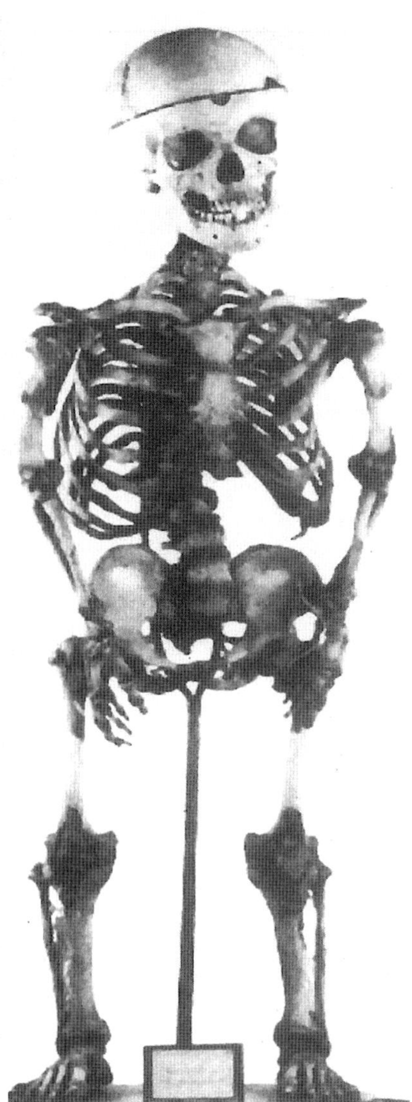

Figure 2
A child with achondroplasia. Note the spinal deformity, short limbs, abnormal feet and hands, and enlarged skull.

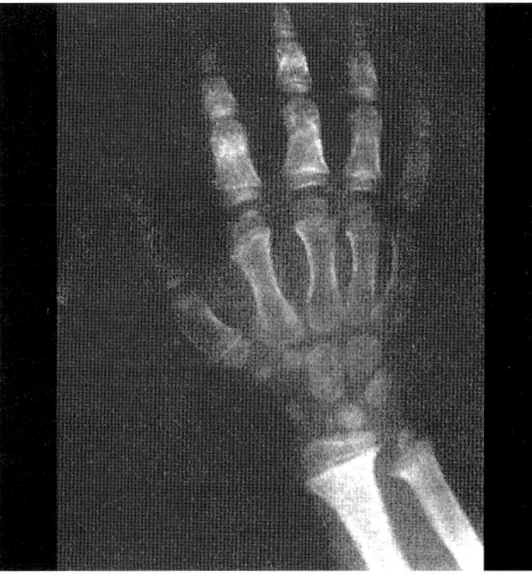

Figure 3
Radiograph of a hand of patient with achondroplasia, showing shortened digits and alteration of the distal radial and ulnar epiphyses.

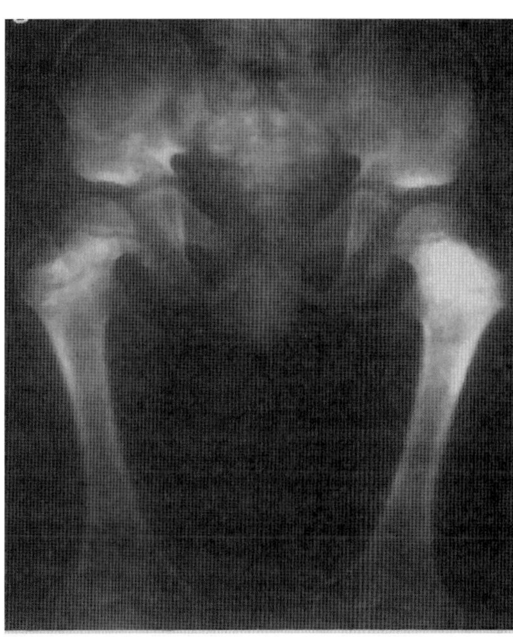

Figure 4
Radiograph of the pelvis and femora of a patient with achondroplasia demonstrates narrowing of the pelvis. The hips and acetabulae are enlarged and the femoral shafts are short, somewhat distorted in structure, widened, and bowed.

deformity[1-3,19,20,29-31] (Figure 1, 2, 4, and 5).

Histologic examination of the epiphysis and adjacent metaphysis shows a deficiency and disorder of cartilage cell proliferation. The zone of proliferating cartilage has fewer cells than normal and the hypertrophic and radial zone cells are in very short and sometimes distorted columns[1-3,19,20,30] (Figure 6). The calcified zone has less calcification than normal, and the "tidemark" is sometimes absent or distorted.[1,2,20] The epiphysis is wider than normal and somewhat distorted in structure because bone formation is diminished. Examination of the skull bones reveals that the major component of the calvarium is well developed and ossified and larger than normal, while the base of the bone that originates from cartilage is poorly structured and developed and diminished in size, especially in the region of the foramen magnum.[1,2,19,20]

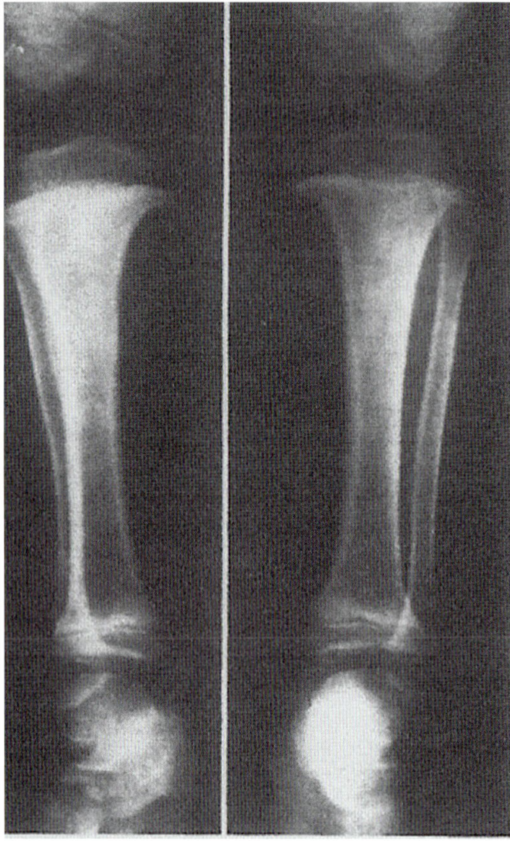

Figure 5
Radiographs of the lower extremities show short, wide tibiae with increased density in the proximal portion.

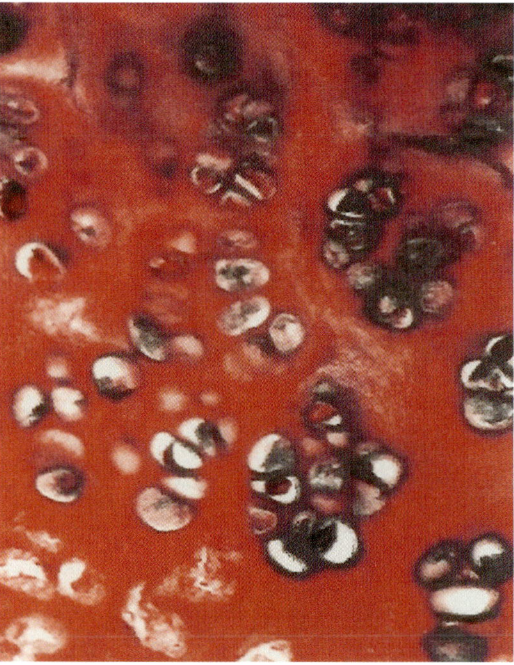

Figure 6
Histologic pattern for the epiphyseal plates demonstrates gross distortion and irregularity of the structure, with limited ossification.

Clinical Features
Birth and Infancy
Achondroplastic children are born with a reduction in birth length but usually a normal birth weight.[1,4,5,15,29,32,33] The extremities show total limb shortening more marked in the upper arms and thighs, a condition known as rhizomelia.[1,3,5,29] Examination of the head shows facial retrusion resulting in a saddle-nose deformity ("Parrot nose"), prognathism, and sometimes marked frontal bossing.[1,3,29] The chest is small and the abdomen and buttocks are protuberant. Dentition is somewhat retarded. Children generally do well in their early stages, although a series of complications may occur, including obstructive hydrocephalus[34] and delayed ambulation.[1,3] Despite the changes in body structure, the children are for the most part mentally normal and once they start to ambulate (usually by 20 months), they can develop good communication skills.[1,3,15,35] Examination of the limbs often shows a lack of full elbow extension and forearm supination.[1,3,5,29,36] Patients are often unable to approximate fully extended fingers (trident hand) and the middle finger is often reduced in length.[1,3,5]

Childhood
Craniofacial abnormalities often become more pronounced as the child ages, and flaring of the chest becomes noticeable.[1,3] The hyperlordotic spine seems to cause the markedly protuberant abdomen and midback kyphosis.[1,3,5,37-39] Genu varum is common when walking begins, along with an external rotation position of the hips.[1,3,37,40] A varus foot deformity is common.[1,3] Cardiorespiratory and sleep dysfunction are often major problems.[1,3,41-44] The sleep problems appear to be related to a relative adenotonsillar hypertrophy or jugular foramen stenosis or muscular upper airway obstruction.[3,41,43,44] Apnea and difficulty with sleep may require the use of nighttime oxygen administrative systems to avoid major problems with respiratory function.[42-47]

Adolescence
Obesity is one of the common problems in young people with achondroplasia and sometimes results in pulmonary and cardiac

disease[1,32,48,49] and even early death.[50] Early arthritis and knee pain may occur and can be disabling.[1,3] Scoliosis is common and not only decreases the child's height but can interfere with pulmonary function.[1,3,5,15,38,51] Psychiatric issues begin to be a problem for the adolescent child, particularly female patients who are concerned with their appearance in school and social settings.[1,51,52]

Adulthood

The adult patient is very prone to neurologic disturbances in addition to the skeletal disturbances described above.[3,13,17,34,41,51,53,54] Paraparesis or paraplegia may develop, and many patients have pain and sensory problems in the extremities in relation to the narrow spinal canal and constriction of the foramen magnum.[13,34,53,54] Female patients and their unborn infant children are at high risk during pregnancy.[1,55] Psychological problems are sometimes major and particularly related to competitive activities in high school and college, sexual activities, marriage, pregnancy, maintaining employment, and communicating with others regarding their personal problems.[1,3,52,55]

Imaging Studies

Changes in the skull show early closure of calvarial ossification centers and brachycephaly, with increased vertical diameter and reduced size of the foramen magnum.[1,29] The vertebrae are normal in shape, but one can note widened disk spaces and caudal narrowing of the interpedicular distances, reduced pedicular length, and a narrowing of the sacrosciatic notch.[29,37,38] The sacrum is narrow and short and articulates low, between the iliac wings. The inferior margin of the ilium is horizontal.[1,37] Lumbar lordosis, thoracic kyphosis and scoliosis are frequently encountered and quite characteristic in appearance.[3,29,38]

Appendicular bones are short and relatively thick.[1,3,5] Epiphyses in the growing child are somewhat larger than normal and sometimes slightly distorted in contour.[1,19,29] Epiphyseal space is normally wide.[19] Rhizomelic changes result in peculiarly shaped hips and shoulders and sometimes early arthritic changes in the knees and hips.[1,3,36,40] Hand radiographs frequently show shortening of the third meta-

carpal, and imaging of the ankles may disclose relative elongation of the fibula, causing a varus deformity of the foot.[1,29]

Recently, CT and MRI have been declared very useful in relation to cranial or spinal problems, and these studies help to define the cause of paralysis or sensory loss, or even hearing loss.[3,38,54,56]

Treatment

Patients with achondroplasia should be carefully evaluated on a regular basis for growth measurement and head circumference. Patients should have a neurologic examination (including CT, MRI, electromyography, and sonography) at regular intervals, particularly if they are symptomatic.[1,3] Respiratory studies, including CT of the lungs, should be done regularly and if sleep apnea develops, nasal-mask continuous positive airway pressure (CPAP) should be introduced to compensate for the problem.[42-44,46-48] Prevention of angular kyphosis is sometimes greatly aided by bracing.[10] Management of obesity is essential.[1,48,49] The death rate from excessive weight gain in these patients is quite high and careful nutritional support is mandatory.[48-50] Delivery of pregnant women should be by cesarean section, and prenatal study of the fetus should be performed by ultrasound to assess the likelihood of achondroplastic changes in the infant.[57]

Surgical procedures have been introduced, but have not been entirely successful.[1,58] Limb lengthening using Ilizarov or other techniques has been proposed and is sometimes successful but is difficult to perform and may lead to neurologic problems in the limb.[1,59] Osteotomies of the tibia or fibula are helpful in correcting bow legs or varus deformity of the foot.[1,5,40,58] Osteotomies of the radius or ulna are sometimes useful in improving elbow function.[1,36] Correction of spinal deformities by laminectomy for stenosis or surgical correction of lordosis or scoliosis is sometimes very useful and life-saving.[1,39,60,61] Enlarging the foramen magnum is sometimes helpful as well.[1,3]

In recent years, several authors have indicated that recombinant human growth hormone can change the status of patients with achondroplasia but the results have been somewhat disappointing in that the amount of growth that occurs is small and the results highly variable.[28,62-68] The most important potential addition to treatment protocol is that proposed by Horton,[62] who suggested that there are three possible ways of interfering with the action of FGFR3. The first protocol proposes to downregulate the tyrosine kinase activity of FGFR3. The second proposes to introduce blocking antibodies to interfere with binding of FGF ligands to FGFR3. The third protocol involves C-type natriuretic peptide (CNP), which appears to downregulate FGF-induced activation of mitogen-activated protein (MAP) kinase signaling pathways in chondrocytes and thus counteract the effects of the achondroplasia mutation.

Patients with achondroplasia have normal intelligence and hence can understand their disease and the psychological and social problems that they may have. Of great importance to patients and their families is a support system for the sometimes severe psychological problems that can occur. The patients are often not treated well or appropriately by normally sized persons in the world and hence sometimes become depressed and angered. If the cause of the problem is a spontaneous mutation, the parents should be tested before considering additional pregnancies and seek opinions regarding the issues of having siblings with achondroplasia. If one or both of the parents have achondroplasia, they should be made aware of the high likelihood that a child will have the disorder (well over 50% probability).[1,3]

Psychiatric help is sometimes very useful for the patients and their families.[52] In addition there are several societies, which the patients and their families may join or consult with to help improve their psychological and social outlook on the disease. These organizations include Little People of America, the Magic Foundation, and the Human Growth Foundation.

References

1. Bailey JA II: *Disproportionate Short Stature: Diagnosis and Management*. Philadelphia, PA, WB Saunders Co, 1973, pp 59-89.

2. Jaffe HL: *Metabolic, Degenerative and Inflammatory Diseases of Bone and Joint*. Philadelphia, PA, Lea and Febiger, 1972, pp 193-206.

3. Rimoin DL, Lachman RS: Genetic disorders of the osseous skeleton, in Beighton P (ed): *McKusick's Heritable Disorders of Connective Tissue*, ed 5. St Louis, MO, Mosby, 1993, pp 557-689.

4. Bailey JA II : Forms of dwarfism recognizable at birth. *Clin Orthop Relat Res* 1971;76:150-159.

5. Kopits S: Orthopedic complications of dwarfism. *Clin Orthop Relat Res* 1976;114:153-179.

6. Stoll C, Dott B, Roth MP: Birth prevalence rates of skeletal dysplasias. *Clin Genet* 1989;35:88-92.

7. Kozma C: Dwarfs in ancient Egypt. *Am J Med Genet A* 2006;140:303-311.

8. Parrot JM: Sur les malformations achondroplasiques et le dieu Ptah. *Bull Soc Anthrop Paris* 1878;1:296-308.

9. Kaufmann E: *Untersuchungen uber die Sogenannte Foetale Rachitis (Chondrodystrophia Foetalis)*. Berlin, Germany, Georg Reimer, 1892.

10. Pauli RM, Breed A, Horton VK, Glinski LP, Reiser CA: Prevention for fixed, angular kyphosis in achondroplasia. *J Pediatr Orthop* 1997;17:726-733.

11. Bowen P: Achondroplasia in two sisters with normal parents. *Birth Defects Orig Artic Ser* 1974;10:31-36.

12. Chiari H: Ueber familaere chondrodystrophia foetalis. *Muench Med Wschr* 1913;60:248-249.

13. Cohen ME, Rosenthal AD, Matson DD: Neurologic abnormalities in achondroplastic children. *J Pediatr* 1967;71:367-376.

14. Donath J, Vogl A: Untersuchungen uber den chondrodystrophischen zwergwuchs. Das verhalten der wirbelsaule beim chondrodystrophischen zwerg. *Wien Arch Finn Med* 1925;10:1-44.

15. Hall JG: The natural history of achondroplasia. *Basic Life Sci* 1988;48:3-9.

16. Maroteaux P, Lamy M: Achondroplasia in man and animals. *Clin Orthop Relat Res* 1964;33:91-103.

17. Vogl A: The fate of the achondroplastic dwarf (neurologic complications of achondroplasia). *Exp Med Surg* 1962;20:108-117.

18. Zelweger H, Taylor B: Genetic aspects of achondroplasia. *J Lancet* 1965;85:8-16.

19. Ponseti IV: Skeletal growth in achondroplasia. *J Bone Joint Surg Am* 1970;52:701-716.

20. Maynard JA, Ippolito EG, Ponseti IV, Mickelson MR: Histochemistry and ultrastucture of the growth plate in achondroplasia. *J Bone Joint Surg Am* 1981;63:969-979.

21. Bellus GA, Hefferon TW, Ortiz de Luna RI, et al: Achondroplasia is defined by recurrent G380R mutations of FGFR3. *Am J Hum Genet* 1995;56:368-373.

22. Cho JY, Guo C, Torello M, et al: Defective lysosomal targeting of activated fibroblast growth factor receptor 3 in achondroplasia. *Proc Natl Acad Sci USA* 2004;101:609-614.

23. Deng C, Wynshaw-Boris A, Zhou F, Kuo A, Leder P: Fibroblast growth factor receptor 3 is a negative regulator of bone growth. *Cell* 1996;84:911-921.

24. Rousseau F, Bonaventure J, Legeai-Mallet L, et al: Mutations in the gene encoding fibroblast growth factor receptor-3 in achondroplasia. *Nature* 1994;371:252-254.

25. Su YN, Lee CN, Chien SC, et al: Rapid detection of FGFR3 gene mutation in achondroplasia by DHPLC system-coupling heteroduplex and fluorescence-enhanced primer-extension analysis. *J Hum Genet* 2004;49:399-403.

26. Shiang R, Thompson LM, Zhu YZ, et al: Mutations in the transmembrane domain of FGFR3 cause the most common genetic form of dwarfism, achondroplasia. *Cell* 1994;78:335-342.

27. Heselson NG, Cremin BJ, Beighton P: Psuedo-achondroplasia: A report of 13 cases. *Br J Radiol* 1977;50:473-482.

28. Tanaka N, Katsumata N, Horikawa R, Tanaka T: The comparison of the effects of short-term growth hormone treatment in patients with achondroplasia and with hypochondroplasia. *Endocr J* 2003;50:69-75.

29. Bailey JA II: Orthopaedic aspects of achondroplasia. *J Bone Joint Surg Am* 1970;52:1285-1301.

30. Horton WA, Hood OJ, Machado MA, Campbell D: Growth plate cartilage studies in achondroplasia. *Basic Life Sci* 1988;48:81-89.

31. Rimoin DL, Hughes GN, Kaufman RL, et al: Endochondral ossification in achondroplastic dwarfism. *N Engl J Med* 1970;283:728-735.

32. Hunter AG, Hecht JT, Scott CI: Standard weight for height curves in achondroplasia. *Am J Med Genet* 1996;62:255-261.

33. Langer LO Jr , Baumann PA, Gorlin RJ: Achondroplasia. *Am J Roentgenol Radium Ther Nucl Med* 1967;100:12-26.

34. Pierre-Kahn A, Hirsch JF, Renier D, et al: Hydrocephalus and achondroplasia: A study of 25 observations. *Childs Brain* 1980;7:205-219.

35. Hecht JT, Thompson NM, Weir T, Patchell L, Horton WA: Cognitive and motor skills in achondroplastic infants: Neurologic and respiratory correlates. *Am J Hum Genet* 1991;41:208-211.

36. Kitoh H, Kitakoji T, Kurita K, Katoh M, Takamine Y: Deformities of the elbow in achondroplasia. *J Bone Joint Surg Br* 2002;84:680-683.

37. Caffey J: Achondroplasia of pelvis and lumbosacral spine. *AJR Am J Roentgenol* 1958;80:449-457.

38. Misra SN, Morgan HW: Thoracolumbar spinal deformity in achondroplasia. *Neurosurg Focus* 2003;14:e4.

39. Park HW, Kim HS, Hahn SB, et al: Correction of lumbosacral hyperlordosis in achondroplasia. *Clin Orthop Relat Res* 2003;414:242-249.

40. Stanley G, McLoughlin S, Beals RK: Observations on the cause of bowlegs in achondroplasia. *J Pediatr Orthop* 2002;22:112-116.

41. Nelson FW, Hecht JT, Horton WA, et al: Neurological basis of respiratory complications in achondroplasia. *Ann Neurol* 1988;24:89-93.

42. Stokes DC, Phillips JA, Leonard CO, et al: Respiratory complications of achondroplasia. *J Pediatr* 1983;102:534-541.

43. Tasker RC, Dundas I, Laverty A, et al: Distinct patterns of respiratory difficulty in young children with achondroplasia: A clinical, sleep and lung function study. *Arch Dis Child* 1998;79:99-108.

44. Zucconi M, Bruni O: Sleep disorders in children with neurologic disorders. *Semin Pediatr Neurol* 2001;8:258-275.

45. Elwood ET, Burstein FD, Graham L, Williams JK, Paschal M: Midface distraction to alleviate upper airway obstruction in achondroplastic dwarfs. *Cleft Palate Craniofac J* 2003;40:100-103.

46. Pauli RM, Scott CI, Wassman ER Jr, et al: Apnea and sudden unexpected death in infants with achondroplasia. *J Pediatr* 1984;104:342-348.

47. Waters KA, Everett F, Sillence DO, Fagan ER, Sullivan CE: Treatment of obstructive sleep apnea in achondroplasia: Evaluation of sleep, breathing and somatosensory-evoked potentials. *Am J Med Genet* 1995;59:460-466.

48. Hecht JT, Hood OJ, Schwartz RJ, et al: Obesity in achondroplasia. *Am J Med Genet* 1988;31:597-602.

49. Hunter AG, Bankier A, Rogers JG, Sillence D, Scott CI Jr: Medical complications of achondroplasia: A multicentre patient review. *J Med Genet* 1998;35:705-712.

50. Hecht JT, Francomano CA, Horton WA, Annegers JF: Mortality in achondroplasia. *Am J Hum Genet* 1987;41:454-464.

51. Haga N: Management of disabilities associated with achondroplasia. *J Orthop Sci* 2004;9:103-107.

52. Gollust SE, Thompson RE, Gooding HC, Biesecker BB: Living with achondroplasia: Attitudes toward population screening and correlation with quality of life. *Prenat Diagn* 2003;23:1003-1008.

53. Gordon N: The neurological complications of achondroplasia. *Brain Dev* 2000;22:3-7.

54. Hecht JT, Butler IJ: Neurologic morbidity associated with achondroplasia. *J Child Neurol* 1990;5:84-97.

55. Lattanzi DR, Harger JH: Achondroplasia and pregnancy. *J Reprod Med* 1982;27:363-366.

56. Lachman RS: Neurologic abnormalities in the skeletal dysplasias: A clinical and radiological perspective. *Am J Med Genet* 1997;69:33-43.

57. Ruano R, Molho M, Roume J, Ville Y: Prenatal diagnosis of fetal skeletal dysplasias by combining two-dimensional and three-dimensional ultrasound and intrauterine three-dimensional helical computer tomography. *Ultrasound Obstet Gynecol* 2004;24:134-140.

58. Beals RK, Stanley G: Surgical correction of bowlegs in achondroplasia. *J Pediatr Orthop B* 2005;14:245-249.

59. Yasui N, Kawabata H, Kojimoto H, et al: Lengthening of the lower limbs in patients with achondroplasia and hypochondroplasia. *Clin Orthop Relat Res* 1997;344:298-306.

60. Ain MC, Shirley ED: Spinal fusion for kyphosis in achondroplasia. *J Pediatr Orthop* 2004;24:541-545.

61. Thomeer RT, van Dijk JM: Surgical treatment of lumbar stenosis in achondroplasia. *J Neurosurg* 2002;96:292-297.

62. Horton WA: Recent milestones in achondroplastic research. *Am J Med Genet A* 2006;140:166-169.

63. Kanazawa H, Tanaka H, Inoue M, et al: Efficacy of growth hormone therapy for patients with skeletal dysplasia. *J Bone Miner Metab* 2003;21:307-310.

64. Key LL Jr , Gross AJ: Response to growth hormone in children with chondrodysplasia. *J Pediatr* 1996;128:S14-S17.

65. Mehta A, Hindmarsh PC: The use of somatotropin (recombinant growth hormone) in children of short stature. *Paediatr Drugs* 2002;4:37-47.

66. Shohat M, Tick D, Barakat S, et al: Short-term recombinant human growth hormone treatment increases growth rate in achondroplasia. *J Clin Endocrinol Metab* 1996;81:4033-4037.

67. Stamoyannou L, Karachaliou F, Neou P, et al: Growth and growth hormone therapy in children with achondroplasia: A two year experience. *Am J Med Genet* 1997;72:71-76.

68. Weber G, Prinster C, Meneghel M, et al: Human growth hormone treatment in prepubertal children with achondroplasia. *Am J Med Genet* 1996;61:396-400.

Chapter 16

Camurati-Engelmann Disease (Progressive Diaphyseal Dysplasia)

Camurati-Engelmann disease is a rare autosomal dominant genetic disorder that occurs in young people and is characterized orthopaedically by marked increase in bone density, osteitis, periostitis, and hyperostosis in the diaphyseal regions of the long bones and often the calvarium. The children are tall and have normal intelligence, but have tender, swollen, and knock-kneed legs; generalized muscular weakness; and problems with nerve damage, ocular abnormalities, and mandibular bony changes when the calvarium is severely affected. The disorder is progressive and leads to generalized functional loss and disability in terms of ambulation and personal capabilities. The disease appears with equal frequency in males and females and is panethnic in occurrence. A recent finding for many patients, which appears to be causative, is a mutational error in the production of transforming growth factor–beta 1 (TGF-β1).

Nomenclature and History

The rare genetic abnormality now known as Camurati-Engelmann disease or Engelmann's disease is also known as progressive diaphyseal dysplasia, craniodiaphyseal dysplasia, diaphyseal sclerosis, osteopathia hyperostotica scleroticans multiplex infantilis, periostitis hyperplastica, and polyostotic infantilia.[1-7] Most of the international literature now uses the eponymic forms of either Camurati-Engelmann or Englemann's disease.

The disorder was first described in 1920 by Cockayne,[8] who attributed the abnormal diaphyseal sclerotic changes to congenital syphilis. In 1922, Mario Camurati,[9] a Bolognese physician described the entity in some detail and suggested its autosomal dominant character as two of his patients were father and son. Seven years later, Gerhardt Engelmann[10] of Vienna further described the disease and outlined the progressive character of the bony changes and the painful myopathic alterations in an 8-year-old child. He called the entity osteopathia hyperostotica scleroticans multiplex infantilis. Subsequent reports over the next 4 decades from various countries included those of Lauterberg,[11] Fritsch,[12] Bingold,[1] Lavine and Koven,[13] Chipps and associates,[3] Cohen and States,[14] Griffiths,[5] Singleton and associates,[15] Girdany,[16] Lennon and associates,[17] and Clawson and Loop.[18] All of these signal studies helped to define aspects of the highly variable clinical presentation, the genetic nature of the disorder, the findings on imaging studies, and the difficulty in establishing a treatment protocol.

Causation

Camurati-Engelmann disease has been demonstrated to be an autosomal dominant genetic disorder that is equally present in males and females.[4,6,7,16-28] It occurs in approximately 50% of the progeny of individuals who may be asymptomatic but carry the gene.[29] The disorder is believed to affect 1 in 100,000 individuals, but because many of the patients are asymptomatic, the incidence may be considerably greater.[7,29] The disorder is also panethnic, affecting individuals in all parts of the world.[6,17,20-27]

The localization of the gene error has been shown by several investigators to be assigned to the chromosomal region 19q13.1-q13.3.[6,22,30-33] Subsequently, the mutations were found in the TGF-β1 gene, which is located within this interval.[22,30,34-40] The mutations reported in patients with Camurati-Engelmann disease and their sometimes asymptomatic family members include R218H, R218C, Y81H, LLL12-13 insertion, C225R, R156C, and H222D.[15,29,34,37-39] There does not appear to be any correlation between the nature of the mutation and the severity of the syndrome or the clinical or radiographic manifestations.

As is well known, TGF-β1 helps regulate bone remodeling by stimulating osteoprogenitor cells to differentiate into osteoblasts.[29,40,41] It also stimulates collagen production and its incorporation into the extracellular matrix. Increased levels of active TGF-β1 may disrupt the balance between bone formation and bone resorption, leading to progressive hyperostosis, such as is seen in patients with Camurati-Engelmann disease.[29,40-42] Most of the pathologic cells in the affected patients secrete TGF-β1 as a large latent complex of TGF-β1/LAP (latency-associated peptide), which materially increases osteoblast production but inhibits osteoclast activity, hence the increased bone formation.[42] In some patients, the TGF-β1/LAP may affect muscle as well, causing the muscle fibrosis characteristic of progressive Camurati-Engelmann disease.[15,29,39,42]

The pathologic characteristics of the disorder are a marked increase in the density of the diaphyseal part of the long bones, with thickening of the cortices and irregularity of bone structure.[3,27,43,44] The cranium is also usually involved and shows a moderate to marked increase in bone density in the base, with involvement of the maxillae and sometimes mandibles.[3,14,16,22,33,45] Histologically, the bone is normal in appearance but the overall structural design shows loss of medullary trabecular architecture and thickening of the cortices. The periosteum is usually markedly thickened and irregular in structure. The periosteal changes are believed to be the cause of pressure on nerve and vascular structures and may be the cause of the frequently encountered local pain and bone tenderness.[14,16,22,33,45] Muscular tissue may show fibrous replacement and scarring.[46,47]

Clinical Characteristics

The average age of onset of symptoms in most series of patients with Camurati-Engelmann disease is 14 years, with a range from birth to 76 years of age.[7,20-22,24-26] Affected individuals may have no symptoms or complaints, but show some quite characteristic features on physical examination. Most patients have decreased muscle mass and weakness in the proximal lower limbs and have difficulty rising from a sitting position.[16,22,26,33,46,47] A wide-based waddling gait is found in more than 60% of patients, and joint contractures are present in almost 50% of patients.[22,26,33,47] Patients may be taller than normal and quite thin, thus at least in body habitus resembling those with Marfan's disease.[2,22] The shafts of the long bones are thicker than normal, which can be noted in children or in thin adults, and the bones are often tender to touch. Pain is the presenting complaint for most patients and is constant, aching, and intense in cold weather.[16,22,46,48] Nonsteroidal anti-inflammatory drugs are occasionally helpful. Pain can be severe and increases with activity and exercise. Most patients have pain, tenderness, swelling, erythema, and warmth in their extremities. Although the bones are more dense than normal, they may be susceptible to fracture.

Orthopaedic problems include varying degrees of lumbar lordosis, kyphosis, scoliosis, coxa valga, genu valgum (a characteristic feature is the knock-knee deformity), and flat feet.[5,7,13,16,18,22-24,48] The patients frequently have intractable distress in their extremities related to the above problems, as well as the marked tenderness and swelling over the shafts of the bones.[5,13,18,48] Delayed dentition, mandibular and maxillary deformities, and teeth problems are common.[3,7,22,49]

In terms of neurologic disease, most patients have normal mentation, but because of the disabilities associated with their disease states, they are sometimes depressed and emotionally impaired.[7,27,43,50] Many patients have cranial abnormalities, and sclerosis of the cranial nerve foramina can lead to neurovascular compromise.[7,22,27,43,50-52] Cerebellar ataxia may be present in some patients who are severely affected.[51] Almost 40% of patients have cranial nerve abnormalities that include hearing loss and visual disturbances, such as proptosis, papilledema, glaucoma, and subluxation of the globe.[22,26,53-56] Facial paralysis is also common. Patients may have profound anemia,[19] and cardiomyopathy has been reported.[26,29,57]

Imaging Studies

Often, the correct diagnosis of Camurati-Engelmann disease is based almost entirely

on imaging studies. The bones are nearly always intensely positive on bone scan.[23,58-60]
The femora and tibiae and often humeri
show widening of the diaphyseal areas, increased density at the medullary sites, and
some alteration in the cortical structure (Figure 1). The external rims of the long bones
are irregular, related to periosteal bone
formation.[5,13,15,17,18,20-24,33,44,45] When the
cranium is involved, there is often progressive and marked enlargement of the midline
cranial bones, causing a distinct facial deformity (Figure 2). This finding is best seen on
CT or MRI, particularly in terms of orbital
disease and, specifically, proptosis and subluxation of the globe.[22,33,43,45,61] Both the
metaphyses and diaphyses of the skull may
be affected. The spinal deformities can be
clearly evidenced by radiologic studies but
can be further identified, particularly as to
potential damage to neurologic structures,
by CT or MRI studies.[22,33,45] MRI of
muscles over the bony sites may show scarring and structural change.[22]

Differential Diagnosis

There are several disorders in which the
bones appear more dense on imaging; these
must be distinguished from Camurati-
Engelmann disease.[7,62] The disorders include the following:

• Ribbing disease. Ribbing disease, originally described in 1949 by Ribbing,[63] is a
very rare osteosclerotic disease of the long
bones presenting after puberty. The bones
are classically widely hyperostotic, although
usually asymmetrical, in contrast with
Camurati-Engelmann disease.[6,63-66] The inheritance pattern is usually considered autosomal recessive.[7] As yet, there are no published reports on TGF-β1 mutation analysis
in these patients.

• Kenny-Caffey dysplasia. This uncommon entity is characterized by dwarfism,
craniofacial anomalies, hypocalcemia, and
hypoparathyroidism, and can be readily distinguished from Camurati-Engelmann disease.[7]

• Juvenile Paget's disease, otherwise
known as hyperphosphatasia, has markedly
coarser bone structure and a profound increase in serum alkaline phosphatase.[7]

• Sclerosteosis and von Buchem's disease. Both of these disorders are autosomal
recessive; although the bones are more

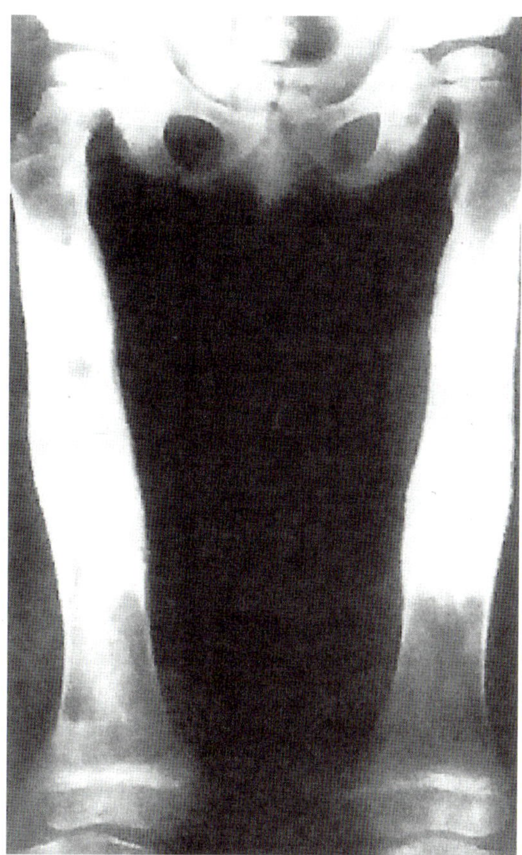

Figure 1
Radiograph of the shafts of the femora showing a
marked increase in bone density in the diaphyseal
region and some deformity. Patients may be notably disabled as a result of these changes.

dense than normal, the appearance is one of
endosteal hyperostosis without the classic
periostitis seen in patients with Camurati-
Engelmann disease. Digital deformities are
more common in these disorders.[6,7,67,68]

Clinical and Laboratory Evaluation

Initial studies should include a thorough
neurologic examination and a genetic counseling evaluation of the patient's family.
Standard laboratory studies are important to
some extent, to rule out other disorders.
Hearing and ophthalmic analyses are also
important. Repeated imaging studies, particularly over sites of increased pain or deformity, are essential. The gene error can be detected by appropriate studies.[29,36,42]

Treatment

The principal agents used in the treatment of
patients with Camurati-Engelmann disease
are corticosteroids, which were first introduced as a treatment for Camurati-

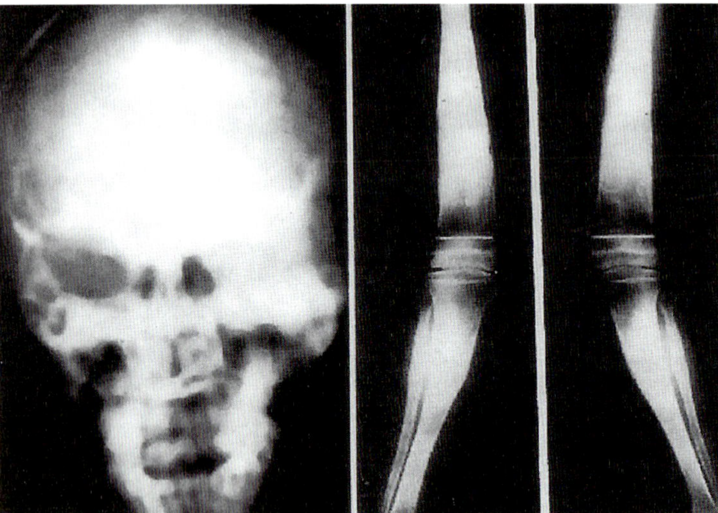

Figure 2

Radiographs of the skull and lower extremities of a patient with Camurati-Engelmann disease. Both sites show a remarkable increase in bone density. The changes in the skull often lead to difficulties with vision, hearing, and other nerve functions. The changes in the lower extremities cause disability and pain. The patient shows a marked degree of genu valgum, which is also disabling.

Engelmann disease by Allen and associates in 1970.[69] Since then, numerous presentations have indicated a modest to moderate degree of success in reducing the patient's complaints and, to some extent, diminishing the progression of the disease.[59,69-75] Nonsteroidal anti-inflammatory agents are useful in reducing some of the discomfort for patients. Bisphosphonates and phosphates have been introduced but thus far are not considered to be effective and may cause complications.[59,76,77] Long-term follow-up studies are essential with the various drug agents to be certain that the disease does not progress and that anemia, hepatosplenom-

egaly, headaches, and cranial nerve disorders do not increase. Patients and their families should have genetic counseling.[21,22,24,58] Orthopaedic, surgical, and neurosurgical care may be necessary for fractures and abnormal spinal or bony alignment or nerve or vascular compression.[5,18,21,48] Ophthalmic, otolaryngologic, and oral surgery may also be necessary to deal with complications.[3,22,49,53-56]

Comments and Conclusions

Patients and their physicians are fortunate that Camurati-Engelmann disease is a very unusual entity and certainly one that is rarely seen by orthopaedic surgeons. There are, however, some fascinating features to the disorder that are noteworthy. First, it is one of the genetic diseases associated with increased bone formation and in an unusual way. Most of the increased bone problems are metaphyseal or diffuse, but in this disease they are diaphyseal, which makes the diagnosis by radiology relatively easy. Second, a sizeable number of individuals who have the disease and can pass it on to their progeny have very few or no symptoms. This suggests some degree of variation in the genetic problem. Third, the studies have very clearly identified and characterized the role of TGF-β1 in bone formation. Equally important is the finding of the problems that arise when its role in osteoclastic resorbtion are limited by a mutational error. With this information, it should be possible, perhaps in the not too distant future, to biologically change this pattern and restore these children to good health and a happier life.

References

1. Bingold AC: Engelmann's disease: Osteopathia hyperostotica (sclerotisans) multiplex infantilis: Progressive diaphyseal dysplasia. *Br J Surg* 1950;37:266-274.

2. Braham RL: Multiple congenital anomalies with diaphyseal dysplasia (Camurati-Engelmann's syndrome): Report of a case. *Oral Surg Oral Med Oral Pathol* 1969;27:20-26.

3. Chipps JE, Penner RS, Travis LO: Mandibular involvement in osteopathia hyperostotica sclerotisans multiplex infantilis (Engelmann's disease). *Oral Surg Oral Med Oral Pathol* 1954;7:1306-1310.

4. Fairbanks T: *An Atlas of General Affections of the Skeleton*. Edinburgh, Livingtone, 1951, pp 184-187.

5. Griffiths DL: Engelmann's disease. *J Bone Joint Surg Br* 1956;38:312-326.

6. McKusick VA: *Mendelian Inheritance in Man: Catalogs of Autosomal Dominant, Autosomal Recessive and X-Linked Phenotypes*, ed 11. Baltimore, MD, The Johns Hopkins University Press, 1994.

7. Wynne-Davies R, Hall CM, Apley AG: Engelmann's disease, in *Atlas of Skeletal Dysplasias*. Edinburgh, Scotland, Churchill Livingstone, 1985, pp 488-484.

8. Cockayne EA: Case for diagnosis. *Proc R Soc Med* 1920;13:132-136.

9. Camurati M: Di uno raro caso di osteite simmetrica ereditaria degli arti inferiori. *Chir Organi Mov* 1922;6:662-665.

10. Engelmann G: Ein fall von osteopathia hyperostica (sclerotisans) multiplex infantilis. *Fortschr Roentgenstr* 1929;39:1101-1106.

11. Lauterberg W: Über zwei fälle von familiärer genalisierter osteosklerose. *Deutsche Ztschr f Chir* 1931;230:308-315.

12. Fritsch H: Ein fall von generalisterterter osteoskelerose. *Wien Arch Finn Med* 1932;23:247-256.

13. Lavine LS, Koven MT: Engelmann's disease (progressive diaphyseal dysplasia). *J Pediatr* 1952;40:235-239.

14. Cohen J, States JD: Progressive diaphyseal dysplasia: Report of a case with autopsy findings. *Lab Invest* 1956;5:492-508.

15. Singleton EB, Thomas JR, Worthington WW, Hild JR: Progressive diaphyseal dysplasia (Engelmann's disease). *Radiology* 1956;67:233-241.

16. Girdany BR: Engelmann's disease (progressive diaphyseal dysplasia): A non-progressive familial form of muscular dystrophy with characteristic bone changes. *Clin Orthop* 1959;14:102-109.

17. Lennon EA, Schechter MM, Hornabrook RW: Engelmann's disease: Report of a case with a review of the literature. *J Bone Joint Surg Br* 1961;43:273-284.

18. Clawson DK, Loop JW: Progressive diaphyseal dysplasia (Engelmann's disease). *J Bone Joint Surg Am* 1964;46:143-150.

19. Ghosal SP, Mukherjee AK, Mukherjee D, Ghosh AK: Diaphyseal dysplasia associated with anemia. *J Pediatr* 1988;113:49-57.

20. Grey AC, Wallace R, Crone M: Engelmann's disease: A 45-year follow-up. *J Bone Joint Surg Br* 1996;78:488-491.

21. Hundley JD, Wilson FC: Progressive diaphyseal dysplasia: Review of the literature and report of seven cases in one family. *J Bone Joint Surg Am* 1973;55:461-474.

22. Janssens K, Vanhoenacker F, Bonduelle M, et al: Camurati-Engelmann disease: Review of the clinical, radiological, and molecular data of 24 families and implications for diagnosis and treatment. *J Med Genet* 2006;43:1-11.

23. Kumar B, Murphy WA, Whyte MP: Progressive diaphyseal dysplasia (Engelmann disease): Scintographic-radiographic-clinical correlations. *Radiology* 1981;140:87-92.

24. Naveh Y, Kaftori JK, Alon U, Ben-David J, Berant M: Progressive diaphyseal dysplasia: Genetics and clinical and radiologic manifestations. *Pediatrics* 1984;74:399-405.

25. Saraiva JM: Progressive diaphyseal dysplasia: A three-generation family with markedly variable expressivity. *Am J Med Genet* 1997;71:348-352.

26. Sparkes RS, Graham CB: Camurati-Engelmann disease: Genetics and clinical manifestations with a review of the literature. *J Med Genet* 1972;9:73-85.

27. Tucker AS, Klein L, Antony GJ: Craniodiaphyseal dysplasia: Evolution over a five year period. *Skeletal Radiol* 1976;1:47-53.

28. Hundley JD, Wilson FC: Progressive diaphyseal dysplasia: Review of the literature and report of seven cases in one family. *J Bone Joint Surg Am* 1973;55:461-474.

29. Wallace SE, Lachman S, Mekikian PB, Bui KK, Wilcox WR: Marked phenotypic variability in progressive diaphyseal dysplasia (Camurati-Engelmann disease): Report of a four-generation pedigree, identification of a mutation in TGFB1, and review. *Am J Med Genet A,* 2004;129A:235-247.

30. Fujii D, Brissenden JE, Derynck R, Francke U: Transforming growth factor beta gene maps to human chromosome 19 long arm and mouse chromosome 7. *Somat Cell Mol Genet* 1986;12:281-288.

31. Ghadami M, Makita Y, Yoshida K, et al: Genetic mapping of the Camurati-Engelmann disease locus to chromosome 19q13.1-q13.3. *Am J Hum Genet* 2000;66:143-147.

32. Janssens K, Gershoni-Baruch R, Van Hul E: Localization of the gene causing diaphyseal dysplasia Camurati-Engelmann to chromosome 19q13. *J Med Genet* 2000;37:245-249.

33. Vanhoencker FM, Janssens K, Van Hul W, Gershonoi-Baruch R, Brik R, De Schepper AM: Camurati-Engelmann disease: Review of radioclinical features. *Acta Radiol* 2003;44:430-434.

34. Campos-Xavier B, Saraiva JM, Savarirayan R, et al: Phenotypic variability at the TGF-beta1 locus in Camurati-Engelmann's disease. *Hum Genet* 2001;109:653-658.

35. Gentry LE, Lioubin MN, Purchio AF, Marquardt H: Molecular event in the processing of recombinant type 1 pre-pro-transforming growth factor beta to the mature polypeptide. *Mol Cell Biol* 1988;8:4162-4168.

36. Hecht JT, Blanton SH, Broussard S, Scott A, Rhoades Hall C, Milunsky JM: Evidence for locus heterogeneity in the Camurati-Engelmann (DPD1) syndrome. *Clin Genet* 2001;59:198-200.

37. Janssens K, ten Dijke P, Ralston SH, Bergmann C, Val Hul W: Transforming growth factor-beta 1 mutations in Camurati-Engelmann disease lead to increased signaling by altering either activation or secretion of the mutant protein. *J Biol Chem* 2003;278:7718-7724.

38. Kinoshita A, Saito T, Tomita H, et al: Domain-specific mutations in TGFB1 result in Camurati-Engelmann disease. *Nat Genet* 2000;26:19-20.

39. Mumm SR, Obrecht TS, Podgornik MN, Whyte MP: Camurati-Engelmann disease: New mutations in the latency-associated peptide of the transforming growth factor type beta1. *J Bone Miner Metab* 2001;16(Suppl 1):S223.

40. Saito T, Kinoshita A, Yoshiura K, et al: Domain specific mutations of the transforming growth factor (TGF)-beta 1 latency-associate peptide cause Camurati-Engelmann disease because of the formation of a constitutively active form of TGF-beta 1. *J Biol Chem* 2001;276:11469-11472.

41. Noda M, Camilliere JJ: In vivo stimulation of bone formation by transforming growth factor-beta. *Endocrinology* 1989;124:2991-2994.

42. Kinoshita A, Fukumaki Y, Shirahama S, et al: TGFB1 mutations in four new families with Camurati-Engelmann disease: Confirmation of independently arising LAP-domain-specific mutations. *Am J Med Genet A* 2004;127:104-107.

43. Applegate LJ, Applegate GR, Kemp SS: MR of multiple cranial neuropathies in a patient with Camurati-Engelmann disease: Case Report. *AJNR Am J Neuroradiol* 1991;12:557-559.

44. Nishimura G, Nishimura H, Tanaka Y, et al: Camurati-Engelmann disease type II: Progres-

sive diaphyseal dysplasia with striations of the bones. *Am J Med Genet* 2002;107:5-11.

45. Kaftori JK, Kleinhaus U, Naveh Y: Progressive diaphyseal dysplasia (Camurati-Engelmann): Radiographic follow-up and CT findings. *Radiology* 1987;164:777-782.

46. Naveh Y, Ludatshcer R, Alon U, Sharf B: Muscle involvement in progressive diaphyseal dysplasia. *Pediatrics* 1985;76:944-949.

47. Yoshioka H, Mino M, Kiyosawa N, et al: Muscular changes in Engelmann's disease. *Arch Dis Child* 1980;55:716-719.

48. Schapira D, Militeanu D, Israel O, Misselevich I, Scharf Y: Progressive diaphyseal dysplasia masquerading as shoulder capsulitis in an adult. *Clin Rheumatol* 1995;14:582-585.

49. Ramon Y, Buchner A: Camurati-Engelmann's disease affecting the jaws. *Oral Surg Oral Med Oral Pathol* 1966;22:592-599.

50. Hellier WP, Brookes GB: Vestibular nerve dysfunction and decompression in Engelmann's disease. *J Laryngol Otol* 1996;110:462-465.

51. Kormas N, Diamond T, Shnier R: Camurati-Englemann disease: Two case reports describing metadiaphyseal dysplasia associated with cerebellar ataxia. *J Bone Miner Res* 1998;13:1203-1207.

52. Mineta Y, Kakigi R, Oda K, Okue A, Shibasaki H: Case of progressive diaphyseal dysplasia (Engelmann) presenting with trigeminal neuropathy and hearing disorder. *Rinsho Shinkeigaku* 1983;23:700-705.

53. Brodrick JD: Luxation of the globe in Engelmann's disease. *Am J Ophthalmol* 1977;83:870-873.

54. Kim CH, Oh DE, Kim YD: Bilateral visual loss in craniodiaphyseal dysplasia. *Am J Ophthalmol* 2006;141:398-399.

55. Morse PH, Walsh FB, McCormick JR: Ocular findings in hereditary diaphyseal dysplasia (Engelmann's disease). *Am J Ophthalmol* 1969;68:100-104.

56. Wright M, Miller NR, McFadzean RM et al: Papilloedema, a complication of progressive diaphyseal dysplasia: A series of three case reports. *Br J Ophthalmol* 1998;82:1042-1048.

57. Choudhury P, Batra V, Batra B, Gandhi D: Engelmann's disease with cardiomyopathy. *Indian Pediatr* 2000;37:1373-1376.

58. Clybouw C, Desmyttere S, Bonduelle M, Piepsz A: Camurati-Engelmann disease: Contribution of bone scintigraphy to genetic counseling. *Genet Couns* 1994;5:195-198.

59. Inoaka T, Shuke N, Sato J, et al: Scintigraphic evaluation of pamidronate and corticosteroid therapy in a patient with progressive diaphyseal dysplasia (Camurati-Engelmann disease). *Clin Nucl Med* 2001;26:680-682.

60. Vidal-Sicart S, Pns F, Guanabens N, Herranz R: Bone scan in Camurati-Engelmann disease. *Clin Nucl Med* 1997;23:791-792.

61. Marden FA, Wippold FJ II: MR imaging features of craniodiaphyseal dysplasia. *Pediatr Radiol* 2004;34:167-170.

62. Crisp AJ, Brenton DP: Engelmann's disease of bone—a systemic disorder? *Ann Rheum Dis* 1982;41:183-188.

63. Ribbing S: Hereditary, multiple diaphyseal sclerosis. *Acta Radiol* 1949;31:522-536.

64. Makita Y, Nishimura G, Ikegawa S, Ishii T, Ito Y, Okuno A: Intrafamilial phenotypic variability in Engelmann Disease (ED): Are ED and Ribbing disease the same entity? *Am J Med Genet* 2000;91:153-156.

65. Seeger LL, Hewel KC, Yao L, et al: Ribbing's disease (multiple diaphyseal sclerosis): Imaging and differential diagnosis. *AJR Am J Roentgenol* 1996;167:689-694.

66. Shier CK, Karasicky GA, Ellis BI, Kottamasu SR: Ribbing's disease: Radiographic-scintigraphic correlation and comparative analysis with Engelmann's disease. *J Nucl Med* 1987;28:244-248.

67. Eastman JR, Bixler D: Generalized cortical hyperostosis (Van Buchem disease): Nosologic considerations. *Radiology* 1977;125:297-304.

68. Van Buchem FS, Hadders HN, Hansen JF, Woldring MG: Hyperostosis corticalis generalisata: Report of seven cases. *Am J Med* 1962;33:387-397.

69. Allen DT, Saunders AM, Northway WH Jr, Williams GF, Schafer IA: Corticosteroids in the treatment of Engelmann's disease: Progressive diaphyseal dysplasia. *Pediatrics* 1970;46:523-531.

70. Baş F, Darendeliler F, Petorak I, et al: Deflazacort treatment in progressive diaphyseal dysplasia (Camurati-Engelmann disease). *J Paediatr Child Health* 1999;35:401-405.

71. Bourantas K, Tsiara S, Drosos AA: Successful treatment with corticosteroid in a patient with progressive diaphyseal dysplasia. *Clin Rheumatol* 1995;14:485-486.

72. Heymans O, Gebhart M, Alexiou J, Sokolow Y: Camurati-Engelmann disease: Effect of corticosteroids. *Acta Clin Belg* 1998;53:189-192.

73. Lindstrom JA: Diaphyseal dysplasia (Engelmann) treated with corticosteroids. *Birth Defects Orig Artic Ser* 1974;10:504-507.

74. Low LC, Stephenson JB, Stuart-Smith DA: Progressive diaphyseal dysplasia mimicking childhood myopathy: Clinical and biochemical response to prednisolone. *Aust Paediatr J* 1985;21:193-196.

75. Minford AM, Hardy GJ, Forsythe WI, Fitton JM, Rowe VL: Engelmann's disease and the effect of corticosteroids: A case report. *J Bone Joint Surg Br* 1981;63:597-600.

76. Castro GR, Apenzeller S, Marques-Neto JF, Bértolo MB, Samara AM, Coimbra I: Camurati-Engelmann disease: Failure of response to bisphosphonates. Report of two cases. *Clin Rhematol* 2005;24:398-401.

77. Chérié-Lignière G, Santalena G, Parafioriti A: Pamidronate in the treatment of progressive diaphyseal dysplasia (Camurati-Engelmann disease). *Clin Exp Rheumatol* 1999;17:264.

Chapter 17

Cartilage-Hair Hypoplasia

In 1964, Victor McKusick[1] described a very unusual genetic disease occurring quite commonly in the Amish people in Pennsylvania. Soon thereafter, the disease was also found to occur with comparable frequency in Finnish people, but remained very rare in the rest of the world. The disorder, now known as cartilage-hair hypoplasia, is characterized by short stature; very thin, colorless hair; and bone deformities, especially of the spine, lower extremities, and hands. Patients are not mentally retarded, but some have a frightening array of complications, including immune deficiencies, anemia and leukopenia, cancers, and increased mortality. The disorder appears to occur in relation to chromosome 9 and is believed to result from mutations in ribonuclease mitochondrial RNA processing.

Nomenclature and History

Cartilage-hair hypoplasia is also known as CHH; metaphyseal chondrodysplasia, McKusick type; spondyloepiphyseal dysplasia; and metaphyseal dysplasia.

The disorder was first described in Old Order Amish families by Victor Almon McKusick,[1-3] a well-known professor at Johns Hopkins who has received numerous awards and has written several articles and books describing genetic disorders.[4] In 1931, Pyle[5] had described a similar patient. In 1963, Theodorou and Adams[6] reported another patient as having a form of metaphyseal dysplasia but noted that the child had strange hair. In 1970, Halle and associates[7] reported on the disorder in a child. Lowry and associates[8,9] further described the syndrome, and the abnormality of the hair in particular. Lux and associates[10] first described neutropenia in patients with the disorder, and in 1974, Mancini and Morabito[11] described two Italian children with the syndrome. In 1978, Wilson and associates[12] and, independently, Virolainen and associates[13] described patients with the disorder and various aspects of immunodeficiency. In 1980, Kaitila and Perheentupa[14] described 33 cases of cartilage-hair hypopla-

sia in 28 families in Finland. In the early 1990s, Mäkitie and associates[15-17] expanded the description of the disease in the Finnish population and described several complications. These studies established Finland as another site for frequent appearance of this truly rare genetic disorder. Because the genetic error appears to be nearly identical for the Old Order Amish and Finnish patients,[18] it is interesting to try to relate these two populations; however, there is little evidence to support such a proposal. The Old Order Amish apparently first lived in The Netherlands and then moved to Switzerland and then on to Pennsylvania and Canada. It is certainly possible, however, that in quite ancient times, a genetic error occurred in one family who then became divided, with one group moving to Finland and the other to The Netherlands.

Pathophysiology

The genetic defect for patients with cartilage-hair hypoplasia is now well established. The gene map locus has been identified as occurring at 9p21-p12.[4,19,20] The disease is inherited as an autosomal recessive disorder with no gender preference.[2,4,15] As noted above, there are two major ethnic groups affected—the Old Order Amish and Finnish populations. A smaller number of patients from Japan have been identified as well.[21,22]

The genetic error has been identified as a mutation in the gene in chromosome 9 for ribonuclease mitochondrial RNA processing (RMRP).[23-26] RMRP is a ribonucleoprotein present in the nucleus and mitochondria that has two functions: cleavage of RNA in mitochondrial DNA synthesis and nucleolar cleaving of preribosomal RNA.[23-26] The agent also plays a role in ribosomal RNA production and may also act in some capacity in nuclear DNA replications.[24] It is required for cell growth, and with mutational changes, defects in cell growth are observed in T cells, B cells, and fibroblasts.[1,23,27,28] This effect appears to be caused by impairment of ribosomal assembly and by alter-

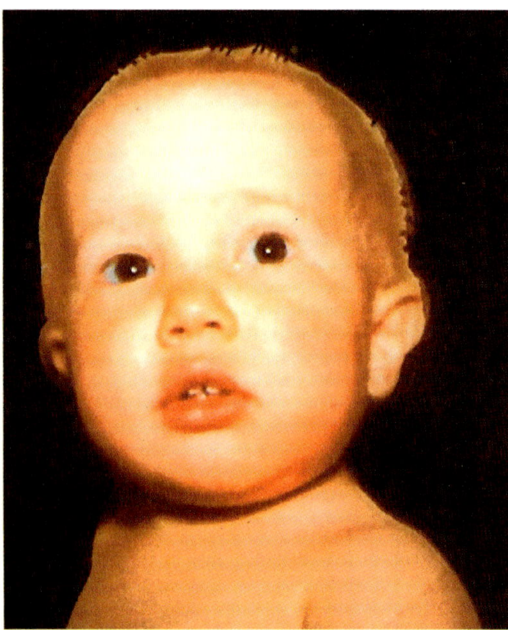

Figure 1

Photograph of a 3-year-old boy showing the classic hair abnormality. The hairs are short and soft, and the color is either yellow or light brown.

ation in cyclin-dependent cell-cycle regulation.[23,26,29] RMRP mutations can be detected by Northern blot analysis.[23]

Although there are several different mutations of RMRP, they tend to fall into two general types.[26,27,30] The first consists of insertions or duplication of 6 to 30 nucleotides that reside in the region between the TATA box and the transcription initiation site.[26,27,30,31] Both of these interfere with the transcription of the RMRP gene. The second type of mutation consists of single nucleotide substitutions and other changes that involve one or two nucleotides in highly conserved regions of the gene.[21,27,30] The most commonly found mutation in patients with cartilage-hair hypoplasia is 70A > G, which causes an alteration in ribosomal processing.[32] The mutations found in Old Order Amish and Finnish patients with cartilage-hair hypoplasia are very similar, while those found in patients from Japan, Spain, Switzerland, and other countries differ.[18,21,22,25,31] Of some importance is the presentation of the clinical syndrome, which sometimes varies widely with different mutational errors,[33] but (at least currently) this is not always predictable on the basis of genetic studies.

Histologic studies of the epiphyseal plates show abnormal cartilage structure with a reduction in the height and sometimes marked irregularity of the columns.[4] The trabeculae of the primary spongiosa are also disordered and irregular in size and structure.[4,17]

Histologic examination of hair fibers from the scalp, eyebrows, and eyelashes of patients with the syndrome display an extraordinarily thin caliber and lack a central core.[9,34] The color differs from that of unaffected siblings and is usually either light brown or darkish blond[4,9,34] (Figure 1).

Clinical Presentation

Patients with cartilage-hair hypoplasia have considerable variation in their clinical presentation, ranging from mild structural alterations without systemic disease to severe changes in immune systems, increased susceptibility to infection, marked anemia and leukopenia, frequent malignancies, and early demise.[4,15] As noted, the disease is very uncommon in the general population of the United States and most other countries, but much more frequent among Old Order Amish people (1 per 1,340 population) and Finns (1 per 23,000 live births in Finland).[2,15] It is transmitted as an autosomal recessive disorder, so there is no gender preference.[4] There is almost always evidence of the disease in children at birth, particularly in terms of their skeletal characteristics and hair color and structure.[3,4,17] Within a short time, they are found to grow less rapidly than unaffected children and almost always display a substantial reduction in height, which has been described as short-limb dwarfism.[4,7,16,17]

Mentation is normal in patients with this disease and the head, facial, and dental features are unaffected with the exception of the incisors, which are often smaller than normal and notched.[4,8,14] The hands and feet are "pudgy" and the skin hypopigmented.[15,17,35] The hands are short and the fingers are frequently bent but can be easily extended.[2,4,35] The nails show foreshortening and a mild dysplasia.[4] The large joints are for the most part flexible, but the limbs are short and the legs are often bowed.[4] The elbows sometimes cannot be extended. The fibula is excessively long, which in some patients results in ankle deformities.[4] The spine often shows a lumbar lordosis and sometimes scoliosis.[4,36] Flaring of the lower

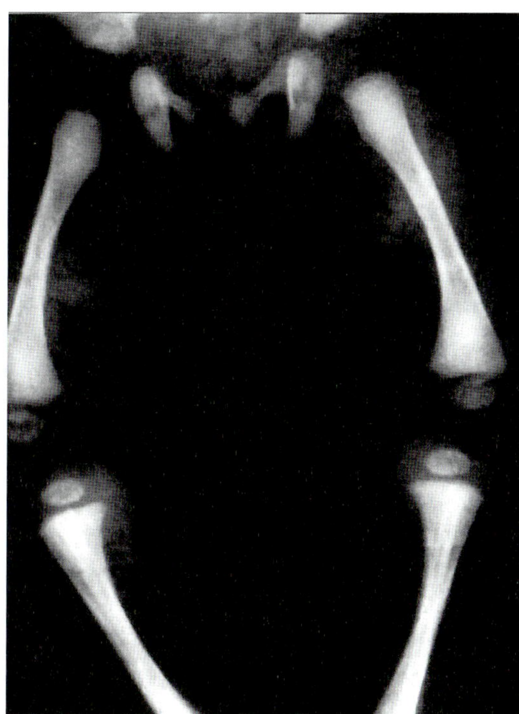

Figure 2
Radiograph of the lower extremities of a child with cartilage-hair hypoplasia. Note the deformity related to bowing and the increased density of the metaphyseal regions.

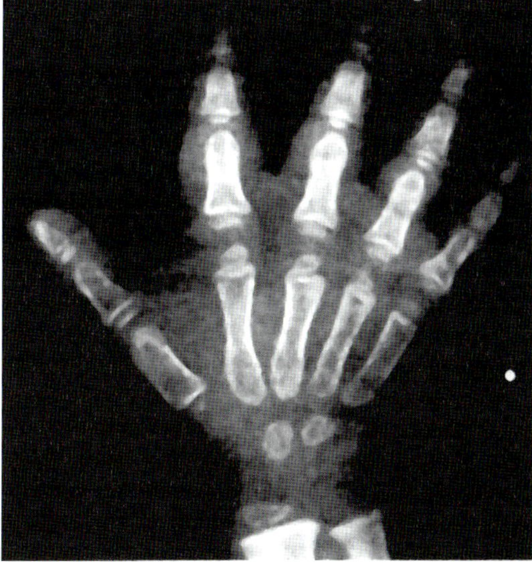

Figure 3
Hand changes in a child with cartilage-hair hypoplasia. The hands are short, particularly the metacarpals and phalanges. The fingers are frequently bent, but can be easily extended.

rib cage is sometimes present and a "Harrison's groove" is often seen.[4] This abnormality is defined as a horizontal line in the lower margin of the thorax where the diaphragm attaches to the ribs.

Several other features may be present in patients with this rare condition. First, and most important, are the chemical and biologic abnormalities. These include anemia, leukopenia, and a T cell or B cell immunodeficiency.[12,31,37-41] The two immunodeficient states sometimes result in susceptibility to infection, particularly with viruses.[39] A special susceptibility to varicella infection (chicken pox) can be very serious and cause death.[42] Gastrointestinal disorders, especially Hirschsprung's disease (an intestinal obstruction resulting from neural failure and causing major enlargement of the bowel), can be an enormous problem for patients with cartilage-hair hypoplasia.[4,43] Male patients may have reduced spermatogenesis,[44] and female patients may be less likely to become pregnant.[4]

Another great concern for patients and their families is the frequency of malignancy. Hodgkin's lymphoma appears to be more frequent, as is basal cell carcinoma.[4,45-49]

Radiographic manifestations include flaring, cupping, fragmentation, and scalloping of the metaphyses of the tubular bones[16,36] (Figure 2). Cyst-like irregularities may extend into the diaphyses.[3,4,36] Shortening is present in the long bones, but also in the metacarpals, metatarsals, and phalanges[35] (Figure 3). The costochondral junctions are often enlarged and resemble the "rachitic rosary."[4] The sternum is short and the ribs are flared. The vertebrae are small and have mild irregularity at the end plates. Scoliosis and lordosis are commonly seen.[4,14,16]

Treatment

Many patients with cartilage-hair hypoplasia do not require treatment. They are normal mentally and, aside from short stature and some characteristic skeletal alterations, they have few problems. The exceptions include concerns about infection, particularly with varicella virus.[42] This may require prophylaxis with varicella-zoster immune globulin and/or acyclovir.[4] Antibody immunodeficiency is a second problem, which may require bone marrow transplantation.[4,50-52] This may help the B cell or T cell immunodeficiency, but has no effect on the skeletal abnormalities. Granulocyte colony-stimulating factor may be useful in the treatment of neutropenia and prevention of infection.[37] Growth hormone has been tried for these children in an attempt to reduce their skeletal growth retardation, but thus far the results are inconclusive.[4,17] Treatment of bowel distress can be an important issue; some patients may need resective surgery, possibly as an emergency.[43] Orthopaedic problems may require bracing or corrective surgery, including possible spinal instrumentation for scoliosis.[4,36]

Discussion

Cartilage-hair hypoplasia is a rare disorder in most of the world and is rarely encountered by pediatricians or orthopaedists in the United States. Children with this disorder are short of stature but normal mentally, and many of them have few problems. However, serious problems can occur, including anemia, leukopenia, immunodeficiency, bowel obstruction, tumors, or some difficulties with the skeleton. What is quite striking about the disorder is that the cause, in terms of the mutations in the RMRP material from chromosome 9, has been clearly identified for about 15 years and yet we have had no major success at trying to alter the gene error. Children may be aided by our current methods of therapy, but they still remain dwarfs and are still at risk for a variety of disorders. It seems reasonable for physicians and scientists working with Old Order Amish and Finnish individuals to try their best to solve this problem with stem cells or enzyme treatment or other possibilities to reverse the process. Their families, friends, and physicians would be overjoyed!

References

1. McKusick VA: Metaphyseal dysostosis and thin hair: A "new" recessively inherited syndrome? *Lancet* 1964;1:832-833.

2. McKusick VA: *Medical Genetics of the Amish: Selected Papers.* Baltimore, MD, Johns Hopkins University Press, 1978.

3. McKusick VA, Eldridge R, Hostetler JA, Ruangwit U, Egeland JA: Dwarfism in the Amish: II. Cartilage-hair hypoplasia. *Bull Johns Hopkins Hosp* 1965;116:285-326.

4. Rimoin DL, Lachman RS: Metaphyseal dysplasia, McKusick type (cartilage–hair dysplasia), in Beighton P (ed): *McKusick's Heritable Disorders of Connective Tissue*, ed 5. St. Louis, MO, Mosby, 1993, pp 631-634.

5. Pyle E: A case of unusual bone development. *J Bone Joint Surg Am* 1931;13:874-876.

6. Theodorou SD, Adams J: An unusual case of metaphyseal dysplasia. *J Bone Joint Surg Br* 1963;45:364-369.

7. Halle MA, Collipp PJ, Roginsky M: Cartilage-hair hypoplasia in childhood. *N Y State J Med* 1970;70:2705-2708.

8. Lowry RB, Wood BJ, Birkbeck JA, Padwick PH: Cartilage-hair hypoplasia: A rare and recessive cause of dwarfism. *Clin Pediatr (Phila)* 1970;9:44-46.

9. Coupe RL, Lowry RB: Abnormality of the hair in cartilage-hair hypoplasia. *Dermatologica* 1970;141:329-334.

10. Lux SE, Johnston RB Jr , August CS, et al: Chronic neutropenia and abnormal cellular immunity in cartilage-hair hypoplasia. *N Engl J Med* 1970;282:231-236.

11. Mancini R, Morabito F: La condrodisplasia metafisaria, tipo McKusick, o 'cartilage-hair hypoplasia': Studio di due casi. *Acta Med Auxol (Milano)* 1974;6:131-148.

12. Wilson WG, Aylsworth AS, Folds JD, Whisnant JK: Cartilage-hair hypoplasia (metaphyseal chondrodysplasia, type McKusick) with combined immune deficiency: Variable expression and development of immunologic functions in sibs. *Birth Defects Orig Artic Ser* 1978;14:117-129.

13. Virolainen M, Savilahti E, Kaitila I, Perheentupa J: Cellular and humoral immunity in cartilage-hair hypoplasia. *Pediatr Res* 1978;12:961-966.

14. Kaitila IJ, Perheentupa J: Cartilage-hair dysplasia (CHH), in Eriksson AW, Forsius HR, Nevanlinna HR, Workman PL, Norio RK (eds): *Population Structure and Genetic Disorders*. New York, NY, Academic Press, 1980, pp 588-591.

15. Mäkitie O, Kaitila I: Cartilage-hair hypoplasia— clinical manifestations in 108 Finnish patients. *Eur J Pediatr* 1993;152:211-217.

16. Mäkitie O, Marttinen E, Kaitila I: Skeletal growth in cartilage-hair hypoplasia: A radiological study of 82 patients. *Pediatr Radiol* 1992;22:434-439.

17. Mäkitie O, Perheentupa J, Kaitila I: Growth in cartilage-hair hypoplasia. *Pediatr Res* 1992;31:176-180.

18. Ridanpää M, Jain P, McKusick VA, Francomano CA, Kaitila I: The major mutation in the RMRP gene causing CHH among the Amish is the same as that found in most Finnish cases. *Am J Med Genet C Semin Med Genet* 2003;121:81-83.

19. Ridanpää M, Sulisalo T, de la Chapelle A, Kaitila I: Genetic and physical mapping of the cartilage-hair hypoplasia locus on 9p13. *Am J Hum Genet* 1995;57:A201.

20. Sulisalo T, Sistonen P, Hästbacka J, et al: Cartilage-hair hypoplasia gene assigned to chromosome 9 by linkage analysis. *Nat Genet* 1993;3:338-341.

21. Hirose Y, Nakashima E, Ohashi H, et al: Identification of novel RMRP mutations and specific founder haplotypes in Japanese patients with cartilage-hair hypoplasia. *J Hum Genet* 2006;51:706-710.

22. Nakashima E, Mabuchi A, Kashimada K, et al: RMRP mutations in Japanese patients with

cartilage-hair hypoplasia. *Am J Med Genet A* 2003;123:253-256.

23. Bonafé L, Schmitt K, Eich G, Gideion A, Superti-Furga A: RMRP gene sequence analysis confirms a cartilage-hair hypoplasia variant with only skeletal manifestations and reveals a high density of single-nucleotide polymorphisms. *Clin Genet* 2002;61:146-151.

24. Chu S, Archer RH, Zengel JM, Lindahl L: The RNA of RNase MRP is required for normal processing of ribosomal RNA. *Proc Natl Acad Sci USA* 1994;91:659-663.

25. Martin AN, Li Y: RNase MRP RNA and human genetic diseases. *Cell Res* 2007;17:219-226.

26. Ridanpää M, van Eenennaam H, Pelin K, et al: Mutations in the RNA component of RNase MRP cause a pleiotropic human disease, cartilage-hair hypoplasia. *Cell* 2001;104:195-203.

27. Hermanns P, Bertuch AA, Bertin TK, et al: Consequences of mutations in the non-coding RMRP RNA in cartilage-hair hypoplasia. *Hum Mol Genet* 2005;14:3723-3740.

28. Thiel CT, Horn D, Zabel B, et al: Severely incapacitating mutations in patients with extreme short stature identify RNA–processing endoribonuclease RMRP as an essential cell growth regulator. *Am J Hum Genet* 2005;77:795-806.

29. Nakashima E, Tran JR, Welting TJ, et al: Cartilage hair hypoplasia mutations that lead to RMRP promoter inefficiency or RNA transcript instability. *Am J Med Genet A* 2007;143:2675-2681.

30. Hermanns P, Tran A, Munivez E, et al: RMRP mutations in cartilage-hair hypoplasia. *Am J Med Genet A* 2006;140:2121-2130.

31. Kuijpers TW, Ridanpää M, Peters M, et al: Short-limbed dwarfism with bowing, combined immune deficiency, and late onset aplastic anaemia caused by novel mutations in the RMPR gene. *J Med Genet* 2003;40:761-766.

32. Ridanpää M, Sistonen P, Rockas S, Rimoin DL, Mäkitie O, Kaitila I: Worldwide mutation spectrum in cartilage-hair hypoplasia: Ancient founder origin of the major 70A→G mutation of the untranslated RMRP. *Eur J Hum Genet* 2002;10:439-447.

33. Thiel CT, Mortier G, Kaitila I, Reis A, Rauch A: Type and level of RMRP functional impairment predicts phenotype in the cartilage hair hypoplasia-anauxetic dysplasia spectrum. *Am J Hum Genet* 2007;81:519-529.

34. Kelling C, Goldsmith LA, Baden HP: Biophysical and biochemical studies of the hair in cartilage-hair hypoplasia. *Clin Genet* 1973;4:500-506.

35. Giedion A: Phalangeal cone-shaped epiphyses of the hand: Their natural history, diagnostic sensitivity, and specificity in cartilage hair hypoplasia and the trichorhinophalangeal syndromes I and II. *Pediatr Radiol* 1998;28:751-758.

36. Glass RBJ, Tifft CJ: Radiologic changes in infancy in McKusick cartilage hair hypoplasia. *Am J Med Genet* 1999;86:312-315.

37. Ammann RA, Duppenthaler A, Bux J, Aebi C: Granulocyte colony-stimulating factor-responsive chronic neutropenia in cartilage-hair hypoplasia. *J Pediatr Hematol Oncol* 2004;26:379-381.

38. Mäkitie O, Juvonen E, Dunkel L, Kaitila I, Siimes MA: Anemia in children with cartilage-hair hypoplasia is related to body growth and to the insulin-like growth factor system. *J Clin Endocrinol Metab* 2000;85:563-568.

39. Mäkitie O, Kaitila I, Savilahti E: Deficiency of humoral immunity in cartilage-hair hypoplasia. *J Pediatr* 2000;137:487-492.

40. Pierce GF, Polmar SH: Lymphocyte dysfunction in cartilage-hair hypoplasia: Evidence for an intrinsic defect in cellular proliferation. *J Immunol* 1982;129:570-575.

41. Williams MS, Ettinger RS, Hermanns P, et al: The natural history of severe anemia in cartilage-hair hypoplasia. *Am J Med Genet A* 2005;138:35-40.

42. Mäkitie O, Kaitila I, Savilahti E: Susceptibility to infections and in vitro immune functions in cartilage-hair hypoplasia. *Eur J Pediatr* 1998;157:816-820.

43. Mäkitie O, Kaitila I, Rintala R: Hirschsprung disease associated with severe cartilage-hair hypoplasia. *J Pediatr* 2001;138:929-931.

44. Mäkitie OM, Tapanaimen PJ, Dunkel L, Siimes MA: Impaired spermatogenesis: An unrecognized feature of cartilage-hair hypoplasia. *Ann Med* 2001;33:201-205.

45. Eisner JM, Russell M: Cartilage hair hypoplasia and multiple basal cell carcinomas. *J Am Acad Dermatol* 2006;54:S8-S10.

46. Francomano CA, Trojak JE, McKusick VA: Cartilage hair hypoplasia in the Amish: Increased susceptibility to malignancy. *Am J Hum Genet* 1983;35:89A.

47. Gorlin RJ: Cartilage-hair-hypoplasia and Hodgkin disease. *Am J Med Genet* 1992;44:539.

48. Mäkitie O, Pukkala E, Kaitila I: Increased mortality in cartilage-hair dysplasia. *Arch Dis Child* 2001;84:65-67.

49. Mäkitie O, Pukkala E, Teppo L, Kaitila I: Increased incidence of cancer in patients with cartilage-hair hypoplasia. *J Pediatr* 1999;134:315-318.

50. Bocca G, Weemaes CM, van der Burgt I, Otten BJ: Growth hormone treatment in cartilage-hair hypoplasia: Effects on growth and the immune system. *J Pediatr Endocrinol Metab* 2004;17:47-54.

51. Guggenheim R, Somech R, Grunebaum E, Atkinson A, Roifman CM: Bone marrow transplantation for cartilage-hair-hypoplasia. *Bone Marrow Transplant* 2006;38:751-756.

52. Matsumoto S, Ozono K, Yamamoto T, et al: Treatment with recombinant IL-2 for recurrent respiratory infection in a case of cartilage-hair hypoplasia with autoimmune hemolytic anemia. *J Bone Miner Metab* 2000;18:36-40.

Chapter 18

Diffuse Idiopathic Skeletal Hyperostosis

Diffuse idiopathic skeletal hyperostosis (DISH) is a common condition of unknown cause, occurring principally in elderly men. It consists of bone proliferation in the fibrous membranes located in the anterior aspects of the thoracic and, less commonly, cervical or lumbar vertebrae. The disorder may be asymptomatic or cause limitation of movement, pain, dysphagia, and sometimes severe cervical arthropathic symptoms and signs. Although some biochemical abnormalities have been noted, there is no evidence to support a specific genetic or biologic cause. Of some concern clinically is that the disorder bears resemblance to at least two other forms of cervical hyperostosis, ankylosing spondylitis and ossification in the posterior longitudinal ligament (OPLL).

In neither of these is the ossific tissue confined to the anterior aspect of the vertebrae, and both have more effect on the canal and its contents.

History and Nomenclature

Although Oppenheimer[1] first described ossification in the anterior longitudinal ligament of the thoracic spine in 1942, it was Forestier and Rotes-Querol[2] who proposed that this was a distinct clinical entity and named it senile ankylosing hyperostosis of the spine. In 1975, Resnick and associates[3] introduced the term diffuse idiopathic skeletal hyperostosis and the classical acronym DISH.

As a result of these publications, the disorder is now commonly known as Forestier syndrome or DISH, but it has also been named senile ankylosing hyperostosis,[4] spondylorheostosis, spondylosis hyperostotica,[5] spondylitis ossificans ligamentosa,[1] and vertebral ankylosing hyperostosis.[6,7]

Presentation and Biology

DISH consists of proliferation of bone, sometimes relatively thick, arising from the fibrous membrane on the anterior aspects of the spinal segments, mostly thoracic but sometimes cervical or lumbar[5,6,8-16] (Figure 1). The following three characteristic features should be present to make the diagnosis of DISH.[5]

- Flowing calcification or ossification along the anterolateral aspects of at least four contiguous vertebrae and relative preservation of the intervertebral disk height in the involved vertebrae[5,8,12,16-18] (Figure 2).
- Absence of apophyseal joint ankylosis or ossification within the canal (OPLL). The lesions of the thoracic spine are usually located slightly more to the right side, related to the presence of the aorta on the left. The vertebrae are often

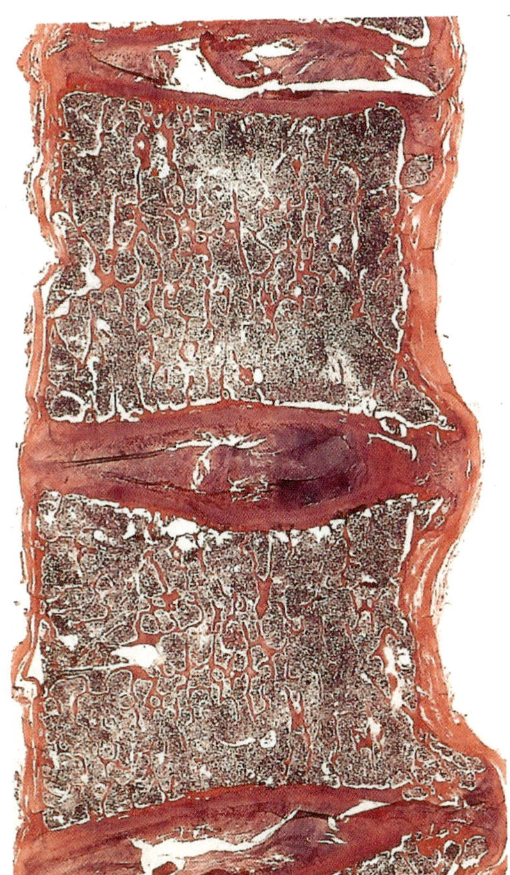

Figure 1

Histologic pattern for diffuse idiopathic skeletal hyperostosis. Note that the anterior fibrous envelope on the vertebrae show ossification, but no changes are noted posteriorly.

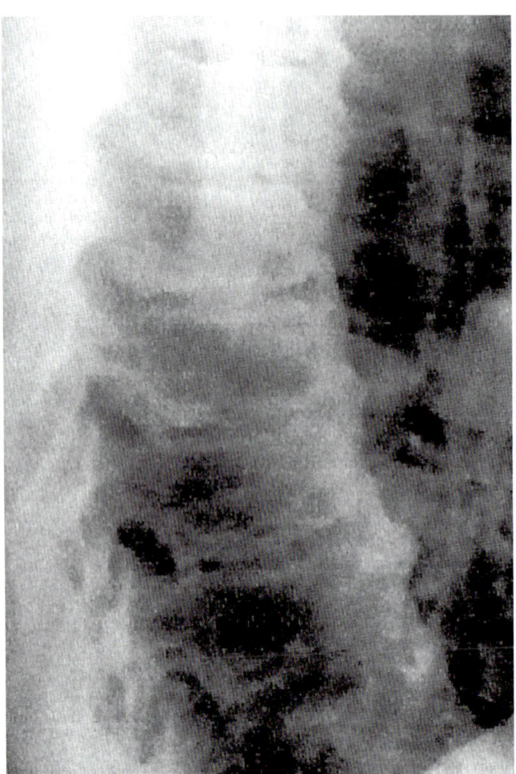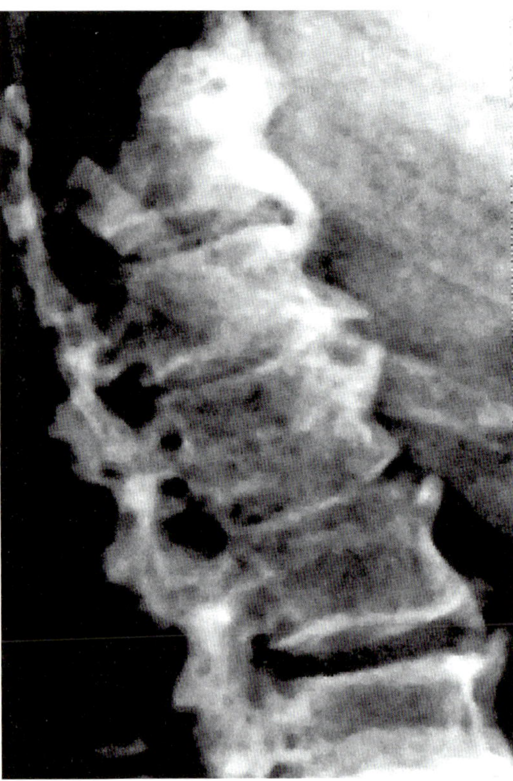

Figure 2

An elderly male reported back pain and limitation of motion. **A,** Radiograph of the thoracic spine shows diffuse idiopathic hyperostosis of the anterior aspects of the adjacent vertebrae without changes on the posterior side. **B,** Similar changes in the lumbar spine.

bound together so that they present with an anterior arthrodesis-like pattern for T2 to T10 or even lower.[5,8,13,14,16-18] Bone scan is positive.[5,13,18]

- The disk space and the canal are usually not invaded, but the roots, particularly on the right side, may be partially obstructed, producing sometimes painful and distressing limitation of motion.[5,13,18]

The complications of the thoracic lesions may include compression of the inferior vena cava, arthrodesis, limitation of motion, and pain in the lower extremities.[5,17,19] Spontaneous pseudarthrosis or fracture may occur and cause severe symptoms.[5,16,20,21] Lesions of the cervical spine are equally productive of new bone, but are centrally placed and sometimes quite extensive. They may produce not only profound limitation of motion but also dysphagia, dysphonia, stridor, myelopathy, sleep apnea, esophageal obstruction, and tracheal compression.[5,7,10,22-30] Fractures of the cervical spine are common and may lead to quadriplegia.[5,21]

Causation

There is no known cause for DISH. The disorder is much more common in elderly individuals and more particularly males, with estimates of frequency of more than 25% for men more than 70 years of age.[5,17,31] Women are much less frequently affected, even at advanced age, with an estimated occurrence of less than 10%. Some female patients with DISH seem to have less osteopororosis and higher bone mineral density than controls.[5,13,16,32]

Although obesity appears to be the most closely related disorder to the presence of DISH, factors such as type II diabetes, hypercholesterolemia, hyperuricemia, acromegaly, and hypertension are also reported, but are less frequently encountered.[6,13,31,33-35] Insulin growth factor-1 also seems to play a role but is not commonly observed.[36] Increased frequency of DISH has been noted in archeologic studies of both paleologic specimens of elderly persons, prehistoric animals, Egyptian mummies, and ancient clergymen.[37-39] On the basis of the last-mentioned study, it is proposed that a monastic way of life could actually be a cause![39]

For DISH, no genetic cause has been detected.[5] It has been suggested that the disorder is of vascular origin and that the new segments arise in relation to anterior vertebral vessel overgrowth.[34] It is essential to point out that a very similar lesion on the posterior aspect of the skeletal body seems to have some biochemical causations, including COL6A1, the candidate gene for OPLL.[40] The same gene is occasionally associated with DISH in Japanese patients but not in those from Czechoslovakia.[40] Similarly, the nucleotide pyrophosphate gene (NPPS) appears to relate the OPLL process, particularly in animals.[5] Another feature of OPLL appears to be the presence of prostaglandin I2, but there is no consistent evidence for the presence of the prostaglandin in the anterior disorder. A recent report has suggested that bone morphogenetic protein-2 may play a role in the pathologic process of the spinal ligament in the OPLL, but no evidence is presented for a similar abnormality in DISH.[41]

Current Concepts for Treatment

Very little information has been provided regarding treatment of aged patients with DISH. Thus far, most treatment protocols are proposed for the complications (specifically fractures, vascular injury, neural damage, etc) for thoracolumbar lesions.[5,21,31,42,43] The cervical problems are much more potentially damaging and include fracture, spinal cord compression, nerve injury, profound limitation of motion and dysphagia, dysphonia, stridor, myelopathy, sleep apnea, and tracheal compression.[5,10,13,22-25,29,30,43] Currently, most treatments available to elderly patients consist of physiotherapeutic measures such as exercises, bracing, sleep adjustments, and respiratory assistance.[5,23,24] Surgery is reserved for patients with fractures, neural damage, paralysis, respiratory impairment, and canal impairment,[5,22,25,42] There currently are no biologic or pharmaceutical approaches other than pain medication, such as aspirin and acetaminophen or cyclooxygenase-2 (COX-2) inhibitors.

Discussion

DISH is one of the most common orthopaedic disorders. It occurs with high frequency in older males and less frequently in females. The principal site is the thoracic spine. It causes limitation of movement of the thoracic and lumbar spine and is a source of pain and disability in older patients. Cervical DISH disease is much more severe at times and causes an array of symptoms and signs, many of which are disabling and some even life-threatening. No biologic origin has been established and no medicinal treatment is available. Patients must be watched closely for evidence of impending complications that threaten function or life. It does seem extraordinary that with apparent biologic control of all sorts of bone-forming and bone-destroying lesions of other causes, none of those agents seem appropriate for treatment of these patients.

References

1. Oppenheimer A: Calcification and ossification of vertebral segments (spondylitis ossificans ligamentosa): Roentgen study of pathogenesis and clinical significance. *Radiology* 1942;38:160-173.

2. Forestier J, Rotes-Querol J: Senile ankylosing hyperostosis of the spine. *Ann Rheum Dis* 1950;9:321-330.

3. Resnick D, Shaul SR, Robins JM: Diffuse idiopathic skeletal hyperostosis (Forestier's disease) with extraspinal manifestations. *Radiology* 1975;115:513-524.

4. Russell AS: Ankylosing spondylitis or DISH in ancient mummies. *Can Assoc Radiol J* 2004;55:335.

5. Weismann BN, Resnick D, Kaushik S, et al: Imaging, in Ruddy S, Harris ED Jr, Sledge CB (eds): *Kelley's Textbook of Rheumatology*, ed 6. Philadelphia, WB Saunders Company, 2001, pp 674-680.

6. Bick EM: Vertebral osteophytosis: Pathologic basis of its roentgenology. *Am J Roentgenol Radium Ther Nucl Med* 1955;73:979-983.

7. Meyer PR Jr: Diffuse idiopathic skeletal hyperostosis in the cervical spine. *Clin Orthop Relat Res* 1999;359:49-57.

8. de Vlam K, Lories RJ, Luyten FP: Mechanisms of pathologic new bone formation. *Curr Rheumatol Rep* 2006;8:332-337.

9. DiFranco M, Mauceri MT, Sili-Scavalli A, Iagnocco A, Ciocci A: Study of peripheral bone mineral density in patients with diffuse idiopathic skeletal hyperostosis. *Clin Rheumatol* 2000;19:188-192.

10. Kobayashi T, Hida K, Iwasaki Y, et al: Dysphagia due to ossification of anterior longitudinal ligament with diffuse idiopathic skeletal hyperostosis

(DISH): Two cases report. *Spinal Surg* 1999;13:197-201.

11. Mizuno J, Nakagawa H, Song J: Symptomatic ossification of the anterior longitudinal ligament with stenosis of the cervical spine. *J Bone Joint Surg Br* 2005;87:1375-1379.

12. Resnick D, Niwayama G: Radiographic and pathologic features of spinal involvement in diffuse idiopathic skeletal hyperostosis (DISH). *Radiology* 1976;119:559-568.

13. Scutellari PN, Orzincolo C, Princivalle M, Franceschini F: Diffuse idiopathic skeletal hyperostosis: Review of diagnostic criteria and analysis of 915 cases. *Radiol Med* 1992;83:729-736.

14. Smith CF, Pugh DG, Polley HF: Physiologic vertebral ligamentous calcification: An aging process. *Am J Roentgenol Radium Ther Nucl Med* 1955;74:1049-1058.

15. Suzuki K, Ishida Y, Ohmorik K: Long term followup of diffuse idiopathic skeletal hyperostosis in the cervical spine: Analysis of progression of ossification. *Neuroradiology* 1991;33:427-431.

16. Tsukomoto Y, Onitsuka H, Lee K: Radiologic aspects of idiopathic skeletal hyperostosis in the spine. *ARJ Am J Roentgenol* 1977;129:913-918.

17. Mata S, Fortin PR, Fitzcharles MA, et al: A controlled study of diffuse idiopathic skeletal hyperostosis: Clinical features and functional status. *Medicine (Baltimore)* 1997;76:104-117.

18. Schwartz JB, Rackson M: Diffuse idiopathic skeletal hyperostosis causes artificially elevated lumbar bone mineral density measured by dual X-ray absorbtiometry. *J Clin Densitom* 2001;4:385-388.

19. Scapinelli R: Compression of the inferior vena cava due to diffuse idiopathic skeletal hyperostosis. *Rev Rheum Engl Ed* 1997;64:198-201.

20. Miyamoto K, Shimizu K, Arimoto R, et al: Spontaneous symptomatic pseudoarthrosis of the T11-T12 intervertebral space with diffuse idiopathic skeletal hyperostosis: A case report. *Spine* 2003;28:E320-E322.

21. Paley D, Schwartz M, Cooper P, Harris WR, Levine AM: Fracture of the spine in diffuse idiopathic skeletal hyperostosis. *Clin Orthop Relat Res* 1991;267:22-32.

22. Burkus JK: Esophageal obstruction secondary to diffuse idiopathic skeletal hyperostosis. *Orthopedics* 1988;11:717-720.

23. Castellano DM, Sinacori JT, Karakla DW: Stridor and dysphagia in diffuse idiopathic skeletal hyperostosis (DISH). *Laryngoscope* 2006;116:341-344.

24. Ebo DG, Uytterhaegen PJ, Lagae PL, Vander Mijnsbrugge AM, Goffin J: Choking, sore throat with referred otalgia and dysphagia in a patient with diffuse idiopathic skeletal hyperostosis. *Acta Clin Belg* 2005;60:98-101.

25. Epstein NE: Simultaneous cervical diffuse idiopathic skeletal hyperostosis and ossification of the posterior longitudinal ligament resulting in dysphagia or myelopathy in two geriatric North Americans. *Surg Neurol* 2000;53:427-431.

26. Escobar C, Amores A, Gonzalas Moscoso P, Redondo R: Dysphagia as a symptom of diffuse idiopathic skeletal hyperostosis (Forstier-Rotes disease): A case report and literature review. *Acta Otorrinolaringol Esp* 1997;48:161-163.

27. Frederici A, Sgadari A, Savo A, Onder G, Bernabei R: Diffuse idiopathic skeletal hyperostosis: An uncommon cause of dysphagia in an older adult. *Aging Clin Exp Res* 2003;15:343-346.

28. Kritzer RO, Parker WD: DISH: A cause of anterior cervical osteophyte-induced dysphagia. *Spine* 1988;13:130-132.

29. Mader R: Clinical manifestations of diffuse idiopathic skeletal hyperostosis of the cervical spine. *Semin Arthritis Rheum* 2002;32:130-135.

30. Nelson RS, Urquhart AC, Faciszewski T: Diffuse idiopathic skeletal hyperostosis: A rare cause of dysphagia, airway obstruction and dysphonia. *J Am Coll Surg* 2006;202:938-942.

31. Kiss C, Szilagyi M, Paksy A, Poor G: Risk factors for diffuse idiopathic skeletal hyperostosis: A case-control study. *Rheumatology (Oxford)* 2002;41:27-30.

32. Sahin G, Polat G, Bagis S, Milcan A, Erdogan C: Study of axial bone mineral density in postmenopausal women with diffuse idiopathic skeletal hyperostosis related to type 2 diabetes mellitus. *J Womens Health (Larchmt)* 2002;11:801-804.

33. Coaccioli S, Fatiti G, DiCato L, et al: Diffuse idiopathic skeletal hyperostosis in diabctes mellitus, impaired glucose tolerance and obesity. *Panminerva Med* 2000;42:247-251.

34. El Miedany YM, Wassif G, el Baddini M: Diffuse idiopathic skeletal hyperostosis (DISH): Is it of vascular aetiology? *Clin Exp Rheumatol* 2000;18:193-200.

35. Sencan D, Elden H, Nacitarihan V, Sencan M, Kaptanoglu E: The prevalence of diffuse idiopathic skeletal hyperostosis in patients with diabetes mellitus. *Rheumatol Int* 2005;25:518-521.

36. Denko CW, Malemud CJ: Body mass index and blood glucose: Correlations with serum insulin, growth hormone and insulin-like growth factor-1 levels in patients with diffuse idiopathic skeletal hyperostosis (DISH). *Rheumatol Int* 2006;26:292-297.

37. Rothschild BM: Diffuse idiopathic skeletal hyperostosis as reflected in the paleontologic record: Dinosaurs and early mammals. *Semin Arthritis Rheum* 1987;17:119-125.

38. Vidal P: A paleoepidemologic study of diffuse idiopathic skeletal hyperostosis. *Joint Bone Spine* 2000;67:210-214.

39. Verlaan JJ, Oner FC, Maas GJ: Diffuse idiopathic skeletal hyperostosis in ancient clergymen. *Eur Spine J* 2007;16:1129-1135.

40. Tsukahara S, Miyazawa N, Akagawa H, et al: COL6A1, the candidate gene for ossification of the posterior longitudinal is associated with diffuse idiopathic skeletal hyperostosis in Japanese. *Spine* 2005;30:2321-2324.

41. Tanaka H, Nagai H, Murata T, et al: Involvement of bone morphogenetic protein-2 (BMP-2) in the pathologic ossification process of the spinal ligament. *Rheumatology (Oxford)* 2001;40:1163-1168.

42. Hendrix RW, Melany M, Miller F, Rogers LF: Fracture of the spine in patients with ankylosis due to diffuse idiopathic skeletal hyperostosis: Clinical and imaging findings. *AJR Am J Roentgenol* 1994;162:899-904.

43. Mader R: Current therapeutic options in the management of diffuse idiopathic skeletal hyperostosis. *Expert Opin Pharmacother* 2005;6:1313-1318.

Chapter 19

The Ehlers-Danlos Syndromes

The Ehlers-Danlos syndromes are multiple forms of an unusual and sometimes bizarre clinical entity characterized principally by thinning and hyperflexibility of the skin. There are at least nine forms of the disorder, which differ chiefly in terms of severity and degree of disease in various systems other than skin. These presentations include hypermobility and dislocation of joints, arterial and cardiac abnormalities, gastrointestinal and urinary disturbances, ocular structural changes, oral problems, and issues related to pregnancy. Many of the nine sometimes indistinctly defined disorders are autosomal dominant and have been studied carefully to assess the genetic abnormalities affecting collagen types I, III, and V, which appear to be the causative systems. Thus far, there does not appear to be any treatment of this sometimes very distressing and occasionally fatal disorder.

History

The history of Ehlers-Danlos syndrome has been well defined in reports by Victor McKusick[1-3] and subsequently by Peter Beighton and associates;[4-13] both of them were apparently intrigued by a disease that involved patients known as the "India rubber man" and the "elastic lady." Hippocrates probably described some aspects of the entity in the fourth century BC,[14] but it was Job Van Meekeren[15] who first clearly identified the syndrome in a Spanish patient in 1682. In 1888, Gould and Pyle[16] published a photograph of the "India rubber man," and shortly thereafter Kopp described Etta Lake as the "elastic lady."[17] Both of these patients could move their skin away from the body frame to an extraordinary degree and without difficulty or pain. Tschernogobow[18] first described the clinical syndrome of fragility and excessive hyperelasticity of skin, along with hypermobility and luxations of joints, and termed it "cutis laxa" in 1891. Williams[19] and Unna[20] examined the skin of patients with the disorder and described unique histologic changes. In 1900, Morris[21] confirmed these findings and also described

cutaneous nodules. It was however the outstanding contributions by Edvard Ehlers[22] in 1901 and Henri-Alexandre Danlos[23] in 1908 that defined the entity as a specific disease of genetic origin with some very unusual skin, articular, cardiac, vascular, oral, and ocular findings. Based on these studies, in 1936 Weber[24] said the term "cutis laxa" should be abandoned and the entity should now be known as the Ehlers-Danlos syndrome (often abbreviated as EDS). The changes seen in the skin and other parts were further confirmed over the next decade by contributions of Tobias,[25] Bolam,[26] Burrows and Turnbull,[27] Barber and associates,[28] Gordon,[29] and Benjamin and Weiner.[30] Autosomal dominant inheritance was described by McKusick in 1959,[1] and he and others were subsequently able to establish nine forms of the disorder with some variation in genetic causation and clinical presentation.[2,3,5,9,11,29,31,32] Ehlers-Danlos syndrome was originally thought to principally occur in Europeans, and many of the authors who described aspects of the disease are from those countries.[1,2] In recent years, the disorders have been found all over the world including the United States, Asia, Africa, and South America.[9] The disease has also been described in dogs and minks.[33,34]

Pathophysiology and Genetics

As indicated above, there are now believed to be nine forms of EDS. More than half the disorders appear to be autosomal dominant.[9,11,31,35] Despite that, the disease is still rarely encountered, possibly because many of the patients with mild disease do not know they have it. The disorder appears to occur principally as an error in collagen structure, but that has been clearly identified in only half the cases.[9,32,35-39]

According to the revised nosology introduced in 1997,[11] the types of Ehlers-Danlos syndrome include the following:

- Type I (gravis)—inherited as an autosomal dominant form, the clinical features are severe, with fairly pronounced musculoskeletal and skin findings

- Type II (mitis)—also autosomal dominant, but very mild; many patients or their physicians are not aware they have the disease
- Type III (joint hyperextensibility form)—an autosomal recessive form with milder skin changes but also joint changes, that are quite severe and sometimes disabling
- Type IV (ecchymotic or arterial form)—an autosomal recessive form with skin defects, hemorrhages, vascular abnormalities, and sometimes early death from cardiac or vascular issues
- Type V (skin and orthopaedic problems)—autosomal recessive and mild, but may have fairly severe joint changes
- Type VI (ocular form)—also autosomal recessive; patients have very severe ocular changes and hyperextensible skin and joints
- Type VII (arthrochalasis multiplex congenita)—may be either recessive or dominant and principally affects joints with less severe skin changes; dislocations are common
- Type VIII (periodontal form)—autosomal dominant and affects teeth, gums, and temporomandibular joints; produces scars in skin and oral cavity with poor healing
- Type IX (X-linked cutis laxa)—rare; occurs in females, who often have severe skin lesions and gastrointestinal disturbances

It would be valuable if the genetic causes of these nine types of disease could be easily identified so that they could be further classified, but unfortunately, even today, there is limited information. Clearly, the diseases affect collagen—most often types I, III, and V.[9,35,37,38,40-43] Mutations in the COL5A1 and COL5A2 genes located in choromosome 1, and encoding the α1 and α2 chains of type V collagen, respectively, have been discovered in many patients with type I and type II disease.[37-39,44] Type III collagen is affected in a much more aggressive form of EDS (type IV), and the mutation of the COL3A1 gene has been confirmed in several of these patients.[9,35-39,44] An error in COL1A1 is only rarely encountered in EDS, which usually has limited effect on type I collagen chains.[42] Another material that is considered to add materially to the process

is tenascin X, a member of a family of extracellular matrix glycoproteins. Tenascin X is believed to be a major participant in regulating collagen fibrillar spacing and interfibrillar distance.[40,45-47] Some patients with autosomal recessive Ehlers-Danlos syndromes have been found to have a considerable decrease in their tenascin X concentration on the basis of a postulated genetic error in chromosome 6 for the production of this material.[47,48]

Histologic studies have been interpreted in different ways; at this point, the changes in the various involved tissues are not really clearly defined. Elastin abnormalities have been described but are not really well defined, and most pathologists now believe that the defect is not in the elastic fibers but in the collagen.[2,9,36,41,49,50] The collagen fibers are diminished in numbers and, more importantly, there is a fibrous derangement and bundle disorder, particularly evident on electron microscopy. Some irregularity and presence of cystic structures are noted within the collagen of the subcutaneous tissue, vascular structures (especially small arteries), connective tissues in and around joints, tendons, and even cardiac and ocular structures.[2,9,36,41,50] Occasionally, giant cells are noted within abnormal and irregular spaces in what should normally be a dense and well-organized collagen component.[49,50]

Clinical Characteristics
Cutaneous Features
Regardless of the form of disease, all patients with EDS have cutaneous abnormalities; however, the severity varies with the type.[1,3,9,30,31] The skin is velvety in appearance and texture and, at least for the infant, is white in color. The skin is hyperextensible, but usually not lax; if stretched, it springs back to its former position (Figure 1). Sometimes the skin may be lax, particularly in elderly individuals, so as to be pendulous—a disorder that in the past was known as cutis laxa[9,17,18] or cutis hyperelastica.[27,51] The skin is fragile and easily bruised or damaged, and wounds may occur with minor trauma.[9,30,52] The tissue is abnormally friable and when lacerative or rounded injuries occur, they are slow to heal. Some of the forms of the disease may show cysts, or raised spheroidal or even calcareous lesions in the skin and subcutane-

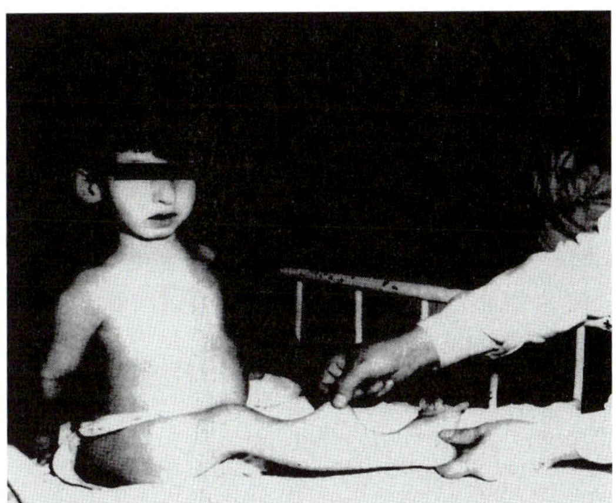

Figure 1

A child with Ehlers-Danlos disease presents marked painless hypermobility of the skin of the lower extremity.

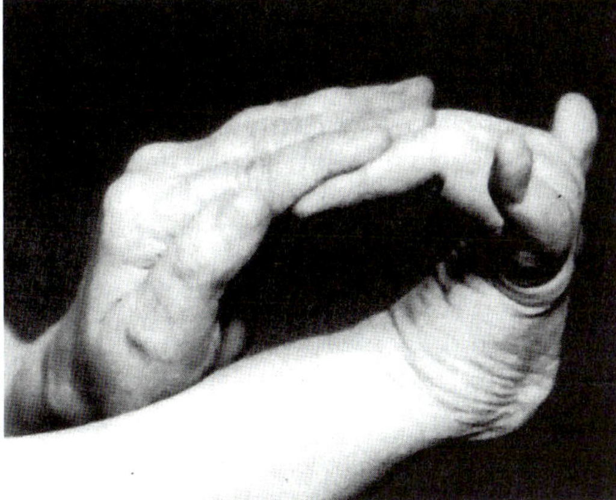

Figure 2

Hyperextension of the wrist and digits can also be done painlessly.

ous tissues.[53] Scarring and vascular anomalies may be present in some of the types, along with gross laxity and extraordinary extensibility.[9,54]

Musculoskeletal Features

Patients are normal in height and generally appear to have normal osseous, articular, and muscular structures. However, hypermobility of joints is characteristic of all forms of Ehlers-Danlos syndrome and some of the problems can lead to considerable disability.[4,9,12,55-62] The range of joint movement is increased as compared with normal individuals, and some of the most striking features are the ability to markedly hyperextend digits (Figure 2), flex the thumb sufficiently to touch the fifth metacarpal, hyperextend the elbows and knees, and forward flex the spine with the knees extended so as to place the palms of both hands on the floor.[2,9,12] Joint effusions, particularly of the knee, are common, and hemarthroses can also be a problem in terms of both pain and reduced function.[12,56,57] Gait is described as "loose-jointed," and dislocations of the radial head, clavicle, or even hip can occur.[12,56] Arthritis may occur, particularly with repeated injuries and dislocations, and this may cause limitation of movement and sufficient pain to require reconstructive surgery.[4,9,12,56,57] Spondylolisthesis occurs in some patients, particularly with type IV disease and in type VI disease may result in sometimes remarkably severe scoliosis. These problems are very difficult to treat

because of the loose structure of the paravertebral connective tissues. Patients with type IV disease are particularly susceptible to bruising of soft tissues, intra-articular bleeding, scarring and discoloration of skin after minor trauma, tendon ruptures, and development of deep wounds that sometimes will not heal even with surgical treatment.[9,12,63-65] All patients with EDS, regardless of type (except perhaps type II), often report easy fatigability and tenderness of limbs to pressure or firm grasp.[2,9]

Vascular Abnormalities

Complications related to arterial fragility, especially the aorta, are principally present in type IV disease but may occur to a lesser extent in other forms of the disease.[6,9,63-67] Type III collagen is the principal component of the vessel walls, and in type IV EDS, this is the most affected biologic structure. Aneurysms of the brain, vertebral arteries, major vascular structures, and even those in the foot or hand can cause serious impairment.[9] Aortic aneurysms are relatively rare but when they occur, they are difficult to repair and represent a major cause of death. Cardiac problems are seen less frequently but may occur, particularly in patients with type III or type IV EDS.[2,6,8,66-69] They can be very severe and life-threatening. These may consist of valve insufficiency, septal defects, aneurysms of the coronary arteries, bundle branch blocks, and aortic incompetence.[9,63,64,70]

Genitourinary and Gastrointestinal Problems

Diverticulae of the bladder are common in patients with EDS and sometimes result in urinary obstruction. Bleeding may occur as well. Eventration of the diaphragm, hiatus hernia, and rectal prolapse can occur and sometimes require emergency surgical procedures.[7,63,71-73] Diverticulae of the stomach, duodenum, or colon may result in serious gastrointestinal impairment. Most of these abnormalities occur in patients with severe disease. Patients with type IV disease may have hemorrhages and bowel perforation, which can be life-threatening.[1,7,9,63,64]

Pulmonary Problems

Emphysema and spontaneous pneumothorax have been reported in patients with EDS but are believed to be rare even in patients with type IV disease.[9,74] Spontaneous bleeding into the lungs and chest are also reported, but this finding is unusual.[1,9]

Neurologic Problems

It is unusual to have nervous system problems in patients with EDS, with the exception of occasional peripheral neuritis occurring with extremity soft-tissue injury or cord or spinal nerve problems associated with spondylolisthesis.[2,9,12,57] Intracranial bleeding can occur along with cerebral vascular accidents, but this is quite uncommon.[2,9] Of concern is the fact that many of the patients with severe forms of the disease have psychiatric problems, mostly related to depression.[75] Mental retardation is almost never seen, even in severely affected children.

Ocular Problems

Changes in the eyes are common findings in patients with type EDS type VI (oculoscoliotic type). Many patients show mild hypertelorism, and blue sclerae is common in all forms of the disease.[2,51] Abnormal epicanthal folds in the skin are often present and internal strabismus is common.[2,9,10] Patients with type VI disease may show alterations in the cornea and occasional retinal changes. Angioid streaks were reported to be present in several groups of patients.[76]

Oral and Dental Problems

Periodontosis is a major issue for patients with EDS type VIII, and patients have progressive gum problems and loss of teeth as they get older. In general, for all forms of the disease there may be temporomandibular abnormalities, including poor placement of underdeveloped teeth.[9,77-81] Both the teeth and the jaw fracture easily and eating hard food can be a problem for children and even some adults. Bleeding can occur even with tooth brushing, and dental work may require transfusions.[77]

Pregnancy Problems

The risks during pregnancy apply to both the mother and the fetus. Intrauterine bleeding is common, and cervical dilatation and uterine structural distortion may be present early in the course.[9,82-84] Premature labor has been reported and fetal (and sometimes maternal) death may be a consequence, particularly for patients with the more aggressive forms of EDS.[84] The fetus may have joint laxity with congenital dislocation of the hips, peripheral nerve palsies, and spinal structural problems.

Diagnostic Measures

A careful family history is essential because many of the diseases are autosomal dominant, so that only one parent may have aspects of the disorder.[9,39] A review of complaints is critical in trying to define the presence of the disease and, more importantly, the type. The key findings are skin hyperextensibility, dystrophic scarring, easy bruising, and joint hypermobility (Figure 3). It would be helpful if one could identify the syndrome by laboratory or imaging properties, but unfortunately that currently cannot be done. We must instead depend on history and physical findings. Patients with type I disease show cardinal manifestations in all systems, many of a severe degree;[3,9,11,31] those with type II and type V have similar but milder disease;[3,9,31] those with type III have more severe problems, particularly in terms of joint disease including dislocations; patients with type IV often have serious difficulty because of very aggressive vascular, cardiac, and bowel disease;[9,11,63,64,72] patients with type VI have eye problems and scoliosis; those with type VII present with mostly osteoarticular difficulties; those with type VIII have many oral and dental problems;[78,79] and female patients with type IX disease have skin and sometimes severe gastrointestinal problems.[85-87]

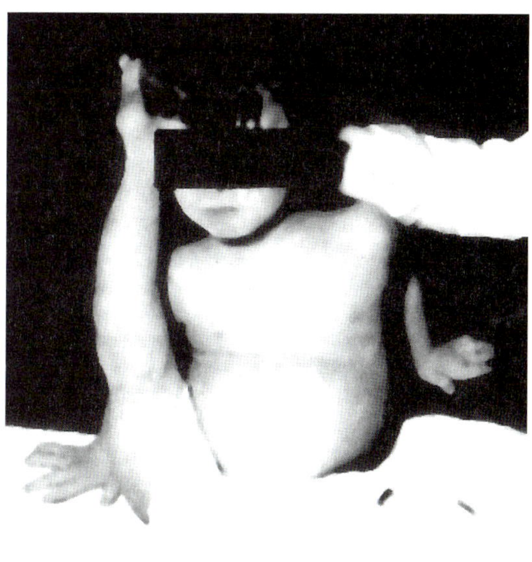

Figure 3
The lower extremity of the child may be flexed to 90° and also rotated to point the toes posteriorly without limitation or pain.

Imaging studies are helpful in terms of the bone and joint difficulties, but the principal studies for the remainder of the clinical problems are ultrasound and echocardiographic studies to assess the existence of vascular, aortic, or cardiac problems.[9,49,54,69,88] Some centers use analyses for the genetic collagen errors and the presence of tenascin X to define the presence of the disease and, at times, the type.[37,40,45] These studies are helpful, but because there is still limited knowledge as to their applicability, they currently are not very useful. Histologic studies, particularly electron microscopic studies of the skin, may be diagnostic.[2,9,36,41,49,50]

Treatment

There are currently no specific treatments of the Ehlers-Danlos disorders. No biochemical agent has been identified that can alter the course of the disease, and genetic approaches are thus far not applicable. The use of laser treatments may be helpful for skin defects,[80] but there are no approaches other than sometimes risky surgical treatment.[13,63,66,67,70,73] Surgical procedures for vascular, aortic, or cardiac abnormalities are sometimes essential but are at times life-threatening because of bleeding and poor wound healing.

Conservative management is sometimes helpful for orthopaedic problems, although bracing may cause skin defects or ecchymoses.[12,55,58,59] Surgery for subluxations of joints; abnormalities of hands and feet; spinal deformities; and dislocated hips, elbows, shoulders, and knees have all been reported.[4,12,55-61] Unfortunately, the procedures are fraught with problems, especially those of anesthesia risks; excessive bleeding; inability of sutures to hold tendons, ligaments, and skin together; wound infections; and difficulties related to postoperative care.

Comments and Conclusions

Ehlers-Danlos syndrome remains an intriguing and, alas, still very confusing clinical entity. The disease was first described more than 300 years ago and captured the imagination of many great contributors. The India rubber man and the elastic lady were described and depicted in texts throughout the world, and the very idea of skin hyperelasticity made physicians and their colleagues in science try their best to cure the disorder. Numerous great clinicians, scientists, and biologists including Anne De Paepe, Peter Byers, Peter Beighton, Victor McKusick, and many more spent much of their scientific lives trying to define the diseases, place them into types I through IX, identify the causation and genetic errors, and hopefully plan for ways to diagnose and effectively treat patients. Although much has been accomplished in terms of defining the genetic causation for some of the disorders, we still cannot fully identify them and have no way of attempting to cure them. The only thing that physicians can do now is wait until complications set in and then hope to be able to treat these to save a life or decrease disability. Fortunately, scientists are still intrigued by the disorder, especially when they see India rubber men and elastic ladies in their practices. Perhaps over time, they will solve some of the patient problems.

References

1. McKusick VA: Hereditary disorders of connective tissue. *Bull N Y Acad Med* 1959;35:143-156.

2. McKusick VA: *Heritable Disorders of Connective Tissue*, ed 3. St. Louis, CV Mosby Company, 1966, pp 179-229.

3. McKusick VA: Editorial: Multiple forms of Ehlers-Danlos syndrome. *Arch Surg* 1974;109:475-476.

4. Beighton P: Articular manifestations of the Ehlers-Danlos syndrome. *Semin Arthritis Rheum* 1972;1:246-261.

5. Beighton P: *The Ehlers-Danlos Syndrome*. London, England, William Heinemann Medical Books, 1970.

6. Beighton P: Cardiac abnormalities in the Ehlers-Danlos syndrome. *Br Heart J* 1969;31:227-232.

7. Beighton P: Gastrointestinal bleeding in the Ehlers-Danlos syndrome. *BMJ* 1968;1:315.

8. Beighton P: Lethal complications of the Ehlers-Danlos syndrome. *BMJ* 1968;3:656-659.

9. Beighton P: *McKusick's Heritable Disorders of Connective Tissue*, ed 5. St. Louis, MO, Mosby, 1993, pp 189-251.

10. Beighton P: Serious ophthalmological complications of the Ehlers-Danlos syndrome. *Br J Ophthalmol* 1970;54:263-268.

11. Beighton P, DePaepe AD, Steinmann B, Tsipouras P, Wenstrup RJ: Ehlers-Danlos syndrome: Revised nosology, Villefranche, 1997. Ehlers-Danlos National Foundation (USA) and Ehlers-Danlos Support Group (UK). *Am J Med Genet* 1998;77: 31-37.

12. Beighton P, Horan F: Orthopaedic aspects of the Ehlers-Danlos syndrome. *J Bone Joint Surg Br* 1969;51:444-453.

13. Beighton P, Horan F: Surgical aspects of the Ehlers-Danlos syndrome: A survey of 100 cases. *Br J Surg* 1969;56:255-259.

14. Adams F: *The Genuine Works of Hippocrates: Air, Waters and Places*. New York, NY, William Wood, 1891, pp 176-178.

15. Van Meekeren JA: De dilatabilitate extraordinaria cutis, in: *Observation Medico-chirugicae*. Amsterdam, Henrici, T. Bloom, 1682.

16. Gould GM, Pyle WL: *Anomalies and Curiosities of Medicine*. Philadelphia, PA, WB Saunders, 1888.

17. Kopp W: Demonstration zweier falle von "cutis laxa." *München Med Wschr* 1888;35:259-260.

18. Tschernogobow A: Cutis laxa (presentation at the first meeting of Moscow Dermatologic and Venerologic Society Nove 13, 1891). *Mhft Prakt Dermatol* 1892;14:76.

19. Williams AW: Cutis laxa. *Monatsschr Prakt Derm* 1892;14:490-501.

20. Unna PG: *The Histopathology of the Diseases of the Skin*. New York, NY, MacMillan, 1896, pp 984-988.

21. Morris M: Case report: Elastic skin and numerous cutaneous nodules. *Br J Dermatol* 1900;12:208-209.

22. Ehlers E: Cutis laxa: Neigung zum haemorrhagien in der haut, lockerung mehrerer artikulationen. *Derm Zschr* 1901;8:173-175.

23. Danlos M: Un cas de cutis laxa avec tumeurs par contusion chronique des coudes et des genoux (xanthome juvenile pseudo-diabetique de MM Halopeau et Mace de Lepinay). *Bull Soc Franc Dermatol Syph* 1908;19:70-72.

24. Weber FP: The Ehlers-Danlos syndrome. *Br J Dermatol Syph* 1936;48:609-617.

25. Tobias N: Danlos syndrome associated with congenital lipomatosis. *Arch Dermatol Syph* 1934;30:540-551.

26. Bolam RM: A case of Ehlers-Danlos syndrome. *Br J Dermatol* 1938;50:174-181.

27. Burrows A, Turnbull HM: Cutis hyperelastica (Ehlers-Danlos syndrome). *Br J Dermatol* 1938;50:648-652.

28. Barber HS, Fiddes J, Benians THC: The syndrome of Ehlers-Danlos. *Br J Dermatol* 1941;53:97-112.

29. Gordon H: Ehlers-Danlos syndrome. *Proc R Soc Med* 1942;35:263-264.

30. Benjamin B, Weiner H: Syndrome of cutaneous fragility and hyperelasticity and articular hyperlaxity. *Am J Dis Child* 1943;65:247-275.

31. Lawrence EJ: The clinical presentation of Ehlers-Danlos syndrome. *Adv Neonatal Care* 2005;5:301-314.

32. Pope FM, Burrows NP: Ehlers-Danlos syndrome has varied molecular mechanisms. *J Med Genet* 1997;34:400-410.

33. Barrera R, Mane C, Curan E, Vives MA, Zaragoza C: Ehlers-Danlos syndrome in a dog. *Can Vet J* 2004;45:355-356.

34. Hegreberg GA: Animal models for human disease: Ehlers-Danlos syndrome. *Am J Pathol* 1975;79:383-386.

35. Byers PH, Holbrook KA: Molecular basis of clinical heterogeneity in the Ehlers-Danlos syndrome. *Ann N Y Acad Sci* 1985;460:298-310.

36. Byers PH: Disorders of collagen biosynthesis and structure, in Scriver CR, Beaudet AL, Sly WS, Valle E (eds): *The Metabolic Basis of Inherited Disease*, ed 6. New York, NY, McGraw–Hill, 1989, pp 2802-2845.

37. Malfait F, Coucke P, Symoens S, et al: The molecular basis of classic Ehlers-Danlos syndrome: A comprehensive study of biochemical and molecular findings in 48 unrelated patients. *Hum Mutat* 2005;25:28-37.

38. Malfait F, De Paepe A: Molecular genetics in classic Ehlers-Danlos syndrome. *Am J Med Genet C Semin Med Genet* 2005;139:17-23.

39. Malfait F, Hakim AJ, De Paepe A, Grahame R: The genetic basis of the joint hypermobility syndromes. *Rheumatology* 2006;45:502-507.

40. Bristow J, Carey W, Egging D, Schalkwijk J: Tenascin-X, collagen, elastin and the Ehlers-Danlos syndrome. *Am J Med Genet C Semin Med Genet* 2005;139:24-30.

41. Kobayasi T: Abnormality of dermal collagen fibrils in Ehlers Danlos syndrome: Anticipation of the abnormality for the inherited hypermobile disorders. *Eur J Dermatol* 2004;14:221-229.

42. Nuytinck L, Freund M, Lagae L, et al: Classical Ehlers-Danlos syndrome caused by a mutation in type I collagen. *Am J Hum Genet* 2000;66:1398-1402.

43. Schwarze U, Atkinson M, Hoffman GG, et al: Null alleles of the COL5A1 gene of type V collagen are a cause of the classic of Ehlers-Danlos

syndrome (types I and II). *Am J Hum Genet* 2000;66:1757-1765.

44. Wenstrup RJ, Langland GT, Willing MC, et al: A splice junction mutation in the region of COL5A1 that codes for carboxyl propeptide of pro alpha I (V) chains results in the gravis form of the Ehlers-Danlos syndrome (type I). *Hum Mol Genet* 1996;5:1733-1736.

45. Burch GH, Gong Y, Liu W, et al: Tenascin-X deficiency is associated with Ehlers-Danlos syndrome. *Nat Genet* 1997;17:104-108.

46. Lindor NM, Bristow J: Tenascin-X deficiency in autosomal recessive Ehlers-Danlos syndrome. *Am J Med Genet A* 2005;135:75-80.

47. Schalkwijk J, Zweers MC, Steijlen PM, et al: A recessive form of the Ehlers-Danlos syndrome caused by tenascin-X deficiency. *N Engl J Med* 2001;345:1167-1175.

48. Peeters AC, Kucharekova M, Timmermans J, et al: A clinical and cardiovascular survey of Ehlers-Danlos syndrome patients with complete deficiency of tenascin-X. *Neth J Med* 2004;62:160-162.

49. Pierard GE, Pierard-Franchimont C, Lapiere CM: Histopathological aid at the diagnosis of the Ehlers-Danlos syndrome, gravis and mitis types. *Int J Dermatol* 1983;22:300-304.

50. Wechsler HL, Fisher ER: Ehlers-Danlos syndrome: Pathologic, histochemical and electron microscopic observations. *Arch Pathol* 1964;77:613-619.

51. Durham DG: Cutis hyperelastica (Ehlers Danlos syndrome) with blue scleras, micro-cornea and glaucoma. *Arch Ophthalmol* 1953;49:220-221.

52. Anstey A, Wilkinson JD, Pope FM: Ehlers-Danlos syndrome with recurrent bruising. *J R Soc Med* 1990;83:800-801.

53. Kahana M, Feinstein A, Tabachnic E, et al: Painful piezogenic pedal papules in patients with Ehlers-Danlos syndrome. *J Am Acad Dermatol* 1987;17:205-209.

54. Eisenbeiss C, Martinez A, Hagedorn-Greiwe M, et al: Reduced skin thickness: A new minor diagnostic criterion for the classical and hypermobility types of Ehlers-Danlos syndrome. *Br J Dermatol* 2003;149:850-852.

55. Badelon O, Bensahel H, Csukonyi Z, Chaumien JP: Congenital dislocation of the hip in Ehlers-Danlos syndrome. *Clin Orthop Relat Res* 1990;255:138-143.

56. Carter CO, Wilkinson J: Persistent joint laxity and congenital dislocation of the hip. *J Bone Joint Surg Br* 1964;46:40-45.

57. Coventry MB: Some skeletal changes in the Ehlers-Danlos syndrome. *J Bone Joint Surg Am* 1961;43:855-860.

58. Gamble JG, Mochizuki C, Rinsky LA: Trapeziometacarpal abnormalities in Ehlers-Danlos syndrome. *J Hand Surg [Am]* 1989;14:89-94.

59. Jerosch J, Castro WH: Shoulder instability in Ehlers-Danlos syndrome: An indication for surgical treatment. *Acta Orthop Belg* 1990;56:451-453.

60. Kornberg M, Aulicino PL: Hand and wrist joint problems in patients with Ehlers-Danlos syndrome. *J Hand Surg [Am]* 1985;10:193-196.

61. Moore JR, Tolo VT, Weiland AJ: Painful subluxation of the carpometacarpal joint of the thumb in Ehlers-Danlos syndrome. *J Hand Surg [Am]* 1985;10:661-663.

62. Rose PS, Johnson CA, Hungerford DS, McFarland EG: Total knee arthroplasty in Ehlers-Danlos syndrome. *J Arthoplasty* 2004;19:190-196.

63. Oderich GS, Panneton JM, Bower TC, et al: The spectrum, management and clinical outcome of Ehlers-Danlos syndrome type IV: A 30 year experience. *J Vasc Surg* 2005;42:98-106.

64. Pepin M, Schwarze U, Superti-Furga A, Byers PH: Clinical and genetic features of Ehlers-Danlos syndrome type IV, the vascular type. *N Engl J Med* 2000;342:673-680.

65. Ruby ST, Kramer J, Cassidy SB, Tsipouras P: Internal carotid aneurysm: A vascular manifestation for type IV Ehlers-Danlos syndrome. *Conn Med* 1989;53:142-144.

66. Karkos CD, Prasad V, Mukhopadhyay U, Thomson GJ, Hearn AR: Rupture of the abdominal aorta in patients with Ehlers-Danlos syndrome. *Ann Vasc Surg* 2000;14:274-277.

67. Krog M, Almgren B, Eriksson I, Nordstrom S: Vascular complications in the Ehlers-Danlos syndrome. *Acta Chir Scand* 1983;149:279-282.

68. Leier CV, Call TD, Fulkerson PK, Wooley CF: The spectrum of cardiac defects in the Ehlers-Danlos syndrome, types I and III. *Ann Intern Med* 1980;92:171-178.

69. McDonnell NB, Gorman BL, Mandel KW, et al: Echocardiographic findings in classical and hypermobile Ehlers-Danlos syndromes. *Am J Med Genet A* 2006;140:129-136.

70. Serry C, Agomuoh OS, Goldin MD: Review of Ehlers-Danlos syndrome: Successful repair of rupture and dissection of abdominal aorta. *J Cardiovasc Surg (Torino)* 1988;29:530-534.

71. Douglas BS, Douglas HM: Rectal prolapse in the Ehlers-Danlos syndrome. *Aust Paediatr J* 1973;9:109-110.

72. Ng SC, Muiesan P: Spontaneous liver rupture in Ehlers-Danlos syndrome type IV. *J R Soc Med* 2005;98:320-322.

73. Silva R, Cogbill TH, Hansbrough JF, et al: Intestinal perforation and vascular rupture in Ehlers-Danlos syndrome. *Int Surg* 1986;71:48-50.

74. Iwama T, Sato H, Matsuzaki T, et al: Ehlers-Danlos syndrome complicated by eventration of the diaphragm, colonic perforation and jejunal perforation: A case report. *Jpn J Surg* 1989;19:376-380.

75. Fehlow P, Tennstedt A: Concomitant neuropsychiatric symptoms in a case of Ehlers-Danlos syndrome [in German]. *Psychiatr Neurol Med Psychol (Leipz)* 1985;37:215-220.

76. Green WR, Friedman-Kien A, Banfield WH: Angioid streaks in Ehlers-Danlos syndrome. *Arch Ophthalmol* 1966;76:197-204.

77. Barabas GM, Barabas AP: The Ehlers-Danlos syndrome: A report of the oral and haematological findings in nine cases. *Br Dent J* 1967;123:473-479.

78. De Coster PJ, Martens LC, De Paepe A: Oral health in prevalent types of Ehlers-Danlos syndromes. *J Oral Pathol Med* 2005;34:298-307.

79. Jones ML: Orthodontic treatment in Ehlers-Danlos syndrome. *Br J Orthod* 1984;11:158-162.

80. Mueller DF, Zimmermann A, Borelli C: The efficiency of laser for the treatment of Ehlers-Danlos

syndrome. *Lasers Surg Med* 2005;36:76-78.

81. Myers DE: Ehlers-Danlos syndrome as a cause of temporomandibular joint disorders. *Anesth Prog* 1985;32:23-24.

82. Atalla A, Page I: Ehlers-Danlos syndrome type III in pregnancy. *Obstet Gynecol* 1988;71:508-509.

83. Mukerji S: Ehlers-Danlos syndrome with pregnancy. *J Indian Med Assoc* 1975;64:149-151.

84. Peaceman AM, Cruikshank DP: Ehlers-Danlos syndrome and pregnancy: Association of type IV disease with maternal death. *Obstet Gynecol* 1987;69:428-431.

85. Hollister DW: Clinical features of Ehlers-Danlos syndrome type VIII and IX, in Akeson WH (ed): *Symposium on Heritable Disorders of Connective Tissue*. St Louis, MO, Mosby Year Book, 1982, pp 102-113.

86. Moore MM, Votava JM, Orlow SJ, Schaffer JV: Ehlers-Danlos syndrome type VIII: Periodontitis, easy bruising, marfanoid habitus and distinctive facies. *J Am Acad Dermatol* 2006;55 (2 Suppl):S41-S45.

87. Nelson DI, King RA: Ehlers-Danlos syndrome type VIII. *J Am Acad Dermatol* 1981;5:297-303.

88. Cremers PT, Busscher DL, MacFarlane JD: Case report: Ultrasound demonstration of a superior mesenteric artery aneurysm in a patient with Ehlers-Danlos syndrome. *Br J Rheumatol* 1990;29:482-484.

Chapter 20

Erdheim-Chester Disease

Erdheim-Chester disease is one of the rarest and most mysterious clinical entities. The first patient with this disease was described by William Chester in an article in *Virchow's Archives* in 1930.[1] At the time, Chester was a pupil of the famous Viennese pathologist and educator Jakob Erdheim. Henry Jaffe, a colleague and great admirer of Erdheim, subsequently named the entity Erdheim-Chester disease.[2] The disease is characterized by development of xanthogranulomatous material in histiocytes in multiple sites including the skin, heart, breast, marrow, kidney, lungs, abdomen, eyes, brain, pituitary gland, and bones. To some extent, the histologic character of the disease resembles Langerhans cell histiocytosis but differs in terms of the age at onset, the biochemical characteristics, a striking difference in the nature of the bone lesions, and the degree of neurologic involvement.[3-5] The disease is so rare that there have been very limited opportunities for research as to causation, but thus far there is no evidence for an infectious, genetic, or biologic cause.

Jakob Erdheim—Pathologist, Collector, Scientist, and Educator

Jakob Erdheim was born in 1874 in Galicia and received his medical degree from the University of Vienna in 1900.[6,7] He became interested in pathology and joined the Pathology Institute of the Municipal Hospital of Vienna. In 1923, he became director of that institution and with great commitment, performed thousands of autopsies and trained hundreds of students in pathology. Included among his revering students were Fritz Schajowicz, Henry Jaffe, Heinrich Karpas, Leo Low-Beer, Ernst Freund, and Fuller Albright.[6-8] His capacity as an investigator is reflected in his remarkable studies of hyperparathyroidism, acromegaly, Paget's disease, pituitary gland abnormalities, action of growth hormone, and a variety of pathologic disorders.[9-12] Erdheim was a recluse. He lived in a room in his hospital, was not married, and was twice hospitalized—once for tuberculosis and later for typhoid fever.[7] He recovered from both but concealed his illnesses from his colleagues and students. According to Dr. Sharon Romm,[7] in 1937, while alone in his hospital residence room, Dr. Erdheim suddenly died of previously unrecognized cardiac disease. There is some doubt as to the cause of his death, although allegedly an autopsy disclosed the occlusion of his left coronary artery. A few months before his death, Erdheim sent his entire collection of pathologic material concealed in a rug to the United States to Ernst Freund, who at the time was working with Henry Jaffe at the Hospital for Joint Diseases. When Freund died, he willed the collection to Jaffe, who in turn, when he died, willed it to Henry Mankin. Erdheim was Jewish, and the reason for his desire to send away this extraordinary collection of pathology may have been related to the Viennese Auschluss, during which many people of various faiths were killed by the Nazis.

Pathophysiology

Erdheim-Chester disease is a rare condition of unknown etiology that infiltrates bone, lung, pituitary gland, orbit, retroperitoneum, and the central nervous system.[13-36] The disease shows some similarity in histologic and biologic characteristics to Langerhans cell histiocytosis, which is much more frequent in occurrence.[2-5,37-40] Studies of patients with Langerhans cell histiocytosis in the early 1990s were thought to show a relationship to Epstein-Barr virus or human herpes virus 6 or 9,[39,41-43] but further studies did not support that finding.[44,45] Attempts to identify a genetic error have also failed to find a consistent abnormality in either disease.[4,29,35,40,41,44,45] Recently, a study of the gene structure for one patient with Erdheim-Chester disease was reported to show a translocation between genes 5 and 12 that appeared to result in platelet-derived growth factor receptor-β, but this could not be confirmed.[46]

In Erdheim-Chester disease, the cytoplasm of the cells is filled with lipid material and is positive for CD68 +, but negative for

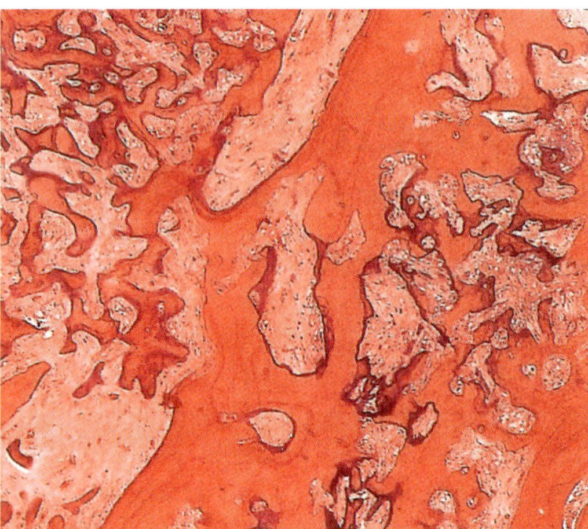

Figure 1

Histologic pattern for the bones of a patient with Erdheim-Chester disease shows extraordinary production of bone, with a marked increase in the number of osteoblasts.

CD1a and only occasionally positive for S-100.[21,29,38,40,46,47] These chemical alterations and the absence of Birbeck granules on electron microscopy and eosinophils on histologic study help to distinguish this disease from Langerhans cell histiocytosis.[3,5,41,48] In addition, the pathologic material often contains some characteristic giant cells, described as Touton-like, which are multinucleated, with the nuclei organized in a wreath-like ring around the xanthomatous cytoplasm.[21,29,38,46] Histologically, the material often shows extensive areas of fibrosis.[5,21,46]

Clinical Syndrome

Erdheim-Chester disease occurs in adults, and it has been suggested that the average age of onset is more than 40 years and that males are more frequently affected than females.[5,15,28,35,40,46] It is believed that the disease may be mild in some, but the majority of patients have extensive disease; the death rate is estimated at more than 50% at an average of 3 or so years after the onset of illness.[5,15,35,40,46] Patients with Erdheim-Chester disease have a highly variable presentation, with some patients having only one or two sites of deposition of the pathologic material and others having extensive disease in multiple sites. In all cases, the cause of the patient's symptomatology and clinical findings is the occurrence of sometimes extensive masses of lipid-laden histiocytes with fibrosis, often in multiple

sites in the entire body. They may occur in the retroperitoneum, the lungs, the cerebrum, and especially the cerebellum, the eyes, the heart, the pituitary gland, and the bones. The material in the bones has two presentations: first, the replacement and depletion of the marrow; and second, the extensive sclerotic bone formation both in the shaft and periosteum (Figure 1).

Because patients with the disease have multiple sites of involvement, they may have an extensive array of complaints and findings. These include the following:

- General health—hypertension, weight loss, fatigue, and occasional fever[5,15,21,26,35,46]

- Ocular findings—exophthalmos, proptosis, periorbital xanthomatous lesions, double vision, and sometimes subsequent blindness[13,14,31,33,47,49]

- Bone lesions—bilateral and often symmetric sclerotic metaphyseal and diaphyseal lesions of tubular bones including the femur, tibia, fibula, radius and ulna. Bone pain, periostitis, jaw lesions, dental abnormalities, fractures, and deformities may be present [5,15,18,20,35,50-54] (Figure 2).

- Abdominal lesions—retroperitoneal collections of xanthogranulomatous masses that may cause obstruction in the intestines and vascular compression, resulting in edematous limbs and sometimes skin ulcerations and soft-tissue changes.[27,34,49,50,55,56]

- Pulmonary and cardiac lesions—extensive pleural and pulmonary involvement that can cause damage to ribs, lungs, blood vessels, and myocardium and result in dyspnea, dysphagia, respiratory failure, cardiac abnormalities, and sometimes death.[14,21,23,24,27,30,32,57,58]

- Cranial and neurologic lesions—headaches, including migraine, diabetes insipidus, cerebellar abnormalities, impaired hearing, extra-axial masses involving the dura, gait disturbances, slurred speech, and confusion.[16,17,19,25,36,46,59-62]

- Other sites— breast nodules, occasionally multiple. Renal disease may occur and often results in enlargement of the kidneys, renal calculi, and sometimes renal failure.[50,63-65]

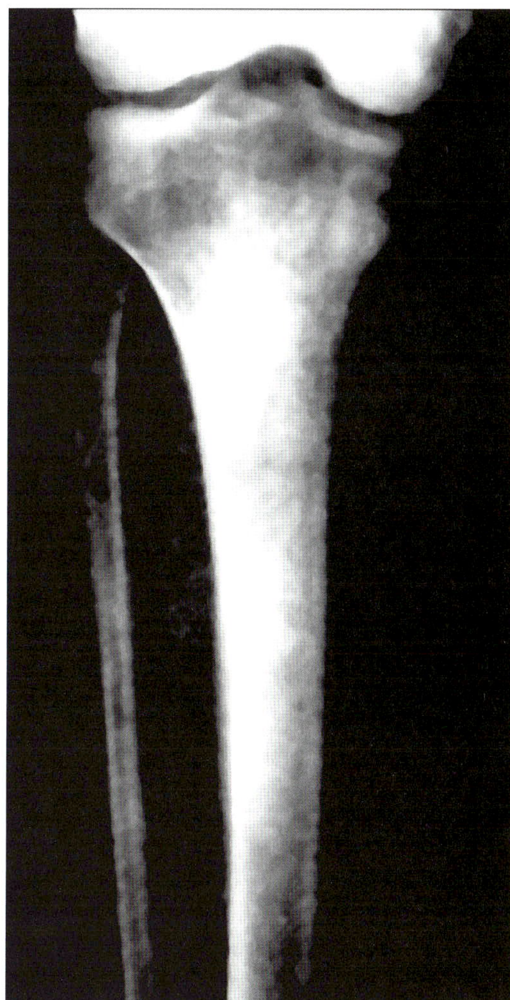

Figure 2
Radiograph of the tibia of a patient with Erdheim-Chester disease showing the marked overproduction of irregular cortical and medullary bone. The bone is deformed.

Laboratory and Imaging Studies

Patients with Erdheim-Chester disease may have evidence of osseous, pituitary, renal, pulmonary, or cardiac disorders, but the findings are not specific. Evidence for diabetes insipidus is common and some patients may have hyperprolactinemia, gonadotrophin deficiency, and decreased insulin-like growth factor levels.[25,29,46] Androgen and estrogen levels are often low or low-normal. Anemia and diminished platelets have been noted, along with a rapid erythrocyte sedimentation rate and increased C-reactive protein.[15,21,29,46,65] Some patients are noted to have increased lipid and cholesterol levels in the blood. Diminished vasopressin and urine concentration failure are found in patients with pituitary dysfunction.[25,29,46]

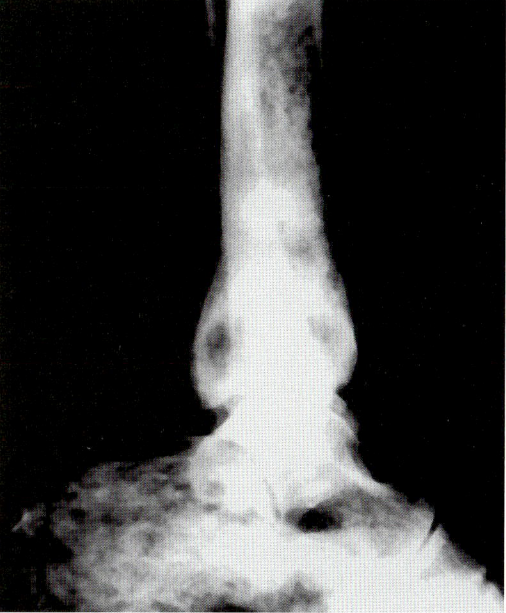

Figure 3
Radiograph of the distal tibia and foot, showing the presence of marked alteration in structure and overproduction of bone in both sites.

Infection of periorbital xanthogranulomatous lesions and skin ulcers is common.

Standard imaging of the bones shows irregular patterns of bone density.[18,20,35,38] Much of the bony tissue shows areas of increased density, with thickening of the cortices and often some periostitis (Figure 3). There are sometimes regions of decreased density associated with cortical irregularity and thinning and bowing deformity.[5,20,35,54] Skull imaging sometimes shows irregularity of structure, and the spine in some cases shows increased density. Bone scans are almost always positive. Osteoarthritis is common in the patient's knee and hip joints, and foci of osteonecrosis are sometimes observed in the shafts. MRI is very useful in defining the extent and nature of the lipoid granulomatous lesions in various places, including the lungs, brain, retroperitoneum, and heart.[19,23,46,47,54,56] The images show that the masses are irregular in shape and size, variable in structure, and usually demonstrate decreased intensity on T1 and a marked increase on T2.[52,54,56]

Treatment

It should be apparent that with so few patients available for study and treatment, no large series can be used for definitive studies of the response to various forms of therapy.

The majority of the therapeutic attempts have involved only one or two patients and these are sometimes in different countries under the care of physicians of different disciplines (eg, hematologists, orthopaedists, cardiologists, pulmonologists, internists, rheumatologists, opthalmologists, etc). It should also be understood that many of the patients with this disorder die within 3 years of the onset of symptoms, and in these patients, the therapy may only be designed to treat cardiac, respiratory, major vascular, or central nervous system compromise or failures.

The earliest agents used for treatment were corticosteroids, which sometimes caused some improvement not only in the patient's symptoms but in the laboratory and imaging findings.[28,30,35,36,46,66] The results, however, were not consistent and the bone problems, including osteonecrosis and lytic areas, seemed to be increased in extent and severity.

Radiation has been used for the treatment of enormous masses, which seem to cause pressure on blood vessels, viscera, or the heart. Despite the use of this treatment, many patients died, but this may have been related to the severity of the disease, rather than the lack of effect of the radiation. In addition, radiation has been suggested for treatment of the brain lesions, and several patients have seemed to improve with this therapy.[36,67]

A series of chemotherapeutic agents has been used over the years. These include vinblastine, vincristine, cyclophosphamide, and doxorubicin, all of which have been used with some success for both Hand-Schüller-Christian disease and children with Letterer-Siwe disease.[3,4,39] For the several patients with Erdheim-Chester disease, the use of some of these agents seemed to be successful for a short period but the complications became a problem for some patients.[36,68] Most recently interferon alpha has been introduced and has been shown to have some success in terms of stabilizing the patient's status and sometimes improving the cardiorespiratory and ocular symptoms.[69,70] One report suggests that introduction of stem cells may have some value for patients who do not respond to other treatment protocols.[71]

Conclusions

Erdheim-Chester disease appears to have only one great advantage for patients and their physicians—its rarity. It is a disease that occurs in very few patients, who are often older than 40 years of age and sometimes present with extensive lesions in the lungs, heart, brain, eyes, bones, blood vessels, and viscera. Most patients seem to fade away over a 3-year period with increasing symptoms and signs of extensive disease.

There does not seem to be a consistently successful treatment, although recently the use of interferon alpha appears to have some effect. If a sufficient number of patients were available to study for evidence of infectious or genetic causes, it is possible another treatment protocol could be used to help them; however, because the disease is so serious, with greater numbers there would be more suffering and greater difficulties for the patients, their families, and their physicians.

References

1. Chester W: Uber lipoidgranulomatose. *Virchow's Arch Patho Anat* 1930;279:561-602.

2. Jaffe HL: Gaucher's disease and certain other inborn metabolic disorders: Lipid (cholesterol) granulomatosis, in Jaffe HL: *Metabolic, Degenerative and Inflammatory Diseases of Bones and Joints.* Philadelphia, PA, Lea and Febiger, 1972, pp 550-560.

3. Campanacci M: *Bone and Soft Tissue Tumors*, ed 2. New York, NY, Springer Verlag, 1999, pp 857-876.

4. Dorfman HD, Czerniak B: *Bone Tumors*. St Louis, MO, Mosby, Inc, 1997, pp 690-701.

5. Mirra JM: Erdheim-Chester disease, in *Bone Tumors: Clinical, Radiologic and Pathological Correlates*. Philadelphia, PA, Lea and Febiger, 1989, pp 1074-1078.

6. Moore RA: Jakob Erdheim (1874-1937). *Cancer* 1952;5:1069.

7. Romm S: Jakob Erdheim: Eminent pathologist of Vienna. *Am J Dermatopathol* 1987;9:447-450.

8. Niederle BE, Schmidt G, Organ CH, Niederle B: Albert J and his surgeon: A historical reevaluation of the first parathyroidectomy. *J Am Coll Surg* 2006;202:181-190.

9. Erdheim J: Morphologische studien über die beziehung der epithelkörperchen zum kalkstoffwechsel. *Frankfurt Zeit Pathol* 1911;7:175-230.

10. Erdheim J: Tetania parathyreopriva. *Mitt Grenzgeb Med Chir* 1906;16:632-644.

11. Erdheim J: Uber die genese der Paget'schen knocheren krankung. *Fortschr Geb Roentgenstrahlen* 1935;52:234-244.

12. Erdheim J: Über epithelkörperchenbefunde bei osteomalacie. *SB Akad Wiss Math Naturw* 1907;116:311-315.

13. Allen TC, Chevez-Barrios P, Shetlar DJ, Cagle PT: Pulmonary and ophthalmic involvement with Erdheim-Chester disease: A case report and review of the literature. *Arch Pathol Lab Med* 2004;128:1428-1431.

14. Alper MG, Zimmerman LE, Piana FG: Orbital manifestations of Erdheim-Chester disease. *Trans Am Ophthalmol Soc* 1983;81:64-85.

15. Athanasou NA, Barbatis C: Erdheim-Chester disease with epiphyseal and systemic disease. *J Clin Pathol* 1993;46:481-482.

16. Babu RP, Lansen TA, Chadburn A, Kasoff SS: Erdheim-Chester disease of the central nervous system: Report of two cases. *J Neurosurg* 1997;86:888-892.

17. Bohlega S, Alwatban J, Tulbah A, Bakheet SM, Powe J: Cerebral manifestations of Erdheim-Chester disease: Clinical and radiologic findings. *Neurology* 1997;49:1702-1705.

18. Breuil V, Brocq O, Pellegrino C, Grimaud A, Euller-Ziegler L: Erdheim-Chester disease: Typical radiological bone features for a rare xanthogranulomatosis. *Ann Rheum Dis* 2002;61:199-200.

19. Caparros-Lefebvre D, Pruvo JP, Remy M, Wallaert B, Petit H: Neuroradiologic aspects of Erdheim-Chester disease. *AJNR Am J Neuroradiol* 1995;16:735-740.

20. Dion E, Graef C, Miquel A, et al: Bone involvement in Erdheim-Chester disease: Imaging findings including periostitis and partial epiphyseal involvement. *Radiology* 2006;238:632-639.

21. Egan AJ, Boardman LA, Tazelaar HD, et al: Erdheim-Chester disease: Clinical, radiologic and histopathologic findings in five patients with interstitial lung disease. *Am J Surg Pathol* 1999;23:17-26.

22. Fink MG, Levinson DJ, Brown NL, et al: Erdheim-Chester disease: Case report with autopsy findings. *Arch Pathol Lab Med* 1991;115:619-623.

23. Gupta A, Kelly B, McGuigan JE: Erdheim-Chester disease with prominent pericardial involvement: Clinical, radiology and histologic findings. *Am J Med Sci* 2002;324:96-100.

24. Haroche J, Amoura Z, Dion E, et al: Cardiovascular involvement, an overlooked feature of Erdheim-Chester disease: Report of 6 new cases and a literature review. *Medicine (Baltimore)* 2004;83:371-392.

25. Kovacs K, Bilbao JM, Fornasier VL, Horvath E: Pituitary pathology in Erdheim-Chester disease. *Endocr Pathol* 2004;15:159-166.

26. Lantz B, Lange TA, Heiner J, Herring GF: Erdheim-Chester disease: A report of three cases. *J Bone Joint Surg Am* 1989;71:456-464.

27. Mergancova J, Kubes L, Elleder M: A xanthogranulomatous process encircling large blood vessels (Erdheim-Chester disease?). *Czech Med* 1988;11:57-64.

28. Molnar CP, Gottschalk R, Gallagher B: Lipid granulomatosis: Erdheim-Chester disease. *Clin Nucl Med* 1988;13:736-741.

29. Ono K, Oshiro M, Uemura K, et al: Erdheim-Chester disease: A case report with immunohis-tochemical and biochemical examination. *Hum Pathol* 1996;27:91-95.

30. Poehling GG, Adair DM, Haupt HA: Erdheim-Chester disease: A case report. *Clin Orthop Relat Res* 1984;185:241-244.

31. Rozenberg I, Wechsler J, Koenig F, et al: Erdheim-Chester disease presenting as malignant exophthalmos. *Br J Radiol* 1986;59:173-177.

32. Rush WL, Andriko JA, Galateau-Salle F, et al: Pulmonary pathology of Erdheim-Chester disease. *Mod Pathol* 2000;13:747-754.

33. Shields JA, Karcioglu ZA, Shields CL, Eagle RC, Wong S: Orbital and eyelid involvement with Erdheim-Chester disease: A report of two cases. *Arch Opthalmol* 1991;109:850-854.

34. Simpson FG, Robinson PJ, Hardy GJ, Losowsky MS: Erdheim-Chester disease associated with ret-roperitoneal xanthogranuloma. *Br J Radiol* 1979;52:232-235.

35. Veyssier-Belot C, Cacoub P, Caparros-Lefebvre D, et al: Erdheim-Chester disease: Clinical and radiologic characteristics of 59 cases. *Medicine (Baltimore)* 1996;75:157-169.

36. Wright RA, Hermann RC, Parisi JE: Neurologic manifestations of Erdheim-Chester disease. *J Neurol Neurosurg Psychiatry* 1999;66:72-75.

37. Brower AC, van den Berg R, Hurst NP, Allen PW: Erdheim-Chester disease: A distinct lipidosis or part of a spectrum of histiocytosis? *Radiology* 1984;151:35-38.

38. Kenn W, Eck M, Allolio B, et al: Erdheim-Chester disease: Evidence for a disease entity different from Langerhans cell histiocytosis? Three cases with detailed radiological and immunohistochemical analysis. *Hum Pathol* 2000;31:734-739.

39. Kilpatrick SE, Wenger DE, Gilchrist GS, et al: Langerhans cell histiocytosis (histiocytosis X) of bone: A clinico-pathologic analysis of 263 pediatric and adult cases. *Cancer* 1995;76:2471-2484.

40. Pertuiset E, Laredo JD, Liote D, et al: Erdheim-Chester disease: Report of a case, review of the literature and discussion of relationships with Langerhans cell histiocytosis. *Rev Rheum* 1993;60L:504-511.

41. Betts DR, Leibundgut KE, Feldges A, Pluss HJ, Niggli FK: Cytogenetic abnormalities in Langerhans cell histiocytosis. *Br J Cancer* 1998;77:552-555.

42. Jensen HB, McClain KL, Leach CT, et al: Evaluation of human herpesvirus type 8 infection in childhood Langerhans cell histiocytosis. *Am J Hematol* 2000;64:237-241.

43. Leahy MA, Krejci SM, Friednash M, et al: Human herpesvirus 6 is present in lesions of Langerhans cell histiocytosis. *J Invest Dermatol* 1993;101:642-645.

44. McClain K, Jin H, Gresik V, Favara B: Langerhans cell histiocytosis: Lack of a viral etiology. *Am J Hematol* 1994;47:16-20.

45. Willman CL, McClain KL: An updated on clonality, cytokines and viral etiology in Langerhans cell histiocytosis. *Hematol Oncol Clin North Am* 1998;12:407-416.

46. Johnson MD, Aulino JP, Jagasia M, Mawn LA: Erdheim-Chester disease mimicking multiple meningiomas syndrome. *AJNR Am J Neuroradiol* 2004;25:134-137.

47. De Abreu MR, Chung CB, Biswal S, et al:

Erdheim-Chester disease: MR imaging, anatomic and histopathologic correlation of orbital involvement. *AJNR Am J Neuroradiol* 2004;25:627-630.

48. Birbeck M, Breathnack A, Everall J: An electron microscope study of basal melanocytes and high-level clear cells (Langerhans cells) in vitiligo. *J Invest Dermatol* 1961;37:51-63.

49. Palmer FJ, Talley NJ: Erdheim-Chester disease with bilateral exophthalmos and liver cell adenoma. *Australas Radiol* 1984;28:305-310.

50. Ivan D, Neto A, Lemos L, Gupta A: Erdheim-Chester disease: A unique presentation with liver involvement and vertebral osteolytic lesions. *Arch Pathol Lab Med* 2003;127:e337-e339.

51. Kim NR, Ko YH, Choe YG, et al: Erdheim-Chester disease with extensive marrow necrosis: A case report and literature review. *Int J Surg Pathol* 2001;9:73-79.

52. Kushihashi T, Munechika H, Sekimizu M, Fujimaki E: Erdheim-Chester disease involving bilateral lower extremities: MR features. *AJR Am J Roentgenol* 2000;174:875-876.

53. Nagatsuka H, Han PP, Taguchi K: Erdheim-Chester disease in a child presenting with multiple jaw lesions. *J Oral Pathol Med* 2005;34:420-422.

54. Olmos JM, Canga A, Velero C, Gonzalez-Macias J: Clinical vignette: Imaging of Erdheim-Chester disease. *J Bone Miner Res* 2002;17:381-383.

55. Eble JN, Rosenberg AE, Young RH: Retroperitoneal xanthogranuloma in a patient with Erdheim-Chester disease. *Am J Surg Pathol* 1994;18:843-848.

56. Yamamoto T, Mizuno K: Erdheim-Chester disease with intramuscular lipogranuloma. *Skeletal Radiol* 2000;29:227-230.

57. Dalinka MK, Turner ML, Thompson JJ, Lee RE: Lipid granulomatosis of the ribs: Focal Erdheim-Chester disease. *Radiology* 1982;142:297-299.

58. Loeffler AG, Memoli VA: Myocardial involvement in Erdheim-Chester disease. *Arch Pathol Lab Med* 2004;128:682-685.

59. Albayram S, Kizilkilic O, Zulfikar Z, et al: Spinal dural involvement in Erdheim-Chester disease: MRI findings. *Neuroradiology* 2002;44:1004-1007.

60. Curgunlu A, Karter Y, Ozturk A: Erdheim-Chester disease: A rare cause of paraplegia. *Eur J Intern Med* 2003;14:53-55.

61. Miyachi S, Kobayashi T, Takahashi T, et al: An intracranial mass lesion in systemic xanthogranulomatosis: Case report. *Neurosurgery* 1990;27:822-826.

62. Tien RD, Kucharcyzak J, Newton TH, Citron JT, Duffy TJ: MR of diabetes insipidus in a patient with Erdheim-Chester disease. *AJNR Am J Neuroradiol* 1990;11:1267-1270.

63. Andre M, Delevaux I, de Fraissinette B, et al: Two enlarged kidneys: A manifestation of Erdheim-Chester disease. *Am J Nephrol* 2001;21:315-317.

64. Barnes PJ, Foyle A, Hache KA, et al: Erdheim-Chester disease of the breast: A case report and review of the literature. *Breast J* 2005;11:462-467.

65. Bellin MF, Cacoub P, Wechsler J, et al: Erdheim-Chester disease associated with renal involvement and thrombocythemia. *Eur J Radiol* 1993;3:266-269.

66. Bourke SC, Nicholson AG, Gibson GJ: Erdheim-Chester disease: Pulmonary infiltration responding to cyclophosphamide and prednisolone. *Thorax* 2003;58:1004-1005.

67. Maschalchi M, Nencini P, Nistri M, Sarti C, Santoni R: Failure of radiation therapy for brain involvement in Erdheim-Chester disease. *J Neurooncol* 2002;59:169-172.

68. Jendro MC, Zeidler H, Rosenthal H, Haller H, Schwarz A: Improvement of Erdheim-Chester disease in two patients by sequential treatment with vinblastine and mycophenolate mofetil. *Clin Rheumatol* 2004;23:52-56.

69. Braiteh F, Boxrud C, Esmaeli B, Kurzrock R: Successful treatment of Erdheim-Chester disease, a non-Langerhans-cell histiocytosis, with interferon-α. *Blood* 2005;106:2992-2994.

70. Esmaeli B, Ahmadi A, Tang R, et al: Interferon therapy of orbital infiltration secondary to Erdheim-Chester disease. *Am J Ophthalmol* 2001;132:945-947.

71. Boissel N, Wechsler B, Leblond V: Treatment of refractory Erdheim-Chester disease with double autologous hematopoietic stem-cell transplantation. *Ann Int Med* 2001;135:844-845.

Chapter 21

Ellis-van Creveld Syndrome

Ellis-van Creveld syndrome was first described in 1940 by two physicians—one British and the other Dutch—who met on a train going to a pediatric society meeting and discovered that they had both seen cases of a very rare disorder. They published their reports regarding the two patients and named the disease chondroectodermal dysplasia based on the extraordinary features. The disorder has some unusual characteristics, including shortness of stature, irregular bone growth and structure, and some remarkable oral findings such as strange teeth and lip ties. The most remarkable feature, however, is polydactyly, the presence of a sixth digit on the ulnar side of the hands and less frequently the fibular side of the feet. Cardiac problem's including a single atrium and a hypoplastic left heart' are major issues with these patients and their lives are threatened quite early in the course. In the last two decades, a genetic autosomal recessive error has been identified, but currently there is no reasonable clinical approach to helping these young children.

Nomenclature and History

Ellis-van Creveld syndrome is also known as chondroectodermal dysplasia, mesoectodermal dysplasia, disproportionate dwarfism, six-fingered dwarfism, and postaxial polydactyly. The gene error and some of the characteristics of the disorder suggest that it is closely related to Weyers syndrome (also known as Curry-Hall syndrome) and Jeune syndrome, which have some similar genetic, dental, polydactylic, and cardiac features.

Richard B. Ellis of Edinburgh and Simon van Creveld of Amsterdam were attending a pediatric society meeting in the late 1930s and met on a train. In their conversation, they each described children with the classical findings of the disorder now known as Ellis-van Creveld syndrome. In 1940, they published a paper in the *Archives of Diseases of Children*,[1] which included not only their two cases but another patient earlier described by Rustin McIntosh[2] in Holt and Howland's 10th edition of *Diseases of Infancy and Childhood*, published in 1933. They named the disorder chondroectodermal dysplasia, but it soon became known as the Ellis-van Creveld syndrome. In 1951, Keizer and Schilder[3] further defined the syndrome, including the skin and cardiac problems, Weller[4] described a classic case of the disorder in England, and Gatto[5] reported another in Switzerland. In 1952, John Caffey[6] cited in detail the clinical characteristics of two patients, and Chauss[7] described the remarkable radiographic features of the disorder in 1955. Gallagher and associates[8,9] focused on the ectodermal changes in their description of patients and noted some of the ocular findings. Around the same time, Metrakos and Fraser[10] pointed out the likelihood that the disorder was genetic. Weiss and Crosett[11] contributed another case in 1955, and then Uehlinger[12] described the pathologic findings in a patient who died of the disease. The genetic nature of the disease was confirmed by Mitchell and Waddell,[13] who in 1958 identified the disease in siblings. Douglas and associates[14] described a larger group of patients, all of whom had the same clinical findings. In 1961, Ferrero and associates[15] described in great detail the orthopaedic changes in a young patient and, in 1962, Ellis and Andrew[16] expanded the description of the syndrome and enumerated the findings and familial nature for all the reported cases up to that point in time.

The most remarkable findings were those of Victor McKusick and associates[17] in 1964. They studied the inbred Amish population of Lancaster County in Pennsylvania in an attempt to define their genetic disorders. They discovered that the disease could be traced to Samuel King and his wife, who emigrated from the Rhineland to Pennsylvania in 1744. As a result, in the year 2000, there were as many as 50 children with Ellis-van Creveld syndrome, despite the evidence at this point that the autosomal recessive disorder was extremely rare in the United States and throughout the world.[18] In 1980, da Silva and associates[19] confirmed the finding by reporting 15 cases in an inbred kindred group of patients, and in 1992, Goldblatt and associates[20] described another collection of inbred patients in a western Australian aboriginal community.

Of some interest is the recent report that cartilage-hair dysplasia, a similar disorder, is quite prevalent among the Amish population as well as in persons living in Finland.[21]

Genetic Characteristics of Ellis-van Creveld Syndrome and Similar Disorders

In 1995, Francomano and associates[22] identified the chromosomal site for genetic error in patients with Ellis-van Creveld syndrome as occurring at 4p16; this finding was confirmed by Polymeropoulos and associates[23] in 1996. Tompson and associates[24] later defined the error as resulting from segmental uniparental disomy of chromosome 4. The actual genetic error that results from the chromosomal syndrome has been named EVC, which is linked to the short arm of chromosome 4; this appears in all of the patients and indeed is diagnostic.[23,24] Studies have defined the site of the gene between D4S3007 and D4S431, and haplotype analysis sublocalizes the gene in the interval between D4S2957 and D4S827.[25,26] Of recent interest is the discovery of a second gene known as EVC2, which is found in the heart, placenta, lung, liver, and skeletal muscle.[27,28] EVC2 shares a common promoter region with EVC, and the majority of patients with the syndrome have one or the other abnormality.[26,27,29,30]

Of interest is the relationship of Ellis-van Creveld syndrome to some other disorders, based at least in part on the changes in chromosome 4 and the EVC genes. The most frequently seen and described entity is known as acrofacial dysostosis, described by Helmut Weyers in 1953.[31] The disease is an autosomal dominant entity, with the error at 4p16 and gene errors at EVC or EVC2.[31] Weyers syndrome is also known as Curry-Hall syndrome, and is characterized by short stature, hypotelorism, an abnormal mandible, teeth abnormalities, polydactyly, and dysplastic nails.[25,31-33] Another entity that "overlaps" with Ellis-van Creveld syndrome is the oral-facial-digital syndrome with short stature, which is also thought to have similar genetic characteristics.[34,35] The cardiothoracic problems that occur in patients with Ellis-van Creveld syndrome are sometimes very similar to those seen in another disorder originally described by Jeune and associates[36] in 1955 which became known as Jeune's asphyxiating thoracic dystrophy.[37,38]

Clinical Presentation

Most patients with Ellis-van Creveld syndrome present with problems at birth and the patients in typical series are all juveniles.[6,16,18,19,39-41] There is an equal gender distribution. As noted above, the disease is rarely encountered; it occurs in roughly 1 per 60,000 live births in the United States.[16,19,40,41] The exceptions noted throughout the world are the increased frequency in Old Order Amish children, some Finnish patients, and a group of Australian aborigines.[18,20,21] The syndromes can now often be identified while the fetus is still in the uterus by special techniques of ultrasound study and fetoscopy.[42,43]

Because cardiorespiratory problems occur in many patients shortly after birth, the death rate in infancy is as high as 50%.[16,18,19,34,39,44] If the children survive, they have a relatively normal life span. Intelligence is usually normal in children with Ellis-van Creveld syndrome, but they almost invariably have growth retardation and remain dwarfed throughout their lives.[6,16,18,19,41]

Chondrodystrophy affects the long bones, resulting in disturbances in epiphyseal growth and alignment and sometimes remarkable degrees of bowing or knock-knee deformities[15,16,29,40] (Figure 1). There are sometimes extraosseous bony masses arising from the tibiae.[45] One of the quite extraordinary characteristics of the disease is the bilateral presence of sixth digits in the hands, arising on the ulnar side[15,16,20,46] (Figure 2). Approximately 10% of the children have similar growths on the fibular side of the feet. Patients usually have fusions of the capitate to the hamate bones in the wrist.[15,16,29,40] The fingernails and toenails are hypoplastic, dystrophic, and friable; in some cases, nails are completely absent.[6,8,15,16,19,29,47]

Hair is often sparse; sometimes children are bald at birth and have very small eyebrows.[8,16,19,29,47] Facial anomalies typically surround and involve the oral cavity.[33,48-51]

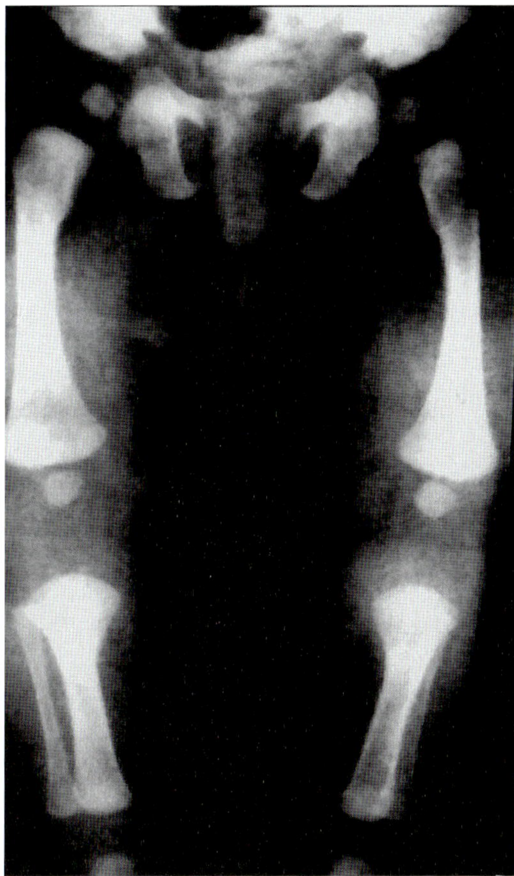

Figure 1
Radiograph of the lower extremities of a patient with Ellis-van Creveld disease showing the sometimes remarkable increase in density and the characteristic bowing deformity. The metaphyseal sites are enlarged.

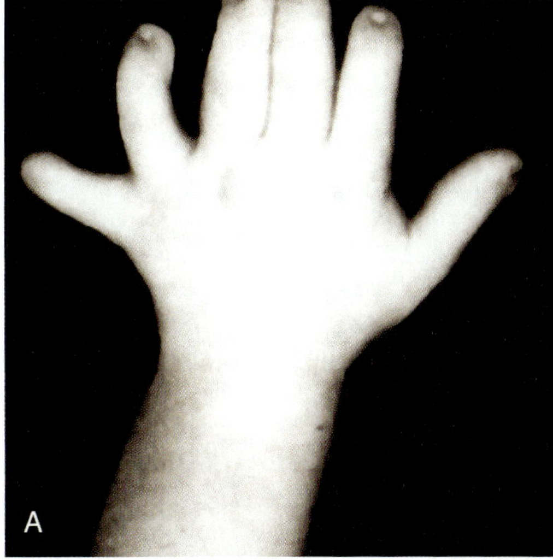

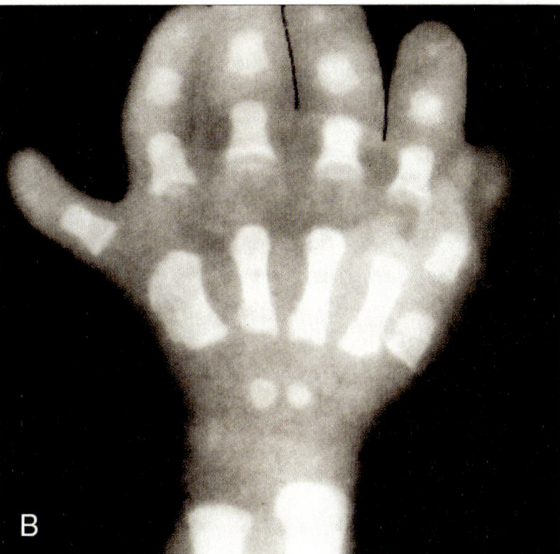

Figure 2
Patients with Ellis-van Creveld disease usually have six digits on the hand. The extra digit is on the ulnar side. Clinical photograph (**A**) and radiograph (**B**) show the irregularity of bony structure that is characteristic for this unusual disorder.

The teeth are small, irregular in structure, and delayed in eruption.[8,28,50] Enamel hypoplasia causes abnormal shape in some of the teeth.[29,48] Pseudocleft lip, also known as lip ties, is a common anomaly.[48] The upper gingivo-labial sulcus is often absent.[28,33,48-51] Ocular problems occur occasionally as well.[9]

Cardiac abnormalities are common. The thorax is narrow. The commonest abnormalities, many of which are present at birth, are a single atrium, defects of the mitral and tricuspid valves, patent ductus, ventricular septal defect, atrial septal defect, and hypoplastic left heart syndrome.[16,34,37,39,44] Death occurs in approximately 50% of patients with these disorders in a matter of weeks, in spite of attempts to treat them.

It should be evident from the description above that similar findings may be present in patients with Weyers syndrome,[31] Curry-Hall syndrome,[32,33] oral-facial-digital syndrome,[32,34,35] and Jeune's asphyxiating thoracic dystrophy;[36,38] in some cases, the genetic error is essentially the same.

Treatment

Patients who are suspected of having Ellis-van Creveld syndrome should be carefully evaluated clinically at the time of birth. Physical examination of the heart, lungs, and oral cavity should be performed to assess the presence of significant abnormalities, and radiographic imaging of the long bones, ribs, hands, and skull is essential. Family history is an important part of the protocol as is biologic assessment for genetic abnormalities.

Once the disease is appropriately diagnosed, the family should be informed of the potential risks and the problems that will possibly ensue in the near future.

The most important care areas are related to problems associated with respiratory distress, infections, and cardiac failure. There is little that can be done once the cardiac failure has begun because surgical procedures to correct the cardiac, aortic, and respiratory anomalies in children of that age are very unlikely to be successful. If the cardiac status is quiescent or limited, some measures can be used to assess the extent of the problems and make simple supportive corrections to improve cardiac and respiratory function.

Dental and facial structural care could be helpful in improving ability to breathe, eat, and speak. The care is complex in view of the size of the oral cavity and the sometimes tight and distorted soft-tissue structure. Crowns are sometimes useful.[15,16,41,48-50]

Orthopaedic surgery may be necessary to correct osseous deformity, with appropriate realignment and sometimes excision of the extra digits.[40,45,46,52] There is no way to change the epiphyseal abnormalities, but sometimes simple bracing may help to keep the lower and upper extremities in reasonable alignment. Spinal curvature can be partly corrected with appropriate physiotherapy and sometimes bracing.

Other problems that may occur include renal failure and hematologic abnormalities; these need to be specifically addressed and treated as necessary.[38,53,54]

Conclusions

The key problems with Ellis-van Creveld syndrome are its rarity, the early and sometimes very severe cardiac and pulmonary problems, and the terribly poor early survival rate. Fifty percent of the patients die within a few months of diagnosis and little can be done to change that prognosis. Survivors are of short stature, have problems with their oral cavities, and unusual orthopaedic findings, all of which make life difficult. There are few solutions available for these patients other than to try to improve their extremity disorders and ability to eat and speak. The disease is so rare that very few physicians, including pediatricians, see enough cases to consider ways to improve the patient's remaining life. There are no genetic approaches currently available; even with intrauterine diagnosis now possible, early treatment with marrow or stem-cell transplant has not yet been used.

References

1. Ellis RW, van Creveld S: A syndrome characterized by ectodermal dysplasia, polydactyly, chondrodysplasia and congenital morbus cordis: Report of three cases. *Arch Dis Child* 1940;15: 65-85.

2. McIntosh R: Ellis-van Creveld disease, in Holt LE, Howland J (eds): *Diseases of Infancy and Childhood*, ed 10. New York, NY, Appleton-Century Co, 1933, p 362.

3. Keizer DP, Schilder JH: Ectodermal dysplasia, achondrodysplasia, and congenital morbus cordis. *AMA Am J Dis Child* 1951;82:341-344.

4. Weller SD: Chondro-ectodermal dysplasia (Ellis-van Creveld syndrome). *Proc R Soc Med* 1951;44:731-732.

5. Gatto I: Ellis-van Creveld syndrome. *Helv Paediatr Acta* 1951;6:437-442.

6. Caffey J: Chondroectodermal dysplasia (Ellis-van Creveld Disease). *Am J Roentgenol Radium Ther Nucl Med* 1952;68:875-886.

7. Chauss JM: Chondroectodermal dysplasia (Ellis-van Creveld disease): A case report. *Radiology* 1955;65:213-217.

8. Gallagher EJ, MacGregor ME, Israelski M: Chondrodystrophy with ectodermal defects. *Arch Dis Child* 1953;28:14-18.

9. Gallagher EJ, MacGregor ME, Israelski M: Chondro-ectodermal dysplasia (Ellis-van Creveld syndrome). *Proc R Soc Med* 1951;44:731-732.

10. Metrakos JD, Fraser FC: Evidence for a hereditary factor in chondroectodermal dysplasia (Ellis-van Creveld syndrome). *Am J Hum Genet* 1954;6:260-269.

11. Weiss H, Crosett AD Jr: Chondroectodermal dysplasia: Report of a case and review of the literature. *J Pediatr* 1955;46:268-275.

12. Uehlinger E: Pathological anatomy of chondroectodermal dysplasia of Ellis van Creveld. *Schweizer Z Pathol Bakteriol* 1957;20:754-766.

13. Mitchell FN, Waddell WW Jr: Ellis-van Creveld syndrome: Report of two cases in siblings. *Acta Paediatr* 1958;47:142-151.

14. Douglas WF, Schonholtz GJ, Geppert LJ: Chondroectodermal dysplasia (Ellis-van Creveld syndrome). *AMA J Dis Child* 1959;97:473-478.

15. Ferrero NA, Pozo OO, Morresi ES: Chondroectodermal dysplasia (Ellis-van Creveld syndrome): Report of a case and review of the literature. *J Bone Joint Surg Am* 1961;43:1230-1236.

16. Ellis RWB, Andrew JD: Chondroectodermal dysplasia. *J Bone Joint Surg Br* 1962;44:626-636.

17. McKusick VA, Egeland JA, Eldridge R, Krusen DE: Dwarfism in the Amish: I. The Ellis-van

Creveld syndrome. *Bull Johns Hopkins Hosp* 1964;115:306-336.

18. McKusick VA: Ellis-van Creveld syndrome and the Amish. *Nat Genet* 2000;24:203-204.

19. da Silva EO, Janovitz D, de Albuquerque SC: Ellis-van Creveld syndrome: Report of 15 cases in an inbred kindred. *J Med Genet* 1980;17:349-356.

20. Goldblatt J, Minutillo C, Pembertons PJ, Hurst J: Ellis-van Creveld syndrome in a western Australian aboriginal community: Postaxial polydactyly as a heterozygous manifestation? *Med J Aust* 1992;157:271-272.

21. Ridanpaa M, Jain P, McKusick VA, Francomano CA, Kaitila I: The major mutation in the RMRP gene causing CHH among the Amish is the same as that found in most Finnish cases. *Am J Med Genet C Semin Med Genet* 2003;121:81-83.

22. Francomano C, Ortiz de Luna R, Ide S, Pyeritz R, Wright, M: The gene for the Ellis-van Creveld syndrome maps to chromosome 4p16. *Hum Genet* 1995;57:a191.

23. Polymeropoulos MH, Ide SE, Wright M, et al: The gene for the Ellis-van Creveld syndrome is located on chromosome 4p16. *Genomics* 1996;35:1-5.

24. Tompson SWJ, Ruiz-Perez VL, Wright MJ, Goodship JA: Ellis-van Creveld syndrome resulting from segmental uniparental disomy of chromosome 4. *J Med Genet* 2001;38:18-19.

25. Ruiz-Perez VL, Ide SE, Strom TM, et al: Mutations in a new gene in Ellis-van Creveld syndrome and Weyers acrodental dysostosis. *Nat Genet* 2000;24:283-286.

26. Ruiz-Perez VL, Tompson SW, Blair HJ, et al: Mutations in two nonhomologous genes in a head to head configuration cause Ellis-van Creveld syndrome. *Am J Hum Genet* 2003;72:728-732.

27. Galdzicka M, Patnala S, Hirshman MG, et al: A new gene EVC2 is mutated in Ellis-van Creveld syndrome. *Mol Genet Metab* 2002;77:291-295.

28. Mostafa MI, Temtamy SA, el-Gaammal MA, Mazen IM: Unusual pattern of inheritance and orodental changes in the Ellis-van Creveld syndrome. *Genet Couns* 2005;16:75-83.

29. Howard TD, Guttmacher AE, McKinnon W, et al: Autosomal dominant postaxial polydactyly, nail dystrophy, and dental abnormalities map to chromosome 4p16 in the region containing the Ellis-van Creveld syndrome locus. *Am J Hum Genet* 1997;61:1405-1412.

30. Tompson SW, Ruiz-Perez VL, Blair HJ, et al: Sequencing EVC and EVC2 identifies mutations in two-thirds of Ellis-van Creveld syndrome patients. *Hum Genet* 2007;120:663-670.

31. Weyers H: Hexadactyly, mandibular fissure and oligodontia: A new syndrome, dysostosis acrofacialis. *Ann Paediat* 1953;181:45-60.

32. Ghosh S, Setty S, Sivakumar A, Pai KM: Report of a new syndrome: Focus on differential diagnosis and review of Ellis-van Creveld, Curry–Hall, acrofacial dysostosis, and orofacial digital syndromes. *Oral Surg Oral Med Oral Pathol Oral Radiol Endod* 2007;103:670-676.

33. Curry CJ, Hall BD: Polydactyly, conical teeth, nail dysplasia and short limbs: A new autosomal dominant malformation syndrome. *Birth Defects Orig Artic Ser* 1979;15:253-263.

34. Digilio M, Marino B, Ammirati A, et al: Cardiac malformations in patients with oral-facial-skeletal syndromes: Clinical similarities with heterotaxia. *Am J Med Genet* 1999;84:350-356.

35. Phadke SR, Pahi J, Pandey A, Agarwal SS: Oral-facial-digital syndrome with acromelic short stature: A new variant—overlap with Ellis-van Creveld syndrome. *Clin Dysmorphol* 1999;8:185-188.

36. Jeune M, Beraud C, Carron R: Asphyxiating thoracic dystrophy with familial characteristics. *Arch Fr Pediatr* 1955;12:886-891.

37. Brueton LA, Dillon MJ, Winter RM: Ellis-van Creveld syndrome, Jeune syndrome, and renal-hepatic-pancreatic dysplasia: Separate entities or disease spectrum? *J Med Genet* 1990;27:252-255.

38. Donaldson MD, Warner AA, Trompeter RS, Haycock GB, Chantler C: Familial juvenile nephrophithisis: Juene's syndrome and associated disorders. *Arch Dis Child* 1985;60:426-434.

39. Husson GS, Parkman P: Chondroectodermal dysplasia (Ellis-van Creveld syndrome) with a complex cardiac malformation. *Pediatrics* 1961;28:285-292.

40. Sergi C, Voightlander T, Zoubaa S, et al: Ellis-van Creveld syndrome: A generalized dysplasia of enchondral ossification. *Pediatr Radiol* 2001;31:289-293.

41. Varela M, Ramos C: Chondroectodermal dysplasia (Ellis-van Creveld syndrome): A case report. *Eur J Orthod* 1996;18:313-318.

42. Dugoff L, Thieme G, Hobbins JC: First trimester prenatal diagnosis of chondroectodermal dysplasia (Ellis-van Creveld syndrome) with ultrasound. *Ultrasound Obstet Gynecol* 2001;17:86-88.

43. Mahoney MJ, Hobbins JC: Prenatal diagnosis of chondroectodermal dysplasia (Ellis-van Creveld Syndrome) with fetoscopy and ultrasound. *N Engl J Med* 1977;297:258-260.

44. Digoy GP, Greenberg M, Magit A: Congenital stridor secondary to an upper airway cyst in a patient with Ellis-van Creveld syndrome. *Int J Pediatr Otorhinolaryngol* 2005;69:1433-1435.

45. Cakir M, Koca L, Gedik Y, et al: Ellis-van Creveld syndrome associated with bilateral tibial exostoses. *Genet Couns* 2006;17:73-75.

46. Okten A, Cakir M, Orhan F, Mungan I: Atypical crossed polydactyly in two siblings with Ellis-van Creveld syndrome and mild clinical manifestations in close relatives. *Pediatr Int* 2004;46:184-187.

47. Qureshi F, Jacques SM, Evans MI, et al: Skeletal histopathology in fetuses with chondroectodermal dysplasia (Ellis-van Creveld syndrome). *Am J Med Genet* 1993;45:471-476.

48. Biggerstaff RH, Mazaheri M: Oral manifestations of the Ellis-van Creveld syndrome. *J Am Dent Assoc* 1968;77:1090-1095.

49. Cahuana A, Palma C, Gonzales W, Gean E: Oral manifestations in Ellis-van Creveld syndrome: Report of five cases. *Pediatr Dent* 2004;26:277-282.

50. Hunter ML, Roberts GJ: Oral and dental anomalies in Ellis-van Creveld syndrome (chondroectodermal dysplasia): Report of a case. *Int J Paediatr Dent* 1998;8:153-157.

51. Susami T, Kuroda T, Yoshimasu H, Suzuki R: Ellis-van Creveld syndrome: Craniofacial mor-

phology and multidisciplinary treatment. *Cleft Palate Craniofac J* 1999;36:345-352.

52. Shibata T, Kawabat H, Yasui N, et al: Correction of knee deformity in patients with Ellis-van Creveld syndrome. *J Pediatr Orthop* 1999;8:282-284.

53. Moudgil A, Bagga A, Kamil ES, et al: Nephronopthisis associated with Ellis-van Creveld syndrome. *Pediatr Nephrol* 1998;12:20-22.

54. Scurlock D, Ostler D, Nguyen A, Wahed A: Ellis-van Creveld Syndrome and dyserythropoiesis. *Arch Path Lab Med* 2005;129:680-682.

Chapter 22

Fibrodysplasia Ossificans Progressiva

Fibrodysplasia ossificans progressiva is a rare genetic disorder in which the fibrous tissues, muscles, and periosteal regions undergo progressive ossification. As a result, beginning at approximately 5 years of age, sometimes massive ectopic osseous collections develop in the muscular regions adjacent to the bones and joints and the patient often becomes extraordinarily disabled by the limitation of movement of joints and alterations in osseous structure. Of note are other extraordinary clinical features, which include shortening and deformity of the great toes and sometimes the thumbs. Patients with the disease are not only disabled, but often do not survive because of functional impairment of the neck and chest, fractures, and damage to cardiac and vascular structures.

Nomenclature and History

The disorder was originally known as myositis ossificans progressiva (MOP), heterotopic osteogenesis, or progressive osseous heterodysplasia.[1] Additional names included Muenchmeyer syndrome,[2] Patin syndrome,[3] exostosis luxurians, myopathia osteoplastica, stiff-man syndrome,[4] and stone-man disease.[5] The term fibrodysplasia ossificans progressiva (FOP) was first suggested by Bauer and Bode[6] in 1940 and is now the most common terminology. Although the disease was first described by Guy Patin[3] in 1692, one of the best early descriptions of a patient is attributed to John Freke,[7] who in 1736 described in some detail a 14-year-old male patient with a massive swelling on his back who was seen in St. Bartholomew's Hospital. Muenchmeyer[2] described 15 cases in 1869; his name was eponymically applied to the disorder but is no longer used. Over the next 5 decades, Hutchinson,[8] Stoneham,[9] Sympson,[10] Rolleston,[11] Michelson,[12] and Garrod[13] added cases and information about the disease. Subsequent contributions by Rosenstirn,[14] Nutt,[15] Smith and associates,[16] van Creveld and Soeters,[17] Fairbank,[18] Koontz,[19] Mather,[20] Mair,[21] and Lutwak[22] established the bizarre nature of the disorder and described the clinical aspects of disease in great detail. A remarkable skeleton of a patient with FOP is on exhibit in the Mutter Museum of the College of Physicians in Philadelphia and certainly supports the monicker stone-man disease.[23] The most comprehensive reviews and descriptions of patient groups were provided in the early 1980s by Connor and Evans,[24-26] who also began an approach to the chemistry and genetics of the disorder. It was not until the 1990s, however, that the genetic aspects and biologic character of the disease were identified. Without question, the greatest contributor to our understanding of FOP has been Frederick S. Kaplan of Philadelphia, who with his colleagues has defined in great detail the nature of the disorder, the genetics, and the causation.[23,27-36]

Biology and Genetics

The nature of this strange genetic disorder is the presence of abnormal heterotopic ossification of the muscle, fascia, and periosteum that appears to be caused by a dysregulation of cell differentiation.[1,24,34] The abnormality causes a sometimes widespread improper induction of bone formation. As stated by Kaplan, "normal bone forms in the wrong place at the wrong time."[23] The disease appears to be genetic and is transmitted as an autosomal dominant disorder but with frequent mutations.[1,23,25] FOP is slightly more common in males, and there is no increased ethnic frequency.[1,23-25,35] The disorder is rare, with perhaps fewer than 1,500 cases reported in the world literature. Of some interest is the fact that FOP has been documented as occurring spontaneously in both cats and pigs.[37-40]

Although numerous studies have been performed, the site of the gene error has not been clearly identified. There have been suggestions that the error occurs in chromo-

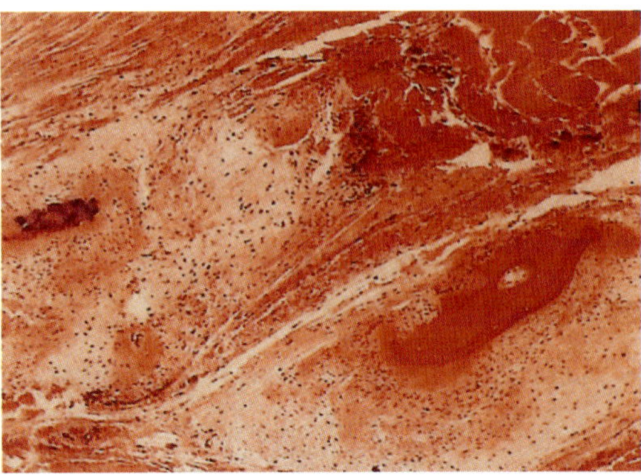

Figure 1

Histologic changes characteristic of FOP show a loose pattern of cellular and fibrous elements with irregular bone formation. Cartilage may be present as well.

somes 4q27-31,[41] 17q21-22,[42] or 2q23-q24.[34] The last seems to be most likely as it is a genetic interval including the ACVR1 gene, which is possibly related to a mutation in the NOG gene.[35] The change in the tissues seems to be caused by an error in the bone morphogenetic protein (BMP)-4 signaling pathway, which is dysregulated and appears to increase bone formation in the soft tissues.[27,29,35,36,43] BMP-4 normally is less active because it upregulates the expression of the BMP antagonist noggin, which in turn establishes an autoregulatory feedback loop.[29,35,36,43] Therefore, a defect in the feedback pathway seems to contribute to the elevated BMP-4 activity, which is believed to be a major cause of the progressive heterotopic bone formation in patients with FOP.[27,29,35,43] The cause of the alteration in the structure of the great toe or the thumb is less clearly understood. New bone formation is not characteristic at those sites. The changes seen in the digits may represent a separate genetic error in patients with FOP and are probably different from the BMP-4 dysregulation process believed to be the cause of the bone formation in the muscle and fibrous tissue.[1,44,45]

Histology

The general pattern for the histologic process associated with FOP is that of a sequential degeneration of skeletal muscle, dysplasia of fibrous tissue, and a subsequent ossification, often occurring at multiple sites[1,30] (Figure 1). Initially, the histologic specimens show loose mxyoid fibrous tissue.[30] The fibrous tissue invades muscle, en-

trapping the myofibrils. Numerous small blood vessels are present, but inflammatory changes are sparse.[30] Staining for vimentin and CD34 is generally positive, and many of the cells are immunoreactive to S-100.[1,24,30] Cartilaginous cells are often present and the tissue seems to undergo endochondral ossification.[30] Woven bone replaces the fibrocartilaginous tissue and, over a short period of time, undergoes conversion to lamellar bone. The marrow spaces between the lamellar segments contain some cellular elements along with fibrocytes and some chondrocytes.[30] The bone that is formed does not have an anatomic orientation and lacks a well-defined cortical structure. None of the changes suggests malignancy. The changes in the great toes and sometimes thumbs show atypical bone formation and abnormal anatomic structure but do not resemble the aggressive osseous-forming changes seen in other tissues, such as the spine, neck, scapula, thorax, or mandible.[1,44,45]

Clinical Presentation

At birth, most patients with FOP show no evidence of osseous deposits in muscle or fascia.[1] The only finding that is sometimes quite evident is the relative shortening and deformity of the great toes and, less frequently, the thumbs[44,45] (Figure 2). The condition is otherwise innocuous at this stage and may remain unrecognized until later childhood when the soft-tissue ossification begins. Patients are usually mentally normal and have no evident discomfort or other problems until the average age of 5 years.[1] At that point, transient localized cystic swellings appear in the neck, thorax, and back[1,17,18,23,24] (Figure 3). The development may be spontaneous or seem to be precipitated by trauma and results in a painful mass, often with an accumulation of fluid.[1,23,24] At times the masses are associated with a fever and elevation of the white count and erythrocyte sedimentation rate.[1,24] As the swelling subsides, ectopic ossification begins to appear on imaging studies. Clinically, the masses are initially soft and tender but subsequently become firm and remain closely adherent to muscular structures, ribs, and bones of the mandible, scapula, and limbs.[1,23,24] Bony bars and bridges occur in relation to the spinal segments and joints and cause sometimes profound limitation of movement of the neck, back, shoulders, elbows, hips, knees, and ankles.[1,5,24,46,47] Based on the extraordinary rigidity of the spine, patients may be unable to sit or, because of almost complete fusion of the shoulder joints, cannot move their arms[4,33,48] (Figure 4). Walking is sometimes difficult and consists of short steps. Falls and fractures are common and can be devastating to the patients and their families.[49] With advancing disease, the jaws often become involved, interfering with normal speech and reducing the ability to eat solid food.[1,24,50-52] Deafness and visual abnormalities develop in many patients, and baldness is common.[1,24,53]

The disease becomes slower in its progression as the child reaches adulthood, but most patients are seriously functionally impaired by the third decade of life. The rib, spine, and scapular limitations induce respiratory problems and pneumonia frequently develops, which is often difficult to treat and may be a cause of early demise.[1,54] With further aging, cardiac and major vascular abnormalities can occur that may also be fatal.[54,55]

Diagnostic Aids

Imaging studies are helpful, particularly early in the course of the disease. They show soft-tissue masses, which slowly become increasingly radiodense, consistent with bone formation in the tissue.[1,31,56] With advancing disease, there are multiple deformities noted in the bones adjacent to the osseous masses, specifically in the spine, mandible, and shoulders.[1,31,56] The ribs and scapula may also become deformed and damaged. Radiographs of the feet and sometimes the hands show shortening and deformities of the great toe and thumb, but rarely show any soft-tissue ossification such as is seen in other sites.[1,44,45] The jaw shows marked alteration in structure related to soft-tissue osseous masses. Bone scans are active over the osseous sites and become progressively more marked with advancing disease.[1,31] CT is quite helpful in defining the soft-tissue masses and is especially useful in distinguishing the evolving lesions from soft-tissue sarcomas.[1,57,58] MRI studies also clearly display the soft-tissue extensions early in the course but may be confusing later as the masses become more calcified

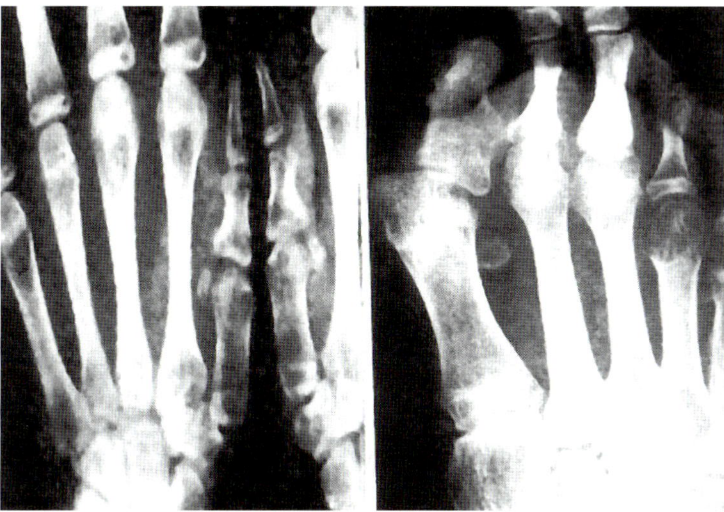

Figure 2

Hand and foot deformities are common and are characterized by shortening and irregularity of the thumb and great toe, with only minimal new bone formation.

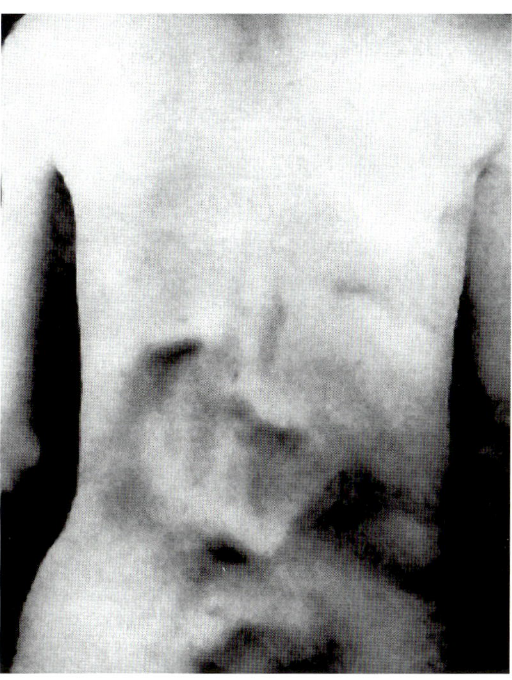

Figure 3

Collections of bone and soft-tissue masses accumulate subcutaneously, as is seen in the back of this child with FOP.

and cause relatively abnormal appearing ossific structures.[59,60]

Laboratory studies are helpful to some extent. In the acute phase, the patient frequently has an increase in leukocyte count and erythrocyte sedimentation rate.[1] The serum alkaline phosphatase is elevated, as is

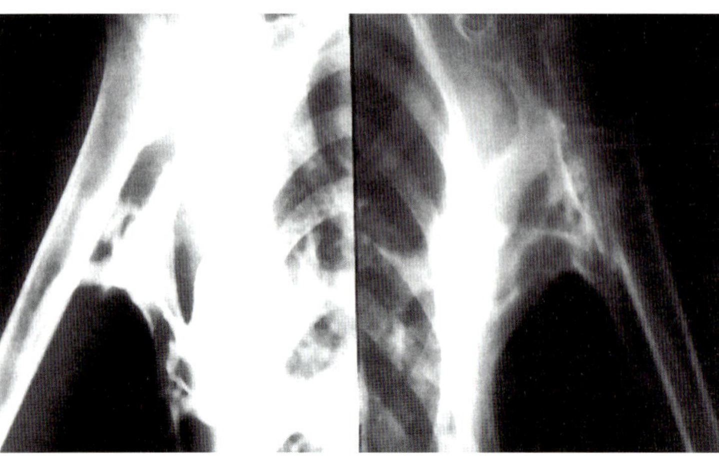

Figure 4
The major deformity and disability occurs in relation to joints. In this case, both scapulae and humeri are attached to the ribs so that the patient was unable to move her arms.

the bone-specific alkaline phosphatase.[1,23,24,26] With advancing disease, the values may diminish somewhat but remain elevated.

Treatment

Despite the long history of recognition of the disease, treatment remains a major problem; for many children and adults with the disorder, there seems to be little if any method of reducing their symptoms or improving their lifestyle. One explanation is that the disease is so rare that, until recently, no group treated sufficient numbers of patients to establish and observe the response to therapeutic trials. The possible future solution to this problem is the development in 1988 of the International Fibrodysplasia Ossificans Progressiva Association (IFOPA) by Frederick Kaplan and his colleagues.

In terms of approaches to therapy, the first was the introduction of beryllium in 1949 by Klemperer and associates[61] in an attempt to inhibit the production of alkaline phosphatase. This approach was ineffective and there were some toxic responses. Radiation was introduced early in the protocols but does not seem to be effective. In view of the sometimes enormous size of the bony lesions, radiation is frequently too difficult to administer. Androgens, corticosteroids, vitamins B and E, ethylenediaminetetraacetic acid (EDTA), and penicillamine were used over the years since the mid-20th century, but none seemed to be effective and the complications were sometimes startling and difficult to manage.[1,22,23] Isotretinoin and diphosphonates (EHDP) were initially thought to be effective but do not seem to have a predictable action and have since been abandoned.[1,23,62-67] Marrow stem cell or transplants from siblings have been attempted without success and most recently, rituximab, a monoclonal anti-CD20 that targets B cells, has been introduced.[1,32]

Surgical resection of the lesions has been proposed but seems to result only in temporary improvement as many seem to grow back rapidly.[1,23,64] Anesthesia is a major problem because of limitation of movement and respiratory problems.[68] Spinal surgery has a particularly high complication rate.[33,47,48] A recent report suggests that indomethacin therapy and radiation following the surgery has resulted in improved function and less difficulty for the patient.[1,69] Surgical procedures for mandibular lesions have often been difficult and have high failure and complication rates.[50,69] A significant problem is the frequency of fractures in patients with FOP and the difficulty in treating them with anesthesia and surgical procedures.[49,68] Of greatest concern is the treatment of patients late in their disease who have respiratory, vascular, or cardiac disorders.[54,55] Antibiotic therapy should be introduced rapidly and maintained for a long period for patients who have had surgery or those with open fractures.

Conclusions

FOP is a terrible problem for patients, their families, and their physicians. Fortunately for the world population, the disease is very rare. Beginning at approximately age 5 years, increasingly enlarging osseous masses develop in patients muscles and fibrous tissue, which cause pain, deformity, and skeletal limitation so that they become "stone men" and end up with fractures and mandibular, cardiac, and pulmonary disorders that cannot be effectively treated either by surgery or drug treatment. There seems to be no approach that has helped us to identify the lesion, define the genetic causation, or introduce trials of management. Many patients die young despite attempts to help them.

However, in the past 2 decades, Dr. Frederick Kaplan and his colleagues accepted the challenge of defining and treating the disorder. FOP is now under very close scrutiny and attempts are being made to not only introduce reasonable biologic treatment approaches but to alter the genetic error and especially the BMP-4 abnormality to alleviate the problem. Let us hope that this will be successful in the near future and help patients and their physicians eliminate one of the true genetic curses for humans (and some animals!).

References

1. Beighton P: Fibrodysplasia ossificans progressive, in Beighton P (ed): *McKusick's Heritable Disorders of Connective Tissue*, ed 5. St. Louis, MO, Mosby, 1993, pp 501-518.

2. Muenchmeyer E: Über myositis ossificans progressiva. *Zeitschrift Ration Med* 1869;34:1-12.

3. Patin G: Letter of 27 August 1648 written to AF, in *Lettres Choisis de Feu M. Guy Patin*. Cologne, France, P du Laurens, 1692, p 28.

4. Naique S, Katakdhond N, Srivastava SK: Stiff man's syndrome. *Indian J Pediatr* 1999;66:145-147.

5. Baysal T, Elmali N, Kutlu R, Baysal O: The stone man: Myositis (fibrodysplasia) ossificans progressiva. *Eur Radiol* 1998;8:479-481.

6. Bauer KH, Bode W: Erbpathologie der Stutzgewebe des Menschen, in Bauer KH (ed): *Handbuch der Erbbiologie*. Berlin, Germany, Julius Springer, 1940, vol 3, p 105.

7. Freke J: A case of an extraordinary exostosis on the back of a boy. *Philo Trans R Soc London* 1736;41:413.

8. Hutchinson J: Case of multiple exostoses with ossification of fascia in various parts and ichthyosis. *Med Times Gazette* 1860;1:March 31.

9. Stoneham C: Myositis ossificans. *Lancet* 1892;2:1485-1492.

10. Sympson T: Case of myositis ossificans. *BMJ* 1886;2:1026-1027.

11. Rolleston HD: Progressive myositis ossificans with references to other developmental diseases of the mesoblast. *Clin J* 1901;17:209-214.

12. Michelson J: Ein Fall von Myositis ossificans progressive. *Z Orthop Chir* 1904;12:424-443.

13. Garrod AE: The initial stage of myositis ossificans. *St. Bartholomew's Hosp Rep* 1907;43:43-49.

14. Rosenstirn J: A contribution to the study of myositis ossificans progressiva. *Ann Surg* 1918;68:485-520, 591-637.

15. Nutt JJ: Report of a case of myositis ossificans progressiva with bibliography. *J Bone Joint Surg* 1923;5:344-359.

16. Smith R, Russell RG, Woods CG: Myositis ossificans progressiva: Clinical features in eight patients and their response to treatment. *J Bone Joint Surg Br* 1976;58:48-57.

17. van Creveld S, Soeters JM: Progressive myositis ossificans. *Am J Dis Child* 1941;62:1000-1013.

18. Fairbank HAT: Myositis ossificans progressiva. *J Bone Joint Surg Br* 1950;32:108-116.

19. Koontz AR: Myositis ossificans progressiva. *Am J Med Sci* 1927;174:406-412.

20. Mather JH: Progressive myositis ossificans. *Br J Radiol* 1931;4:207-210.

21. Mair WF: Myositis ossificans progressiva. *Edinburgh Med J* 1932;39:13-36.

22. Lutwak L: Myositis ossificans progressiva: Mineral metabolic and radioactive calcium studies of the effects of hormones. *Am J Med* 1964;37:269-293.

23. Kaplan FS: Fibrodysplasia ossificans progressiva: An historical perspective. *Clin Rev Bone Mineral Metab* 2005;3:179-181.

24. Connor JM, Evans DA: Fibrodysplasia ossificans progressiva: The clinical features and natural history of 34 patients. *J Bone Joint Surg Br* 1982;64:76-83.

25. Connor JM, Evans DA: Genetic aspects of fibrodysplasia ossificans progressiva. *J Med Genet* 1982;19:35-39.

26. Connor JM, Evans DA: Quantitative and qualitative studies on the skin fibroblast alkaline phosphatase in fibrodysplasia ossificans progressiva. *Clin Chim Acta* 1981;117:355-360.

27. Kaplan FS, Fiori J, De La Pena LS, et al: Dysregulation of the BMP-4 signaling pathway in fibrodysplasia ossificans progressiva. *Ann N Y Acad Sci* 2006;1068:54-65.

28. Kaplan FS, Glaser DL, Shore EM, et al: The phenotype of fibrodysplasia ossificans progressiva. *Clin Rev Bone Mineral Metab* 2005;3:183-188.

29. Kaplan FS, Shore EM, Gupta R, et al: Immunological features of fibrodysplasia ossificans progressiva and the dysregulated BMP-4 pathway. *Clin Rev Bone Mineral Metab* 2005;3:189-193.

30. Kaplan FS, Tabas JA, Gannon FH, et al: The histopathology of fibrodysplasia ossificans progressiva: An endochondral process. *J Bone Joint Surg Am* 1993;75:220-230.

31. Kaplan FS, Stear CM, Zasloff MA: Radiographic and scintographic features of modeling and remodeling in the heterotopic skeleton of patients who have fibrodysplasia ossificans progressiva. *Clin Orthop Relat Res* 1994;304:238-247.

32. Olmsted EA, Kaplan FS, Shore EM: Bone morphogenetic protein-4 regulation in fibrodysplasia ossificans progressiva. *Clin Orthop Relat Res* 2003;408:331-343.

33. Shah PB, Zasloff MA, Drummond D, Kaplan FS: Spinal deformity in patients who have fibrodysplasia ossificans progressiva. *J Bone Joint Surg Am* 1994;76:1442-1450.

34. Shore EM, Feldman GJ, Xu M, Kaplan FS: The genetics of fibrodysplasia ossificans progessiva. *Clin Rev Bone Mineral Metab.* 2005;3:201-204.

35. Shore EM, Xu M, Feldman GJ, et al: A recurrent mutation in the BMP type I receptor ACVR1 causes inherited and sporadic fibrodysplasia ossificans progressive. *Nat Genet* 2006;38:525-527.

36. Shore EM, Xu M, Shah PB, et al: The human bone morphogenetic protein (BMP-4) gene: Molecular structure and transcriptional regulation. *Calcif Tissue Int* 1998;63:221-229.

37. Asano K, Sakata A, Shibuya H, et al: Fibrodyspla-

sia ossificans progressiva-like condition in a cat. *J Vet Med Sci* 2006;68:1003-1006.

38. Seibold HR, Davis CL: Generalized myositis ossificans (familial) in pigs. *Pathol Vet* 1967;4:79-88.

39. Valentine BA, George C, Randolph JF, et al: Fibrodysplasia ossificans progressiva in the cat: A case report. *J Am Vet Med Assoc* 1992;6:335-340.

40. Valentine BA, Kaplan FS: Fibrodysplasia ossificans progressiva in cats: A potentially important animal model of the human disease. *Feline Pract* 1996;24:6.

41. Feldman G, Li M, Martin S, et al: Fibrodysplasia ossificans progressiva, a heritable disorder of severe heterotopic ossification, maps to human chromosome 4q27-31. *Am J Hum Genet* 2000;66:128-135.

42. Lucotte G, Bathelier C, Mercier G, et al: Localization of the gene for fibrodysplasia ossificans progressiva (FOP) to 17q21-22. *Genet Couns* 2000;11:329-334.

43. Groppe J, Greenwald J, Wiater E, et al: Structural basis of BMP signaling inhibition by Noggin, a novel twelve-membrane cystine knot protein. *J Bone Joint Surg Am* 2003;85:52-58.

44. Harrison RJ, Pitcher JD, Mizel MS, et al: The radiographic morphology of foot deformities in patients with fibrodysplasia ossificans progressiva. *Foot Ankle Int* 2005;26:937-941.

45. Schroeder HW Jr, Zasloff M: The hand and foot malformations in fibrodysplasia ossificans progressiva. *Johns Hopkins Med J* 1980;147:73-78.

46. Connor JM, Smith R: The cervical spine in fibrodysplasia ossificans progressiva. *Br J Radiol* 1982;55:492-496.

47. Falliner A, Drescher W, Brossmann J: The spine in fibrodysplasia ossificans progressiva. *Spine* 2003;28:E519-522.

48. Hsu LC, Hsu KY, Leong JC: Severe scoliosis associated with fibrodysplasia ossificans progressiva: A report of two cases. *Spine* 1986;11:643-644.

49. Glaser DL, Rock DM, Kaplan FS: Catastrophic falls in patients who have fibrodysplasia ossificans progressiva. *Clin Orthop Relat Res* 1998;346:110-116.

50. Herford AS, Boyne PJ: Ankylosis of the jaw in a patient with fibrodysplasia ossificans progressiva. *Oral Surg Oral Med Oral Pathol Oral Radiol Endod* 2003;96:680-684.

51. Iriarte JI, Coulon JP, Reychler H: Temporomandibular ankylosis and progressive ossifying myositis: Review of the literature apropos of a case report. *Rev Stomatol Chir Maxillofac* 1990;91:51-55.

52. Renton P, Parkin SF, Stamp TC: Abnormal temporomandibular joints in fibrodysplasia ossificans progressiva. *Br J Oral Surg* 1982;20:31-38.

53. Sorenson MS: Fibrodysplasia ossificans progressiva and hearing loss. *Int J Pediatr Otorhinolaryngol* 1987;14:79-82.

54. Kussmaul WG, Esmail BA, Sagar Y, et al: Pulmonary and cardiac function in advanced fibrodysplasia ossificans progressiva. *Clin Orthop Relat Res* 1998;346:104-109.

55. Jaworski RC, Gibson M: Mitral and aortic valve abnormalities in a patient with fibrodysplasia ossificans progressiva. *Pathology* 1983;15:325-328.

56. Cremin B, Connor JM, Beighton P: The radiological spectrum of fibrodysplasia ossificans progressiva. *Clin Radiol* 1982;33:499-508.

57. Lindhout D, Golding RP, Taets van Amerongen AH: Fibrodysplasia ossificans progressiva: Current concepts and the role of CT in acute changes. *Pediatr Radiol* 1985;15:211-213.

58. Nunnelly JF, Yussen PS: Computed tomographic findings in patients with limited jaw movement due to myositis ossificans progressiva. *J Oral Maxillofac Surg* 1986;44:818-821.

59. Caron KH, Dipietro MAQ, Aisen AM, et al: MR imaging of early fibrodysplasia ossificans progressiva. *J Comput Assist Tomogr* 1990;14:318-321.

60. Hagowara J, Aida N, Machida J, et al: Contrast-enhanced MRI of an early preosseous lesion of fibrodysplasia ossificans progressiva in a 21-month-old boy. *AJR Am J Roentgenol* 2003;181:1145-1147.

61. Klemperer FW, Miller JM, Hill CJ: The inhibition of alkaline phosphatase by beryllium. *J Biol Chem* 1949;180:281-288.

62. Allgrove J: Use of bisphosphonates in children and adolescents. *J Pediatr Endocrinol Metab* 2002;15(Suppl 3):921-928.

63. Alpigiani MG, Puleo MG, Callegarini L, et al: Dichlormethylenbiphosphoric acid in the therapy of myositis ossificans progressiva. *Minerva Pediatr* 1996;48:159-163.

64. Crofford LJ, Brahim J, Zasloff MA, Marini JC: Failure of surgery and isotretinoin to relieve jaw immobilization in fibrodysplasia ossificans progressiva: Report of two case. *J Oral Maxillofac Surg* 1990;48:204-208.

65. Hentzer B, Jacobsen HH, Asboe-Hansen G: Fibrodysplasia (myositis) ossificans progressiva treated with disodium etidronate. *Clin Radiol* 1978;29:69-75.

66. Rogers JG, Dorst JP, Geho WB: Use and complications of high-dose disodium etidronate therapy in fibrodysplasia ossificans progressiva. *J Pediatr* 1977;91:1011-1014.

67. Zasloff MA, Rocke DM, Crofford LJ, et al: Treatment of patients with fibrodysplasia ossificans progressiva with isoretinoin. *Clin Orthop Relat Res* 1998;346:121-129.

68. Tumulo M, Moscatelli A, Sivestri G: Anaesthetic management of a child with fibrodysplasia ossificans progressiva. *Br J Anaesth* 2006;97:701-703.

69. Benetos IS, Mavorgenis AF, Themistocleous GS, et al: Optimal treatment of fibrodysplasia ossificans progressiva with surgical excision of heterotopic bone, indomethacin and irradiation. *J Surg Orthop Adv* 2006;15:99-104.

Chapter 23

Marfan Syndrome

The syndrome originally described by Antoine Bernard-Jean Marfan in 1896 is a common inherited connective tissue abnormality that occurs as an autosomal dominant genetic disorder with frequent mutations. The patients have normal mentation but have as characteristic features excessive height, abnormally long limbs (dolichostenomelia), arachnodactyly (spider-like digits on hands and feet), joint hypermobility, distinctive facial abnormalities, scoliosis, dislocating lenses (ectopia lentis), enlargement of the dural sac (dural ectasia), and an array of aortic and cardiac abnormalities that are frequently life-threatening. The nature of the abnormality has been identified and the genetic cause has been discovered. Some medical treatments are currently available to somewhat protect against cardiac disasters, and surgical approaches can reduce the risk considerably. The orthopaedic problems can be significant and sometimes require surgical intervention, particularly for spinal or hip abnormalities or fractures.

History

Antoine Bernard-Jean Marfan (1858-1942) was born in France; after completing his medical training in Toulouse and some special training in children's diseases, he became Chief of Pediatrics at the University of Paris and the Hopital des Enfants Maladies in 1914, a position he held until his retirement in 1928.[1] He became very involved in defining infectious and other disorders in children and described features of syphilis (Dennie-Marfan syndrome), a red triangle on the tongue characteristic of typhus (Marfan's sign), rachitic epiphyseal swelling of the medial malleous (Marfan's symptom), and a prognostic rule related to tuberculosis of the throat (Marfan's law).[1] In 1896, Marfan presented the case of a 5-year-old girl to the Société Médicale des Hôpitaux de Paris.[2] He pointed out her disproportionately long limbs, asthenic physique, and slender and exceptionally long fingers and toes. She was studied again with radiographs by Henri Mery and Leon Babonneix[3] in 1902, who noted scoliosis and thoracic asymmetry; somewhat later, she was discovered to have cardiovascular abnormalities and dislocations of her lenses. Subsequent reports on other patients by Achard[4] in 1902 defined the familial nature of the disease, and in 1912, Salle[5] reported necropsy findings of changes in the heart and aorta. In 1914, Boerger[6] first clearly defined ectopia lentis in the patients. It was Weve[7] who in 1931 confirmed the hereditary characteristic of the disease and provided the name "dystrophia mesodermalis congenital, type Marfanis;" since then, the disorder has been known as Marfan syndrome. Cardiac and aortic abnormalities in patients were further described by Baer and associates in 1943[8] and shortly thereafter by Etter and Glover.[9] Victor A. McKusick became fascinated with the disease and wrote about it extensively beginning in 1955.[10-11] In the 1960s, both Gordon[12] and Schwartz[13] attempted to establish the likelihood that Abraham Lincoln had had Marfan syndrome, but despite attempts to seek the gene error in his remains, the issue still remains unclear.[14]

Genetic Causation and Frequency

Marfan syndrome is an inherited connective tissue disorder transmitted as an autosomal dominant trait with frequent mutations.[11,14-20] The disorder is equally distributed in ethnic groups, is slightly more frequent in females than males, and occurs worldwide at 1 per 5,000 to 10,000 births.[11,14,15,19,20] The disorder is now known to be caused by mutations in the fibrillin-1 (FBN-1) gene located on chromosome 15q21.1.[14,16,17,21,22] The gene encodes the glycoprotein fibrillin, which is a major building block for microfibrils, including those involved in the skeletal system, the spinal dura, the optic lens supporting system, and the elastin in the aorta and cardiac valvular structures.[14,17,18,21,23,24] It has also been proposed that there is a disturbance of tissue homeostasis of elastic fibers, increased susceptibility of fibrillin to proteolysis, and dysregulation of transforming

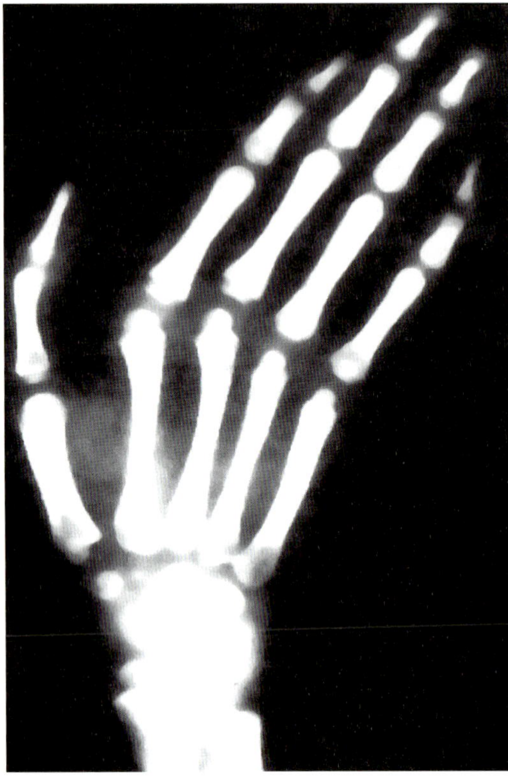

Figure 1

Radiograph of the hand in a patient with Marfan syndrome. The hand is very long and displaced medially. Function is very limited and patients often cannot lift or carry objects.

growth factor-β resulting in increased apoptosis.[17,18,25,26] The gene error can be identified not only in patients with the disorder or their family but in uterine fluids. It is also possible to identify the changes seen in the child in the uterus by appropriate imaging studies.[14,19,27]

Clinical Findings

Patients with Marfan syndrome may have multiple findings, some that occur frequently and some less commonly. In 1986, a committee established the Berlin Criteria, which include diagnostic features that are commonly present and are required to make the diagnosis (major factors) and others that are less commonly present and may be associated with other disorders.[14,15,28] Of some importance in any discussion of Marfan syndrome is a listing of some of the other genetic disorders that may resemble aspects of Marfan syndrome and cause confusion in both diagnosis and treatment protocols. The similar lesions that have some of the characteristics of Marfan syndrome include ho-

mocystinuria,[14] Ehlers-Danlos syndrome,[11,14] Klinefelter syndrome,[29-31] Lujan-Fryns syndrome,[32] van den Ende-Gupta disease,[33,34] Joubert syndrome,[35,36] Shprintzen-Goldberg syndrome,[37-39] Beals disease,[40] Marfanoid hypermobility syndrome,[41] Stickler syndrome,[42] PHACE (posterior fossa malformation, hemangioma, arterial abnormalities, coarctation of the aorta, eye abnormalities) syndrome,[43] and some other disorders that affect the hands, feet, heart, aorta and bones.[9,11,14,35,44] The list of findings included in this chapter are considered important only for the diagnosis of Marfan syndrome and hence are known as "major factors" according to the Berlin Criteria.[15]

General and Orthopaedic Characteristics of Marfan Syndrome

Most patients with Marfan syndrome have normal mentation.[11,14,20,45,46] Children born with Marfan syndrome are often quite tall and in a short time are taller than their normal siblings and peers.[11,14,15,45,47] Some patients as adults may grow to more than 7 feet in height.[19,45-47] An important finding is dolichostenomelia, which is defined as having excessively long limbs, far in excess of the normal relationship of the upper and lower extremities to the rest of the body.[11,14] The bones are generally osteopenic with frequent fractures[15,48-51] and an unusually high occurrence of protrusio acetabuli, which can be very disabling.[49,52-55] The limbs are excessively thin, suggesting that not only are the bones diminished in circumference but that there is less soft tissue surrounding them. The fat content of the soft tissues of the extremities is reduced and there is often muscular underdevelopment so that the extremities are much thinner than those of unaffected individuals.[11,14,15] The hands and feet show very thin and much elongated digits that are described as "arachnodactyly," suggesting that they resemble spider's limbs (Figure 1).[9,15,18-20] Flat feet are common, as are dislocations of joints such as the elbows, wrists, knees, and especially hips.[11,14,18] The great toe is sometimes excessively elongated (Figure 2). The hand digits are excessively mobile and the flexed thumb may extend beyond the four fingers when the hand and digits are flexed (Steinberg thumb sign).[14] In addition, the combination of a thin wrist and long digits

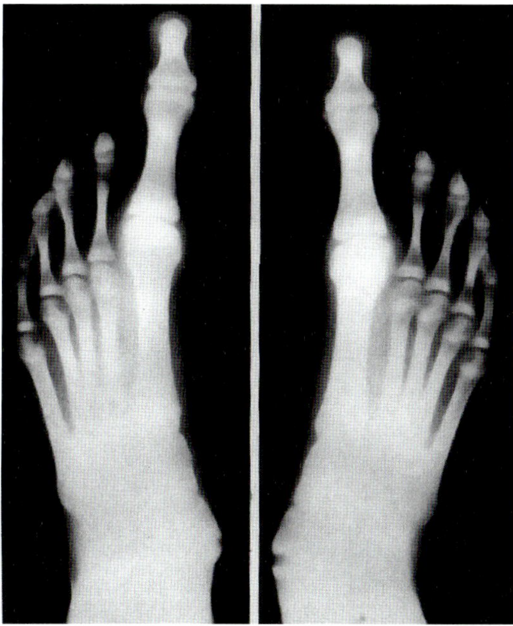

Figure 2
One of the most unusual features of Marfan syndrome is the presence of extraordinary length to the great toe.

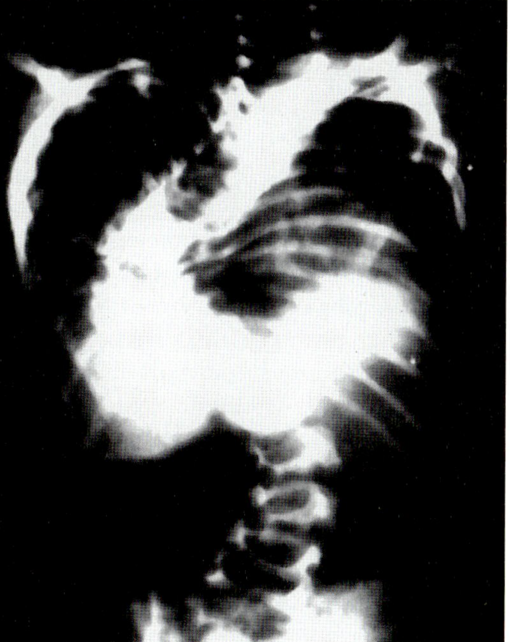

Figure 3
Scoliosis can be very severe and frequently leads to neurologic problems for patients with Marfan syndrome.

may allow an overlap of the thumb and first and fifth fingers when the wrist is grasped (Walker-Murdoch sign).[14] The ribs show abnormal growth and many patients show either a pectus excavatum or a pectus carinatum.[11,14,56]

Scoliosis or kyphoscoliosis occurs in 30% to 60% of patients, is commonly present in even young children, and progresses with advancing years (Figure 3).[11,14,18,19,57] The lesions, along with the pectus changes and facial deformities, are such as to compromise pulmonary function in some patients and may be associated with sometimes severe sleep apnea.[11,56,58,59] Additional findings include spina bifida occulta, hemivertebra, cleft or high-arched palate, and dental crowding,[11,57] and a thin narrow face and prognathism is characteristic.[14,18,19,57] One of the more common entities is dural ectasia, in which the dura becomes moderately or markedly expanded, causing widening of the spinal canal, thinning of the vertebral cortex and pedicles, dilatation of the neural foramina, and protrusion of the dura outside the bony canal.[15,54,57,60-65] These findings may cause loss of nerve function and even paraplegia. Many patients are muscularly impaired and cannot perform exercises or participate in sports.[11,45,46,48,66]

Ocular Findings

Almost all patients with Marfan syndrome have ocular findings and often complaints related to visual alterations and loss. The most frequent problem is "ectopia lentis," partial or complete dislocation of the lens, which occurs in 50% to 80% of patients.[11,14,20,44,67] Tremor of the iris may occur and suggests the likelihood of dislocating lenses. Flattening of the cornea is common; blue sclerae have been reported in patients with the disease and visual loss is common.[11,14,67] Many patients have myopia and loss of visual acuity that requires glasses. Occasional cases of retinal detachment are encountered, and blindness is not unusual in these patients. Despite normal intelligence, some patients have considerable difficulty in a school setting because of inability to read either small print or a distant blackboard.[46,66,67]

Cardiovascular Disorders

Seventy percent of the patients with Marfan syndrome have aortic root dilatation and aortic regurgitation.[8,10,11,14,19,20,35,68] The process may be manifest at an early age and is more common in men.[10,11,14,35,44] A diastolic murmur over the aortic valve may be present.[14] Aortic dissection involving the ascending aorta is a serious problem and can lead to death of the patient. Mitral valve prolapse may occur in 55% to 70% of patients and results in a high-pitched late systolic murmur, shortness of breath, and a rapid pulse rate.[10,11,14,44] Pulmonary artery dilatation may also occur and even a dissecting aneurysm of the pulmonary artery, which can be fatal.[14,20,44,68] Most of these can be diagnosed by electrocardiography, echocardiography, and MRI studies of the heart and the aorta; these studies should be done regularly. In addition, some patients have been found to have other cardiovascular manifestations, including coarctation of the aorta, patent ductus arteriosus, absent pulmonary valve, and interatrial stenosis.[11,14,20,68] Spontaneous pneumothorax or apical blebs may develop.[14,59] Cardiac and aortic disorders are serious and can lead to the patient's death, often unexpectedly and at an early age or even intrapartum.[10,14,27,35,68-70]

Other Findings

Other findings include unusual skin changes such as striae atrophicae (transverse striations often located in the back). Some patients may have spontaneous or incisional herniae.[11,14]

Diagnostic Studies

As indicated above, family history is an essential part of the evaluation of the patient. Studies for the molecular gene error seeking the FBN1 mutation are important to provide a competent system of diagnosis of the disease. Similar studies seeking the genetic error in the patient's parents and siblings may also be helpful.[11,14,16,21,24]

All children or adults thought to have Marfan syndrome should be evaluated by a team of clinicians; this includes individuals interested in genetic diseases, orthopaedic disorders, ocular problems, and cardiac diseases. Both children and adults require imaging studies, which include the spine, pelvis, limbs, hands, feet, chest, skull, heart, and lungs. Some of these should be done regularly. CT and MRI are particularly important in the study of the spine for dural ectasia.[60-62,64,65] Bone densitometry should be performed at least yearly for all patients.[50,51] Frequent evaluation of heart sounds by a competent cardiologist and echocardiography, electrocardiography, and MRI may be useful and lifesaving.[10,11,14,19,20,24] Ocular studies should include slit-lamp evaluation and keratometry.[14,67]

Treatment

Some patients with Marfan syndrome may require no treatment other than frequent observation for ocular, cardiac, or orthopaedic complaints or findings. The majority, however, do require some attempts to alter the progress of the disease, not only to keep them alive but to improve their life status.

Medical Treatment

Recently, beta blockers have been introduced to reduce the cardiac and aortic stress and hopefully reduce some of the commonly developing problems.[14,19,71-73] The drugs include atenolol, propranolol hydrochloride, and verapamil hydrochloride. Estrogen, androgen, and somatostatin have been administered to children to slow their skeletal progression, but at this point the strategy has only limited success and may produce additional problems.[14,47,74]

Cardiac Treatment

Supportive cardiac measures may be helpful for some patients.[24,75] For patients whose lives are threatened, surgery for aortic or mitral valve repair or replacement, aortic arch reconstruction, or composite aortic graft insertion or replacement may be required.[14,24,68,75] A recent report suggests that cardiac transplantation is necessary for some patients.[76]

Ocular Treatment

Myopia is treatable with refraction, and lens defects are best treated by surgical procedures.[62,67]

Orthopaedic Treatment

Bracing of spinal curvature may be helpful and prevent progression of scoliotic and kyphotic changes. It may be necessary to do corrective surgery, especially if dural ectasia or progressive scoliotic deformity develops.[64,75,77-79] Pectus excavatum, if severe, may require surgery to prevent damage to the pulmonary tree and the aorta.[11,14] Surgery to correct protrusio acetabulae is sometimes necessary but may not be effective.[53-55] Surgery for hands, feet, elbows, hips, or knees is occasionally necessary for subluxations or fractures. The use of bisphosphonates in an attempt to decrease the osteopenia of bony segments and reduce the likelihood of fractures may be tried, but as yet has not been reported to be successful.[14,50]

Psychological Treatment

It should be apparent that patients with Marfan syndrome and their families carry great physical and emotional burdens.[46,66] The children are tall and unusually structured and considered strange in appearance by most individuals. The development of eye problems sometimes limits their ability to be educated and their physical problems markedly limit their ability to participate in social and athletic activities. Patients and their parents may need psychiatric support, and they should also consult with geneticists about issues related to having more children.

Discussion

Over the years since Professor Marfan first described his patient in 1896, we have gathered information about the clinical characteristics of the disease and the sometimes life- and limb-threatening complications. We now know the genetic origin of the process and how it causes the disorder, and this is very helpful in diagnosis and familial evaluation. We have catalogued the frequency of the various symptoms and signs and established their value in providing criteria for diagnosis. Although we have also begun a series of medical and surgical protocols for management of these patients, at least to this point we really cannot reverse the process; we can only treat the complications. It is hoped that over the next decade, we will be able to define how best to treat the genetic error, possibly in utero after the diagnosis is made, and thus reduce the effect of this sometimes devastating disorder.

References

1. Enersen OD: Antoine Bernard-Jean Marfan biography, in http://whonamedit.com/doctor.cfm/972.html.2001. Accessed March 11, 2009.

2. Marfan AB: Un cas de deformation congenitale des quatre: Membres plus prononcee aux extremites characterisee par l'allongement des os avec un certain degre d'amincissement. *Bull Mem Soc Med Hop Paris* 1896;13:220-226.

3. Mery H, Babonneix L: Un cas de deformation congenitale des quatre members: Hyperchondroplasie. *Bull Mem Soc Med Hop Paris* 1902;19:671-676.

4. Achard C: Arachnodactylie. *Bull Mem Soc Med Hop (Paris)* 1902;19:834-840.

5. Salle V: Ueber einen Fall von angeborener abnormer Grosse der Extemitaten mit einen Akronemegalia erinnerden Symptomenkomplex. *Jahrb Kinderheilkd* 1912;75:540-550.

6. Boerger D: Uber zwei Falle von arachnodaktylie. *Zeitschrift Kinderheilkd* 1914;12:161-184.

7. Weve H: Ueber Archnodaktylie (dystrophia mesodermalis congenita, typus Marfanis). *Arch Augenheilk* 1931;104:1-46.

8. Baer RW, Taussig HB, Oppenheimer EH: Congenital aneurysmal dilation of the aorta associated with arachnodactyly. *Bull Johns Hopkins Hosp* 1943;72:309-331.

9. Etter LE, Glover LP: Arachnodactyly complicated by dislocated lens and death from rupture of dissecting aneurysm of the aorta. *JAMA* 1943;123:88-89.

10. McKusick VA: The cardiovascular aspects of Marfan's syndrome: A heritable disorder of connective tissue. *Circulation* 1955;11:321-342.

11. McKusick VA: The Marfan syndrome, in *Heritable Disorders of Connective Tissue*, ed 3. St. Louis, MO, CV Mosby Company, 1966, pp 38-149.

12. Gordon AM: Abraham Lincoln: A medical appraisal. *J Ky Med Assoc* 1962;60:249-253.

13. Schwartz H: Abraham Lincoln and the Marfan syndrome. *JAMA* 1964;187:473-479.

14. Godfrey M: The Marfan syndrome, in Beighton P (ed): *McKusick's Heritable Disorders of Connective Tissue*, ed 5. St. Louis, MO, Mosby-Year Book, 1993.

15. Beighton P, de Paepe A, Danks D, et al: International nosology of heritable disorders of connective tissue, Berlin, 1986. *Am J Med Genet* 1988;29:581-594.

16. Boileau C, Jondeau G, Mizuguchi T, Matsumoto N: Molecular genetics of Marfan syndrome. *Curr Opin Cardiol* 2005;20:194-200.

17. Dietz HC, Pyeritz RE: Mutations in the human gene for fibrillin-1 (FBN1) in the Marfan syndrome and related disorders. *Hum Mol Genet* 1995;4:1799-1809.

18. Giampietro PF, Raggio C, Davis JG: Marfan syndrome: Orthopedic and genetic reviews. *Curr Opin Pediatr* 2002;14:35-41.

19. Judge DP, Dietz HC: Marfan's syndrome. *Lancet* 2005;366:1965-1976.

20. Pyeritz RE: The Marfan syndrome. *Annu Rev Med* 2000;51:481-510.

21. Dietz HC, Cutting GR, Pyeritz RE, et al: Marfan syndrome caused by a recurrent de novo missense mutation in the fibrillin gene. *Nature* 1991;352:337-339.

22. Robinson PN, Booms P, Katzke S, et al: Mutations

of FBN1 and genotype-phenotype correlations in Marfan syndrome and related fibrillinopathies. *Hum Mutat* 2002;20:153-161.

23. Gigante A, Chillemi C, Greco F: Changes of elastic fibers in musculoskeletal tissues of Marfan syndrome: A possible mechanism of joint laxity and skeletal overgrowth. *J Pediatr Orthop* 1999;19:283-288.

24. Nollen GJ, Mulder BJ: What is new in the Marfan syndrome? *Int J Cardiol* 2004;97:103-108.

25. Mizuguchi T, Collod-Beroud G, Akiyama T, et al: Heterozygous TGFBR2 mutations in Marfan syndrome. *Nat Genet* 2004;36:855-860.

26. Neptune ER, Frischmeyer PA, Arking DE, et al: Dysregulation of TGF-beta activation contributes to the pathogenesis in Marfan syndrome. *Nat Genet* 2003;33:407-411.

27. Buchanan R, Wyatt GP: Marfan's syndrome presenting as an intrapartum death. *Arch Dis Child* 1985;60:1074-1076.

28. Rose PS, Levy HP, Ahn NU, et al: A comparison of the Berlin and Ghent nosologies and the influence of dural ectasia in the diagnosis of Marfan syndrome. *Genet Med* 2000;2:278-282.

29. Kamischke A, Baumgardt A, Horst J, Nieschlag E: Clinical and diagnostic features of patients with supected Klinefelter syndrome. *J Androl* 2003;24:41-48.

30. Ratcliffe SG, Bancroft J, Axworthy D, McLaren W: Klinefelter's syndrome in adolescence. *Arch Dis Child* 1982;57:6-12.

31. Smyth CM, Bremner WJ: Klinefelter syndrome. *Arch Intern Med* 1998;158:1309-1314.

32. Purandare KN, Markar TN: Pyschiatric symptomatology of Lujan-Fryns syndrome: An X-linked syndrome displaying Marfanoid symptoms with autistic features, hyperactivity, shyness and schizophreniform symptoms. *Psychiatr Genet* 2005;15:229-231.

33. Guerra D, Sanchez O, Richieri-Costa A: van den Ende-Gupta syndrome of blepharophimosis, arachnodactyly, and congenital contractures. *Am J Med Genet A* 2005;136:377-380.

34. Schweitzer DN, Lachman RS, Pressman BD, Graham JM Jr: van den Ende-Gupta syndrome of blepharophimosis, arachnodactyly, and congenital contractures: Clinical delineation and recurrence in brothers. *Am J Med Genet A* 2003;118:267-273.

35. Gleason TG: Heritable disorders predisposing to aortic dissection. *Semin Thorac Cardiovasc Surg* 2005;17:274-281.

36. Morava E, Dinopoulos A, Kroes HY, et al: Mitochondrial dysfunction in a patient with Joubert syndrome. *Neuropediatrics* 2005;36:214-217.

37. Hassed S, Shewmake K, Teo C, Curtis M, Cunniff C: Shprintzen-Goldberg syndrome with osteopenia and progressive hydrocephalus. *Am J Med Genet* 1997;70:450-453.

38. Robinson PN, Neumann LM, Demuth S, et al: Shprintzen-Goldberg syndrome: Fourteen new patients and a clinical analysis. *Am J Med Genet A* 2005;135:251-262.

39. Sood S, Eldadah ZA, Krause WL, McIntosh I, Dietz HC: Mutation in fibrillin-1 and the Marfanoid-craniosynostosis (Shprintzen-Goldberg) syndrome. *Nat Genet* 1996;12:209-211.

40. Takaesu-Miyagi S, Sakai H, Shiroma T, Hayakawa K, Funakoshi Y, Sawaguchi S: Ocular findings of Beals syndrome. *Jpn J Ophthalmol* 2004;48:470-474.

41. Walker BA, Beighton PH, Murdoch JL: The Marfanoid hypermobility syndrome. *Ann Intern Med* 1969;71:349-352.

42. Bennett JT, McMurray SW: Stickler syndrome. *J Pediatr Orthop* 1990;10:760-763.

43. Slavotinek AM, Dubovsky E, Dietz HC, Lacbawan F: Report of a child with aortic aneurysm, orofacial clefting, hemangioma, upper sternal defect, and Marfanoid features: Possible PHACE syndrome. *Am J Med Genet* 2002;110:283-288.

44. Bawle E, Quigg MH: Ectopia lentis and aortic root dilatation in congenital contractural arachnodactyly. *Am J Med Genet* 1992;42:19-21.

45. Erkula G, Jones KB, Sponseller PD, Dietz HC, Pyeritz RE: Growth and maturation in Marfan syndrome. *Am J Med Genet* 2002;109:100-115.

46. Peters K, Apse K, Blackford A, McHugh B, Michalic D, Biesecker B: Living with Marfan syndrome: Coping with stigma. *Clin Genet* 2005;68:6-14.

47. Noordam C, van Daalen S, Otten BJ: Treatment of tall stature in boys with somatostatin analogue 201-995: Effect on final height. *Eur J Endocrinol* 2006;154:253-257.

48. Braverman AC: Exercise and the Marfan syndrome. *Med Sci Sports Exerc* 1998;30:S387-S395.

49. Do T, Giampietro PF, Burke SW, et al: The incidence of protrusio acetabuli in Marfan's syndrome and its relationship to bone mineral density. *J Pediatr Orthop* 2000;20:718-721.

50. Giampietro PF, Peterson M, Schneider R, et al: Assessment of bone mineral density in adults and children with Marfan syndrome. *Osteoporos Int* 2003;14:559-563.

51. Le Parc JM, Plantin P, Jondeau G, Goldschild M, Albert M, Boileau C: Bone mineral density in sixty adult patients with Marfan syndrome. *Osteoporos Int* 1999;10:475-479.

52. Sponseller PD, Jones KB, Ahn NU, Erkula G, Foran JR, Dietz HC III: Protrusio acetabuli in Marfan syndrome: Age-related prevalence and associated hip function. *J Bone Joint Surg Am* 2006;88:486-495.

53. Steel HH: Protrusio acetabuli: Its occurrence in the completely expressed Marfan syndrome and its musculoskeletal component and a procedure to arrest the course of protrusion in the growing pelvis. *J Pediatr Orthop* 1996;16:704-718.

54. Van de Velde S, Fillman R, Yandow S: Protrusio acetabuli in Marfan syndrome: History, diagnosis, and treatment. *J Bone Joint Surg Am* 2006;88:639-646.

55. Yule SR, Hobson EE, Dean JC, Gilbert FJ: Protrusio acetabuli in Marfan syndrome. *Clin Radiol* 1999;54:95-97.

56. Arn PH, Scherer LR, Haller JA Jr, Pyeritz RE: Outcome of pectus excavatum in patients with Marfan syndrome and in the general population. *J Pediatr* 1989;115:954-958.

57. Birch JG, Herring JA: Spinal deformity in Marfan syndrome. *J Pediatr Orthop* 1987;7:546-552.

58. Cistulli PA, Gotsopoulos H, Sullivan CE: Relationship between craniofacial abnormalities and sleep-disordered breathing in Marfan's syndrome. *Chest* 2001;120:1455-1460.

59. Fuleihan FJ, Suh SK, Shepherd RH: Some aspects of pulmonary function in the Marfan syndrome. *Bull Johns Hopkins Hosp* 1963;113:320-329.

60. Ahn NU, Sponseller PD, Ahn UM, et al: Dural ectasia in the Marfan syndrome: MR and CT findings and criteria. *Genet Med* 2000;2:173-179.

61. Ahn NU, Sponseller PD, Ahn UM, Nallamshetty L, Kuszyk BS, Zinreich SJ: Dural ectasia is associated with back pain in Marfan syndrome. *Spine* 2000;25:1562-1568.

62. Foran JR, Pyeritz RE, Dietz HC, Sponseller PD: Characterization of the symptoms associated with dural ectasia in the Marfan patient. *Am J Med Genet A* 2005;134:58-65.

63. Pyeritz RE, Fishman EK, Bernhardt BA, Siegelman SS: Dural ectasia is a common feature of the Marfan syndrome. *Am J Hum Genet* 1988;43:726-732.

64. Stern WE: Dural ectasia and the Marfan syndrome. *J Neurosurg* 1988;69:221-227.

65. Villeirs GM, Van Tongerloo AJ, Verstraete KL, Kunnen MF, De Paepe AM: Widening of the spinal canal and dural ectasia in Marfan's syndrome: Assessment by CT. *Neuroradiology* 1999;41:850-854.

66. Van Tongerloo A, De Paepe A: Psychosocial adaptation in adolescents and young adults with Marfan syndrome: An exploratory study. *J Med Genet* 1998;35:405-409.

67. Maumenee IH: The eye in the Marfan syndrome. *Trans Am Ophthalmol Soc* 1981;79:684-733.

68. Ramirez F, Dietz HC: Therapy insight: Aortic aneurysm and dissection in Marfan's syndrome. *Nat Clin Pract Cardiovasc Med* 2004;1:31-36.

69. Murdoch JL, Walker BA, Halpern BL, Kuzma JW, McKusick VA: Life expectancy and causes of death in the Marfan syndrome. *N Engl J Med* 1972;286:804-808.

70. Silverman DI, Burton KJ, Gray J, et al: Life expectancy in the Marfan syndrome. *Am J Cardiol* 1995;75:157-160.

71. Rios AS, Silber EN, Bavishi N, et al: Effect of long-term beta-blockade on aortic root compliance in patients with Marfan syndrome. *Am Heart J* 1999;137:1057-1061.

72. Rossi-Foulkes R, Roman MJ, Rosen SE, et al: Phenotypic features and impact of beta blocker or calcium antagonist therapy on aortic lumen size in the Marfan syndrome. *Am J Cardiol* 1999;83:1364-1368.

73. Yetman AT, Bornemeier RA, McCrindle BW: Usefulness of enalapril versus propranolol or atenolol for prevention of aortic dilation in patients with the Marfan syndrome. *Am J Cardiol* 2005;95:1125-1127.

74. Rozendaal L, le Cessie S, Wit JM, Hennekam RC, The Dutch Marfan Working Group: Growth-reductive therapy in children with Marfan syndrome. *J Pediatr* 2005;147:674-679.

75. Milewicz DM, Dietz HC, Miller DC: Treatment of aortic disease in patients with Marfan syndrome. *Circulation* 2005;111:e150-e157.

76. Krasemann T, Kotthoff S, Kehl HG, et al: Cardiac transplantation in neonatal Marfan syndrome—a life-saving approach. *Thorac Cardiovasc Surg* 2005;53:S146-S148.

77. Di Silvestre M, Greggi T, Giacomini S, et al: Surgical treatment for scoliosis in Marfan syndrome. *Spine* 2005;30:E597-E604.

78. Lipton GE, Guille JT, Kumar SJ: Surgical treatment of scoliosis in Marfan syndrome: Guidelines for a successful outcome. *J Pediatr Orthop* 2002;22:302-307.

79. Sponseller PD, Sethi N, Caameron DE, Pyeritz RE: Infantile scoliosis in Marfan syndrome. *Spine* 1997;22:509-516.

Chapter 24

Osteosclerotic Disorders: Osteopoikilosis, Osteopathia Striata, and Melorheostosis

Osteopoikilosis of Albers-Schönberg, osteopathia striata of Voorhoeve, and melorheostosis of Leri are clinical entities that are all of unknown cause and quite distinct in appearance and structural and histologic abnormalities. The three disorders are generally benign in that some of the patients are asymptomatic and the lesions do not seem to progress. In others, particularly if associated with additional disorders of skin, fibrous tissue, and especially the calvarium, there may be significant disability. The three syndromes, although clinically quite distinct, are somehow related, and having one of them makes the patient prone to having another. The three diseases are ancient; Lester[1] reported findings of melorheostosis in a prehistoric Alaskan skeleton and Canci and associates[2] noted findings of melorheostosis and diffuse idiopathic skeletal hyperostosis in a skeleton of a Greek female from the 6th century BC. In 2005, Amezcua-Guerra and associates[3] described osteopoikilosis in an ancient skeleton.

Nomenclature and History

Osteopoikilosis is otherwise known as "mottled bones," "spotted bones," osteitis condensans generalisata, osteosclerosis disseminata, osteopathia condensans disseminata, osteopoikila familiara, or osteodysplasia enostotica. Patients who in addition have skin and soft-tissue abnormalities are sometimes listed as having Buschke-Ollendorff syndrome.[4-6] Osteopoikilosis was first described in 1915 by Heinrich Albers-Schönberg,[7] and several other authors over the next 50 years further defined aspects of the disease. These works included a description of the clinical entity by Putti in 1927;[8] the findings of skin abnormalities by Curth in 1934;[5] and clinical patient presentations by Funstein and Kotschiew,[9] Erbsen,[10] and Holly[11] in 1936. Hinson[12] defined the familial characteristics, and Berlin and associates[13] described the clinical and genetic characteristics for a series of patients.

Melorheostosis was first described by Leri and Joanny[14] in 1922 and is known as Leri's syndrome. It is also known from its Greek words of origin (melos and rheos) as "melted wax dripping down one side of a candle."[15-18] The disorder is also called flowing hyperostosis, flowing periostitis, osteopathia hyperostica congenita embri unius, or osteosis eburnisans monomelica. Junghagen[19] showed radiographic changes in a patient in 1930; in 1933, Kraft[18] described the histologic abnormalities while Moore and de Lorimier[20] outlined the radiographic findings. Over the next 10 years, Franklin and Matheson[21] defined the clinical changes, Gillespie and Siegling[22] described the disease in a child, and Hall[23] described the bony changes in great detail. Aarseth[24] biopsied the bone of a patient and described the histologic changes in a 1948 article. In a study performed in 1961, Maroteaux and Lamy[25] showed the changes in a newborn infant; in a signal presentation published in 1968, Campbell and associates[16] described 14 cases and, to a large extent, clarified the nature of the disease.

Osteopathia striata was described by Voorhoeve[26] in 1924 and is known as Voorhoeve's dyschondroplasia, osteopathia condensans disseminate, or osteorhabdotosis. This disorder is less commonly encountered than the other two and is believed to be a form of osteopoikilosis, although this is not clear in terms of genetics or clinical characteristics.[15,17,27] In 1953, Hurt[28] described the frequent occurrence of cranial abnormalities with osteopathia striata, and the combined cranial and peripheral disorders were defined as being autosomal dominant in origin, according to a 1978 study by Horan and Beighton.[29] As reported by

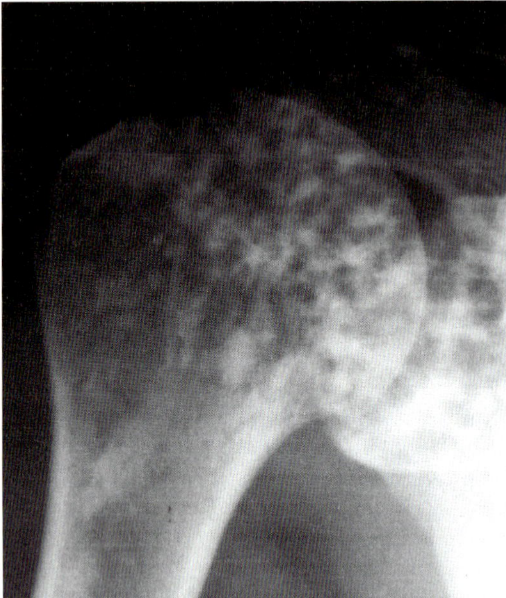

Figure 1
Osteopoikilosis of the proximal humerus. Small bony masses are present in the metaphyseal region. These are generally asymptomatic.

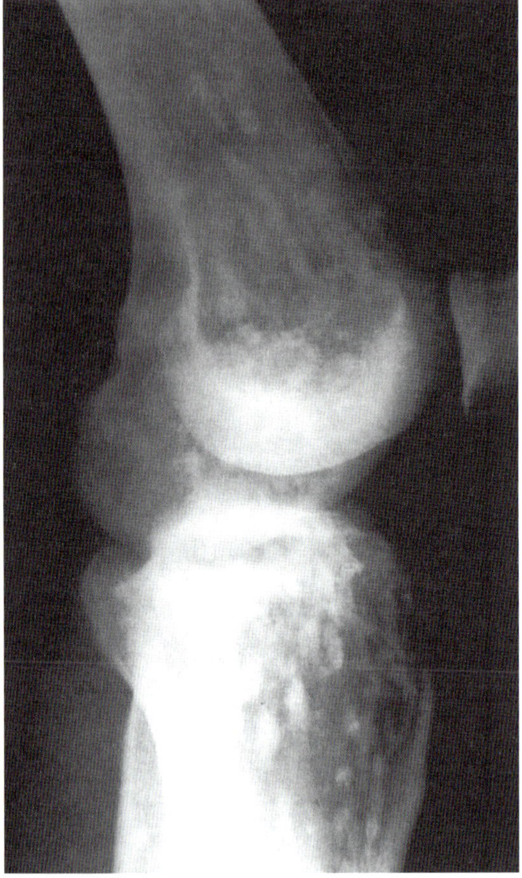

Figure 2
Osteopoikilosis affecting the tibia and distal femur appear as small areas of increased density within the bone.

Knockaert and Dequeker in 1979,[30] the disease may also be associated with focal dermal hypoplasia, a syndrome described earlier by Goltz and associates.[31]

Clinical, Radiographic, and Histologic Features
Osteopoikilosis

Osteopoikilosis is, as described above, "spotted bone disease," consisting of small, round circumscribed nodules of increased density within the bones.[13,15,17,32,33] The disorder is rare in most reported series.[15,17,34] The lesions are believed to be genetic in origin and are thought to be autosomal dominant, with familial occurrences quite common.[11-13,34] In recent years, patients with the disorder were thought to have a loss-of-function mutation of LEMD3,[35,36] but recent studies suggest that this is not always present.[37,38]

Osteopoikilotic lesions occur equally in males and females, and there is no identifiable ethnic predominance.[12,13,15,17,34] The lesions may be found at an early age but do not seem to grow or increase in number rapidly; once adulthood is reached, they remain stable for life. The osteopoikilotic lesions are quite small, usually less than 1 cm in diameter[15,17] (Figure 1). As many as 40 spots may appear in the metaphyseal-diaphyseal portions of the long bones, pelvis, and calca-

neus, but do not appear in the epiphyses[13,15,39] (Figure 2). The sclerotic spots are frequently bilaterally symmetric.[39] The skull and spinal sites are usually spared. Most patients are asymptomatic and the disorder is often discovered incidentally by radiographic examinations. Skin lesions known as dermatofibrosis lenticularis disseminate, originally described by Buschke and Ollendorff[4] in 1928, frequently occur in these patients.[5-6,36,40-43] The skin abnormalities are described as compact, slightly elevated, whitish-yellow, and oval or oblong in outline. The skin lesions are mostly inconspicuous and are usually located on the posterior aspect of the thighs, buttocks, or trunk, but not on the face.[5,41,42] They tend to disappear with advancing age.

Imaging studies are helpful in diagnosing and following patients with osteopoikilosis. Radiographs will show the small, round, dense lesions in the metaphyseal-epiphyseal regions of the long bones and pelvis.[13,15,17,33] These can also be followed with MRI or with CT, but generally they add very little to the plain radiograph images. The bone scan is generally positive over the sites of the nodules, but not very active as compared with the two other disorders.[15,17]

Histologic examination of the rounded segments show that they are composed of lamellar bone with a central area containing Haversian systems (Figure 3). The stratified layers on the surface of the nodules are separated by cement lines.[15,17,39] The lesions are benign and have no features suggestive of neoplastic activity. In terms of complications, Weisz[44] reported a patient with osteopoikilosis in whom spinal stenosis developed. In 1978, Mindell and associates[45] reported an osteosarcoma arising in a patient with osteopoikilosis. In 1988, Ayling and Evans[46] described a giant cell tumor, while Grimer and associates[47] described a chondrosarcoma, both in patients with osteopoikilosis.

Osteopathia Striata

Osteopathia striata receives its name from the presence of longitudinal parallel linear osteosclerotic streaks occurring in the metaphyseal-diaphyseal ends of the long bones.[15,17] Generally, it is believed that there are two forms: a mild, autosomal recessive form with limited presentation of the bony lesions; and a more severe autosomal dominant form that not only has much more extensive bony changes, but very often has marked calvarial involvement and disorders of the palate.[27,29,37,48-55] The disease is less common and far less severe in women, which strongly suggests that the lesion is X-linked.[52,56] The frequent association of this disorder with Goltz disease of the skin, which is also X-linked, makes this a likely probability.[31]

The majority of patients with the autosomal recessive form or women with osteopathia striata are relatively asymptomatic.[15,17,27] Patients with the more aggressive autosomal dominant form of the disorder often have multiple complaints and problems. By definition, all patients have thin linear osteosclerotic parallel streaks arising from the region of the metaphysis and extending into the diaphysis; these are quite evident on radiographs[15,17,27] (Figure 4). Lesions may cause some expansion of bone and, in fact, lead to Erlenmeyer-flask abnormalities,

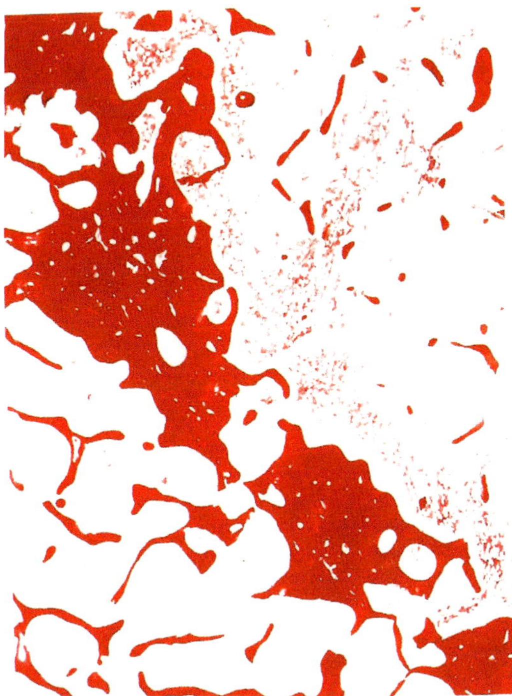

Figure 3
Histologic appearance of osteopoikilosis. The lesions are small, round, dense areas of normal bone.

but not as marked as in patients with Gaucher's or Pyle's disease. Of importance, patients with extensive disease may present with syndactyly, oligodactyly, polydactyly, rib anomalies, and segmentation errors of the vertebrae.[15,27,30,49,54] Increased bone density is often seen in the ribs, vertebrae, pelvis, and carpal and tarsal bones.

Patients with cranial sclerosis will show evidence of exuberant periosteal bone formation that results in sometimes profound narrowing of neural outlets, leading to hearing and sight loss and facial abnormalities, such as hypertelorism, frontal bossing, broad nasal bridge, and cleft palate.[15,29,30,48-53,55-57] Patients with the severe form of the disorder may have bone fragility resulting in fractures that are often difficult to treat.[15]

Imaging studies show the linear parallel, osteosclerotic streaked bony structures in the metaphyseal and diaphyseal region.[15,17,27,32,34,48] Bone scans are almost always active over the sites of the lesions.[58] Histologic evaluation of tissue from both the bones and the calvarium for those patients who have very active disease show exten-

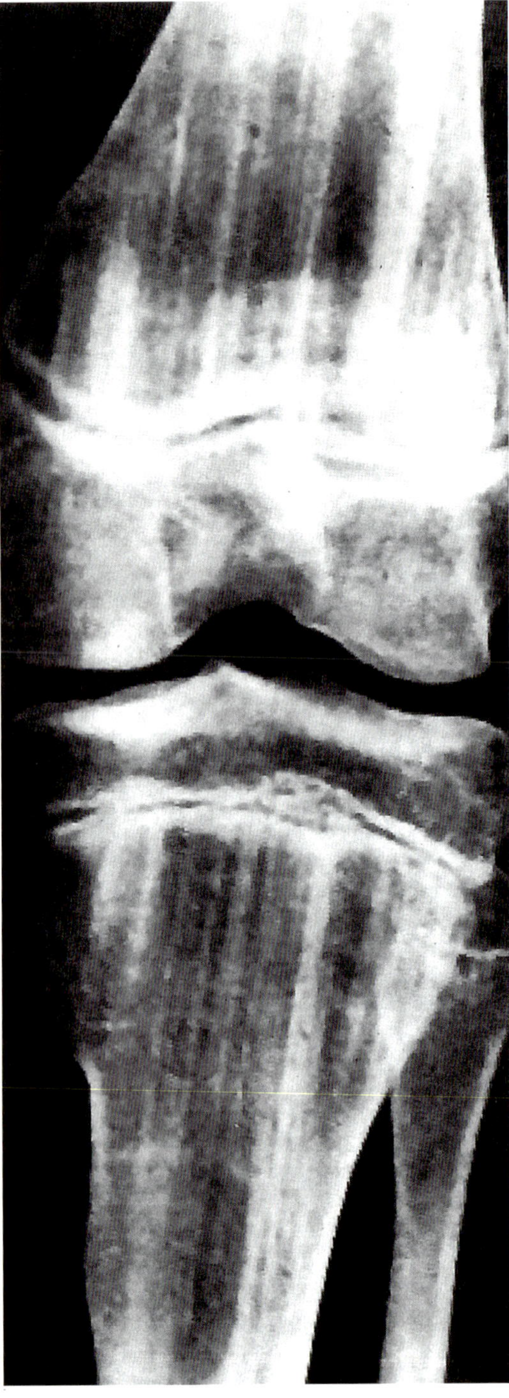

Figure 4

Osteopathic striata of the distal femur and proximal tibia in a growing child. The lesions are in the metaphysis and do not occur in the epiphysis. The lesions are elongated and always parallel to the long axis of the bone.

sive amounts of trabecular bone in the striated lesions and a generalized osteosclerosis in the calvarium.[15,17,48,49,52,53]

Melorheostosis

As indicated in the introduction to this chapter, melorheostosis is a rare entity in which extensive lesions develop on the external surface of one side of usually a long bone, such as the femur, tibia, or even the upper extremities ("melted wax dripping down one side of a candle")[2,15,17,59,60] (Figure 5). The lesions may occur in a single site or in several bones, and may be small or sufficiently large so as to greatly interfere with the structure of the limb and its function.[16,59-66] Melorheostosis is a sporadic lesion that has been reported to occur in family members; although a genetic error has been suspected, there is only limited evidence to support that concept.[36,38,67,68] The lesions occur equally in males and females, and children may be born with the disease or it may appear with advancing years.[15,16,22,59,60]

Clinically, the lesions occur usually on one side of a long bone and sometimes several bones in the same extremity.[15-17,69] The lower limb is more frequently affected than the upper limb.[15,16,69] The bony sclerosis typically affects the diaphyses of the long bones, the pelvis, and the carpal and tarsal bones. One side of the body is more often affected.[16,69] Tubular bones show endosteal bone formation, along with the periosteal osteoblastic changes[16,17] (Figure 5). Soft tissues overlying the site of the bony lesions may show some changes including fibrosis, muscle atrophy, contractures, angular deformities, limb shortening, and scleroderma.[16,23,65,69,70] Vascular abnormalities including lymphedema, hyperpigmentation, hemangiomas, glomus tumors, and aneurysms have been reported but are uncommon.[71-73]

Imaging studies are often striking, showing large masses of bone on the outside of one side of the femur or tibia that may extend into the soft tissues.[15,16,74] The lesions may be within the bone in some settings, particularly in the smaller bones and especially hands and feet. The lesions are usually very dense on radiographs and show considerable soft-tissue abnormality on CT or MRI.[58,59,69,72,75] Bone scans are almost always very positive. Histologic studies of the bone show irregularly arranged Haversian systems with dense, thick trabeculae and prominent cement lines[16,18,24,69] (Figure 6). Several patients are reported to have melorheostosis in unusual sites, including

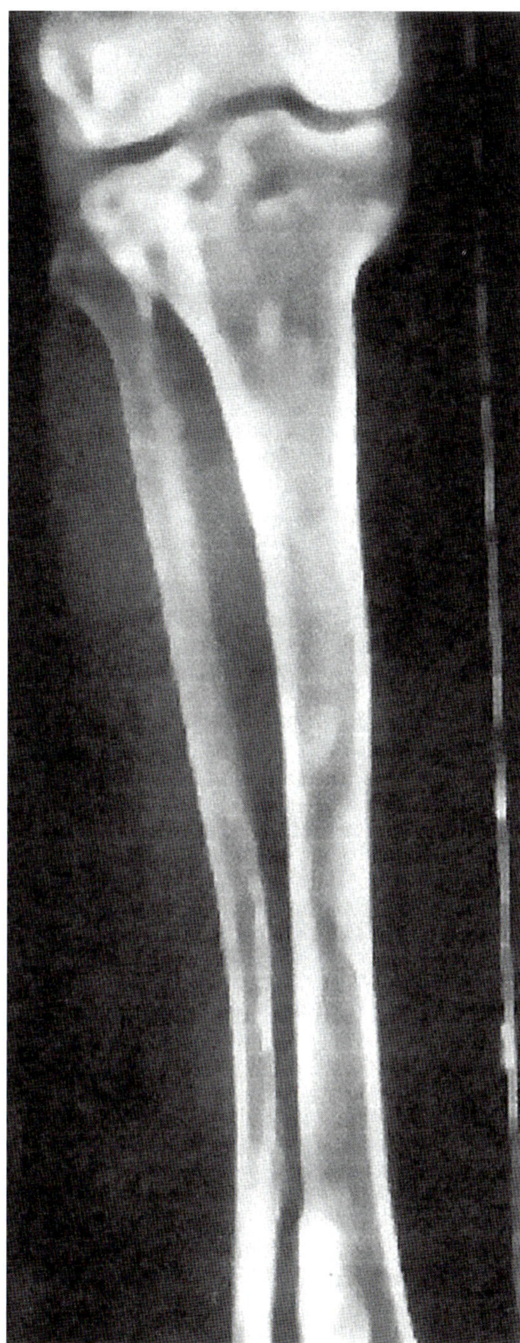

Figure 5
Melorheostosis affecting the tibia. Usually the material is attached to the surface of the bone and runs from one end to the other. It may produce limitation of movement.

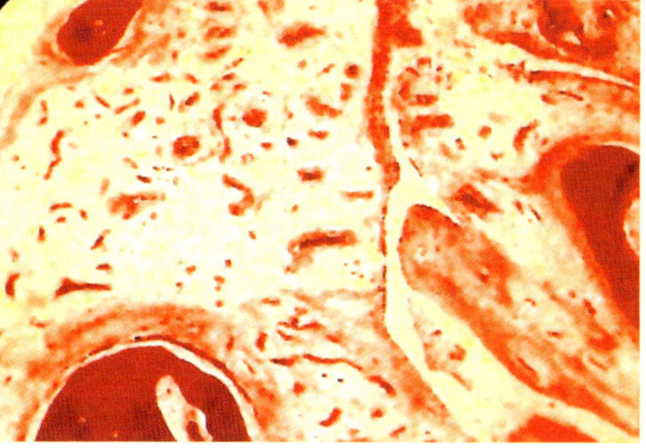

Figure 6
Histologic study of melorheostosis shows endosteal bone formation, often with periosteal new bone formation. The bone that is formed is normal in appearance.

the upper limb,[62] in association with subclavian and axillary artery aneurysms,[70] the hand,[61,63] the craniofacial skeleton,[64,76] the axial skeleton,[65] with scleroderma and hypertrichosis,[71,73] and with a desmoid tumor.[66] There are two reports of osteosarcoma arising in patients with melorheostosis: one by Bostman and associates[77] in 1987, and a second by Brennan and associates[78] in 2002, in which the patient also had osteopathia striata.

Treatment

Many patients with any of the three entities do not require treatment. In recent years, bisphosphonates have been introduced for melorheostosis or extensive osteopathia striata, but little is known regarding the results.[79] Surgery for complications remains the treatment of choice. Vascular disturbances, skin problems, jaw abnormalities, calvarial lesions with damage to neural routes, fractures, limitations of movement, and joint malfunction may require surgical corrective procedures. The success of such surgery is dependent on the extent of the disease and the patient's ability to deal with the limitations imposed.[15-17,59]

The Relationship of the Three Disorders

If all three of these osteogenetic disorders were completely independent of one another, they would represent a collection of benign rare diseases, presumably of thus far unknown genetic origin. They were present in historic populations, occur in all ethnic groups, and can be present in childhood or appear in young adults. They all have familial relationships in that there are frequent reports of members of the same family having the disease. There are no known treatments, although surgery may help improve function or repair fractures.

The problem is that the three disorders not only relate to other disorders such as skin lesions and cranial problems, but also to each other; there are numerous reports of two or sometimes even three clinical presentations representing the trio of disorders. In 1968, Abrahamson[80] reported on an asymptomatic patient with all three syndromes; Green and associates,[81] Butkus and associates,[82] Nevin and associates,[83] Debeer and associates,[84] and Happle[68] identified patients with melorheostosis who also had familial osteopoikilosis. In 1991, Cantatore and associates[32] presented a patient who had both osteopoikilosis and osteopathia striata. Verbov and Graham,[43] Happle,[40] and Kotulska and Kucharz[6] described the relationship of the Buschke-Ollendorff syndrome to osteopoikilosis. In 2004, Hellemans and associates[36] described a disorder consisting of Buschke-Ollendorff syndrome in a patient with both osteopoikilosis and melorheostosis. In 1979, Knockaert and Dequeker[30] described the relationship of the Goltz skin and soft-tissue abnormality to osteopathia striata. Further studies have identified multiple osseous and soft-tissue alterations, including digital abnormalities, short or deformed limbs, joint contractures, and abnormal facial structure.[49,55,61-64,76] In addition, some authors have described an array of skin, soft-tissue, and neurologic disorders that appear to occur in relation to one or several of these disorders. These include scleroderma, fibromatosis, desmoid tumors, tuberous sclerosis, craniostenosis, vascular malformations, jaw abnormalities, deafness, and ocular disturbances.[23,29,34,42,48-51,53,56,65,70,71,73]

Thus the problem is that without genetic structural identities and clearly defined clinical syndromes, how do we distinguish melorheostosis from osteopathia striata or from osteopoikilosis? Furthermore, even if some forms of therapy were available for one of these, how do we treat the disease if we are not sure what the disorder actually is? These are clearly serious problems for the clinician. Fortunately, however, the majority of the presentations are benign, and all three of the diseases are rarely encountered.

References

1. Lester CW: Melorheostosis in a prehistoric Alaskan skeleton. *J Bone Joint Surg Am* 1967;49:142-143.

2. Canci A, Marchi D, Caramella D, et al: Coexistence of melorheostosis and DISH in a female skeleton from Magna Graecia (Sixth Century BC). *Am J Phys Anthropol* 2005;126:305-310.

3. Amezcua-Guerra LM, Mansilla-Lory J, Fernandez-Tapia S, et al: Osteopoikilosis in an ancient skeleton: More than a medical curiosity. *Clin Rheumatol* 2005;24:502-506.

4. Buschke A, Ollendorff H: Ein fall von dermatofibrosis lenticularis disseminata und osteopathia condensans disseminata. *Dermatol Wochenschr* 1928;86:257-262.

5. Curth HO: Dermatofibrosis lenticularis disseminata and osteopoikilosis. *Arch Dermatol Syph* 1934;30:552-560.

6. Kotulska A, Kucharz EJ: Osteopoikilosis and Buschke-Ollendorff syndrome. *Case Rep Clin Pract Rev* 2002;3:290-293.

7. Albers-Schönberg H: Eine seltene, bisher nicht becante Strukturanomalie des Skelettes. *Fortschr Geb Roengenstr* 1915;23:174-177.

8. Putti V: L'osteosi eburneizzante monomelica: Una nuova sindrome osteopatica. *Chir Organi Mov* 1927;11:335-361.

9. Funstein L, Kotschiew K: Uber die osteopoikilie. *Fortsch Roentgenstr* 1936;54:595-603.

10. Erbsen H: Die osteopoikilie (osteopathia condensans disseminata). *Ergebn Med Strahlenforsch* 1936;7:137-174.

11. Holly LE: Osteopoikilosis: Five year study. *AJR Am J Roentgenol* 1936;36:512-517.

12. Hinson A: Familial osteopoikilosis. *Am J Surg* 1939;45:566-573.

13. Berlin R, Hedensio B, Lilja B, Linder L: Osteopoikilosis—a clinical and genetic study. *Acta Med Scand* 1967;18:305-314.

14. Leri A, Joanny J: Une affection non decrite des os hyperostose " en coulee" sur toute la longuer d' un membre ou "melorheostose". *Bull Mem Soc Med Hop Paris* 1922;46:1141-1145.

15. Beighton P: *McCusick's Heritable Disorders of Connective Tissue*, ed 5. St. Louis, CV Mosby, 1993, pp 657-659.

16. Campbell CJ, Papademetriou T, Bonfiglio M: Melorheostosis: A report of the clinical, roentgenographic and pathological findings in fourteen cases. *J Bone Joint Surg Am* 1968;50:1281-1304.

17. Jaffe HL: *Metabolic, Degenerative and Inflammatory Diseases of Bones and Joints*. Philadelphia, Lea and Febiger, 1972, pp 226-236.

18. Kraft E: The pathology of monomelic flowing hyperostosis or melorheostosis. *Radiology* 1933;20:47-55.

19. Junghagen S: Sur la melorheostose. *J Radiol Electrol* 1930;14:495-500.

20. Moore JJ, de Lorimier AA: Melorheostosis Leri: Review of the literature and report of a case. *AJR Am J Roentgenol* 1933;29:161-171.

21. Franklin EL, Matheson I: Melorheostosis: Report of a case with review of the literature. *Br J Radiol* 1942;15:1273-1279.

22. Gillespie JB, Siegling JA: Melorheostosis Leri. *Am J Dis Child* 1938;55:1273-1279.

23. Hall GS: A contribution to the study of melorheostosis: Unusual bone changes associated with tuberose sclerosis. *Q J Med* 1943;12:77-100.

24. Aarseth S: Melorheostosis: A case with biopsy. *Acta Med Scand* 1948;131:394-402.

25. Maroteaux P, Lamy M: La melorheostoses chez l'infant. *Ann Pediatr (Paris)* 1961;8:570-575.

26. Voorhoeve N: L'image radiologique non encore decrite d'une anomalie du squelette. *Acta Radiol* 1924;3:407-427.

27. Bass HN, Weiner JR, Goldman A, et al: Osteopathia striata syndrome. *Clin Pediatr (Phila)* 1980;19:369-373.

28. Hurt RL: Osteopathia striata-Voorhoeve's disease: Report of a case presenting the features of osteopathia striata and osteopetrosis. *J Bone Joint Surg Br* 1953;35:89-96.

29. Horan F, Beighton PH: Osteopathia striata with cranial sclerosis: An autosomal dominant entity. *Clin Genet* 1978;13:201-206.

30. Knockaert D, Dequeker J: Osteopathia striata and focal dermal hypoplasia. *Skeletal Radiol* 1979;4:223-227.

31. Goltz RW, Peterson WC, Gorlin RJ, Ravits HG: Focal dermal hypoplasia. *Arch Dermatol* 1962;86:708-717.

32. Cantatore FP, Carrozzo M, Lopefidon MC: Mixed sclerosing bone dystrophy with features resembling osteopoikilosis and osteopathia striata. *Clin Rheumatol* 1991;10:191-195.

33. Kransdorf MU, Meis JM: From the archives of the AFIP: Extraskeletal osseous and cartilaginous tumors of the extremities. *Radiographics* 1993;13:853-884.

34. Gunal I, Kiter E: Disorders associated with osteopoikilosis: 5 different lesions in a family. *Acta Orthop Scand* 2003;74:497-499.

35. Ben-Asher E, Zelzer E, Lancet D: LEMD3: The gene responsible for bone density disorders (osteopoikilosis). *Isr Med Assoc* 2005;7:273-274.

36. Hellemans J, Preobrzhenska O, Willaert A, et al: Loss-of-function mutations in LEMD3 result in osteopoikilosis, Buschke-Ollendorff syndrome and melorheostosis. *Nat Genet* 2004;36:1213-1218.

37. Hall CM: International nosology and classification of constitutional disorders of bone (2001). *Am J Med Genet* 2002;113:65-77.

38. Hellemans J, Debeer P, Wright M, et al: Germline LEMD3 mutations are rare in sporadic patients with isolated melorheostosis. *Hum Mutat* 2006;27:290.

39. Chigara M, Kato K, Mashio K, Shozaki T: Symmetry of bone lesions in osteopoikilosis: Report of 4 cases. *Acta Orthop Scand* 1991;62:495-496.

40. Happle R: Buschke-Ollendorf syndrome: Early, unilateral and pronounced involvement may be explained as type 2 segmental manifestation. *Eur J Dermatol* 2001;11:505.

41. Raque CJ, Wood MG: Connective-tissue nevus: Dermatofibrosis lenticularis disseminata with osteopoikilosis. *Arch Dermatol* 1970;102:390-396.

42. Schorr WF, Optiz JM, Reyes CN: The connective tissue nevus-osteopoikilosis syndrome. *Arch Dermatol* 1972;106:208-214.

43. Verbov K, Graham R: Buschke-Ollendorff syndrome: Disseminated dermatofibrosis with osteopoikilosis. *Clin Exp Dermatol* 1986;11:17-26.

44. Weisz GM: Lumbar spinal canal stenosis in osteopoikilosis. *Clin Orthop Relat Res* 1982;166:89-92.

45. Mindell ER, Northup CS, Douglass HO: Osteosarcoma associated with osteopoikilosis. *J Bone Joint Surg Am* 1978;60:406-408.

46. Ayling RM, Evans PEL: Giant cell tumor in a patient with osteopoikilosis. *Acta Orthop Scand* 1988;59:74-76.

47. Grimer RJ, Davies AM, Starkie CM, Sneath RS: Chondrosarcoma in a patient with osteopoikilosis: Apropos of a case. *Rev Chir Orthop Reparatrice Appar Mot* 1989;75:188-190.

48. Gay BB Jr, Elsas LJ, Wyly JB, Pasquiali M: Osteopathia striata with cranial sclerosis. *Pediatr Radiol* 1994;24:56-60.

49. Kornreich L, Grunebaum M, Ziv N, Shuper A, Mimouni M: Osteopathia striata, cranial sclerosis with cleft palate and facial nerve palsy. *Eur J Pediatr* 1988;147:101-103.

50. Paling MR, Hyde I, Dennis NR: Osteopathia striata with sclerosis and thickening of the skull. *Br J Radiol* 1981;54:344-348.

51. Rabinow M, Unger F: Syndrome of osteopathia striata, macrocephaly and cranial sclerosis. *Am J Dis Child* 1984;138:821-823.

52. Viot G, Lacombe D, David A, et al: Osteopathia striata cranial sclerosis: Non-random X-inactivation suggestive of X-linked dominant inheritance. *Am J Med Genet* 2002;107:1-4.

53. Ward LM, Rauch F, Travers R, et al: Osteopathia striata with cranial sclerosis: Clinical, radiological and bone histological findings in an adolescent girl. *Am J Med Genet A* 2004;129:8-12.

54. Whyte MP, Murphy WA: Osteopathia striata associated with familial dermopathy and white forelock: Evidence for postnatal development of osteopathia striata. *Am J Med Genet* 1980;5:227-234.

55. Winter RM, Crawfurd MD'A, Meire HB, Mitchell N: Osteopathia striata with cranial sclerosis: Highly variable expression within a family including cleft palate in two neonatal cases. *Clin Genet* 1980;18:462-474.

56. Pellegrino JE, McDonald-McGinn DM, Schneider A, Markowitz RI, Zackai EH: Further clinical delineation and increased morbidity in males with osteopathia striata with cranial sclerosis: An X-linked disorder? *Am J Med Gen* 1997;70:159-165.

57. Berenholz L, Lippy W, Harrell M: Conductive hearing loss in osteopathia striata-cranial sclerosis. *Otolaryngol Head Neck Surg* 2002;127:124-126.

58. Whyte MP, Murphy WA, Siegel BA: 99m-Tc-pyrophosphate bone imaging in osteopoikilosis, osteopathia striata and melorheostosis. *Radiology* 1978;127:439-443.

59. Freyschmidt J: Melorheostosis: A review of 23 cases. *Eur Radiol* 2001;11:474-479.

60. Greenspan A, Azouz EM: Bone dysplasia series: Melorheostosis: Review and update. *Can Assoc Radiol J* 1999;50:324-330.

61. Ameen S, Nagy L, Gerich U, Anderson SE: Melorheostosis of the hand with complicating bony spur formation and bursal inflammation:

Diagnosis and treatment. *Skeletal Radiol* 2002;31:467-470.

62. Campbell CS: Melorheostosis of the upper limb: Report of a case. *J Bone Joint Surg Br* 1955;37:471-473.

63. Caudle RJ, Stern PJ: Melorheostosis of the hand: A case report with long-term follow-up. *J Bone Joint Surg* 1987;69:1229-1231.

64. Ethunandan M, Khosla N, Tilley E, Webb A: Melorheostosis involving the craniofacial skeleton. *J Craniofac Surg* 2004;15:1062-1065.

65. Garver P, Resnick D, Hahighi P, Guerra J: Melorheostosis of the axial skeleton with associated fibrolipomatous lesions. *Skeletal Radiol* 1982;9:41-44.

66. Ippolito V, Mirra JM, Motta C, et al: Case report 771: Melorheostosis in association with desmoid tumor. *Skeletal Radiol* 1993;22:284-288.

67. Endo H, Katsumi A, Kuroda K, et al: Increased procollagen alpha 1(I) mRNA expression by dermal fibroblasts melorheostosis. *Br J Dermatol* 2003;148:799-803.

68. Happle R: Melorheostosis may originate as a type 2 segmental manifestation of osteopoikilosis. *Am J Med Genet A* 2004;125:221-223.

69. Rozencwaig R, Wilson MR, Mc Farland GJ: Melorheostosis. *Am J Orthop* 1997;26:83-89.

70. Applebaum RE, Camono DA, Sun CC, Azizkhan RA, Queral LA: Synchronous left subclavian and axillary artery aneurysms associated with melorheostosis. *Surgery* 1986;99:249-253.

71. Miyachi Y, Horio T, Yamada A, Ueo T: Linear melorheostotic scleroderma with hypertrichosis. *Arch Dermatol* 1979;115:1233-1234.

72. Murray RO, McCredie J: Melorheostosis and sclerotomes: A radiologic correlation. *Skeletal Radiol* 1979;4:57-71.

73. Wagers LT, Young AW Jr, Ryan SF: Linear melorheostotic scleroderma. *Br J Dermatol* 1972;86:297-301

74. Morris JM, Samilson RI, Corley CL: Melorheostosis: Review of the literature and report of an interesting case with nineteen year follow-up. *J Bone Joint Surg Am* 1963;45:1191-1206.

75. Judkiewicz AM, Murphey MD, Resnik CS, et al: Advanced imaging of melorheostosis with emphasis on MRI. *Skelet Radiol* 2001;30:447-453.

76. Williams JW, Monoghan D, Barrington NA: Cranio-facial melorheostosis: Case report and review of the literature. *Br J Radiol* 1991;64:60-62.

77. Bostman OM, Holmstrom T, Riska EB: Osteosarcoma in a melorheostotic femur. *J Bone Joint Surg Am* 1987;69:1232-1237.

78. Brennan DD, Bruzzi JF, Thakore H, O'Keane JC, Eustace S: Osteosarcoma arising in a femur with melorheostosis and osteopathia striata. *Skeletal Radiol* 2002;31:471-474.

79. Donath J, Poor G, Kiss C, Fornet B, Genant H: Atypical form of active melorheostosis and its treatment with bisphosphonate. *Skeletal Radiol* 2002;31:709-713.

80. Abrahamson MN: Disseminated asymptomatic osteosclerosis with features resembling melorheostosis, osteopoikilosis and osteopathia striata: Case report. *J Bone Joint Surg Am* 1968;50:991-996.

81. Green AE Jr, Ellwood WH, Collins JR: Melorheostosis and osteopoikilosis: With a review of the literature. *Am J Roentgenol Radium Ther Nucl Med* 1962;87:1096-1111.

82. Butkus CE, Michels VV, Lindor NM, Cooney WP III: Melorheostosis in a patient with familial osteopoikilosis. *Am J Med Genet* 1997;72:43-46.

83. Nevin NC, Thomas PS, Davis RI, Cowie GH: Melorheostosis in a family with autosomal dominant osteopoikilosis. *Am J Med Genet* 1999;82:409-414.

84. Debeer P, Pykels E, Lammens J, et al: Melorheostosis in a family with autosomal dominant osteopoikilosis: Report of a third family. *Am J Med Genet A* 2003;119:188-193.

Chapter 25

Nail-Patella Syndrome: Hereditary Onycho-osteodysplasia

Nail-patella syndrome is a rare autosomal dominant hereditary disorder that was first described in the 19th century. Its characteristics are unusual in that four sites are principally affected. The fingernails and, less commonly, toenails show marked structural changes; the patellae are small, dislocated, or sometimes absent; the proximal radial heads are absent or dislocated; and bony growths on the iliac wings known as "horns" are characteristic and virtually diagnostic. The patients have normal intelligence, are often thin with poor musculature, and have some irregular facial features. They may have several other areas of involvement, the most threatening of which is renal failure; in addition, eye abnormalities are commonly observed. The genetic error has been well defined, but thus far there have been no methods of treatment for patients with the problem other than care for specific orthopaedic, renal, or ocular abnormalities.

Terminology and History

Nail-patella syndrome has many other names. These include onycho-osteodysplasia, iliac horn disease, Fong disease, Turner syndrome, Turner-Kieser syndrome, Österreicher-Fong syndrome, and Trauner-Rieger syndrome.

Historically, according to a report by Wolfgang Roeckerath,[1] a case of nail- patella syndrome was described by Chatelain in 1820. In 1897, Little[2] described several patients with absent or delayed development of the patellae. In 1925, Trauner and Rieger[3] reported on six members of one family over four generations with radial subluxations and anomalies of the fingernails. In 1929, Österreicher[4] described several patients with strange fingernails and skeletal anomalies. In the 1930s, Turner,[5] Lester,[6] and Kieser[7] described in great detail familial dyschondroplasia associated with anonychia and other deformities.

It was Fong,[8] however, who in 1946 described the "iliac horns" that are virtually diagnostic for nail-patella syndrome and rarely occur in any other anomaly. In the 2 decades following Fong's report, several authors from various countries described in great detail the clinical findings, radiographic imaging, and familial frequency of nail-patella syndrome.[9-16]

Genetic Causation

A number of clinical studies have determined that nail-patella syndrome is familial and is transmitted as an autosomal dominant trait with a high degree of penetrance but variable expression.[17-20] The chromosomal location for the error has been identified as the long arm of chromosome 9 (9q34.1),[19,21] and the disorder appears to be caused by mutations in transcription factor LMX1B.[19,20,22-27] LMX1B is a member of the LIM-homeodomain family of transcription factors that are involved in body-pattern formation during development, including dorsoventral patterning of the limb, differentiation of some neurons, patterning of the skull, and normal development of the kidneys and eyes. The locus for nail-patella syndrome is linked to the locus for the alpha-1 chain of type IV collagen.[26] There are at least 18 mutational modifications of the LMX1B factor that affect the hand and fingernail appearances, osseous alignment and structure, the kidneys, the eyes, some forms of collagen, and the general body habitus.[19,24,25,27-31]

Clinical Presentation

Nail-patella syndrome has a variable clinical pattern; for some patients, it is clearly present at birth, while for others the findings are much delayed and may in fact not be

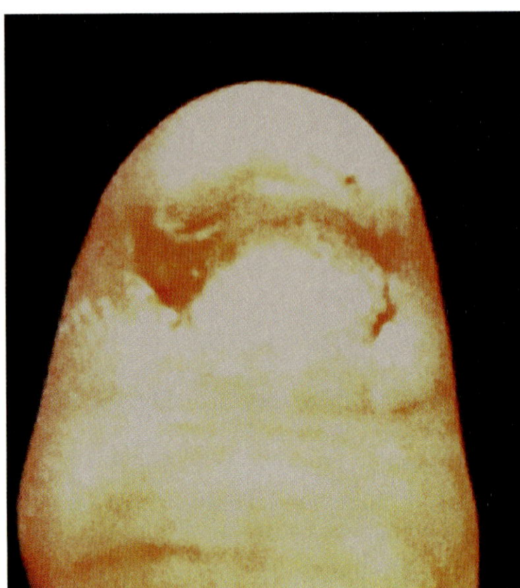

Figure 1
Classic appearance of the nail in a child with nail-patella syndrome. There is only a small amount of nail present, it is irregular in structure, and the color is usually yellow or light brown.

hypoplastic, or dystrophic[14,15,17,20,34-37] (Figure 1). They are sometimes ridged longitudinally or horizontally, pitted, or even separated into two halves by a cleft or a ridge of skin. The thumbnails are the most severely affected. The changes may show as triangular lunules. As a rule, the changes in the toenails are less marked. The skin over the distal phalanges shows a loss of creases, particularly over the index fingers.[14,15,35,36] The hand may show a diminished capacity for flexion or hyperextension of the joints, which may produce a characteristic swan-neck deformity and a mild functional impairment.[20]

Patellar abnormalities are one of the key features of the disorder. The patellae may be absent or very small and laterally displaced[17,18,20,38,39] (Figure 2). The result is a knock-knee deformity and sometimes limitation of movement and osteoarthritic changes with advancing age. Patients report instability and occasionally dislocation or locking of the small patellae.[18,38] Elbow involvement, like the knee, may be asymmetric. There may be limitation of motion, especially flexion, pronation, and supination.[18,20,37,40,41] On radiographs, the radial head may be very small or even absent and the humeral-ulnar joint distorted and osteoarthritic. Foot deformities are often present as well, most often representing varus or equinus position. Pes planus is quite common.[19]

The most striking feature of the disorder is the presence of iliac horns. These are bilateral conical bony processes that project posteriorly and laterally from the center of the ilium[16,42-44] (Figure 3). They are often palpable on physical examination and can even be diagnosed in the third trimester of fetal life using ultrasound.[45,46] The presence of iliac horns is considered pathognomonic for nail-patella syndrome.[19,44] A recent report described horns arising from the clavicle.[47]

Additional skeletal involvement includes lumbar lordosis, scoliosis, and pectus excavatum.[19] Back pain develops in many older patients. Coxa valga may be a problem, and in early childhood hip dislocations can occur.[48]

noted for most of the patient's life.[12,17-20,32] Because it is autosomal dominant in occurrence, the disease may be identified in an asymptomatic patient based on the presence of the disorder in relatives.[17,19,20,32] The disease is rarely encountered and appears to occur in fewer than 1 in 50,000 births.[20] There is no gender or ethnic preference; in some cases, the disease may be evident at birth, while in others not until the patient is 50 years of age or older.[17,18,20,32] Patients with nail-patella syndrome usually have normal intelligence.[19]

Patients with nail-patella syndrome most frequently have a lean body habitus and have difficulty putting on weight despite increased dietary intake.[19,20] In many patients, there is a fairly marked decrease in muscle mass in the proximal upper and lower extremities. The biceps, triceps, quadriceps, and gluteal muscles may be markedly diminished in size, while the forearm and leg musculature appears normal.[13,18,19,32,33] Lumbar lordosis is frequently present. The forehead is high and the hairline appears to be receding, even in young children or women.[19] Occasionally, an affected child is bald for several years after infancy.[20]

One of the most striking characteristics of the disease is the nails, which may be absent,

Renal involvement is the most serious consequence of nail-patella syndrome and virtually the only cause of death.[19,41,49,50] Proteinuria and hematuria may be the first

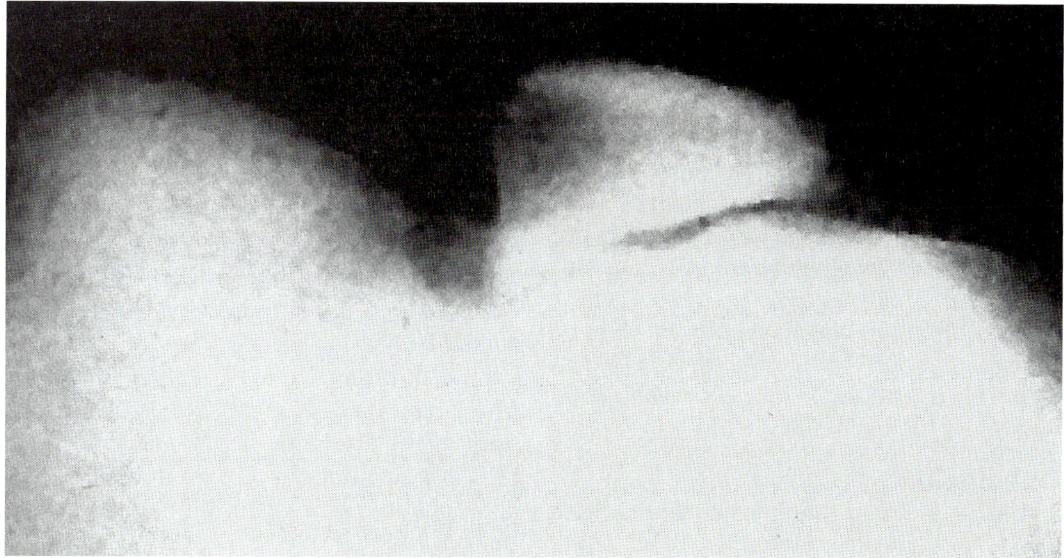

Figure 2
Anteroposterior view of the knee joint, demonstrating that only about half the patella is present and it is displaced laterally.

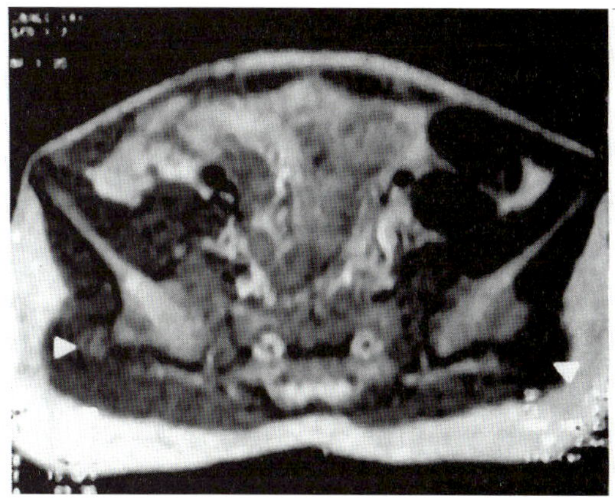

Figure 3
Iliac horns are evident in this imaging study. They are located in the lateral aspect of the upper portion of the ilium and project sufficiently to be palpable.

findings, and some patients subsequently progress to nephritic syndrome, nephritis, and renal failure.[19,40,50]

Ophthalmic changes occur in many patients. Glaucoma may be a major finding, but is present in only 10% of patients.[51-53] Almost all patients are likely to demonstrate an unusual finding, Lester's sign, which consists of a cloverleaf-like darker pigmentation around the central part of the iris.[54] Patients with this finding are asymptomatic, and the sign may be present in normal individuals and those with other disorders as well.[19,54]

Occasionally, patients with nail-patella syndrome present with gastrointestinal complaints or some neurologic disorders. The latter usually present as numbness and tingling in the hands and feet related to the nail and bone structural problems.[19] Sometimes patients may present with hearing loss.[55]

Imaging studies are helpful principally in identifying the iliac horns, which are virtually diagnostic for the disease.[43,56] The patellar size and placement are also of value, as few other diseases include absent or displaced small patellae as a characteristic. Dislocation and deformity of the radial head is also helpful in defining the extent of the patient's functional difficulties. Histologic studies are of limited value because there are no diagnostic findings.[10,19,20] Genetic studies may provide information regarding the syndrome and possibly may be of value in identifying familial issues.[19]

Treatment

Currently, there is no treatment that can alter the course of the disease. The patients must be carefully studied as soon as the diagnosis is made to assess the extent of the orthopaedic problems. Correction of displaced patellae is sometimes helpful as is corrective muscle surgery for absent radial heads or patellae.[38,39,57] Corrective realignment of femora, tibiae, and forearms may be necessary to help improve function and prevent arthritic changes in the joints or fractures of the bones.[20,48] Most often, the iliac horns are asymptomatic and there is little reason to resect them. The principal concerns that physicians should have for these patients regard renal function and glaucoma. Laboratory studies should be done regularly, seeking evidence for nephritic problems, and ocular studies for glaucoma are important. The renal problems can be treated effectively with renal transplant surgery. Genetic therapy has not been employed, nor has stem cell treatment or marrow transplantation.

Conclusion

Nail-patella syndrome is a rare entity with some very unusual features. It can affect anyone in the world and has no ethnic or gender selectivity. It is characterized by thin body structure, proximal limb muscle atrophy, markedly abnormal fingernails, small displaced or absent patellae and radial heads, and horns growing in the ilium. Aside from orthopaedic disorders, renal failure and glaucoma are the only real problems for patients. The remarkable genetic findings are quite striking and now thoroughly understood. They quite clearly identify the cause for this disorder, but may be related to other problems as well. Unfortunately, the knowledge of the causation and some quite spectacular animal research have not yielded an approach to treating children or adults with the syndrome.

References

1. Roeckerath W: Hereditaire osteo-onycho-dysplasie. *Fortschr Geb Röntgenstr* 1951;75:700-712.

2. Little EM: Congenital absence or delayed development of the patella. *Lancet* 1897;2:781-784.

3. Trauner R, Rieger H: Eine familie mit 6 fällen von luxation radii congenita mit übereinstimmenden anomalien der finger-und kniegelenke sowie der nagelbildung in 4 generationen. *Arch Klin Chir* 1925;137:659-666.

4. Österreicher W: Nägel und skelettanomalien. *Wien Klin Wschr* 1929;43:632.

5. Turner JW: A hereditary arthrodysplasia associated with hereditary dystrophy of nails. *JAMA* 1933;100:882-884.

6. Lester AM: A familial dyschondroplasia associated with anonychia and other deformities. *Lancet* 1936;2:1519-1521.

7. Kieser W: Die sogennante flughaut beim menschen ihre beziehung zum status dysraphicus und ihre erblichkeit (darustellung an der Sippe Fr). *Zschr Menschl Vererb Konstit* 1939;32:594-619.

8. Fong EE: "Iliac horns" (symmetrical bilateral central posterior iliac processes). *Radiology* 1946;47:517-518.

9. Beals RK, Eckhardt AL: Hereditary onycho-osteodysplasia (nail-patella syndrome): A report of nine kindreds. *J Bone Joint Surg Am* 1969;51:505-516.

10. Darlington D, Hawkins CF: Nail-patella syndrome with iliac horns and hereditary nephropathy: Necropsy report and anatomical dissection. *J Bone Joint Surg Br* 1967;49:164-174.

11. Duncan JG, Souter WA: Hereditary onycho-osteodysplasia: The nail-patella syndrome. *J Bone Joint Surg Br* 1963;45:242-258.

12. Duthie RB, Hecht F: The inheritance and development of the nail-patella syndrome. *J Bone Joint Surg Br* 1963;45:259-267.

13. Love WH, Beiler DD: Osteo-onychodysplasia. *J Bone Joint Surg Am* 1957;39:645-650.

14. Maini PS, Mittal RL: Hereditary onycho-osteo-arthrodysplasia. *J Bone Joint Surg Am* 1966;48:924-930.

15. Mino RA, Mino VH, Livingstone RG: Osseous dysplasia and dystrophy of the nails: Review of the literature and report of a case. *Am J Roentgenol Radium Ther* 1948;60:633-641.

16. Thompson EA, Walker ET, Weens HS: Iliac horns: An osseous manifestation of hereditary arthrodysplasia associated with dystrophy of the fingernails. *Radiology* 1949;53:88-92.

17. Bongers EM, Gubler MC, Knoers NV: Nail-patella syndrome: Overview on clinical and molecular findings. *Pediatr Nephrol* 2002;17:703-712.

18. Guidera KJ, Satterwhite Y, Ogden JA, Pugh L, Ganey T: Nail patella syndrome: A review of 44 orthopaedic patients. *J Pediatr Orthop* 1991;11:737-742.

19. Sweeney E, Fryer A, Mountford R, Green A, McIntosh I: Nail patella syndrome: A review of the phenotype aided by developmental biology. *J Med Genet* 2003;40:153-162.

20. Towers AL, Clay CA, Sereika SM, McIntosh I, Greenspan SL: Skeletal integrity in patients with nail patella syndrome. *J Clin Endocrinol Metab* 2005;90:1961-1965.

21. McIntosh I, Clough MV, Schäffer AA, et al: Fine mapping of the nail-patella syndrome locus at 9q34. *Am J Hum Genet* 1997;60:133-142.

22. Bongers EM, Huysmans FT, Levtchenko E, et al: Genotype-phenotype studies in nail-patella syndrome show that LMX1B mutation location is involved in the risk of developing nephropathy. *Eur J Hum Genet* 2005;13:935-946.

23. Bongers EM, van Kampen A, van Bokhoven H, Knoers NV: Human syndromes with congenital patellar anomalies and the underlying gene defects. *Clin Genet* 2005;68:302-319.

24. Dreyer SD, Morello R, German MS, et al: LMX1B transactivation and expression in nail-patella syndrome. *Hum Mol Genet* 2000;9:1067-1074.

25. Dreyer SD, Zhou G, Baldini A, et al: Mutations in LMX1B cause abnormal skeletal patterning and

renal dysplasia in nail patella syndrome. *Nat Genet* 1998;19:47-50.

26. Morello R, Zhou G, Dreyer SD, et al: Regulation of glomerular basement membrane collagen expression by LMX1B contributes to renal disease in nail patella syndrome. *Nat Genet* 2001;27:205-208.

27. Sato U, Kitanaka S, Sekine T, Takahashi S, Ashida A, Igarashi T: Functional characterization of LMX1B mutations associated with nail-patella syndrome. *Pediatr Res* 2005;57:783-788.

28. Dunston JA, Hamlington JD, Zaveri J, et al: The human LMX1B gene: Transcription unit, promoter and pathogenic mutations. *Genomics* 2004;84:565-576.

29. Dunston JA, Lin S, Park JW, Malbroux M, McIntosh I: Phenotype severity and genetic variation at the disease locus: An investigation of nail dysplasia in the nail patella syndrome. *Ann Hum Genet* 2005;69:1-8.

30. Hamlington JD, Jones C, McIntosh I: Twenty-two novel LMX1B mutations identified in nail patella syndrome (NPS) patients. *Hum Mutat* 2001;18:458.

31. Knoers NV, Bongers RN, van Beersum SE, Lommen EJ, van Bokhoven H, Hol FA: Nail-patella syndrome: Identification of mutations in LMX1B gene in Dutch families. *J Am Soc Nephrol* 2000;11:1762-1766.

32. Beguiristáin JL, de Rada PD, Barriga A: Nail-patella syndrome: Long term evolution. *J Pediatr Orthop B* 2003;12:13-16.

33. Burkhart CG, Bhumbra R, Iannone AM: Nail-patella syndrome: A distinctive clinical and electron microscopic presentation. *J Am Acad Dermatol* 1980;3:251-256.

34. Itin PH, Eich G, Fistarol SK: Missing creases of distal finger joints as a diagnostic clue of nail-patella syndrome. *Dermatology* 2006;213:153-155.

35. Ogden JA, Cross GL, Guidera KJ, Ganey TM: Nail patella syndrome: A 55 year follow-up of the original description. *J Pediatr Orthop B* 2002;11:333-338.

36. Schulz-Butulis BA, Welch MD, Norton SA: Nail-patella syndrome. *J Am Acad Dermatol* 2003;49:1086-1087.

37. Seitz CS, Hamm H: Congenital brachydactyly and nail hypoplasia: Clue to bone-dependent nail formation. *Br J Dermatol* 2005;152:1339-1342.

38. Doughty KS, Richmond JC: Arthroscopic findings in the knee in nail-patella syndrome: A case report. *Arthroscopy* 2005;21:e1-e5.

39. Mavrodontidis AN, Zalavras CG, Papadonikolakis A, Soucacos PN: Bilateral absence of the patella in nail-patella syndrome: Delayed presentation with anterior knee instability. *Arthroscopy* 2004;20:e89-e93.

40. Lee JJ, Chiu YW, Kuo YT, Chen HC, Hwang SJ: Nail-patella syndrome with renal involvement and antecubital pterygia. *J Formos Med Assoc* 2002;101:655-660.

41. Rizzo R, Pavone L, Micali G, Hall JG: Familial bilateral antecubital pterygia with severe renal involvement in nail-patella syndrome. *Clin Genet* 1993;44:1-7.

42. Goshen E, Schwartz A, Zilka LR, Zwan ST: Bilateral accessory iliac horns: Pathognomonic findings in Nail-Patella syndrome. Scintigraphic evidence on bone scan. *Clin Nucl Med* 2000;25:476-477.

43. Karabulut N, Aryurek M, Erol C, Tacal T, Balkanci F: Imaging of "iliac horns" in nail-patella syndrome. *J Comput Assist Tomogr* 1996;20:530-531.

44. Sartoris DJ, Reznick D: The horn: A pathognomonic feature of paediatric bone dysplasias. *Aus Paediatr J* 1987;23:347-349.

45. McIntosh I, Clough MV, Gak E, Frydman M: Prenatal diagnosis of nail-patella syndrome. *Prenat Diagn* 1999;19:287-288.

46. Pinette MG, Ukleja M, Blackstone J: Early prenatal diagnosis of nail-patella syndrome by ultrasonography. *J Ultrasound Med* 1999;18:387-389.

47. Yarali HN, Erden GA, Karaalarsen F, Bilgiç SC, Cumhur T: Clavicular horn: Another bony projection in nail-patella syndrome. *Pediatr Radiol* 1995;29:549-550.

48. Jacofsky DJ, Stans AA, Lindor NM: Bilateral hip dislocation and pubic diastasis in familial nail-patella syndrome. *Orthopedics* 2003;26:329-330.

49. Bennett WM, Musgrave JE, Campbell RA, et al: The nephropathy of the nail-patella syndrome: Clinicopathologic analysis of 11 kindred. *Am J Med* 1973;54:304-319.

50. Gao X, Miyai T, Tahara T, et al: IgA nephropathy associated with nail-patella syndrome in a 7-year-old girl. *Pediatr Int* 2001;43:434-436.

51. Lichter PR, Richards JE, Downs CA, Stringham HM, Boehnke M, Farley FA: Cosegregation of open-angle glaucoma and the nail-patella syndrome. *Am J Ophthalmol* 1997;124:506-515.

52. Mimiwati Z, Mackey DA, Craig JE, et al: Nail-patella syndrome and its association with glaucoma: A review of eight families. *Br J Ophthalmol* 2006;90:1505-1509.

53. Millá E, Hernan I, Gamundi MJ, Martínez-Gimeno M, Carballo M: Novel LMX1B mutation in familial nail-patella syndrome with variable expression of open angle glaucoma. *Mol Vis* 2007;13:639-648.

54. Flickinger RR, Spivey BE: Lester's line in hereditary osteo-onychodysplasia. *Arch Ophthalmol* 1969;82:700-703.

55. Hussain SS, Hope GA: Sensorineural hearing loss and nail patella syndrome. *Arch Otolaryngol Head Neck Surg* 1994;120:674-675.

56. Tuncbilek N, Karakas HM, Okten OO: Imaging of nail-patella syndrome. *Hong Kong Med J* 2005;11:116-118.

57. Marumo K, Fujii K, Tanaka T, Takeuchi H, Saito H, Koyano Y: Surgical management of congenital permanent dislocation of the patella in nail patella syndrome by Stanisavljevic procedure. *J Orthop Sci* 1999;4:466-469.

Chapter 26

Kniest Dysplasia

Kniest dysplasia is a rare disorder that was first described by Wilhelm Kniest in 1952, while he was a chief resident at the Children's Hospital at the University of Jena in Thuringia, Germany. The disorder consists of a chondrodysplasia caused by an autosomal dominant genetic error in the synthesis of type II collagen. The findings are present at birth and consist of short trunk dwarfism, platyspondyly, small iliac bones, short and often bowed extremity bones, flat feet, and deformed hands. Facial abnormalities, auditory problems, and visual disturbances are commonly seen and sometimes have serious consequences. The patients have normal intelligence and for the most part have a normal life span.

Terminology and History

Kniest dysplasia is also known as metatropic dwarfism type II, metatropic dysplasia type II, pseudometatropic dwarfism, Kniest syndrome, Kniest chondrodystrophy, and Swiss cheese cartilage syndrome.

Kniest dysplasia was first described by Wilhelm Kniest[1] in 1952, when he was a resident in pediatrics at the University of Jena in Germany. His original patient was a 3.5-year-old girl with "skeletal changes showing a certain relationship to classical chondrodystrophy but differing in many of its manifestations." The child had short stature involving the trunk and extremities, marked joint contractures, and moderate kyphoscoliosis. She became blind and had hearing loss, but was of normal intelligence and lived a full life despite her disabilities.[2] Patients with similar findings were reported by Roaf and associates[3] in 1967, Larose and Gay in 1969,[4] and Maroteaux and Spranger in 1973.[5] Lachman and associates[6] added cases with special emphasis on the radiologic aspects in 1975, and in the same year, Brill and associates[7] further defined the imaging aspects and on that basis tried to establish the pathologic changes. Kniest extended his observations with two descriptive articles in 1977 and 1979.[8,9] In 1976, Rimoin and associates[10] described the bone and joint abnormalities in a detailed and well-illustrated publication in *Clinical Orthopaedics and Related Research*. In addition, Horton and Rimoin[11] described the histologic features of both bone and cartilage in 1979. In the same year, Frayha and associates[12] introduced the term "Swiss cheese cartilage" as a characteristic of Kniest dysplasia. David Rimoin has over the years become greatly involved in descriptions of the syndrome and especially the radiologic, histologic, and ultrastructural findings, and he still remains an active contributor.[10,13,14]

Physiology, Biology, and Genetics

Kniest dysplasia is clearly an autosomal dominant genetic error that for the most part is equally divided among males and females, except for a small number of male patients who seem to have an X-linked gene error.[13-17] There is no known ethnic preponderance.[14] The gene error principally affects the synthesis and maintenance of type II collagen and, far less commonly, type XI collagen.[15,18-23] As is well known, type I collagen is present in skin and bone, but type II is principally located in articular and epiphyseal cartilage.[14] The effect of damage to these structures is principally in bone formation in the fetus or infant and results in the changes in the shape and structure of long bones, small bones of the hands and feet, ribs, and especially the spine.[7,13,14,16,24] Growth is slowed, and the cartilage-forming structures are deformed as a result of the Swiss cheese cartilage changes and substitution by other forms of cartilage.[11,12,14,15,19,21,25]

The mechanism by which the cartilage is altered has been thoroughly studied. Mutations in the gene that encodes type II collagen (COL2A1) have recently been identified.[14,18-21,26] At least nine mutations have been described in patients with Kniest dysplasia, two of which are missense.[14,20,27-29] All of these are located between exons 12 and 24 in the COL2A1 gene.[20,26-30] Six different arginine and cys-

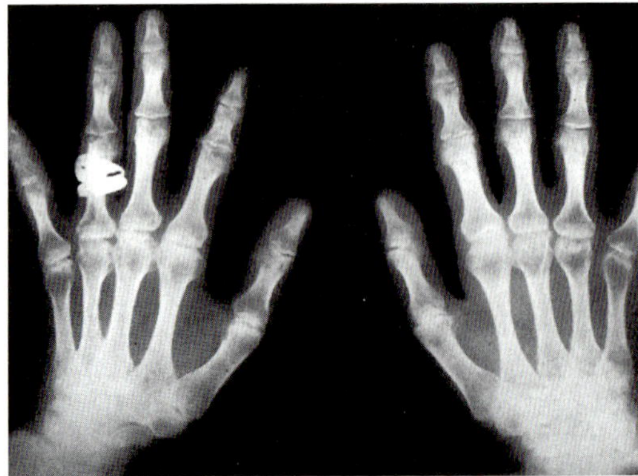

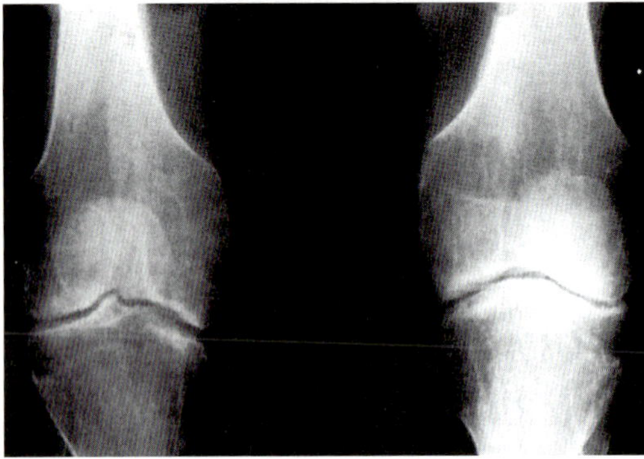

Figure 1

Radiographs of the hands and knees of an adult with Kniest syndrome. There is marked splaying of the long bone metaphyses, "dumbbell morphology" and loss of normal trabecular bone pattern, and mild osteoporosis. Narrowing of the joint space is noted in the knees.

teine mutations (occurring at R75C, R365C, R519C, R704C, R789C, R1076C) are located in 11 unrelated probands.[14,23,28,30,31] R365C and R789C are also found in the Stickler dysplasia and spondyloepiphyseal dysplasia congenita syndrome.[32-34] Type XI collagen is a minor component of cartilage but peculiar changes, including ocular abnormalities, occur with mutations in this gene in both the Kniest and Stickler dysplasias.[22,30]

Clinical, Histologic, and Imaging Findings

The clinical appearance of Kniest dysplasia is somewhat confusing, chiefly because there are several other syndromes that closely resemble it. The closest in comparison is Stickler dysplasia,[14,32,35] which is also present at birth but has far less dwarfism or extremity shortening, yet more spinal abnormalities and problems with facial structure, vision, and hearing. The other source of confusion is that the Stickler dysplasia is also caused by mutational errors in either the COL2A1 or COL11A1 genes, with some similarities to the Kniest errors.[22,23,30,32]

Despite the resemblance to other syndromes, Kniest dysplasia has some characteristic features that make it possible to diagnose without confusion. The diagnostic clinical features for Kniest dysplasia include the following:

- Disproportionate dwarfism (the limbs are more severely affected than the trunk)[14,24,33]
- Kyphoscoliosis and lumbar lordosis, sometimes severe[6,10,13,33]
- Short and bell-shaped thorax[10,13,14]
- Flat facies, prominent forehead, and wide-set eyes[13,14,36]
- Cleft palate, otitis media, and hearing loss[14]
- Proptosis and severe myopia, which can lead to retinal detachment[2,37,38]
- Early cataract development[2,37,38]
- Short and bowed long bones, with moderately enlarged joints[10,14]
- Hip flexion contractures and limitation of motion in knees, elbows, and shoulders[10,14]
- Long knobby fingers, which make it difficult for the patient to form a fist[4]
- Limitation of movement of feet and ankles, with occasional clubfoot deformity.[10,13,14]

Stickler dysplasia is the closest in terms of similarity of genetic problems, but most of those patients are taller and actually sometimes resemble patients with Marfan's disease. They have limited skeletal changes, but often fairly severe oral and ocular problems.[32,35]

Imaging of patients with Kniest dysplasia shows the following features[17,36,39-42]:

- Splaying of the long bone metaphyses and "dumbbell morphology" (Figure 1)
- Irregular punctate epiphyses
- Fluffiness and irregularity of growth plates (Figure 2).
- Loss of normal trabecular bone pattern with mild osteoporosis (Figure 1)
- Flattened and squared-off epiphyses of tubular bones of hands and feet (Figure 2)
- Narrowing of joint spaces
- Trefoil-shaped pelvis with marked coxa vara (Figure 3)

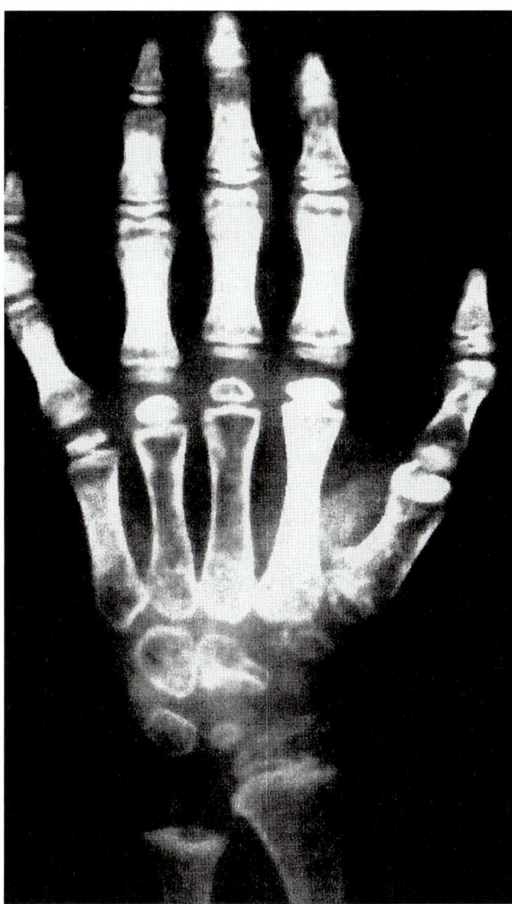

Figure 2
Radiograph of the hand of a child with Kniest syndrome showing irregular punctate epiphyses and fluffiness and irregularity of growth plates.

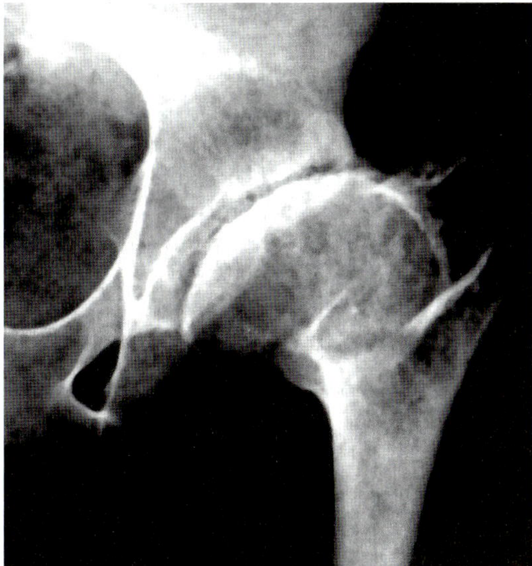

Figure 3
Radiographs of the hips and pelvis show narrowing of the joint space and a trefoil-shaped hemipelvis with coxa vara.

- Sometimes severe platyspondyly
- Radial head dislocations

Histologic changes show abnormal structure in cartilaginous tissue described as Swiss cheese cartilage.[11,12,14,39,41] In addition, the collagen fibers are abnormal in structure and shape with irregularity of contour. Joints show an early osteoarthritic change. Medullary bone shows osteopenic changes.[14,39,41] Ocular changes suggest early retinal alterations and cataract formation.[36-38]

Treatment

Early cardiac or respiratory symptoms develop in some patients with Kniest dysplasia, and they may die before the age of 3 or 4 years.[43] These patients may require emergency therapy. Regrettably, there are no genetic or pharmacologic agents to treat patients with Kniest dysplasia. The majority of patients who survive may have serious and

significant problems with ocular function and orthopaedic difficulties. The ocular issues are difficult to treat. Treatment measures are usually not successful in preventing retinitis, cataracts, or blindness and may require drug therapy or surgery.[36-38] Orthopaedic bracing or surgical procedures are sometimes required for spinal disorders and hip, shoulder, or radial dislocations.[13-15,41] Early development of knee arthritis is common and may require treatment. The clubfoot deformity may require corrective surgery, including arthrodesis.[14,15]

Discussion

Kniest dysplasia is a strange clinical entity that is rarely encountered. Despite being an autosomal dominant genetic disorder (and occasionally X-linked), the disease is very infrequently encountered even in pediatric hospitals or institutions, in which patients with genetic disorders are most often seen. Most frequently, the children appear without a family history of Kniest dysplasia, so the disorder is seemingly an isolated occurrence. The striking feature is the genetic changes, which occur in the COL2A1 gene and damage articular and especially epiphyseal cartilage. This causes alterations in bone and joint structure, and problems with the spine and oral cavity. Patients often exhibit shortness of stature; have problems with hands, feet, and major joints; and may in fact become blind or deaf early in the course of the disease. They have normal intelligence and, if they do not have cardiovascular problems, can live a long life. Currently, surgery can help the bones and joints and sometimes the eyes, but full functional status really cannot be achieved. These children have short, bowed extremities and a damaged spine and fairly rapidly lose their sight. It would be very advantageous for physicians to collect sufficient patients and for scientists to develop ways to deal with the malformed collagen molecule so that these children can be treated effectively shortly after birth and be restored to a normal life.

References

1. Kniest W: Differential diagnosis between dysostosis enchondralis and chondrodystrophy. *Z Kinderheilkd* 1952;70:633-670.

2. Spranger J, Winterpacht A, Zabel B: Kniest dysplasia: Dr W. Kniest, his patient, the molecular defect. *Am J Med Genet* 1997;69:79-84.

3. Roaf R, Longmore JB, Forrester RM: A childhood syndrome of bone dysplasia, retinal detachment and deafness. *Dev Med Child Neurol* 1967;9:464-473.

4. Larose JH, Gay BB Jr: Metatropic dwarfism. *J Roentgenol Radium Ther Nucl Med* 1969;106:156-161.

5. Maroteaux P, Spranger J: Kniest's disease. *Arch Fr Pediatr* 1973;30:735-750.

6. Lachman RS, Rimoin DL, Hollister DW, et al: The Kniest syndrome. *Am J Roentgenol Radium Ther Nucl Med* 1975;123:805-814.

7. Brill PW, Kim HJ, Beratis NG, Hirschhorn K: Skeletal abnormalities in the Kniest syndrome with mucopolysacchariduria. *Am J Roentgenol Radium Ther Nucl Med* 1975;125:731-738.

8. Kniest W, Leiber B: Kniest syndrome (author's transl). *Monatsschr Kinderheilkd* 1977;125:970-973.

9. Kniest W: Das Kniest syndrome und seine differential diagnose. *Dt Gesundh Wesen* 1979;34:1317-1321.

10. Rimoin DL, Siggers DC, Lachman RS, Silberberg R: Metatropic dwarfism, the Kniest syndrome and the pseudoachondroplastic dysplasias. *Clin Orthop Relat Res* 1976;114:70-82.

11. Horton WA, Rimoin DL: Kniest dysplasia: A histochemical study of the growth plate. *Pediatr Res* 1979;13:1266-1270.

12. Frayha R, Melhem R, Idriss H: The Kniest (Swiss cheese cartilage) syndrome: Description of a distinct arthropathy. *Arthritis Rheum* 1979;22:286-289.

13. Rimoin DL, Hollister DW, Siggers DC, et al: Clinical, radiographic, histologic and ultrastructural definition of Kniest Syndrome. *Pediatr Res* 1979;13:1266-1270.

14. Rimoin DL, Lachman RS: Genetic disorders of the osseous skeleton: Kniest-Stickler dysplasia group, in Beighton P (ed): *McKusick's Heritable Disorders of Connective Tissue*, ed 5. St. Louis, MO, Mosby, 1993, pp 601-605.

15. Cole WG: Abnormal skeletal growth in Kniest dysplasia caused by type II collagen mutations. *Clin Orthop Relat Res* 1997;341:162-169.

16. Gilbert-Barnes E, Langer LO Jr, Opitz JM, Laxova R, Sotelo-Arila C: Kniest dysplasia: Radiologic, histopathological, and scanning electronmicroscopic findings. *Am J Med Genet* 1996;63:34-45.

17. Kim HJ, Beratis NG, Brill P, Raab E, Hirschhorn K, Matalon R: Kniest syndrome with dominant inheritance and mupolysacchariduria. *Am J Hum Genet* 1975;27:755-764.

18. Bogaert R, Wilkin D, Wilcox WR, et al: Expression, in cartilage, of a 7-amino-acid deletion in type II collagen from two unrelated individuals with Kniest dysplasia. *Am J Hum Genet* 1994;55:1128-1136.

19. Fernandes RJ, Wilkin DJ, Weis MA, et al: Incorporation of structurally defective type II collagen into cartilage matrix in kniest chondrodysplasia. *Arch Biochem Biophys* 1998;355:282-290.

20. Nishimura G, Haga N, Kitoh H, et al: The phenotypic spectrum of COL2A1 mutations. *Hum Mutat* 2005;26:36-43.

21. Poole AR, Pidoux I, Reiner A, et al: Kniest dysplasia is characterized by an apparent abnormal processing of the C-propeptide of type II cartilage resulting in imperfect fibril assembly. *J Clin Invest* 1988;81:579-589.

22. Spranger J: The type XI collagenopathies. *Pediatr Radiol* 1998;28:745-750.

23. Spranger J, Menger H, Mundlos S, Winterpacht A, Zabel B: Kniest dysplasia is caused by dominant collagen II (COL2A1) mutations: Parental somatic mosaicism manifesting as Stickler phenotype and mild spondyloepiphyseal dysplasia. *Pediatr Radiol* 1994;24:431-435.

24. Kozi S, Sestan B, Matovinovi D: Kniest dysplasia: Patient's growth progress and development— evolution of abnormalities, 30 year follow-up. *Acta Med Okayama* 1997;51:285-294.

25. Chan D, Cole WG, Chow CW, Mundlos S, Bateman JF: A COL2A1 in achondrogenesis type II results in the replacement of type II collagen by type I and III collagens in cartilage. *J Biol Chem* 1995;270:1747-1753.

26. Wilkin DJ, Artz AS, South S, et al: Small deletions in the type II collagen triple helix produce Kniest dysplasia. *Am J Med Genet* 1999;85:105-112.

27. Chen L, Yang W, Cole WG: Alternative splicing of exon 12 of the COL2A1 gene interrupts the triple helix of type–II collagen in the Kniest form of spondyloepiphyseal dysplasia. *J Orthop Res* 1996;14:712-721.

28. Weis MA, Wilkin DJ, Kim HJ, et al: Structurally abnormal type II collagen in a severe form of Kniest dysplasia caused by an exon 24 skipping mutation. *J Biol Chem* 1998;273:4761-4768.

29. Wilkin DJ, Bogaert R, Lachman RS, Rimoin DL, Eyre DR, Cohn DH: A single amino acid substitution (G103D) in the type II collagen triple helix

produces Kniest syndrome. *Hum Mol Genet* 1994;3:1999-2003.

30. Winterpacht A, Superti-Furga A, Schwarze U, et al: The deletion of six amino acids at the C-terminus of the alpha 1 (II) chain causes over-modification of type II and type XI collagen: Further evidence for the association between small deletions in COL2A1 and Kniest dysplasia. *J Med Genet* 1996;33:649-654.

31. Hoornaert KP, Dewinter C, Vereecke I, et al: The phenotypic spectrum in patients with arginine to cysteine mutations in the COL2A1 gene. *J Med Genet* 2006;43:406-413.

32. Liberfarb RM, Levy HP, Rose PS, et al: The Stickler syndrome: A genotype/phenotype correlation in 10 families with Stickler syndrome resulting from seven mutations in the type II collagen gene locus COL2A1. *Genet Med* 2003;5: 21-27.

33. Spranger J, Winterpacht A, Zabel B: The type II collagenopathies: A spectrum of chondrodysplasias. *Eur J Pediatr* 1994;153:56-65.

34. Winterpacht A, Hilbert M, Schwarze U, Mundlos S, Spranger J, Zabel BU: Kniest and Stickler dysplasia phenotypes caused by collagen type II gene (COL2A1) defect. *Nat Genet* 1993;3:323-326.

35. Stickler GB, Belau PG, Farrell FJ, et al: Hereditary progressive arthro-opthalmopathy. *Mayo Clin Proc* 1965;40:433-455.

36. Friede H, Matalon R, Harris V, Rosenthal IM: Craniofacial and mucopolysaccharide abnormalities in Kniest dysplasia. *J Craniofac Genet Dev Biol* 1985;5:267-276.

37. Chalam KV, Tripathi RC, Tripathi BJ, Shah VA, Yee D, Pakalnis VA: Cataract in Kniest dysplasia: Clincopathologic correlation. *Arch Ophthalmol* 2004;122:913-915.

38. Yokoyama T, Nakatani S, Murakami A: A case of Kniest dysplasia with retinal detachment and the mutation analysis. *Am J Ophthalmol* 2003;136:1186-1188.

39. Dwek JR: Kniest dysplasia: MR correlation of histologic and radiographic peculiarities. *Pediatr Radiol* 2005;35:191-193.

40. Maldjian C, Chew FS, Klein R, et al: Kniest dysplasia: New radiographic features in the skeleton. *Radiology Case Report* 2007;2:72-77.

41. Oestreich AE, Prenger EC: MR demonstrates cartilaginous megaepiphyses of the hips in Kniest dysplasia of the young child. *Pediatr Radiol* 1992;22:302-303.

42. Westvik J, Lachman RS: Coronal and sagittal clefts in skeletal dysplasias. *Pediatr Radiol* 1998;28:764-770.

43. Hicks J, De Jong A, Barrish J, Zhu SH, Popek E: Tracheomalacia in a neonate with kniest dysplasia: Histopathologic and ultrastructural features. *Ultrastruct Pathol* 2001;25:79-83.

Chapter 27

Mucopolysaccharidosis Type I

The term mucopolysaccharidosis (MPS), type I describes several types of rare disorders resulting from an autosomal recessive genetic error. The entity along with six other mucopolysaccharidoses, are broadly classified as lysosomal storage diseases and are caused by enzyme deficiencies that, in the case of patients with type I disease, result in a failure to degrade the glycosaminoglycans (GAGs) dermatan sulfate and heparan sulfate. The material necessary to destroy the two GAGs is alpha-L-iduronidase, and the failure to produce it appears to relate to a series of as many as 15 mutations that cause a decrease in the production of the enzyme. The presence of excessive amounts of the two GAGs cause neurologic, ocular, skeletal, pulmonary, and cardiac abnormalities that may, at least for one of the forms of the disease, be so severe as to be recognizable shortly after birth and can cause early death.

History

The first description of a patient with MPS was by William Osler[1] in 1897. In 1907, Berkhan[2] described a child with what subsequently became known as Hurler syndrome, and in 1917 Charles Hunter[3] presented a paper at the Royal Society of Medicine in which he described two brothers who were dwarfed and deformed and were subsequently known to have Hunter's disease or MPS type II. In 1919, Gertrud Hurler (1889-1965),[4] a pediatrician in Munich, described in great detail a child with marked skeletal deformity, mental retardation, cardiac disease, and corneal clouding. Based on her extensive description, the disease become known as Hurler syndrome or, more recently, as MPS type I–H.[5-7] In 1936, Richard Ellis and his associates[8] suggested the name gargoylism for MPS type I–H, but soon thereafter, mostly at the request of the patients' families, the term was abandoned.[9] Another term proposed by assessment of bone disease was "dysostosis multiplex congenita;" this was also abandoned.[7,10,11] In 1936, Fratantoni and associates[12] identified the material that accumulated in the tissues in Hurler and Hunter syndromes as GAGs. Other contributors to the descriptions and definitions of the various syndromes included Luis Morquio[13] and James Brailsford,[14] both of whom in 1929 independently described a disorder that has now become known as Morquio-Brailsford syndrome or MPS type IV.[7,11] In 1963, Sylvester Sanfilippo[15] described another syndrome, which became known as MPS type III,[7,11] and in 1965, Pierre Maroteaux and Maurice Lamy[16] described yet another disorder, which was classified as MPS type VI.[7,11] In 1973, Sly and associates[17] described a new MPS that was labeled MPS type VII.[7,11] One of the key contributors to the syndrome of MPS type I, however, was an ophthalmologist, Harold Scheie (1909-1990),[18] who, with his associates, described patients with a mild form of MPS who have a normal or near-normal intellect but some facial and skeletal changes and progressive corneal clouding. Initially, this syndrome was known as Scheie's disease and was defined as MPS type V;[7,11] however, because the genetic enzyme defect for Scheie's disease was found to be identical to that of Hurler syndrome, the nomenclature was changed and MPS type V became known as type I–S (or type I mild), to be distinguished from type I–H (or type I severe).[5-7,11,19-23] Today, there are three forms of MPS type I: H (severe disease), S (mild disease), and HS (intermediate disease). All have similar genetic errors but different degrees of enzymatic deficit, which produces the three syndromes differing in extent and severity of the resultant disease and the outcome.[5-7,11,19-22]

Genetic Error, Histology, and Biologic Problems

All of the MPS type I disorders are rare, with possibly as few as 1,000 current patients in the United States.[7,24] The disorders are distinctly autosomal recessive in transmission, with only occasional spontaneous mutations. Several sources have suggested that the genetic errors for all three forms of MPS I are located on the 4p16.3 gene.[7,11] Af-

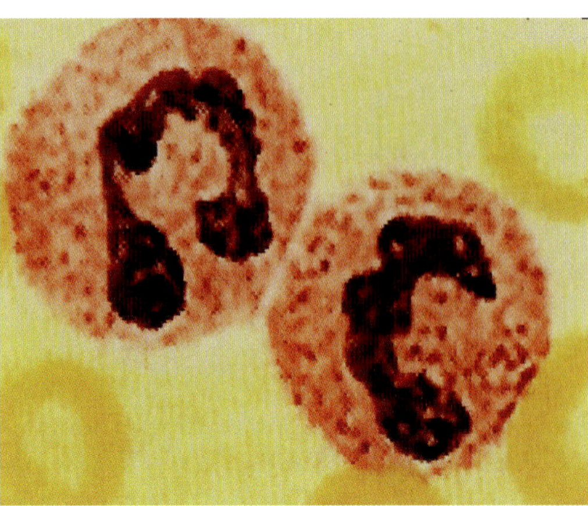

Figure 1

Histologic picture of two leukocytes showing MPS granules in the lysosomal bodies. The entity, known as Reilly granules, is characteristic for many of the mucopolysaccharidoses.

fected patients have an error in GAG metabolism, and increased amounts of these materials in the blood, urine, and reticuloendothelial cells appear to be the cause of the findings.[5,7,11,12,25] For the type I group, excessive amounts of heparan and dermatan sulfates accumulate, and both become lodged in the lysosomal bodies of the reticuloendothelial cells and cause a variety of cell, tissue, and organ dysfunctions.[5-7,11] Because the GAGs may also be present in excessive amounts in the urine, this was once a clinical test for the disorder.[25] The cause of this overproduction of GAGs appears to be related to a decrease in the amount of alpha-L-iduronidase resulting from a series of mutations in well over 15 codons.[7,19,22,26-32] The two most prevalent of these premature stop codons are located at Q70X and W402X; these account for up to 70% of the defects that occur.[7,19,26,27,29-31] The decrease in the amount of alpha-L-iduronidase appears to vary with the type and extent of the stop codon involved, which accounts for the variability in clinical presentation of the syndromes.[5,7,19,26,29,31] Clinically, the assessment of the presence and extent of the disease may be determined by analysis of body fluids for alpha-L-iduronidase, which is usually very low.[7,11] Serum and urinary GAG concentration are usually high as well.[25] The same studies have recently been demonstrated to be possible to perform on cultured amniocytes or chorionic villae obtained by analysis of prenatal uterine materials.[7,33]

Histologic studies of patients with MPS type I show the intracellular accumulations of mucopolysaccharides, causing increased cell size.[34] The cytoplasm of macrophagic or reticuloendothelial cells show a distinctive granular appearance, presumably caused by the presence of the mucopolysaccharides in the lysosomal bodies.[7,11,34-36] When the collections of material are located in leukocytes, they appear as small nodular collections that are known as Reilly granules, as described by Reilly[37] in 1941 (Figure 1). The original description was for patients with Hurler syndrome, but these granules may be present in other forms of the mucopolysaccharidoses.[7,34] Chondrocytes in the epiphyseal plates show collections of mucopolysaccharides in the cells; these changes are probably responsible for the growth abnormalities, which may be quite striking.[34] Collections of granular material are also found in the brain and spinal cord and are presumed responsible for the mental and neurologic problems displayed by children with MPS I–H.[7,34,35,38,39]

Clinical Presentation
MPS Type I–H, Hurler's Disease

Infants with MPS I–H seem normal at birth but may have inguinal or umbilical hernias, a large head, and seem somewhat heavier than normal. The mean time to diagnosis is 9 months and virtually all are diagnosed by 18 months. Death, most often by cardiorespiratory failure, usually occurs by the tenth year of life.[5,7,11,20]

The affected children are usually dwarfed and have progressive mental deterioration, most often in association with hydrocephalus.[5,7,11,20,22,35] The craniofacial appearance is quite striking. The children have large heads with mask-like facies[20] (Figure 2). The hair on their heads and eyebrows is coarse, bristly, and straight. The nose is flat and wide, and the nares are large and upturned. The ears are large, with thick lobes. The lips are patulous, considerably larger than normal, and the tongue protrudes.[40] The teeth are late to erupt and may be small and malformed.[40] A child with the extensive disease commonly has a short neck and a short thorax, with a prominent gibbus usually occurring in the dorsolumbar junction region. The neck problem sometimes endangers the spinal cord and

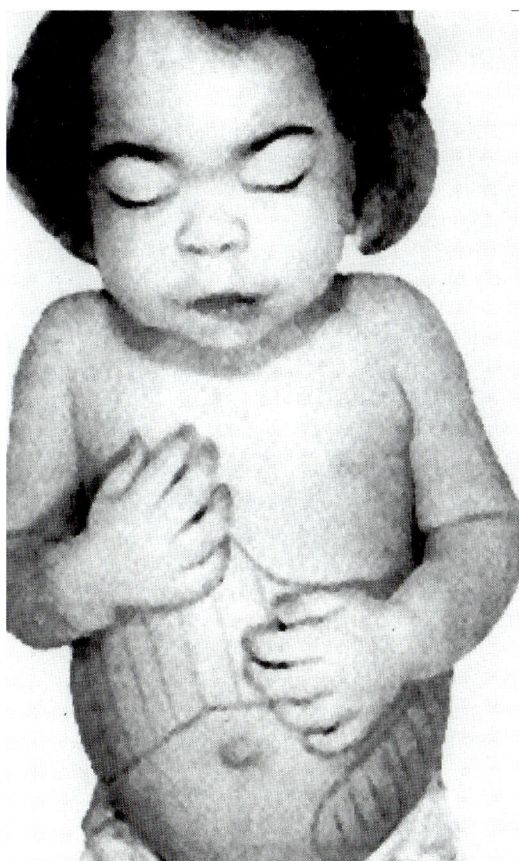

Figure 2
Photograph of a child with Hurler's disease (MPS I–H). Her spleen and liver are enlarged.

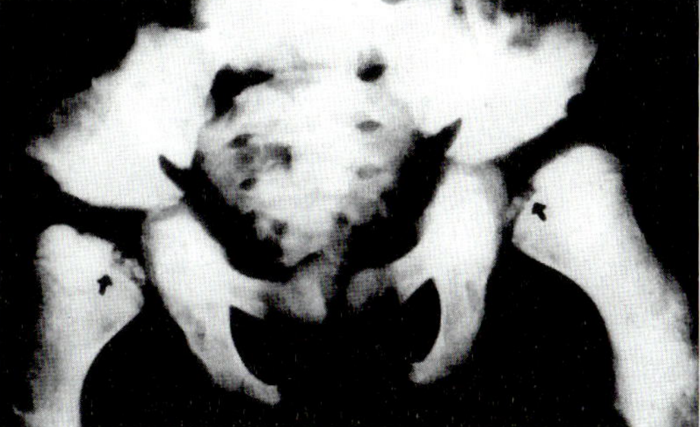

Figure 3
Radiograph of the pelvis of a child with Hurler's disease, demonstrating deformity of both pelvis and femoral heads and coxa valga.

leads to quadriparesis. The abdomen is usually prominent on the basis of splenomegaly and hepatomegaly and hernias are common (Figure 2). Many patients with MPS I–H have chronic diahrrea.

Hypertelorism and early photophobia are the rule, and corneal clouding occurs in all patients.[7,11,20,34,41] Progression of the visual problems may lead to retinal degeneration and, ultimately, blindness. Hearing loss is frequent and often related to infection or scarring of the tympanic membrane and damage to the eighth nerve.[39] Children with MPS I–H frequently have difficulty sleeping due to coarse breathing, and apnea may greatly increase the problems they encounter with their defective mental status.[7,20,42-44]

The skeletal changes are quite severe and are present at birth or soon thereafter. Mild irregularity of the hips is usually present at birth and quite characteristically consists of coxa valga, acetabular hypoplasia, and enlargement and flaring of the iliac wings[5,7,11,34,45] (Figure 3). Widening of the anterior and lateral ribs with narrowing of the posterior portions is frequently present, and the chest contours are often quite irregular. The vertebral segments are usually ovoid in shape, with wedge-shaped vertebrae at T12 or L1; this is the cause of the malformed shortened spine and gibbus formation[38,39,45] (Figure 4). The phalanges are wide but are proximally pointed, and there is a V-shaped deformity of the distal radius and ulna based on oblique deformity of both bones at their terminal ends[46] (Figure 5). The digits usually fail to completely extend, causing a "claw hand," and carpal tunnel syndrome is a frequent finding.[46,47]

Cardiac involvement is seen in all patients with MPS I–H.[7,11,48,49] Murmurs are present early in the disease and reflect the progressive thickening and stiffening of the valve leaflets, which often lead to mitral and aortic regurgitation. Cardiomyopathy becomes more severe with advancing age and leads to coronary artery disease, arrhythmia, and sometimes sudden death.[7,48,49] Pulmonary problems related to structural change and fibrosis may increase the cardiac complications.[48-50] The life for children with MPS I–H is hardly a happy one; the same is true for their families, who watch the terrible series of events occur.

MPS Type I–S or Type I–HS

Patterns of clinical findings for MPS I–S or MPS I–HS are not nearly as well documented as for type I–H.[5-7,11,18,22,23,30,31,48] Both forms are less severe, the patients have considerably less physical compromise, and they are usually not at risk for an early death. The mild disease (MPS I–S) may not

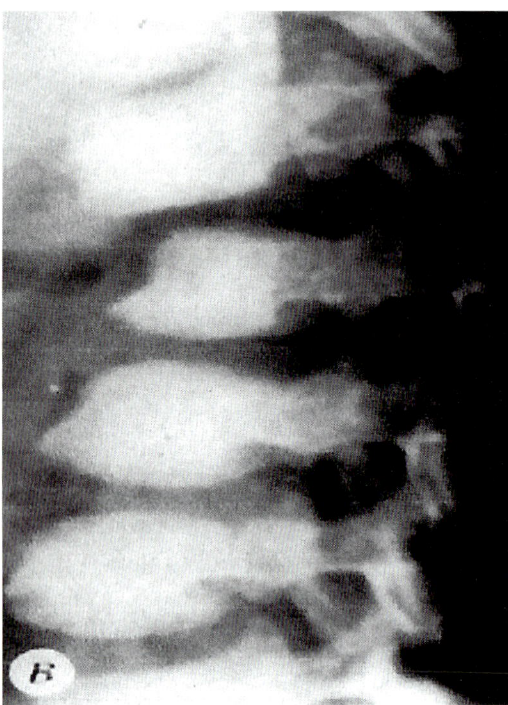

Figure 4
Radiograph of the spine of a child with Hurler syndrome, showing the characteristic wedge-shaped vertebral segment.

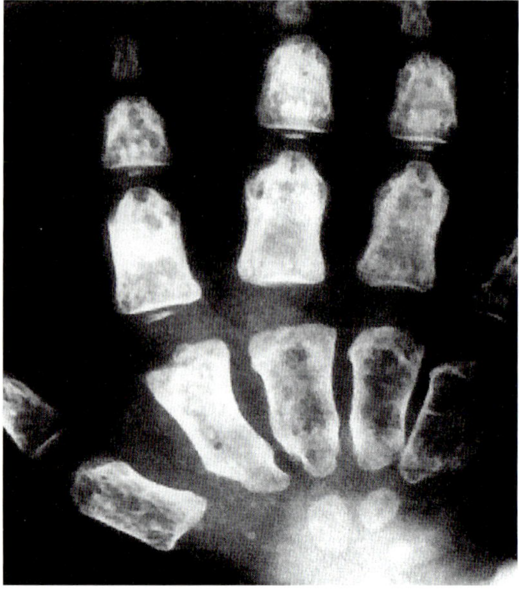

Figure 5
Hand deformity in a patient with Hurler's disease, showing the proximal pointing of the metacarpals and the wide, shortened phalanges.

be diagnosed until patients are 15 years of age or older.[7,18,23] Mentation is normal or near normal, and stature is also relatively normal. Patients have some facial deformities, with somewhat coarse features, a flat nose, and upturned nostrils, and their lips are thicker than normal (Figure 6). Despite these findings, the patient's breathing is usually not impaired, hearing is normal, and, although the neck is somewhat shorter than normal, the risk of cord damage is very small.[43] The principal problem these patients face is ocular, in that corneal clouding is present in all patients; for some, progressive glaucoma, retinal degeneration, and blindness may occur[5,7,18,22,23,41] (Figure 7).

Although liver and spleen involvement is far less than for MPS I-H, patients with mild disease may have a larger abdomen than normal.[7] Cardiac involvement with mild disease is uncommon early in the course but may occur later in life.[7,49]

Progressive arthropathy is common. Kyphosis, scoliosis, and severe back pain are often the principal complaints, even for patients with mild disease.[5,7,38] Poor hand function is sometimes quite striking, and claw hands and carpal tunnel disease are

frequent causes of disability[7,23,46,47] (Figure 8).

Patients with moderate disease (MPS I-HS) show many of the features of the severe form, but they occur at a later age and are less damaging or disabling.[5,7,41,49] Patients have relatively normal or a moderately impaired intellect and, although their facial features are more deforming, with the exception of their visual problems, they are much more functional than patients with severe disease. The risk of cardiac disease is higher and the skeletal changes considerably more deforming than with the mild form, and most patients are shorter than normal. Many of them have problems with breathing and also have sleep apnea.[42,44] Chronic diarrhea is not uncommon in both the mild and moderate forms of the disorder.[7,11]

Treatment

Until relatively recently, only very limited treatments were available for patients with MPS type I.[5,7,11] Children with the severe form of the disease required respiratory aid, particularly at night when apnea developed. In most cases, treatment of cardiac problems such as heart failure or coronary occlusion is essential. Bowel disease was treated symptomatically, and little could be done to alter the progressive blindness associated

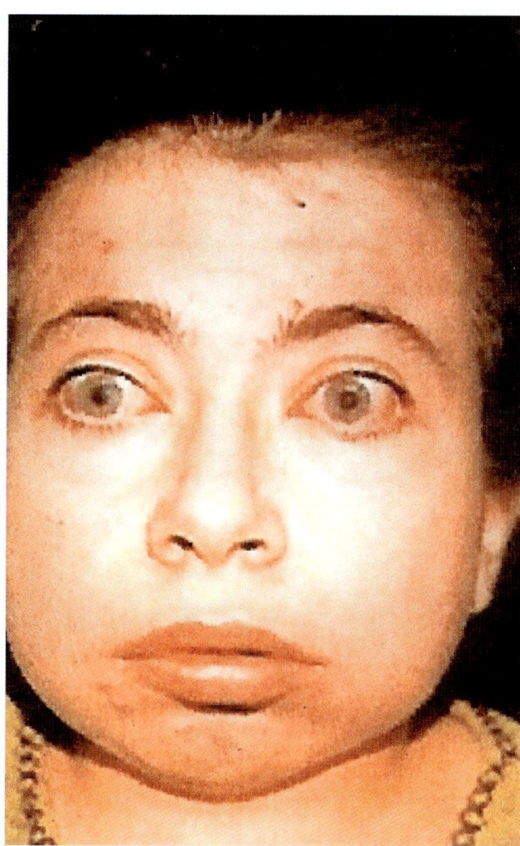

Figure 6

Characteristic facial deformity in a patient with MPS I–S (Scheie's disease), showing coarse features, a flat nose, upturned nostrils, and thick lips.

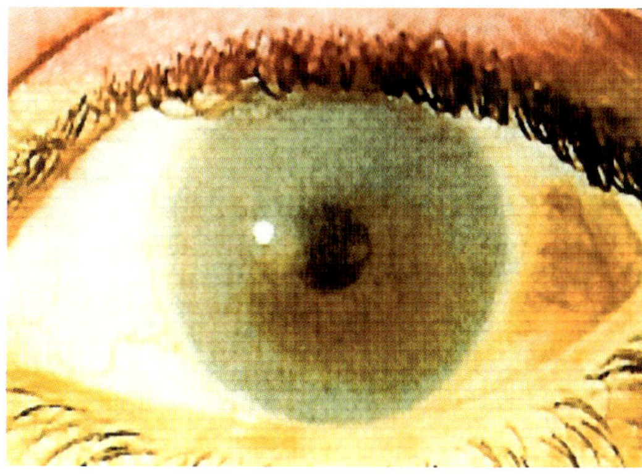

Figure 7

Ocular changes in a patient with MPS type I–S, showing marked corneal clouding. Glaucoma may develop.

with visual damage in either MPS I–H or MPS I–S. In recent years, corneal transplants have been useful for patients with mild or moderate disease and have considerably improved vision problems.[41]

The finding of the genetic character of the diseases inspired physicians to introduce marrow transplants as a possible solution for some of the problems. This was at least in part successful in reducing symptomatology and slowing the progress of the bone disease.[51] If the transplant is performed early in the child's life, hepatomegaly and obstructive airway disease are both reduced, as are bone abnormalities. Marrow transplants, even when provided by a sibling, are not without complications and some fragile children have died as a result.[6,7,38,45,50,52,53] Transplants from closely matched or mismatched individuals have an even higher death rate and have been abandoned as a treatment system. More recently, the introduction of stem cells has appeared to be successful in reducing mental and neurologic problems and decreasing the size of the liver and spleen.[6,7,54] Similarly, attempts at altering the uterine genetic abnormality are still currently under study.

The major contribution over the past 10 years has been the introduction of treatment with alpha-L-iduronidase, which can alter the problems associated with deposition of GAGs. The method of improving the transport of the alpha-L-iduronidase into the lysosomal body of the cell is based on adding a mannose-6-phosphate recognition signal to the material, allowing it to enter the cell membrane and attack and destroy the lysosomal structure containing the GAGs, in a similar fashion to the method used to introduce β-glucosidase into the cells of patients with Gaucher disease.[7,21,55] This treatment has been found to reverse some patients' disabling features, including improving mental impairment, decreasing neurologic problems, changing cardiac abnormalities, diminishing visual alterations, and modestly improving bone structure.[6,7,21,56-60] However, administration of this agent does not alter the natural history of the musculoskeletal disease and, over time, most patients continue to have deformity and disability. The material must be administered weekly through an intravenous port. A recent report suggests that the combination of enzyme replacement and stem cell transplant is even more successful for patients with MPS I–H than either given separately and that the complications are less marked than for either treatment given individually.[57]

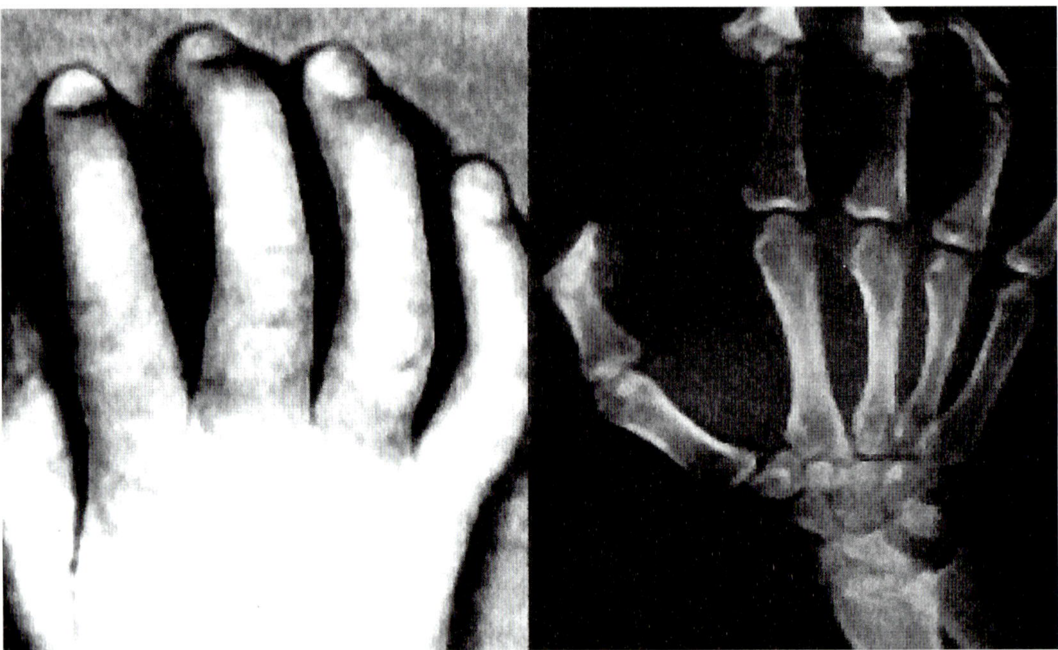

Figure 8
Classic appearance of the hands of a patient with MPS I–S, illustrating the structural clawing of the digits. Function is only moderately impaired.

Conclusions

MPS type I is a rare complex genetic entity, with a vast array of findings and three distinct forms of presentation. The severe form, MPS I–H, includes skeletal, cardiac, and corneal abnormalities, as well as mental retardation, and leads to an early demise. This disorder, still known as Hurler syndrome, is closely related to two other clinical syndromes, however, one of which is mild and mostly associated with ocular problems and the other more severe but still less of a problem clinically than MPS I–H. Physicians who treat the patients and the scientists who have studied the disorders have made some major discoveries that have greatly advanced our approaches to these patients, as well as to some other genetic disorders. Specifically, they have discovered the nature of the entity in terms of excessive amounts of GAGs stored in lysosomal bodies of the reticuloendothelial cells; the failure of the synthesis of alpha-L-iduronidase as the cause; the sites and nature of the gene error; and, most recently, the use of marrow transplant, stem cell administration, and enzyme treatment to alleviate some of the problems. In that respect, despite the rarity of the diseases, patients with MPS I, Gaucher disease, Fabry disease, and several other genetic disorders can be helped. This represents major progress in the field of genetic disorders and provides a true window of opportunity to help patients with these diseases.

References

1. Osler W: Sporadic cretinism in America. *Trans Congr Am Phys Surg* 1897;4:169-206.

2. Berkhan O: Zwei falle von skaphokephalie. *Arch Anthrop* 1907;34:8.

3. Hunter C: A rare disease in two brothers: Evaluation of scapula, limitation of movement of joint and other abnormalities. *Pr R Soc Med* 1917;10:104-116.

4. Hurler G: Uber einen typ mutipler abartungen, vorwiegend am skelettsystem. *Z Kinderheilk* 1919;24:220-234.

5. Muenzer J: The mucopolysaccharidoses: A heterogeneous group of disorders with variable pediatric presentations. *J Pediatr* 2004;144:S27-S34.

6. Muenzer J, Fisher A: Advances in the treatment of mucopolysaccharidosis type I. *N Engl J Med* 2004;350:1932-1934.

7. Whitly CB: The mucopolysaccharidoses, in Beighton P (ed): *McKusick's Heritable Disorders of Connective Tissue*, ed 5. St. Louis, MO, Mosby, 1993, pp 367-499.

8. Ellis RWB, Sheldon W, Capon NB: Gargoylism (chondro-osteo-dystrophy, corneal opacities, hepatosplenomegaly, and mental deficiency). *Q J Med* 1936;5:119-139.

9. Brante G: Gargoylism: A mucopolysaccharidosis. *Scand J Clin Lab Invest* 1952;4:43-46.

10. Gasteiger H, Liebenam L: Beitrag zur dysostosis multiplex unter besonderer Beruchsichtigung des augenbefundes. *Klin Monastbl Augenheilkd* 1937;99:433-447.

11. Wynne-Davies R, Fairbank TJ: *Fairbank's Atlas of General Affections of the Skeleton*, ed 2. Edinburgh, Scotland, Churchill Livingstone, 1976, pp 166-177.

12. Fratantoni JC, Hall CW, Neufeld EF: The defect in Hurler's and Hunter's syndromes: Faulty degradation of mucopolysaccharide. *Proc Natl Acad Sci USA* 1968;60:699-706.

13. Morquio L: Sur une forme de dystrophie osseuse familiale. *Arch Med Enf* 1929;32:129-140.

14. Brailsford JF: Chondro-osteo-dystrophy: Roentgenographic and clinical features of a child with dislocation of vertebrae. *Am J Surg* 1929;7:404-410.

15. Sanfillippo SJ: Mental retardation associated with acid mucopolysacchariduria (heparitin sufate type). *J Pediatr* 1963;63:837-838.

16. Maroteaux P, Lamy M: Hurler's disease, Morquio's disease and related mucopolysaccharidoses. *J Pediatr* 1965;67:312-323.

17. Sly WS, Quinton BA, McAlister WH, Rimoin DL: Beta-glucuronidase deficiency: Report of clinical, radiological and biochemical features of a new mucopolysaccharidosis. *J Pediatr* 1973;82:249-257.

18. Scheie HG, Hambrick GW Jr, Barness LA: A newly recognized forme fruste of Hurler's disease (gargoylism). *Am J Ophthalmol* 1962;53:753-769.

19. Bach G, Friedman R, Weissman B, Neufield EF: The defect in the Hurler and Scheie syndromes: Deficiency of -L-iduronidase. *Proc Natl Acad Sci USA* 1972;69:2048-2051.

20. Cleary MA, Wraith JE: The presenting features of mucopolysaccharidosis type IH (Hurler syndrome). *Acta Paediatr* 1995;84:337-339.

21. Pastores GM, Meere PA: Musculoskeletal complications associated with lysosomal storage disorders: Gaucher disease and Hurler Scheie syndrome (mucopolysaccharidosis type I). *Curr Opin Rheumatol* 2005;17:70-78.

22. Roubicek M, Gehler J, Spranger J: The clinical spectrum of alpha-L-iduronidase deficiency. *Am J Med Genet* 1985;20:471-481.

23. Vijay S, Wraith JE: Clinical presentation and follow-up of patients with the attenuated phenotype of mucopolysaccharidosis type I. *Acta Paediatr* 2005;94:872-877.

24. Lowry RB, Renwick DH: Relative frequency of the Hurler and Hunter syndromes. *N Engl J Med* 1971;284:221-222.

25. Dorfman A, Lorincz AE: Occurrence of urinary acid mucopolysaccharides in the Hurler syndrome. *Proc Natl Acad Sci USA* 1957;43:443-446.

26. Beesley CE, Meaney CA, Greenland G, et al: Mutational analysis of 85 mucopolysaccharidosis type I families: Frequency of known mutations, identification of 17 novel mutations and in vitro expression of missense mutations. *Hum Genet* 2001;109:503-511.

27. Gort L, Chabás A, Coll MJ: Analysis of five mutations in 20 mucopolysaccharidosis type 1 patients: High prevalence of the W402X mutation. Mutations in brief no. 121: Online. *Hum Mutat* 1998;11:332-333.

28. Hein LK, Bawden M, Muller VJ, Sillence D, Hopwood JJ, Brooks DA: Alpha-L-iduronidase premature stop codons and potential read-through in mucopolysaccharidosis type I patients. *J Mol Biol* 2004;338:453-462.

29. Hein LK, Hopwood JJ, Clements PR, Brooks DA: The alpha-L-iduronidase mutations R89Q and R89W result in an attenuated mucopolysaccharidosis type I presentation. *Biochim Biophys Acta* 2003;1639:95-103.

30. Lee-Chen GJ, Lin SP, Chen IS, Chang JH, Yang CW, Chin YW: Mucopolysaccharidosis type I: Identification and characterization of mutations affecting alpha-L-iduronidase activity. *J Formos Med Assoc* 2002;101:425-428.

31. Lee-Chen GJ, Sin SP, Tang YF, Chin YW: Mucopolysaccharidosis type I: Characterization of novel mutations affecting alpha-L-iduronidase activity. *Clin Genet* 1999;56:66-70.

32. Scott HS, Litjens T, Nelson PV, et al: Identification of mutations in the alpha-L-iduronidase gene (IDUA) that cause Hurler and Scheie syndromes. *Am J Hum Genet* 1993;53:973-986.

33. Young EP: Prenatal diagnosis of Hurler disease by analysis of alpha-iduronidase in chorionic villi. *J Inherit Metab Dis* 1992;15:224-230.

34. Jaffe HL: *Metabolic, Degenerative and Inflammatory Diseases of Bones and Joints*. Philadelphia, PA, Lea and Febiger, 1972, pp 542-552.

35. Ashby R, Stewart RM, Watkin IH: Chondro-osteodystrophy of Hurler type (gargoylism): A pathologic study. *Brain* 1937;60:149-179.

36. Berry HK: Screening for mucopolysaccharide disorders with the Berry spot test. *Clin Biochem* 1987;20:365-371.

37. Reilly WA: The granules in leukocytes in gargoylism. *Am J Dis Child* 1941;62:489-491.

38. Kachur E, Del Maestro R: Mucopolysaccharidoses and spinal cord compression: Case report and review of the literature with implications of bone marrow transplantation. *Neurosurgery* 2000;47:223-229.

39. Tandon V, Williamson JB, Cowie RA, Wraith JE: Spinal problems in mucopolysaccharidosis I (Hurler syndrome). *J Bone Joint Surg Br* 1996;78:938-944.

40. Gardner DG: The oral manifestations of Hurler's syndrome. *Oral Surg Oral Med Oral Pathol* 1971;32:46-57.

41. Ashworth JL, Biswas S, Wraith E, Lloyd IC: Mucopolysaccharidoses and the eye. *Surv Ophthalmol* 2006;51:1-17.

42. Leighton SE, Papsin B, Vellodi A, Dinwiddie R, Lane R: Disordered breathing during sleep in patients with mucopolysaccharidoses. *Int J Pediatr Otorhinolaryngol* 2001;58:127-138.

43. Peters ME, Ary S, Langer LO, Gilbert EF, Carlson R, Adkins W: Narrow trachea in mucopolysaccharidoses. *Pediatr Radiol* 1985;15:225-228.

44. Shih SL, Lee YJ, Lin SP, Sheu CY, Blickman JG: Airway changes in children with mucopolysaccharidoses. *Acta Radiol* 2002;43:40-43.

45. Weisstein JS, Delgado E, Steinbach LS, Hart K, Packman S: Musculoskeletal manifestations of Hurler syndrome: Long-term follow-up after bone marrow transplantation. *J Pediatr Orthop* 2004;24:97-101.

46. Haddad FS, Jones DH, Vellodi A, Kane N, Pitt MC: Carpal tunnel syndrome in the mucopolysaccharidoses and mucolipidoses. *J Bone Joint Surg Br* 1997;79:576-582.

47. Gschwind C, Tonkin MA: Carpal tunnel syndrome in children with mucopolysaccharidosis and related disorders. *J Hand Surg Am* 1992;17:44-47.

48. Dangel JH: Cardiovascular changes in children with mucopolysaccharide storage diseases and related disorders—clinical and echocardiographic changes in 64 patients. *Eur J Pediatr* 1998;157:534-538.

49. Fischer TA, Lehr HA, Nixdorff U, Meyer J: Combined aortic and mitral stenosis in mucopolysaccharidosis type I-S (Ullrich-Scheie syndrome). *Heart* 1999;81:97-99.

50. Gassas A, Sung L, Doyle JJ, Clarke JT, Saunders EF: Life-threatening pulmonary hemorrhages post bone marrow transplantation in Hurler syndrome: Report of three cases and review of the literature. *Bone Marrow Transplant* 2003;32:213-215.

51. Braunlin EA, Stauffer NR, Peters CH, et al: Usefulness of bone marrow transplantation in the Hurler syndrome. *Am J Cardiol* 2003;92:882-886.

52. Guffon N, Souillet G, Maire I, Straczek J, Guibaud P: Follow-up of nine patients with Hurler syndrome after bone marrow transplantation. *J Pediatr* 1998;133:119-125.

53. Peters C, Shapiro EG, Anderson J, et al: Hurler syndrome: II. Outcome of HLA-genotypically identical sibling and HLA-haploidentical related donor bone marrow transplantation in fifty-four children: The Storage Disease Collaborative Study Group. *Blood* 1998;91:2601-2608.

54. Souillet G, Guffon N, Maire I, et al: Outcome of 27 patients with Hurler's syndrome transplanted from either related or unrelated haematopoietic stem cell sources. *Bone Marrow Transplant* 2003;31:1105-1117.

55. Ghosh P, Dahms NM, Kornfeld S: Mannose 6-phosphate receptors: New twists in the tale. *Nat Rev Mol Cell Biol* 2003;4:202-212.

56. Brooks DA: Alpha-L-iduronidase and enzyme replacement therapy for mucopolysaccharidosis I. *Expert Opin Biol Ther* 2002;2:967-976.

57. Grewal SS, Wynn R, Abdenur JE, et al: Safety and efficacy of enzyme replacement therapy in combination with hematopoietic stem cell transplantation in Hurler syndrome. *Genet Med* 2005;7:143-146.

58. Kakkis ED, Muenzer J, Tiller GE: Enzyme-replacement therapy in mucopolysaccharidosis I. *N Engl J Med* 2001;344:182-188.

59. Miebach E: Enzyme replacement therapy in mucopolysaccharidosis type I. *Acta Paediatr Suppl* 2005;94:58-60.

60. Wraith JE, Clarke LA, Beck M, et al: Enzyme replacement therapy for mucopolysaccharidosis-I: A randomized, double-blinded, placebo-controlled, multinational study of recombinant human alpha-L-iduronidase (laronidase). *J Pediatr* 2004;144:581-588.

Chapter 28

Hunter's Disease: Mucopolysaccharidosis Type II

The mucopolysaccharidoses are inherited lysosomal storage diseases that cause extraordinary changes in the biology, physical structure, mental status, and survival of affected children. There are now seven forms of these rare genetic abnormalities, and one of these is known as Hunter's disease, based on the first description of the disorder by Charles Hunter in 1917.[1] Hunter's disease is now further identified as mucopolysaccharidosis (MPS) type II. This entity is similar to MPS type I, known as Hurler's disease or syndrome, but with some distinct differences. Although both are causes of dwarfism and mental retardation, MPS type II is generally less destructive, usually does not involve the eyes, and is less lethal. The disorder is genetic, transmitted as a sex-linked autosomal recessive disorder, and is present at birth in male children. There are two forms of the disease—severe (type A) and mild (type B). Children with severe disease have multiple problems early in life and most die before the age of 15 years, while those with the milder form have a much less affected life and usually survive sometimes into late adulthood.

Nomenclature and History

As noted above, Hunter's disease or Hunter's syndrome is also known as MPS type II, severe (type A) and mild (type B), or simply as MPS II. The terms gargoylism and dysostosis multiplex congenita were proposed for both Hunter's and Hurler's syndromes, but have since been abandoned. The disorder is also known as iduronate-2-sulfatase deficiency or sulfoiduronate deficiency.

The first description of patients with MPS was attributed to William Osler in 1897.[2] These patients most likely had MPS I, or Hurler's syndrome, which was later described by Gertrud Hurler in 1919.[3] The definition of the MPS II disorder, however, was in the form of a spectacular presentation by Charles Hunter (1873-1955) in 1917 at the Royal Society of Medicine.[1] Hunter

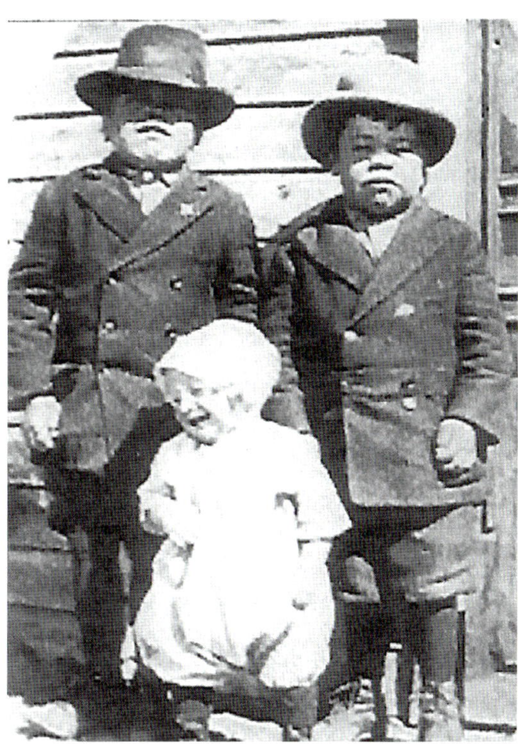

Figure 1
The patients described by Hunter. The photograph originally obtained by Hunter was submitted by Drs. Gemmell and Bell of the University of Manitoba in Winnipeg. (Reproduced with permission from Whitley CB: The mucopolysaccharidoses, in Beighton P (ed): *McKusick's Heritable Disorders of Connective Tissue*, ed 5. St. Louis, MO, Mosby, 1993, p 368.)

was born in Scotland and, after receiving his degree in internal medicine in London, moved to Winnipeg, Manitoba, Canada, where he became known as a leading medical diagnostician. In his presentation, Hunter described two dwarfed and deformed brothers whose photographs appear in the chapter by Whitley[4] in Beighton's 5th edition of *McKusick's Heritable Disorders of Connective Tissue*. The pictures originally obtained by Hunter were submitted by Gemmell and Bell of the University of Manitoba in Winnipeg[4] (Figure 1). Patients with Hunter's disease are dwarfs and are believed to be irritable; it is possible that they may have been the people encountered in the Catskills as described by Washington Irving in his short story "Rip Van Winkle"!

In 1936, Fratantoni and associates[5] identified the material that accumulated in the tissue of patients with both Hurler's and Hunter's diseases as glycosaminoglycans. The earliest pedigree study on patients with Hunter's disease was by Wolff in 1942,[6] but he did not stress the gender linkage. In 1946, Nja[7] defined the sex-linked pedigree. The best definition of all of the mucopolysaccharidoses over the next several years was by clinician-scientist Victor A. McKusick,[8-11] who not only clearly defined the clinical aspects of the first six disorders but contributed meaningfully to our understanding of their genetic origins.

Genetics and Biology

Hunter's disease is an X-linked autosomal recessive disorder for which the gene map locus is Xq27.3-q28.[4,12-15] The syndrome results from an iduronate-2-sulfatase deficiency.[4,12,14,16] Most often the disease occurs in males and is present at birth, although it may not be apparent for a year or two.[4,7,15,16] There are several reports regarding the occasional occurrence of the disorder in females,[17-20] and one description of occurrence in a golden retriever.[21] Description of the frequency varies, but it is suggested that the disease is rare and occurs in fewer than 1 in 70,000 live births.[4,16] In regard to ethnic frequency, several authors have proposed that the disorder is more frequent in Ashkenazi Jews,[22,23] but increased frequency is also reported in Russian, Spanish, Japanese, Korean, and western Australian populations.[16,24-29]

Hunter's disease is caused by a deficiency of iduronate-2-sulfatase, which hydrolyses terminal iduronate-2-sulfate ester on the glycosaminoglycans heparan sulfate and dermatan sulfate.[13-15,27,30] This results in the accumulation of these two glycosaminoglycans in osseous, hepatic, cardiovascular, orofacial, and intracranial tissues, which causes structural and functional damage.[4,15,16,31] Clinical presentation shows a spectrum of mild to severe forms as a result of more than 250 different mutations in the functional gene. The mutations include missense and nonsense mutations, mutations affecting splicing, small insertions and deletions, partial gene deletions, and deletions or rearrangements of the entire iduronate-2-sulfate gene.[4,12-15,25,27] As a result of the changes in the iduronate-2-sulfatases, the heparan and dermatan sulfates cannot be destroyed and accumulate in many sites. They have an effect on the organs and tissues in these sites, which produce the syndromes of both severe and mild Hunter's disease.[4,16,31] In addition, the materials found in the urine can be considered a diagnostic study.[4,15,16,31] A report by Dean and associates[32] in 2006 described a more secure detection of MPS type II by measurement of iduronate-2-sulfatase in blood spots and plasma.[33]

Clinical Presentations for Severe and Mild Types

Differentiation between the severe and mild forms of Hunter's disease is not always simple, particularly early in the child's life.[4,15,16,31,34,35] The severe form is characterized by early mental deterioration and a rapid advance to cachexia, with death occurring usually before 15 years of age.[4,15,34] The mild form is diagnosed somewhat later, with patients typically living into adulthood.[4,35] The mild form is much more rare and is sometimes difficult to clinically distinguish from other MPS disorders. The changes in the severe form resemble those seen in patients with Hurler's syndrome (MPS I–S).[4,15,16,31] Prenatal diagnosis is now possible for patients with Hunter's disease using a new fluorometric enzyme assay, which can detect iduronate-2-sulfatase in uncultured chorionic villae.[36]

Children with Hunter's disease have large heads with hydrocephaly.[4,15,16,31] Their facies are coarse, with a large flattened nose and depressed nasal bridge, frontal bossing, hypertelorism, and a thickened tongue.[4,37] The teeth are widely spaced and drooling is often excessive.[4,31,34,37] Cysts in the teeth are frequently seen. Hydrocephalus may develop as the disease progresses.[4,16,38]

For patients with the severe form, mental impairment is usually evident by 4 years of age and increases progressively with advancing years.[15,16,39] The progressive neuronal degeneration seems to result from storage of dermatan and heparan sulfate in the nervous system.[16,38] Dilatation of the ventricles

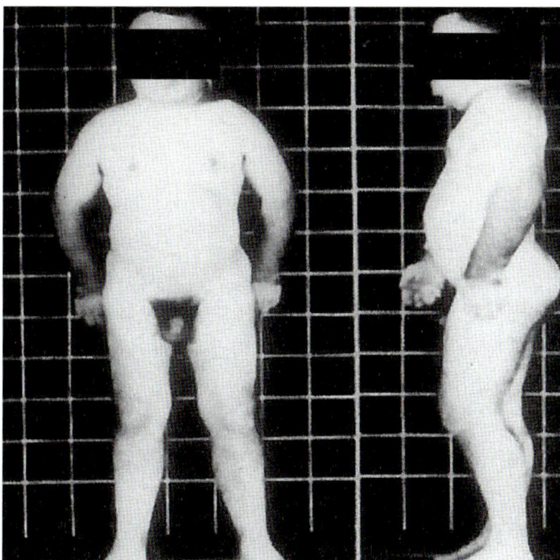

Figure 2
Photograph of a male patient with Hunter's disease. Note the short stature, enlarged cranium, and prominent abdomen.

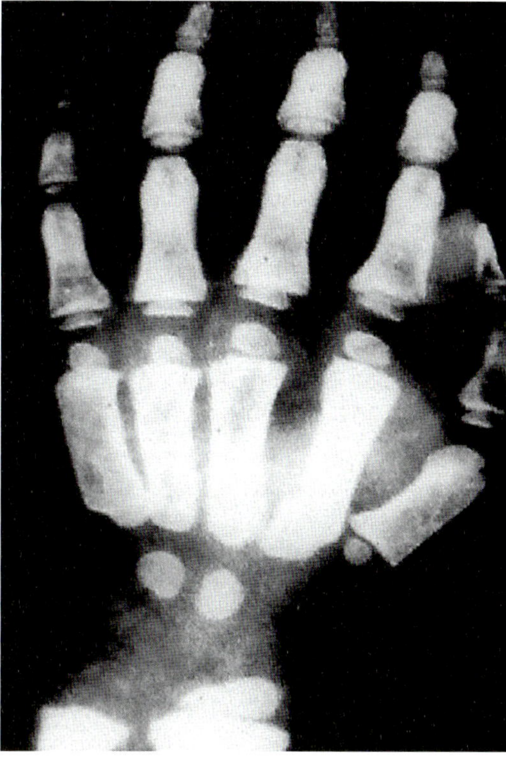

Figure 3
Radiograph of the hand of a patient with Hunter's disease. Note the thickened and somewhat dense bones. The hands are often deformed and clawed.

and low density of white matter are evident on MRI studies.[40] Compressive myelopathy may occur from cervical spine injury and subluxation as a result of progressive thickening of the dura with glycosaminoglycan deposition.[4,38,41]

Carpal tunnel compression is commonly present in patients with severe and even mild disease.[42-44] Hearing loss is common in Hunter's disease, relating to recurrent otitis media as a result of glycosaminoglycan deposition.[4,31] A distinguishing feature of Hunter's disease from Hurler's is the absence of corneal clouding, although some changes related to the deposition of glycosaminoglycans in the eye structures may develop late in the course in patients with severe disease.[34,45,46]

Respiratory problems are common in patients with Hunter's disease and result from adenoid hypertrophy, nasal congestion, and thick rhinorrhea.[4,16,47-49] Sonorous breathing and obstructive sleep apnea are common.[31,47,50] Tracheal stenosis and collapse have been described and may lead to sudden death.[47,51] Cardiac disease is present in many patients, mostly related to valve problems that can lead to congestive heart failure and death.[15,31,49,52,53] Aortic stenosis is common, and the heart is often enlarged even without other findings.[39] Despite hepatomegaly, which is commonly seen, there is usually no abdominal distress, except for diarrhea that is sometimes frequent and profuse.[4]

All patients with Hunter's disease are short in stature (Figure 2), but the cause is not well understood.[15,16,31] Attempts to study pituitary function and growth hormone production are not conclusive, and there are no findings to support thyroid or other endocrine disorders as the cause.[4] Skeletal changes show that the limbs are all held in partial flexion, and hands are described as "clawed"[15,16] (Figure 3). Carpal tunnel syndrome develops in many patients, which limits their ability to use their hands.[42-44] Fractures of the femoral neck and precocious osteoarthritis in the hips are sometimes encountered, and the bones of the limbs and spine are sometimes distorted in shape and structure[54] (Figure 4). Examination of the foot often discloses a pes cavus deformity.[4]

Skin changes are sometimes quite striking. Hypertrichosis is common and eyebrows may be confluent.[4,37] Papular structures known by the term "pebbling" may be seen in many sites.[55] "Mongolian blue spots" can be quite large and are located in the buttocks and posterior thighs.[56,57]

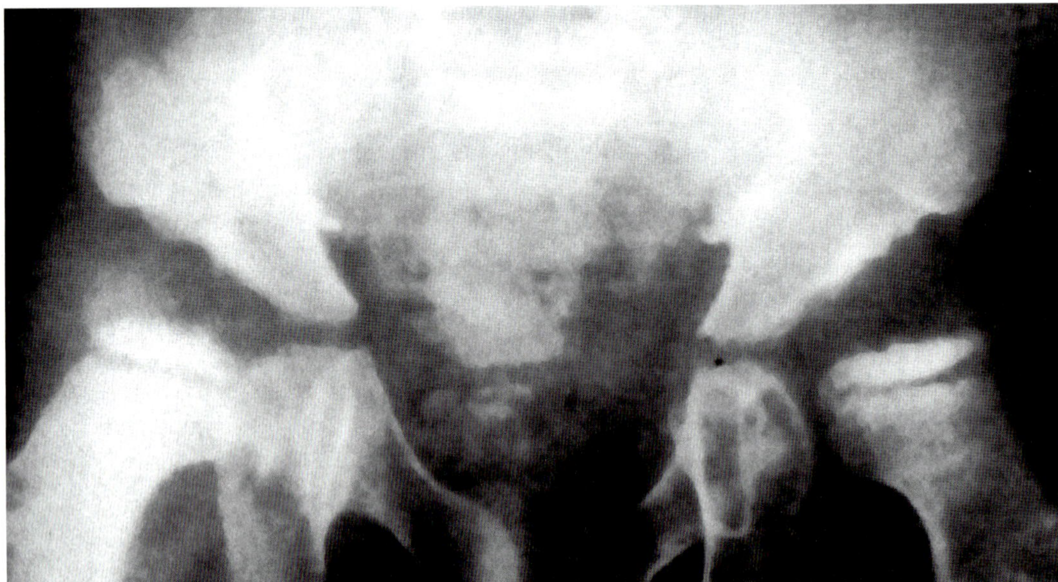

Figure 4
Radiograph of the pelvis and hips of a child with Hunter's disease. The pelvis is widened, epiphyses are dense, and the hips are already osteoarthritic.

Imaging studies support the findings as described. MRI and echocardiogram studies are particularly helpful in identifying cardiac structural abnormalities.[15,52,53] Imaging of the skull and brain show sometimes marked changes with advancing age, reflecting the deterioration of mentation and the changes in facial and oral structures.[40] Histologic studies using special stains show increased concentrations of glycosaminoglycans in the form of Berry spots[58] and alteration of cellular and fibrous structure in various organs.[4,15,16,59]

Treatment

Patients with the mild form of Hunter's disease often require only supportive care, although such problems as sleep apnea, cardiac enlargement, and respiratory impairment may require specific clinical assistance as the patient ages.[35,49] Patients who require the greatest care have the severe form, and the lives of these individuals are often threatened by the age of 10 years.[4,15,16,31,52] They frequently require supplemental oxygen while sleeping, and sometimes tonsillectomy and adenoidectomy are helpful.[4] With progressive narrowing, a tracheostomy and continuous positive pressure oxygen therapy may be required.[4] Cardiac disease development can be detected by frequent monitoring and, if necessary, cardiac surgery to treat valve disease.[16,31,52] Anesthesia

is sometimes a severe problem in these patients.[4] Surgical treatment of carpal tunnel syndrome is usually successful, and sometimes braces for lower extremity problems and shoe orthotics for structural alterations are helpful for ambulation.[42,43,54]

The modern approaches to treatment include marrow transplants, which at times have been helpful in improving the physical status of the patients,[60] and, more recently, the use of allogeneic stem cells.[61,62] This type of treatment has helped reduce the clinical finding of pebble skin and improved respiratory problems and sleep apnea. A more direct approach under clinical trial is the use of recombinant human iduronate-2-sulfatase (idursulfase), which has been shown to be of value, particularly in preventing disastrous complications.[63,64]

Conclusions

Hunter's disease is a rare disorder; many physicians have never encountered patients with this or some of the other mucopolysaccharidoses. Even the severe form of the disease is less of a problem to the patient than Hurler's syndrome, but is still much more devastating than some of the other mucopolysaccharidoses. The patients are short in stature, with mental impairment, cardiac, and respiratory problems, and have a great deal of difficulty with even simple activities of daily living. Until relatively recently, nothing could be done to improve the patient's condition other than awaiting respiratory, cardiac, neurologic, or orthopaedic disorders and then trying to deal with them. Remarkably, in recent years, stem cells, marrow replacement, and, most importantly, enzyme therapy with idursulfase show promise in providing these children with a better life. This is what science can contribute to the practice of medicine and improving the quality of life of our patients and their families.

References

1. Hunter C: A rare disease in two brothers: Evaluation of scapula, limitation of movement of joint and other abnormalities. *Proc R Soc Med* 1917;10:104-106.

2. Osler W: Sporadic cretinism in America. *Trans Cong Am Phys* 1897;4:169-206.

3. Hurler G: Uber einen typ multiplex abartungen, vorwiegend am skelettsystem. *Z Kinderheilk* 1919;24:220-234.

4. Whitley CB: The mucopolysaccharidoses, in Beighton P (ed): *McKusick's Heritable Disorders of Connective Tissue*, ed 5. St. Louis, MO, Mosby, 1993, pp 367-499.

5. Fratantoni JC, Hall CW, Neufeld EF: The defect in Hurler's and Hunter's syndromes: Faulty degradation of mucopolysaccharide. *Proc Natl Acad Sci USA* 1968;60:699-706.

6. Wolff D: Microscopic study of the temporal bones in dysotosis multiplex (gargoylism). *Laryngoscope* 1942;52:218-223.

7. Nja A: Sex-linked type of gargoylism. *Acta Paediatr* 1946;93:267-286.

8. McKusick VA: *Heritable Disorders of Connective Tissue*, ed 1. St Louis, MO, Mosby-Year Book, 1956, pp 152-183.

9. McKusick VA: On the X chromosome of man. *Q Rev Biol* 1962;37:69-175.

10. McKusick VA: The nosology of the mucopolysaccharidoses. *Am J Med* 1969;47:730-747.

11. McKusick VA, Kaplan D, Wise D, et al: The genetic mucopolysaccharidoses. *Medicine (Baltimore)* 1965;44:445-483.

12. Hopwood JJ, Bunge S, Morris CP, et al: Molecular basis of mucopolysaccharidosis type II: Mutations in the iduronate-2-sulphatase gene. *Hum Mutat* 1993;2:435-442.

13. Jonsson JJ, Aronovich EL, Braun SE, Whitley CB: Molecular diagnosis of mucopolysaccharidosis type II (Hunter syndrome) by automated sequencing and computer-assisted interpretation: Toward mutation mapping of the iduronate-2-sulfatase gene. *Am J Hum Genet* 1995;56:597-607.

14. Li P, Bellows AB, Thompson JN: Molecular basis of iduronate-2-sulphatase gene mutations in patients with mucopolysaccharidosis type II (Hunter syndrome). *J Med Genet* 1999;36:21-27.

15. Neufeld EF, Muenzer J: The mucopolysaccharidoses, in Scriver CR, Beaudet AL, Sly WS, Valle D (eds): *The Metabolic Bases of Inherited Diseases*, ed 8. New York, NY, McGraw-Hill, 2001, pp 3421-3452.

16. Muenzer J: The mucopolysaccharidoses: A heterogeneous group of disorders with variable pediatric presentations. *J Pediatr* 2004;144:S27-S34.

17. Broadhead DM, Kirk JM, Burt AJ, Gupta V, Ellis PM, Besley GT: Full expression of Hunter's disease in a female with an X-chromosome deletion leading to non-random inactivation. *Clin Genet* 1986;30:392-398.

18. Clarke JT, Willard HF, Teshima I, Chang PL, Skomorowski MA: Hunter disease (mucopolysaccharidosis type II) in a karyotypically normal girl. *Clin Genet* 1990;37:355-362.

19. Neufeld EF, Liebaers I, Epstein CJ, Yatziv S, Milunsky A, Migeon BR: The Hunter syndrome in females: Is there an autosomal recessive form of iduronate sulfatase deficiency? *Am J Hum Genet* 1977;29:455-461.

20. Tuschl K, Gal A, Paschke E, Kircher S, Bodamer OA: Mucopolysaccharidosis type II in females: Case report and review of literature. *Pediatr Neurol* 2005;32:270-272.

21. Wilkerson MJ, Lewis DC, Marks SL, Prieur DJ: Clinical and morphologic features of mucopolysaccharidosis type II in a dog: Naturally occurring model of Hunter syndrome. *Vet Pathol* 1998;35:230-233.

22. Schaap T, Bach G: Incidence of mucopolysaccharidoses in Israel: Is Hunter disease a "Jewish disease"? *Hum Genet* 1980;56:221-223.

23. Zlotogora J, Schaap T, Zeigler M, Bach G: Hunter syndrome in Jews in Israel: Further evidence for prenatal selection favoring the Hunter allele. *Hum Genet* 1991;86:531-533.

24. Isogai K, Sukegawa K, Tomatsu S, et al: Mutation analysis in the iduronate-2-sulphatase gene in 43 Japanese patients with mucopolysaccharidosis type II (Hunter disease). *J Inherit Metab Dis* 1998;21:60-70.

25. Kim CH, Hwang HZ, Song SM, et al: Mutational spectrum of the iduronate 2 sulfatase gene in 25 unrelated Korean Hunter syndrome patients: Identification of 13 novel mutations. *Hum Mutat* 2003;21:449-450.

26. Nelson J, Crowhurst J, Carey B, Greed L: Incidence of the mucopolysaccharidoses in Western Australia. *Am J Med Genet A* 2003;123:310-313.

27. Sukegawa K, Tomatsu S, Fukao T, et al: Mucopolysaccharidosis type II (Hunter disease): Identification and characterization of eight point mutations in the iduronate-2-sulfatase gene in Japanese patients. *Hum Mutat* 1995;6:136-143.

28. Gort L, Chabás A, Coll MJ: Hunter disease in the Spanish population: Molecular analysis in 31 families. *J Inherit Metab Dis* 1998;21:655-661.

29. Karsten S, Voskoboeva E, Tishkanina S, Pettersson U, Krasnopolskaja X, Bondeson ML: Mutational spectrum of the iduronate-2-sulfatase (IDS) gene in 36 unrelated Russian MPS II patients. *Hum Genet* 1998;103:732-735.

30. Vafiadaki E, Cooper A, Heptinstall LE, Hatton CE, Thornley M, Wraith JE: Mutation analysis in 57 unrelated patients with MPS II (Hunter's

disease). *Arch Dis Child* 1998;79:237-241.

31. Schwartz IV, Ribeiro MG, Mota JG, et al: A clinical study of 77 patients with mucopolysaccharidosis type II. *Acta Paediatr Suppl* 2007;96:63-70.

32. Dean CJ, Bockmann MR, Hopwood JJ, Brooks DA, Meikle PJ: Detection of mucopolysaccharidosis type II by measurement of iduronate-2-sulfatase in dried blood spots and plasma samples. *Clin Chem* 2006;52:643-649.

33. Parkinson EJ, Muller V, Hopwood JJ, Brooks DA: Iduronate-2-sulphatase protein detection in plasma from mucopolysaccharidosis type II patients. *Mol Genet Metab* 2004;81:58-64.

34. Young ID, Harper PS: The natural history of the severe form of Hunter's syndrome: A study based on 52 cases. *Dev Med Child Neurol* 1983;25:481-489.

35. Young ID, Harper PS, Newcombe RG, Archer IM: A clinical and genetic study of Hunter's syndrome: 2. Differences between the mild and severe forms. *J Med Genet* 1982;19:408-411.

36. Keulemans JL, Sinigerska I, Garritsen VH, et al: Prenatal diagnosis of the Hunter syndrome and the introduction of a new fluorimetric enzyme assay. *Prenat Diagn* 2002;22:1016-1021.

37. Finlayson LA: Hunter syndrome (mucopolysaccharidosis II). *Pediatr Dermatol* 1990;7:150-152.

38. Banna M, Hollenberg R: Compressive meningeal hypertrophy in mucopolysaccharidoses. *AJNR Am J Neuroradiol* 1987;8:385-386.

39. Bax MC, Colville GA: Behaviour in mucopolysaccharide disorders. *Arch Dis Child* 1995;73:77-81.

40. Parsons VJ, Hughes DG, Wraith JE: Magnetic resonance imaging of the brain, neck and cervical spine in mild Hunter's syndrome (mucopolysaecharidoses Type II). *Clin Radiol* 1996;51:719-723.

41. Vinchon M, Cotten A, Clarisse J, Chiki R, Christiaens JL: Cervical myelopathy secondary to Hunter syndrome in an adult. *AJNR Am J Neuroradiol* 1995;16:1402-1403.

42. Gschwind C, Tonki MA: Carpal tunnel syndrome in children with mucopolysaccharidosis and related disorders. *J Hand Surg Am* 1992;17:44-47.

43. Haddad FS, Jones DH, Vellodi A, Kane N, Pitt MC: Carpal tunnel syndrome in the mucopolysaccharidoses and mucolipidoses. *J Bone Joint Surg Br* 1997;79:576-582.

44. Wraith JE, Alani SM: Carpal tunnel syndrome in the mucopolysaccharidoses and related disorders. *Arch Dis Child* 1990;65:962-963.

45. Anawis MA: Hunter syndrome (MPS II-B): A report of bilateral vitreous floaters and maculopathy. *Ophthalmic Genet* 2006;27:71-72.

46. Ashworth JL, Biswas S, Wraith E, Lloyd IC: Mucopolysaccharidoses and the eye. *Surv Ophthalmol* 2006;51:1-17.

47. Sasaki CT, Ruiz R, Gaito R Jr , Kirchner JA, Seshi B: Hunter's syndrome: A study in airway obstruction. *Laryngoscope* 1987;97:280-285.

48. Shih SL, Lee YJ, Lin SP, Sheu CY, Blickman JG: Airway changes in children with mucopolysaccharidoses. *Acta Radiol* 2002;43:40-43.

49. Young ID, Harper PS: Long-term complications in Hunter's syndrome. *Clin Genet* 1979;16:125-132.

50. Leighton SE, Papsin B, Vellodi A, Dinwiddie R, Lane R: Disordered breathing during sleep in patients with mucopolysaccharidoses. *Int J Pediatr Otorhinolaryngol* 2001;58:127-138.

51. Peters ME, Arya S, Langer LO, Gilbert EF, Carlson R, Adkins W: Narrow trachea in mucopolysaccharidoses. *Pediatr Radiol* 1985;15:225-228.

52. Dangel JH: Cardiovascular changes in children with mucopolysaccharide storage diseases and related disorders—clinical and echocardiographic changes in 64 patients. *Eur J Pediatr* 1998;157:534-538.

53. Kettles DI, Sheppard M, Liebmann RD, Davidson C: Left ventricular aneurysm, aortic valve disease and coronary narrowing in a patient with Hunter's syndrome. *Cardiovasc Pathol* 2002;11:94-96.

54. Ichikawa T, Nishimura G, Tsukune Y, Dezawa A, Miki H: Progessive bone resorption after pathological fracture of the femoral neck in Hunter's syndrome. *Pediatr Radiol* 1999;29:914-916.

55. Thappa DM, Singh A, Jaisankar TJ, Rao R, Ratnaker C: Pebbling of the skin: A marker of Hunter's syndrome. *Pediatr Dermatol* 1998;15:370-373.

56. Ochiai T, Ito K, Okada T, Chin M, Shichino H, Mugishima H: Significance of extensive Mongolian spots in Hunter's syndrome. *Br J Dermatol* 2003;148:1173-1178.

57. Sapadin AN, Friedman IS: Extensive Mongolian spots associated with Hunter's disease. *J Am Acad Dermatol* 1998;39:1013-1015.

58. Berry HK: Screening for mucopolysaccharide disorders with the Berry spot test. *Clin Biochem* 1987;20:365-371.

59. Voznyi YV, Keulemans JL, van Diggelen OP: A fluorimetric enzyme assay for the diagnosis of MPS II (Hunter's disease). *J Inherit Metab Dis* 2001;24:675-680.

60. Vellodi A, Young E, Cooper A, et al: Long-term follow-up following bone marrow transplantation for Hunter disease. *J Inherit Metab Dis* 1999;22:638-648.

61. Ito K, Ochiai T, Suzuki H, Chin M, Shichino H, Mugishima H: The effect of haematopoietic stem cell transplant on papules with 'pebbly' appearance in Hunter's syndrome. *Br J Dermatol* 2004;151:207-211.

62. Krivit W: Allogeneic stem cell transplantation for the treatment of lysosomal and peroxisomal metabolic diseases. *Springer Semin Immunopathol* 2004;26(1-2):119-132.

63. Muenzer J, Lamsa JC, Garcia A, Dacosta J, Garcia J, Treco DA: Enzyme replacement therapy in mucopolysaccharidosis type II (Hunter syndrome): A preliminary report. *Acta Paediatr Suppl* 2002;91:98-99.

64. Muenzer J, Gucsavas-Calikoglu M, McCandless SE, Schuetz TJ, Kimura A: A phase I/II clinical trial of enzyme replacement therapy in mucopolysaccharidosis II (Hunter syndrome). *Mol Genet Metab* 2007;90:329-337.

Chapter 29

Morquio Syndrome: Mucopolysaccharidosis Type IV

Morquio syndrome is an unusual autosomal recessive genetic disorder that comes in two forms: mucopolysaccharidosis (MPS) type IVA, which is more severe and is caused by a deficiency of N-acetylgalactosomine-6-sulfate sulfatase; and type IVB, which is milder and is caused by a deficiency of β-galactosidase. The defects for both forms of the disease result in a diminished capacity to degrade keratan sulfate. Compared to many of the other mucopolysaccharidoses, Morquio syndrome is clinically less severe and patients usually have normal mentation and facies. The more unique findings are those of spondyloepiphyseal dysplasia, ligamentous laxity, platyspondyly, flared ribs, pectus carinatum, ligamentous laxity, and odontoid hypoplasia. Ocular involvement is sometimes present, and cardiac problems are common and sometimes fatal.

Nomenclature and History

As noted above, Morquio syndrome is commonly referred to as MPS types IVA and IVB. In addition, the disorder is sometimes known as Morquio-Brailsford syndrome or Morquio-Ullrich syndrome. Other, less common names associated with reports of patients include atypical chondrodystrophy, chondrodystrophia tarda, dysostosis enchondralis metaepiphysaria, scaphocephaly, familial skeletal dystrophy, chondro-osteo-dystrophy, hereditary chondrodysplasia, keratosulfaturia, and KS (keratan sulfate)–mucopolysaccharidosis.

Patients with features characteristic of the Morquio syndrome were first described by Sir William Osler[1] in 1897; Osler suggested the name of sporadic cretinism. In 1909, Voison and Voison[2] reported an unusual case of achondroplasia; in 1925, Putnam and Pelkan[3] called the syndrome scaphocephaly. All three groups of patients were considered to have unusual forms of achondroplasia by these authors. In 1929, Professor Luis Morquio[4] of Uruguay first described a form of "familial skeletal dystro-phy" in four Swedish children and defined the syndrome as quite novel and distinctly different from achondroplasia. Professor Morquio (1867–1935) was a famous pediatrician in Montevideo who had a distinguished career; his face even appears on a postage stamp from Uruguay![5] Also in 1929, British radiologist James Brailsford[6] reported the clinical and radiographic findings in a child with a disorder he called "chondro-osteo-dystrophy." All these cases were subsequently identified as forms of MPS type IV. As a result of their publications, the disease became known as Morquio-Brailsford syndrome, a name that is now less commonly used.[7] Two subsequent reports, those by Ruggles[8] in 1931 and by Gasteiger and Liebenam[9] in 1937, further defined the clinical features of the disease. In a comprehensive analysis of multiple genetic disorders published in 1943, Ullrich[10] further defined the Morquio syndrome and added the component of ocular abnormality, which may occur somewhat later in the patient's life. This led to another name for the disorder—Morquio-Ullrich syndrome. Further studies over the next several decades, including those by Whiteside and Cholmeley[11] in 1952, Robinow[12] in 1958, Zellweger and associates[13] in 1961, and Anderson and associates[14] in 1962, defined the clinical and imaging characteristics and established the autosomal recessive character of the disorder. Maroteaux and Lamy[15,16] described the corneal opacities in patients with the disorder and the clinical and radiologic characteristics in the early 1960s. Pedrini and associates[17] first isolated and identified the presence of keratan sulfate in the urine in 1962, and thus helped establish the biochemical causation of the syndrome. As reported by Goidanich and Lenzi[18] in 1964, the orthopaedic spinal problems were sometimes extraordinary in extent and threatening to the patient's function and survival. One of the largest groups of patients was reported by Gadbois and as-

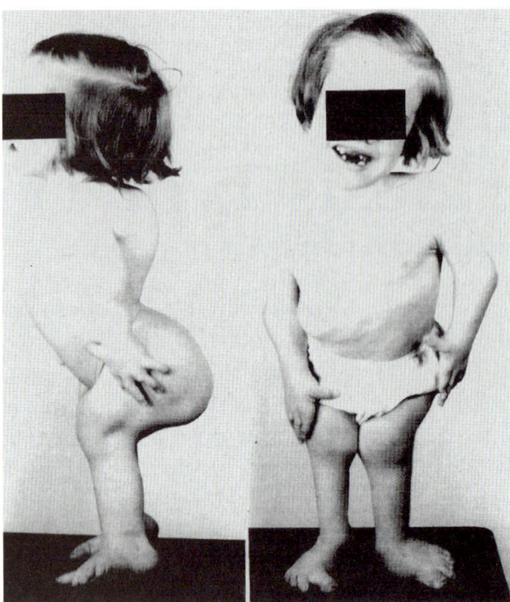

Figure 1
Photograph of an 8-year-old girl with Morquio syndrome. Note the short stature, hand and foot deformities, spinal abnormalities, and poor teeth.

sociates,[19] who described the syndrome in 48 patients in Quebec in 1973. In 1974, Matalon and associates[20] defined an enzyme deficit in β galactosidase sulfatase, which resulted in a defect in both keratan and chondroitin sulfates (type B disease). In 1978, Di Ferrante and associates[21] defined another error in the deficiency of N-acetylgalactosamine 6-sulfate sulfatase (type A disease).

Biology and Genetics

The two forms of Morquio syndrome are MPS type IVA and type IVB.[7,22-24] Both lesions are autosomal recessive errors and occur equally in both sexes.[7,22,23,25] No specific ethnic frequency has been identified, although reports have suggested a high frequency in Canada, Sweden, Australia, and among gypsies.[4,7,19,22,26,27] The chromosomal site for type A is 16q24.3[28] and for type B, 3p21.33.[7] The material that accumulates in both disorders is keratan sulfate,[29] as a result of errors in the synthesis of two degradative enzymes N-acetylgalactosamine-6-sulfate sulfatase for type A[7,20,23,25,30-34] and β-galactosidase sulfatase for type B disease.[7,21,23,25,35,36]

The N-acetylgalactosamine-6-sulfate sulfatase encodes a 522 amino acid protein that is stabilized in a complex with two other lysosomal enzymes (β-galactosidase and α-neurominidase) and a protective protein cathepsin A.[7,32,37] More than 148 unique mutations have been reported for this enzyme.[23,27,30,33,37-41] The β-galactosidase responsible for type B disease occurs in chromosomal site 3p21.33 and encodes a 677 active amino acid protein.[7,23,36,42] At least 50 novel mutations have also been reported for this lesion as well.[26,42-44] Both the type A and type B genetic errors result in the retention of large amounts of keratan sulfate in lysosomal structures within certain cellular sites in the body and the presence of extraordinary concentrations of the material in the serum and urine.[7,23,25,29,30] As a result of the defects, increased urinary excretion of keratan sulfate is an important diagnostic finding for both forms of the disease.[7,17,23,30]

Clinical Findings

Patients with Morquio syndrome type A or B appear normal at birth.[7,16,25,35] Their intellect is not impaired and their body weight and height are essentially normal.[22-25,35,45] The first abnormal physical findings for these patients occur at approximately 2 years of age. Unlike many of the other mucopolysaccharidoses, the patient's facial features are relatively normal and there is no significant organomegaly.[23,24,35,45] In the second or third year of life, the patients are noted to have an awkward gait, retarded growth, knock knees, sternal bulging, flaring of the rib cage, flat feet, and a dorsal kyphosis.[7,18,23,24,35] Although patients with Morquio syndrome are not as reduced in stature as patients with some of the other mucopolysaccharidoses, they are most often shorter than normal and usually are less than 5 feet in height[7,23] (Figure 1).

The patient's cervical spine is abnormal and odontoid hypoplasia is commonly present.[7,18,23,24,46] As the child gets older, the cervical problems may become complex and severe. Atlantoaxial laxity and subluxation may result in high spinal cord compression and is a major complication, especially with type A disease.[7,18,23,46,47] Ligamentous laxity in the lower extremities increases with advancing age and legs tend to buckle. Patients have difficulty walking up and down stairs; much of this problem results from genu valgum, which is sometimes severe[7,18,23,24,45] (Figure 2). Marked deformity may be present in the patient's hands (Figure 3) and feet (Figure 4).

Dental changes are quite distinctive and, as reported by Gardner,[48] may help to identify patients with Morquio syndrome. They also may help to clinically distinguish type A disease from type B. Children with type A disease show abnormalities in both deciduous and permanent teeth. The changes consist of thinness of enamel, fractures and flaking, and a dull, gray color to the crowns of the teeth.[7,22,48-50] Molars are sharp, and all the teeth are subject to caries as the children get older.[48-50] Dental abnormalities in type B disease are usually far less evident.

Ocular changes are sometimes severe, particularly for patients with type A disease. Corneas become progressively opacified, but clouding is not clinically evident much before 10 years of age.[7,15,22,51,52] Glaucoma may occur, presumably because of accumulation of keratan sulfate in the trabecular meshwork.[53] Retinal problems have also been reported.[51]

Progressive deafness usually has its onset in the teens and gradually increases.[7,47]

Cardiac involvement and aortic valve incompetence are well-recognized occurrences in patients with Morquio syndrome.[7,22,23,54] These seem to occur primarily in relation to spinal deformity, thoracic malalignment, and aortic structural abnormality.[7,54] Respiratory paralysis may occur in relation to cervical cord compression.[22,24,46,54,55] The cardiorespiratory complications are most often the cause of early demise for patients, particularly those with type A disease.[7]

Histology and Radiographic Changes

The histologic findings in children with Morquio syndrome are quite distinctive. Many cells have membrane-bound inclusions containing keratan sulfate.[7,34] Cartilage cells from epiphyseal plates or from articular surfaces also may show accumulation of glycosaminoglycans and vacuolation.[14] The cartilage in the calcified zone of the articular cartilage is reduced in concentration.[14,45,56] Bone quantity appears to be normal in long bones but markedly reduced in the abnormal vertebrae, particularly in the cervical spine.[46,57]

The radiographic changes are chiefly no-

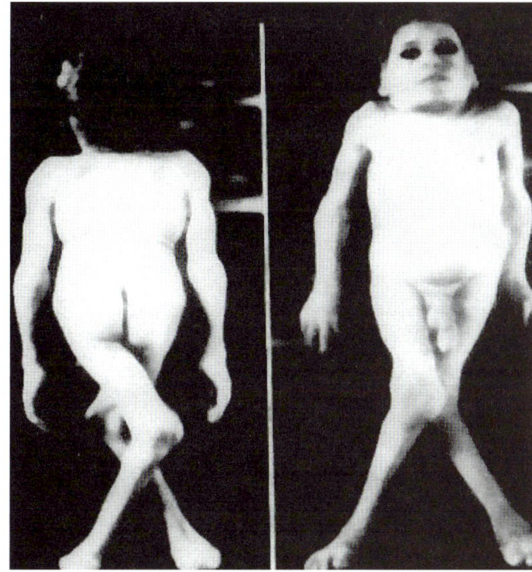

Figure 2

A 16-year-old male with short stature, facial abnormality, marked genu valgum, and foot deformity.

ticeable in the spine, which shows marked platyspondyly with kyphosis and thoracic deformity.[7,16,22,58] The vertebral bodies are flattened and rectangular, with widened disk spaces.[18,46,47,58] The odontoid process is hypoplastic or absent.[7,23,47] Flaring of the iliac wings is typical and, although the hips are normal in appearance early in the course, they often show coxa valga and progressive flattening and fragmentation of the joint surface with advancing years.[18,23,59] The distal radius and ulna are inclined toward each other, and knock-knee deformity is common and associated with early destructive changes in both ankles and knees.[7,18] Carpal and tarsal centers are small and retarded in development.[23]

Treatment

Patients with Morquio type B are, as a rule, less severely affected than those with type A and sometimes do not require treatment other than periodic observation.[60]

No medications are currently used to reverse the development of the disorder. Specifically, although enzyme treatment has been devised and used for other types of lysosomal storage diseases including several mucopolysaccharidoses, none is currently available for patients with Morquio syndrome. Bone marrow transplantation has been suggested, but there is very limited information regarding the value of this protocol.[61]

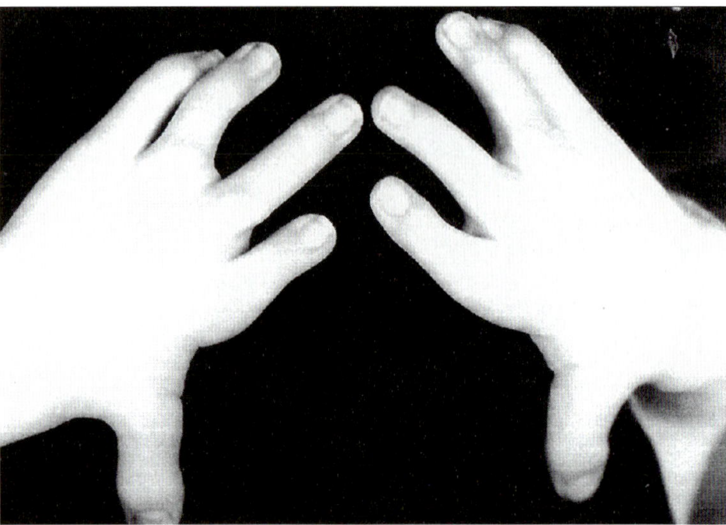

Figure 3
Malformation of the hand with an abnormal thumb in a patient with Morquio syndrome.

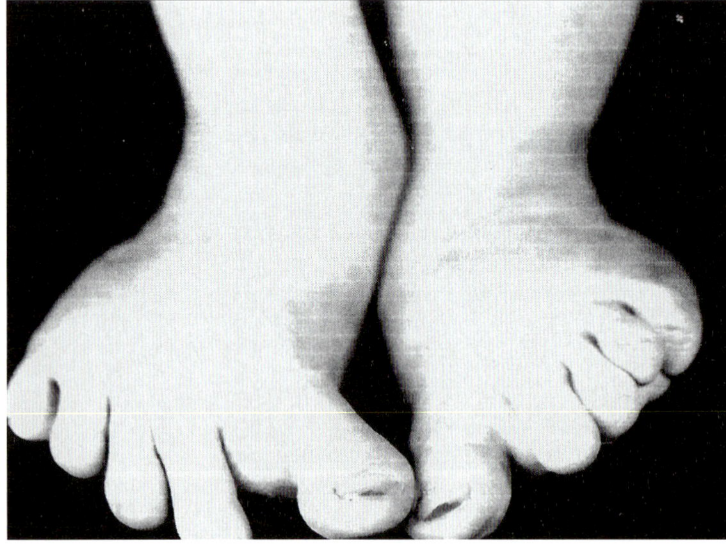

Figure 4
Irregularity of the structure of the foot seen in a patient with Morquio syndrome.

The cervical and thoracic spines of children with Morquio syndrome must be carefully and frequently evaluated for evidence of cord compression. Arthrodeses of C1 and C2 to the occiput may be necessary to decrease potential damage to the central nervous system.[46] The cardiac and aortic status is also critical. These areas of complications are most severe and are potentially life-threatening.[46,47,55] Corrective surgery may be required, but anesthesia is sometimes very complex.[7,55]

Ocular problems may require surgery to decrease corneal damage.[51-53,60]

Orthopaedic management is often required to improve quality of life, but is sometimes difficult to apply.[18,45,56,59] Bracing of the spine, wrists, and feet is sometimes helpful.[7] Genu valgum may require surgical correction; coxa vara and other hip difficulties may require osteotomies or, as the patient ages, total joint arthroplasty.[7,18,45,56,59]

Conclusions

Morquio syndrome is an uncommon form of MPS that is quite different from the other members of this family of disorders. Patients are less disabled, have good mentation, and, although short, are initially quite functional. Their problems are principally orthopaedic and more specifically related to severe alterations in the cervical and thoracic spine, which lead to neurologic and cardiac failure. In addition, they become functionally impaired because of ligamentous laxity; poor structure of knees, hips, hands, and feet; and ultimately can become crippled and require difficult surgery to correct their problems.

As is well known, some of the other genetic lysosomal storage diseases—including MPS type I; Pompe, Fabry, and Gaucher diseases; and several others—are currently being treated with enzymes that at least partially improve patients' conditions. It would seem logical to attempt to introduce β-galactosidase or, more logically, N-acetylgalactosamine-sulfate sulfatase in an attempt to alter the Morquio syndrome and restore the patient to better health. If this can be done early in the child's life, the cervical and other orthopaedic disorders may be corrected. What a happy circumstance that might represent!

References:

1. Osler W: Sporadic cretinism in America. *Trans Congr Am Phys Surg* 1897;4:169-206.

2. Voison J, Voison R: Un cas d'achondroplasie. *Encephale* 1909;4:221-227.

3. Putnam MC, Pelkan KF: A case of scaphocephaly with malformation of skeleton and other tissues. *Am J Dis Child* 1925;29:51-58.

4. Morquio L: Sur une forme de dystrophie osseuse familiale. *Arch Med Enf* 1929;32:129-140.

5. Chudley AE, Chakrovorty C: Genetic landmarks through philately: Luís Morquio 1867-1935. *Clin Genet* 2002;62:438-439.

6. Brailsford JF: Chondro-osteo-dystrophy: Roentgenographic and clinical features of a child with dislocation of vertebrae. *Am J Surg* 1929;7:404-410.

7. Whitly CB: Mucopolysaccharides Type IV, in Beighton P (ed): *McKusick's Heritable Disorders of Connective Tissue*, ed 5. St. Louis, MO, Mosby, 1993, pp 431-441.

8. Ruggles HE: Dwarfism due to disordered epiphyseal development. *AJR Am J Roentgenol* 1931;25:91-94.

9. Gasteiger H, Liebenam L: Beitrag zur dysostosis multiplex unter besonderer beruchsichtigung des augenbefundes. *Klin Monastbl Augenheilkd* 1937;99:433-447.

10. Ullrich O: Die Pfaundler-Hurlersche Krankheit. Dysotosis multiplex (Hurler)-Dysostotische idiotie (Hassler)-familiar-dysostotischer zwergwuchs; typ-Pfaundler-Hurler (De Ridder)-Gargoylismus (Ellis-Sheldon und Capon). Ein beitrag zum problem pleiotroper Gerwirkung in der erbpathologie des menschen. *Erg Inn Med Kidnerh* 1943;63:929-1000.

11. Whiteside JD, Cholmeley JA: Morquio's disease: Review of the literature with a description of four cases. *Arch Dis Child* 1952;27:487-497.

12. Robinow M: Morquio's disease. *Clin Orthop Relat Res* 1958;11:138-153.

13. Zellweger H, Ponseti IV, Pedrini V, Stamler FS, von Noorden G: Morquio-Ullrich's disease: Report of 2 cases. *J Pediatr* 1961;59:549-561.

14. Anderson CE, Crane JT, Harper HA, Hunter TW: Morquio's disease and dysplasia epiphysealis multiplex: A study of epiphyseal cartilage in seven cases. *J Bone Joint Surg Am* 1962;44:295-306.

15. Maroteaux P, Lamy M: Corneal opacities and metabolic disorders in Morquio's disease. *Rev Franc Etud Clin Biol* 1961;6:481-483.

16. Maroteaux P, Lamy M, Foucher M: Morquio's disease: Clinical, radiological and biological study. *Presse Med* 1963;71:2091-2094.

17. Pedrini V, Lennzi L, Zambotti V: Isolation and identification of keratosulphate in urine of patients affected by Morquio-Ullrich disease. *Proc Soc Exp Biol Med* 1962;110:847-849.

18. Goidanich IF, Lenzi L: Morquio-Ullrich disease: A new mucopolysaccharidosis. *J Bone Joint Surg Am* 1964;46:734-746.

19. Gadbois P, Moreau J, Laberge C: Morquio's disease of the province of Quebec. *Union Med Can* 1973;102:602-607.

20. Matalon R, Arbogast B, Justice P, Brandt IK, Dorfman A: Morquio's syndrome: A deficiency of chondroitin sulfate N-acetylhexosamine sulfate sulfatase. *Biochem Biophys Res Commun* 1974;61:759-765.

21. Di Ferrante N, Ginsburg LC, Donnelly PV, Di Ferrante DT, Caskey CT: Deficiences of glucosamine–6-sulfate or galactosamine–6-sulfatases are responsible for different mucopolysaccharidoses. *Science* 1978;199:79-81.

22. Montaño AM, Tomatsu S, Gottesman GS, Smith M, Orii T: International Morquio A Registry: Clinical manifestations and natural course of Morquio A disease. *J Inherit Metab Dis* 2007;30:165-174.

23. Neufeld EF, Muenzer J: The mucopolysaccharidoses, in Scriver CR, Beaudet AL, Sly WS (eds): *The Metabolic and Molecular Bases of Inherited Disease*, ed 8. New York, NY, McGraw-Hill, 2001, pp 3421-3452.

24. Northover H, Cowie RA, Wraith JE: Mucopolysaccharidoses type IVA (Morquio syndrome): A clinical review. *J Inherit Metab Dis* 1996;19:357-365.

25. McKusick VA: The nosology of the mucopolysaccharidoses. *Am J Med* 1969;47:730-747.

26. Santamaria R, Chabás A, Coll MJ, Miranda CS, Vilageliu L, Grinberg D: Twenty-one novel mutations in the GLB1 gene identified in a large group of GM1-gangliosidosis and Morquio B patients: Possible common origin for the prevalent p.R59H mutation among gypsies. *Hum Mutat* 2006;27:1060.

27. Yamada N, Fukuda S, Tomatsu S, et al: Molecular heterogeneity in mucopolysaccharidosis IVA in Australia and Northern Ireland: Nine novel mutations including T312S, a common allele that confers a mild phenotype. *Hum Mutat* 1998;11:202-208.

28. Baker E, Guo XH, Osborn AM, et al: The Morquio A syndrome (mucopolysaccharidosis IVA) gene maps to 16q24.3. *Am J Hum Genet* 1993;52:96-98.

29. Funderburgh JL: Keratan sulfate: Structure, biosynthesis and function. *Glycobiology* 2000;10:951-958.

30. Ogawa T, Tomatsu S, Fukuda S, et al: Mucopolysaccharidosis IVA: Screening and identification of mutations of the N-acetylgalactosamine-6-sulfate sulfatase gene. *Hum Mol Genet* 1995;4:341-349.

31. Parkinson-Lawrence EJ, Muller VJ, Hopwood JJ, Brooks DA: N-acetylgalactosamine-6-sulfatase protein detection in MPS IVA patient and unaffected samples. *Clin Chim Acta* 2007;377:88-91.

32. Tomatsu S, Nishioka T, Montaño AM, et al: Mucopolysaccharidosis IVA: Identification of mutations and methylation study in GALNS gene. *J Med Genet* 2004;41:e98-e104.

33. Tomatsu S, Montaño AM, Nishioka T, et al: Mutation and polymorphism spectrum of the GALNS gene in mucopolysaccharidosis IVA (Morquio A). *Hum Mutat* 2005;26:500-512.

34. Yuen M, Fensom AH: Diagnosis of classical Morquio's disease: N-acetylgalactosamine 6-sulphatase activity in cultured fibroblasts, leukocytes, amniotic cells and chorionic villi. *J Inherit Metab Dis* 1985;8:80-86.

35. Beck M, Petersen EM, Spranger J, Beighton P: Morquio disease type B (beta-galactosidase deficiency) in three siblings. *S Afr Med J* 1987;72:704-707.

36. Okumiya T, Sakuraba H, Kase R, Sugiura T: Imbalanced substrate specificity of mutant beta-galactosidase in patients with Morquio B disease. *Mol Genet Metab* 2003;78:51-58.

37. Sukegawa K, Nakamura H, Kao Z, et al: Biochemical and structural analysis of missense mutations in N-acetylgalactosamine-6-sulfate sulfatase causing mucoplysaccharidosis IVA phenotypes. *Hum Mol Genet* 2000;9:1283-1290.

38. Bunge S, Kleijer WJ, Tylki-Szymanska A, et al: Identification of 31 novel mutations in the N-acetylgalactosamine-6-sulfatase gene reveals excessive allelic heterogeneity among patients with Morquio A syndrome. *Hum Mutat* 1997;10:223-232.

39. Kato Z, Fukuda S, Tomatsu S, et al: A novel common missense mutation G301C in the N-acetylgalactosamine-6-sulfate sulfatase gene in mucopolysaccharidosis IVA. *Hum Genet* 1997;101:97-101.

40. Tomatsu S, Fukuda S, Cooper A, et al: Fifteen polymorphisms in N-acetylgalactosamine-sulfate sulfatase (GALNS) gene: Diagnostic implications in Morquio disease. *Hum Mutat* 1998;1:S42-S46.

41. Tomatsu S, Montaño AM, Lopez P, et al: Determinant factors of spectrum of missense variants in mucopolysaccharidosis IVA gene. *Mol Genet Metab* 2006;89:139-149.

42. Bagshaw RD, Zhang S, Hinek A, et al: Novel mutations (Asn 484 Lys, Thr 500 Ala, Gly 438 Glu) in Morquio B disease. *Biochim Biophys Acta* 2002;1588:247-253.

43. Oshima A, Yoshida K, Shimmoto M, Fukuhara Y, Sakuraba H, Suzuki Y: Human beta-galactosidase gene mutations in morquio B disease. *Am J Hum Genet* 1991;49:1091-1093.

44. Paschke E, Milos I, Kreimer-Erlacher H, et al: Mutation analyses in 17 patients with deficiency in acid beta-galactosidase: Three novel point mutations and high correlation of mutation W273L with Morquio disease type B. *Hum Genet* 2001;109:159-166.

45. Kalteis T, Schubert T, Caro WC, Schröder J, Lüring C, Grifka J: Arthroscopic and histologic findings in Morquio's syndrome. *Arthroscopy* 2005;21:233-237.

46. Rigante D, Antuzzi D, Ricci R, Segni G: Cervical myelopathy in mucopolysaccharidosis type IV. *Clin Neuropathol* 1999;18:84-86.

47. Sataloff RT, Schiebel BR, Spiegel JR: Morquio syndrome. *Am J Otol* 1987;8:443-449.

48. Gardner DG: The dental manifestations of the Morquio syndrome (mucopolysaccharidosis type IV): A diagnostic aid. *Am J Dis Child* 1975;129:1445-1448.

49. Barker D, Welbury RR: Dental findings in Morquio syndrome (mucopolysaccharidosis type IVa). *ASDC J Dent Child* 2000;67:431-433.

50. Rølling I, Clausen N, Nyvad B, Sindet-Pedersen S: Dental findings in three siblings with Morquio's syndrome. *Int J Paediar Dent* 1999;9:219-224.

51. Dangel ME, Tsou BH: Retinal involvement in Morquio's syndrome (MPS IV). *Ann Ophthalmol* 1985;17:349-354.

52. Iwamoto M, Nawa Y, Maumenee IH, Young-Ramsaran J, Matalon R, Green WR: Ocular histopathology and ultrastructure of Morquio syndrome (systemic mucopolysaccharidosis IVA). *Graefes Arch Clin Exp Ophthalmol* 1990;228:342-349.

53. Cahane M, Treister G, Abraham FA, Melamed S: Glaucoma in siblings with Morquio syndrome. *Br J Ophthalmol* 1990;74:382-383.

54. Barry MO, Beardslee MA, Braverman AC: Morquio's syndrome: Severe aortic regurgitation and late pulmonary autograft failure. *J Heart Valve Dis* 2006;15:839-842.

55. Shinhar SY, Zablocki H, Madgy DN: Airway management in mucopolysaccharide storage disorders. *Arch Otolaryngol Head Neck Surg* 2004;130:233-237.

56. de Waal Malefijt MC, van Kampen A, van Gemund JJ: Total knee arthroplasty in patients with inherited dwarfism—a report of five knee replacements in two patients with Morquio's disease type A and one with spondylo-epiphyseal displasia. *Arch Orthop Trauma Surg* 2000;120:179-182.

57. Rigante D, Buonuomo PS, Caradonna P: Early-onset osteoporosis with high bone turnover in children with Morquio-Brailsford syndrome. *Rheumatol Int* 2006;26:1163-1164.

58. Langer LO Jr, Carey LS: The roentgenographic features of the KS mucopolysaccharidosis of Morquio (Morquio-Brailsford's disease). *Am J Roentgenol Radium Ther Nucl Med* 1966;97:1-20.

59. Kanazawa T, Yasunaga Y, Ikuta Y, Harada A, Kusaka O, Sukegawa K: Femoral head dysplasia in Morquio disease type A: Bilateral varus osteotomy of the femur. *Acta Orthop Scand* 2001;72:18-21.

60. Onçağ G, Ertan Erdinç AM, Cal E: Multidisciplinary treatment approach of Morquio syndrome (Mucopolysaccharidosis Type IVA). *Angle Orthod* 2006;76:335-340.

61. Hoogerbrugge PM, Brouwer OF, Bordigoni P, et al: Alllogeneic bone marrow transplantation for lysosomal storage diseases: The European Group for Bone Marrow Transplantation. *Lancet* 1995;345:1398-1402.

Maroteaux-Lamy Syndrome: Mucopolysaccharidosis Type VI

The mucopolysaccharidoses are a series of genetic disorders, all caused by the failure to synthesize materials that degrade the glycosaminoglycans (GAGs) keratan sulfate, heparan sulfate, dermatan sulfate, and/or chondroitin sulfate. These large molecules materially affect multiple organ systems in patients and result in an array of sometimes very disabling and life-threatening clinical problems including short stature; mental retardation; and orthopaedic, ocular, oral, neurologic, and cardiovascular abnormalities. Type VI disease was first described in 1965 by Pierre Maroteaux and Maurice Lamy[1] and appears to result from an enzymatic defect in N-acetylgalactosamin-4-sulfatase, also known as arylsulfatase B, which causes persistence of dermatan sulfate and is responsible for the clinical and biologic abnormalities. The disorder is in many ways milder and less threatening than some of the other mucopolysaccharidoses but still materially impairs the life of the patient.

Nomenclature and history of mucopolysaccharidosis type VI

Mucopolysaccharidosis (MPS) type VI is also known as Maroteaux-Lamy syndrome, arylsulfatase deficiency, polydystrophic dwarfism, and MPS VI.

Additional mucopolysaccharidoses other than Hurler's or Hunter's diseases were first identified in 1952 by Brante.[2] Dorfman[3] later defined the cause of these as being related to a failure in the metabolism of mucopolysaccharides. Maroteaux and Lamy[1] described a clinical entity in an article published in 1965 and separated it from Hurler's and Morquio's disorders based on clinical and biologic differences they and their associates first noted in 1963.[4] Patients with this disorder were not mentally retarded and had fewer early ocular, neurologic, or cardiac problems. In 1970, the clinical characteristics of the syndrome were further clarified by Spranger and associates[5]

and Goldberg and associates.[6] Reports by Baron and Neufeld,[7] O'Brien and associates,[8] Kelly,[9] and Pilz and associates[10] later that decade helped to define some of the biologic aspects of this rare disorder.

Pathophysiology

As is well known, the mucopolysaccharidoses are a group of inherited disorders that result from a deficiency of one or more enzymes required for GAG metabolism.[11,12] The GAGs are normally present in connective tissues, especially cartilage and the skeleton, but also within heart valves, ocular structures, and the oral cavity. Hence, any insufficiency in the amount of enzyme required to appropriately destroy the GAGs may lead to a series of systemic disorders known as the mucopolysaccharidoses. The autosomal recessive genetic error may affect dermatan sulfate (type I, type VI, or type VII), heparan sulfate (type I, type III, or type VII), keratan sulfate (type IV), or chondroitin sulfate (type VII).

Maroteaux-Lamy syndrome has been defined as showing an error in gene 5q13.3; the resultant defective enzyme is N-acetylgalactosamine-4-sulfatase (also known as arylsulfatase B), which is required to appropriately degrade dermatan sulfate.[13,14] More than 40 mutations have been discovered in 10 or more separate alleles that affect the degradation to different degrees.[15-22] As a result, various authors have described the disorder as being severe, moderate, or mild.[11,19,23,24] Because of the numbers of mutations, the clinical patterns resulting from the heterogeneity are somewhat variable. The biochemical nature and extent of the disease may be assessed by determination of dermatan sulfate in the urine (a condition known as dermatan sulfaturia), by the presence of Reilly granules in the lysosomal bodies of the white cells,[25-27] or by the Berry spot test.[28]

Of some importance is the presence of an almost identical genetic syndrome in

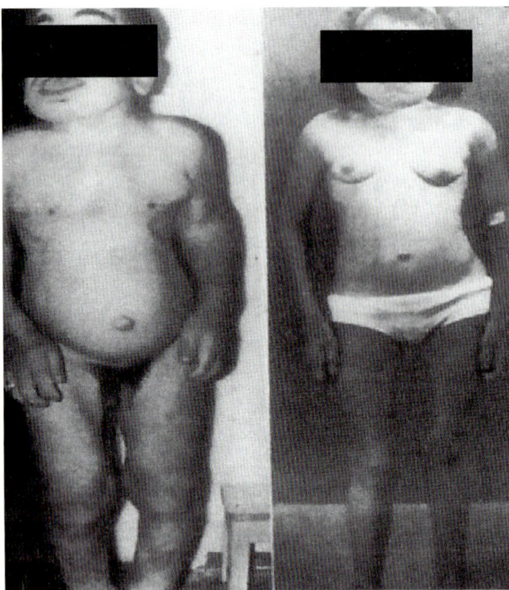

Figure 1

Photographs of two patients with Maroteaux-Lamy syndrome. Both are dwarfed and show lumbar kyphosis, sternal protuberance, and genu valgum, all of which add to the decreased height pattern. All these changes become somewhat worse with advancing age.

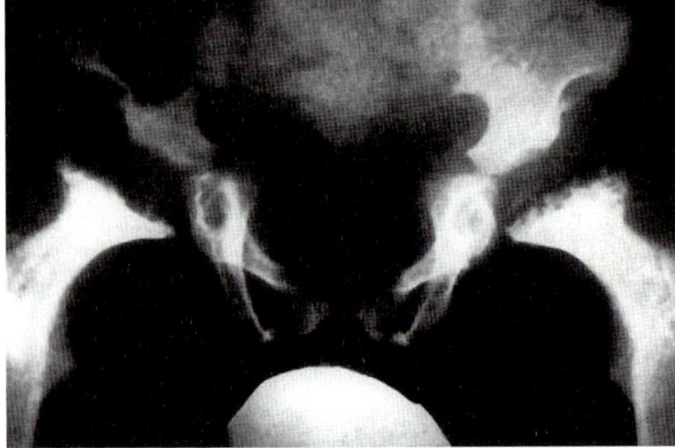

Figure 2

Changes in the pelvis are quite remarkable, with iliac wing flaring, small acetabulae, and irregular ossification of the femoral heads. This patient has modest coxa valga as well.

Siamese cats.[29-31] This has allowed scientists to study some of the biologic features and, as a result, introduce sometimes quite effective treatment protocols in this group of animals.[29,32,33]

Clinical Presentation

Regardless of the type of error and the degree of severity, Maroteaux-Lamy syndrome is transmitted as an autosomal recessive disorder. There is no difference in the relative frequency in males and females. The disease is rare and, although ethnic frequency in South Americans has been proposed, there is little evidence to support this distribution.[11,12,20,23]

Growth retardation is first noted at 2 to 3 years of age and is characterized by stunting of the trunk and limbs.[12,22] Lumbar kyphosis, sternal protuberance, and genu valgum add to the decreased height pattern and become somewhat worse with advancing age[22] (Figure 1). Facial features are moderately distorted, but not nearly as much as in patients with Hurler or Morquio syndrome[22] (Figure 1). Dentiginous cysts are common, as is irregularity of dental structure.[34]

The hands are remarkably involved, with sometimes severe carpal tunnel disease and restricted digital movement.[35-37] The subcutaneous tissues over the volar surface of the hands are thickened, contributing to the poor function of the digits. The skull is often severely involved and is quite similar to the changes seen in patients with MPS type I (Hurler's disease).[12,22] Mild cases have much less facial or oral deformity.[38]

Corneal opacities are common and occur quite early in the child's life.[6,22,39] The cornea is increased in thickness and clouding is noted at the periphery.[6] Glaucoma is frequently seen and must be treated to prevent blindness.[39]

Skeletal problems can be quite striking.[12,22,23,33] The diaphyses of the long bones are moderately expanded and a characteristic constriction at the metaphysis may be noted. Changes in the pelvis are quite remarkable, with iliac wing flaring, small acetabulae, and irregular ossification of the femoral heads[12,22] (Figure 2). As the child ages, the appearance of the hips suggests early subluxation.[11,22] Imaging studies show narrowing of the vertebral ends of the ribs with widening of the anterior aspects.[12] Medial clavicles are expanded and the scapulae are small. Radiographs of the spine show defects in the vertebral segments, producing a pointed compression that can lead to serious spinal impairment (Figure 3).

Serious cardiovascular abnormalities are frequent.[40-42] Patients have murmurs and abnormal valve functions that are detected even quite early in childhood.[42] Cardiac involvement, with myocarditis, aortic and ventricular aneurysms, and heart failure are common causes of death in these pa-

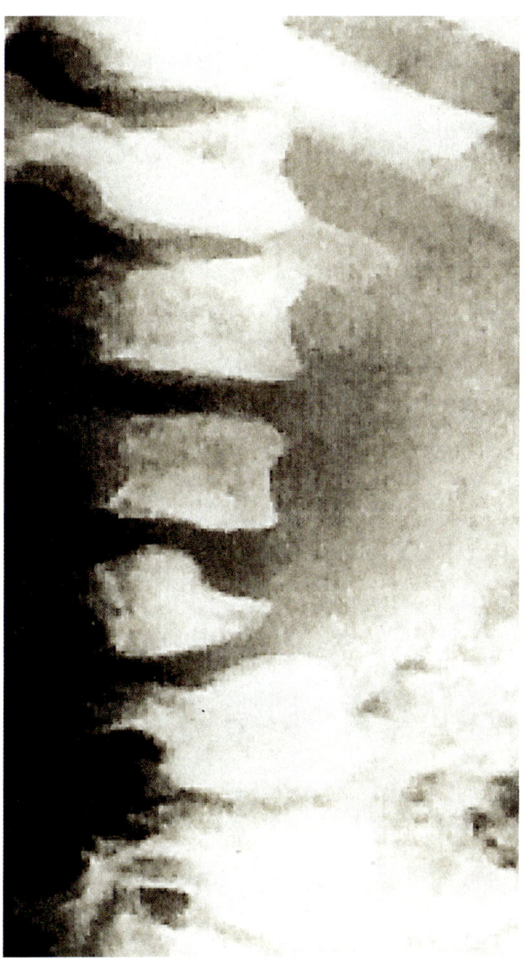

Figure 3

Spinal abnormalities are frequent and sometimes disabling. Radiographs show defects in the vertebral segments, producing a pointed compression that can lead to serious spinal impairment.

tients.[41,43] Airway changes may also occur.[44]

Mentation is most often normal, although with advancing years, children become somewhat demented.[12] However, neurologic abnormalities are quite frequent.[45] These include hydrocephalus, spastic paraplegia, compressive myelopathy, and deafness.[22,46-48]

Treatment

Patients with mild or even moderate forms of Maroteaux-Lamy syndrome may require little treatment. After 2 or more years, they are noted to have normal mentation but begin to undergo changes in their skeletal structure, stature, and ocular function, and have some difficulties with ambulation and neurologic status. Several authors have proposed studies to catalog the patient's disabil-

ities; these can be defined biologically by study of their urinary output of dermatan sulfate, presence of Reilly granules in the peripheral white cells, and, most recently, determination of the serum concentration of arylsulfatase B.[12-14,16,20,23,26-28,49] A recent report suggests that the 6-minute walk test is helpful in defining the extent of the patient's cardiac and pulmonary problems.[49,50]

Corneal dystrophy and glaucoma may require surgical procedures to improve vision,[6,14,22,39] and surgical repair may be necessary for oral and dental structural changes.[12,14,34,38] Cardiac and respiratory changes may be life-threatening and require pharmacologic treatment or sometimes corrective surgery.[14,22,40,42-44] Carpal tunnel surgery may be necessary, along with other orthopaedic procedures to improve function and prevent fractures or dislocations.[12,22,35-37] Hydrocephalus and neurologic problems are sometimes difficult to treat effectively, even with surgery.[22,46,48,51]

Biologic treatment of patients with MPS type VI is perhaps the most extensive for any of the lysosomal diseases. Administration of recombinant arylsulfatase B has been attempted and has shown great success in cats[29,32] and moderate success in human patients.[12,14,52-55] Moderate and more prolonged improvement has resulted from marrow replacement with allogenic cells or cells from a sibling who does not have the disease.[14,56-58] Stem cells, especially those obtained from the umbilical cord, seem to help patients grow and reduce some of the ocular and cardiac abnormalities.[12,14,59,60]

Conclusions

Maroteaux-Lamy syndrome is a form of MPS that has enabled clinicians and scientists to work closely together to not only effectively define the nature of the disease, but more importantly to develop biologic methods of treatment. Because of the feline model, it has been possible to introduce an array of approaches to improving the state of the disease. These have included enzyme replacement, bone marrow transplant, and stem cell treatment; all of these have considerably improved the condition of patients. No treatment has thus far "cured" them, but early utilization of some of the protocols has led to a fairly marked change in the patient's status and survival. It would be of considerable importance to attempt to alter the gene error. Certainly that would be the next approach, but it may be difficult to achieve. In any event, the success with these patients has encouraged physicians and research workers

to approach the other five mucopolysaccharidoses to assess whether they can also be modified in ways that will not only improve the status of the patients but bring some joy to their families.

References

1. Maroteaux P, Lamy M: Hurler's disease, Morquio's disease and related mucopolysaccharidoses. *J Pediatr* 1965;67:312-323.

2. Brante G: Gargoylism: A mucopolysaccharidosis. *Scand J Clin Lab Invest* 1952;4:43-46.

3. Dorfman A: Metabolism of acid mucopolysaccharides. *Biophys J* 1964;4:155-165.

4. Maroteaux P, Leveque B, Marie J, Lamy M: A new dysostosis with urinary elimination of chondroitin sulfate B. *Presse Med* 1963;71:1849-1852.

5. Spranger JW, Koch F, McKusick VA, Natzschka J, Wiedemann HR, Zellweger H: Mucopolysaccharidosis VI (Maroteaux-Lamy's disease). *Helv Paediatr Acta* 1970;25:337-362.

6. Goldberg MF, Scott CI, McKusick VA: Hydrocephalus and papilledema in the Maroteaux-Lamy syndrome (mucopolysaccharidosis VI). *Am J Ophthalmol* 1970;69:969-975.

7. Baron RW, Neufeld EF: A distinct biochemical deficit in the Maroteaux-Lamy syndrome (mucopolysaccharidosis VI). *J Pediatr* 1972;80:114-116.

8. O'Brien JF, Cantz M, Spranger J: Maroteaux-Lamy disease (mucopolysaccharidosis VI) subtype A: Deficiency of N-acetylgalactosamine-4-sulfatase. *Biochem Biophys Res Commun* 1974;60:1170-1177.

9. Kelly TE: The mucopolysaccharidoses and mucolipidoses. *Clin Orthop Relat Res* 1976;114:116-136.

10. Pilz H, von Figura K, Goebel HH: Deficiency of arylsulfatase B in 2 brothers age 40 and 38 years (Maroteaux-Lamy syndrome, type B). *Ann Neurol* 1979;6:315-325.

11. Muenzer J: The mucopolysaccharidoses: A heterogeneous group of disorders with variable pediatric presentations. *J Pediatr* 2004;144:S27-S34.

12. Neufeld EF, Muenzer J: The mucopolysaccharidoses, in Scriver CR, Beaudet AL, Sly WS (eds): *The Metabolic and Molecular Bases of Inherited Disease*, ed 8. New York, NY, McGraw-Hill, 2001, pp 3421-3452.

13. Brooks DA, McCourt PA, Gibson GJ, Ashton LJ, Shutter M, Hopwood JJ: Analysis of N-acetylgalactosamine-4-sulfatase protein and kinetics in mucopolysaccharidosis type VI patients. *Am J Hum Genet* 1991;48:710-719.

14. Giugliani R, Harmatz P, Wraith JE: Management guidelines for mucopolysaccharidosis VI. *Pediatrics* 2007;120:405-418.

15. Bradford TM, Litjens T, Parkinson EJ, Hopwood JJ, Brooks DA: Mucopolysaccharidosis type VI (Maroteaux-Lamy syndrome): A Y210C mutation causes either altered protein handling or altered protein function of N-acetylgalactosamine 4-sulfatase at multiple points in the vacuolar network. *Biochemistry* 2002;41:4962-4971.

16. Isbrandt D, Arlt G, Brooks DA, Hopwood JJ, von Figura K, Peters C: Mucopolysaccharidosis VI (Maroteaux-Lamy syndrome): Six unique arylsulfatase B gene alleles causing variable disease phenotypes. *Am J Hum Genet* 1994;54:454-463.

17. Jin WD, Jackson CE, Desnick RJ, Schuchman EH: Mucopolysaccharidosis type VI: Identification of three mutations in the arylsulfatase B gene of patients with the severe and mild phenotypes provides molecular evidence for genetic heterogeneity. *Am J Hum Genet* 1992;50:795-800.

18. Litjens T, Hopwood JJ: Mucopolysaccharidosis type VI: Structural and clinical implications of mutations in N-acetylgalactosamine-4-sulfatase. *Hum Mutat* 2001;18:282-295.

19. Litjens T, Morris CP, Robertson EF, Peters C, von Figura K, Hopwood JJ: An N-acetyl-galactosamine-4 sulfatase mutation (delta-G238) results in a severe Maroteaux-Lamy phenotype. *Hum Mutat* 1992;1:397-402.

20. Petry MF, Nonemacher K, Sebben JC, et al: Mucopolysaccharidosis type VI: Identification of novel mutations on the arylsulphatase B gene in South American patients. *J Inherit Metab Dis* 2005;28:1027-1034.

21. Villani GR, Balzano N, Vitale D, Saviano M, Pavone V, Di Natale P: Maroteaux-Lamy syndrome: Five novel mutations and their structural localization. *Biochim Biophys Acta* 1999;1453:185-192.

22. Whitly CB: The mucopolysaccharidoses, in Beighton P (ed): *McKusick's Heritable Disorders of Connective Tissue*, ed 5. St. Louis, MO, Mosby, 1993, pp 367-499.

23. Azevedo AC, Schwartz IV, Kalakun L, et al: Clinical and biochemical study of 28 patients with mucopolysaccharidosis type VI. *Clin Genet* 2004;66:208-213.

24. Paterson DE, Harper G, Weston HJ, Mattingley J: Maroteaux-Lamy syndrome, mild form—MPS VI B. *Br J Radiol* 1982;55:805-812.

25. Alder A: Über konstitutionell bedingte Granulationsveraenderungen der Leukocyten. *Dtsch Arch Klin Med* 1939;183:372-378.

26. Levy LA, Lewis JC, Sumner TE: Ultrastructures of Reilly bodies (metachromatic granules) in the Maroteaux-Lamy syndrome (mucopolysaccharidosis VI): A histochemical study. *Am J Clin Pathol* 1980;73:416-422.

27. Reilly WA: The granules in the leukocytes in gargoylism. *Am J Dis Child* 1941;62:489-491.

28. Berry HK: Screening for mucopolysaccharide disorders with the Berry spot test. *Clin Biochem* 1987;20:365-371.

29. Bielicki J, Crawley AC, Davey RC, Varnai JC, Hopwood JJ: Advantages of using same species enzyme for replacement therapy in a feline

model of mucopolysaccharidosis type VI. *J Biol Chem* 1999;274:36335-36343.

30. Crawley AC, Muntz FH, Haskins ME, Jones BR, Hopwood JJ: Prevalence of mucopolysaccharidosis type VI mutations in Siamese cats. *J Vet Intern Med* 2003;17:495-498.

31. Haskins ME: Jezyk PF, Petterson DF: Mucopolysaccharide storage disease in three families of cats with arylsulfatase B deficiency: Leukocyte studies and carrier identification. *Pediatr Res* 1979;13:1203-1210.

32. Crawley AC, Brooks DA, Muller VJ, et al: Enzyme replacement therapy in a feline model of Maroteaux-Lamy syndrome. *J Clin Invest* 1996;97:1864-1873.

33. Simonaro C, D'Angelo M, Haskins ME, Schuchman EH: Joint and bone disease in mucopolysaccharidoses VI and VII: Identification of new therapeutic targets and biomarkers using animal models. *Pediatr Res* 2005;57:701-707.

34. Roberts MW, Barton NW, Constantopoulos G, Butler DP, Donahue AH: Occurrence of multiple dentigerous cysts in a patient with the Maroteaux-Lamy syndrome (mucopolysaccharidosis type VI). *Oral Surg Oral Med Oral Pathol* 1984;58:169-175.

35. Gschwind C, Tonki MA: Carpal tunnel syndrome in children with mucopolysaccharidosis and related disorders. *J Hand Surg Am* 1992;17:44-47.

36. Haddad FS, Jones DH, Vellodi A, Kane N, Pitt MC: Carpal tunnel syndrome in the mucopolysaccharidoses and mucolipidoses. *J Bone Joint Surg Br* 1997;79:576-582.

37. Wraith JE, Alani SM: Carpal tunnel syndrome in the mucopolysaccharidoses and related disorders. *Arch Dis Child* 1990;65:962-963.

38. Alpöz AR, Coker M, Celen E, et al: The oral manifestations of Maroteaux-Lamy syndrome (mucopolysaccharidosis type VI): A case report. *Oral Surg Oral Med Oral Pathol Oral Radiol Endod* 2006;101:632-637.

39. Cantor LB, Disseler JA, Wilson FM II: Glaucoma in the Maroteaux-Lamy syndrome. *Am J Ophthalmol* 1989;108:426-430.

40. Dangel JH: Cardiovascular changes in children with mucopolysaccharide storage diseases and related disorders: Clinical and echocardiographic changes in 64 patients. *Eur J Pediatr* 1998;157:534-538.

41. Oudit GY, Butany J, Willams WG, Clarke JT, Iwanochko RM: Images in cardiovascular medicine: Left ventricular aneurysm associated with mucopolysaccharidosis Type VI syndrome (Maroteaux-Lamy syndrome). *Circulation* 2007;115:e60-e62.

42. Tan CT, Schaff HV, Miller FA Jr, Edwards WD, Karnes PS: Valvular heart disease in four patients with Maroteaux-Lamy syndrome. *Circulation* 1992;85:188-195.

43. Wilson CS, Mankin HT, Pluth JR: Aortic stenosis and mucopolysaccharidosis. *Ann Intern Med* 1980;92:496-498.

44. Shih SL, Lee YJ, Lin SP, Sheu CY, Blickman JG: Airway changes in children with mucopolysaccharidoses. *Acta Radiol* 2002;43:40-43.

45. Peterson DI, Bacchus H, Seaich L, Kelly TE: Myelopathy associated with Maroteaux-Lamy syndrome. *Arch Neurol* 1975;32:127-129.

46. Schwartz GP, Cohen EJ: Hydrocephalus in Maroteaux-Lamy syndrome. *Arch Ophthalmol* 1998;116:400.

47. Walkley SU, Thrall MA, Haskins ME, et al: Abnormal neuronal metabolism and storage in mucopolysaccharidosis type VI (Maroteaux-Lamy) disease. *Neuropathol Appl Neurobiol* 2005;31:536-544.

48. Young R, Kleinman G, Ojemann RG, et al: Compressive myelopathy in Maroteaux-Lamy syndrome: Clinical and pathological findings. *Ann Neurol* 1980;8:336-340.

49. Swiedler SJ, Beck M, Bajbouj M, et al: Threshold effects of urinary glycosaminoglycans and the walk test as indicators of disease progression in a survey of subjects with Mucopolysaccharidosis type VI (Maroteaux-Lamy syndrome). *Am J Med Genet A* 2005;134A:144-150.

50. ATS Committee on Proficiency Standards for Clinical Pulmonary Function Laboratories: ATS statement: Guidelines for the six-minute walk test. *Am J Respir Crit Care Med* 2002;166:111-117.

51. Mut M, Cila A, Varil K, Akalan N: Multilevel myelopathy in Maroteaux-Lamy syndrome and review of the literature. *Clin Neurol Neurosurg* 2005;107:230-235.

52. Auclair D, Hopwood JJ, Brooks DA, Lemontt JF, Crawley AC: Replacement therapy in mucopolysaccharidosis type VI: Advantages of early onset of therapy. *Mol Genet Metab* 2003;78:163-174.

53. Harmatz P, Giugliani R, Schwartz I, et al: Enzyme replacement therapy for mucopolysaccharidosis VI: A phase 3 randomized, double-blind, placebo-controlled, multinational study of recombinant human N-acetylgalactosamine 4-sulfatase (recombinant human arylsulfatase B or rhASB) and follow-on, open-label extension study. *J Pediatr* 2006;148:533-539.

54. Harmatz P, Kramer WG, Hopwood JJ, et al: Pharmacokinetic profile of recombinant human N-acetylgalctosamine 4-sulphatase enzyme replacement therapy in patients with mucopolysaccharidosis VI (Maroteaux-Lamy syndrome): A phase I/II study. *Acta Paediatr Suppl* 2005;94:61-68.

55. Harmatz P, Whitley CB, Waber L, et al: Enzyme replacement therapy in mucopolysaccharidosis VI (Maroteaux-Lamy Syndrome). *J Pediatr* 2004;144:574-580.

56. Herskhovitz E, Young E, Rainer J, et al: Bone marrow transplantation for Maroteaux-Lamy syndrome (MPS VI): Long-term follow-up. *J Inherit Metab Dis* 1999;22:50-62.

57. Krivit W: Maroteaux-Lamy syndrome (mucopolysaccharidosis type VI): Treatment by allogenic bone marrow transplantation in 6 patients and potential for auto-transplantation bone marrow gene insertion. *Int Pediatr* 1992;7:47-52.

58. Krivit W, Pierpont ME, Ayaz K, et al: Bone marrow transplantation in the Maroteaux-Lamy syndrome (mucopolysaccharidosis VI): Biochemical and clinical status 24 months after transplantion. *N Engl J Med* 1984;311:1606-1611.

59. Krivit W: Stem cell bone marrow transplantation in patients with metabolic storage diseases. *Adv Pediatr* 2002;49:359-378.

60. Lee V, Li CK, Shing MM, et al: Umbilical cord blood transplantation for Maroteaux-Lamy syndrome (mucopolysaccharidosis VI). *Bone Marrow Transplant* 2000;26:455-458.

Chapter 31

Clinical Gout and Hyperuricemia

Gout is a series of heterogenous diseases resulting from the deposition of monosodium urate or uric acid crystals in various body parts from hyperuricemic extracellular body fluids. The disease is common and most often consists of deposition in joints (gouty arthritis) or connective tissue elements of the crystalline material (tophi). This frequently causes pain and tenderness (acute gout) or joint damage. The material may also be deposited in the kidney, causing an entity known as gouty nephropathy. The disorder is much more common in men and is often genetically related, particularly in certain ethnic groups. The disorder does not normally occur in creatures other than humans and Dalmatian dogs.

History of Gout

The history of gout is truly a fascinating subject and has resulted in several major contributions by medical historians. Hippocrates described gout in his book written in the 5th century BC, probably the oldest written medical text.[1] Using ancient Greek terminology, he named the foot abnormalities "podagra." Galen first described tophi, occurring particularly around the foot as tender, swollen masses.[2-4] Celsus decided that gout afflicted only the rich and powerful, while other Roman authors stated that the disease was inherited and distinctly familial.[3,4] The term gout comes from the Roman term "gutta," which means "drop," as it was believed that the disease occurred in response to drops of poison falling on the patient's limbs.[2,5-7] In 1679, van Leeuwenhoek, a Dutch scientist, sketched needle-shaped crystals obtained from a gouty tophus.[8] Thomas Sydenham studied the clinical presentation and causation of gout; in 1705, he stated "The gout most commonly seizes such old men, as have lived the most part of their lives tenderly and delicately, allowing themselves freely banquets, wine and by reason of the sloth that attends old age, have quite omitted such exercise as young men are wont to use."[9] Although many famous scientists worked on aspects of the gout syndromes over the years, it is important to mention Wollaston,[10] who in 1797 described concretions in the kidney and joints, and Garrod who first clearly defined the pathogenetic mechanisms for gout and the relationship to the body's uric acid metabolism.[11,12] These works were ignored for more than a century, until McCarty and Hollander[13] found the same materials in the synovial fluid in 1961.

Over the centuries, many famous people have had gout; the reports on these individuals are cited in numerous literature presentations.[2-5,7,14-26] Affected individuals included King Asa of Israel, who reigned from 906 to 867 BC,[15] the Byzantine Emperors (Constantas I, Justinian I, and John V Palaeologus),[23] Nostradamus, Galileo,[27] Charles V of Flanders, Christopher Columbus,[18] Michelangelo,[19,22] King Henry VIII,[9] Samuel Johnson, Alfred Lord Tennyson, Benjamin Franklin, Thomas Jefferson, Kubla Khan, George IV, John Hancock, William Pitt, Benjamin Disraeli, Alexander Hamilton, John Milton, Isaac Newton, and Charles Dickens.[4,6,21] The descriptions of their illnesses and problems related to the disease are quite remarkable and indeed poetic; in some cases, they include medieval paintings of the persons involved with tophaceous bare feet on benches or foot stands.[3,28] One of the most unusual writers on the subject was William Stukeley; in the early 18th century, based on analysis of his personal gout problem, Stukeley extensively described both the disease and a variety of treatment protocols that were used by individuals with gout.[26]

Causes of Hyperuricemia

Gout is a series of heterogeneous disorders including acute gouty arthritis, tophaceous gout, gouty renal disease, and uric acid urolithiasis—all associated with hyperuricemia, a condition in which the serum uric acid concentration is above normal values (greater than 7 mg/dL).[4,6,29-35] Patients with hyperuricemia may be asymptomatic or the uric acid elevation may be associated with renal failure, diabetes, alcoholism, obesity, lead intoxication, cyclosporine treatment, renal transplantation, and/or a series of other unusual disorders.[4,6,29,33-41] Syndromes associated with hyperuricemia include two genetic errors that are characterized by a hypoxanthine-guanine phosphoribosyltransferase (HPRT) deficiency. The first of these, Lesch-Nyhan syndrome, is a complete HPRT deficiency presenting in affected children as choreoathetosis, growth and mental retardation, spasticity, self-mutilation, and marked hyperuricemia.[4,6,33-35,42] The second is the Kelley-Seegmiller syndrome, which is a milder condition with few neurologic problems but often severe hyperuricemia, based on a partial deficiency of HPRT.[4,6] Other unusual causes of secondary hyperuricemia include deficiency of glucose-6-phosphatase (von Gierke's disease), deficiency of fructose-1-phosphate aldolase, or increased degradation of adenosine triphosphate in association with chronic illness.[4,6,29] The other form of hyperuricemia, which is by far the most common, is that associated with classical gout arthritic and tophaceous disease and seems to be ethnically prevalent and familial. Although some recent reports defined a uromodulin gene error as a cause, and another defined a hyperuricemic nephropathy associated with a hepatocyte nuclear factor-1β gene mutation, there is still no classic form of identified gene error to account for the occurrence of hyperuricemic gout.[6,35,41,43-46]

It is important to distinguish gout from another entity known as pseudogout, which is caused by deposition of calcified materials in relation to such disorders as hyperparathyroidism, renal osteodystrophy, alkaptonuric ochronosis, or even diffuse idiopathic skeletal hyperostosis (DISH).[6] All of these show calcification in the soft tissues on imaging studies, whereas urate crystals are not radiopaque.[6,30]

International Incidence of Gout

The ancient history of gout exceeds that of human origin. A recent study has supported the findings of uric acid deposits in a tyran-nosaurus rex.[47] Furthermore, there is ample evidence for the disorder's presence in Dalmatian dogs[48] and, much less commonly, in some great apes.[6]

In humans, hyperuricemia or gout have been described in 2% to 18% of various populations studied.[2,4,6,29,32,33,45,49] People of British origin, including those in Australia and New Zealand, have a higher rate than those from other countries in Europe.[50] The disease seems to be much more prevalent in blacks living in the United States than those living in Africa.[51] The rates among the Maoris in New Zealand, the Chamorros and Carolinians of the Mariana Islands, and the Aborigines in Taiwan are extraordinarily high.[4,6]

The disease is far more common in men than in women. Ninety-five percent of patients with gouty arthritis are males.[4,6] Although females comprise less than 6% in all series, the concentration of serum urate (ordinarily < 6 mg/dL for all women) rises after menopause.[4] Although hyperuricemia is present in approximately 5% of the population and may be found at an earlier age, gout is a disease of the elderly; the average age for patients with tophi, podagra, or renal disease is almost always greater than 50 years.[4,6,29,35,41,45,49]

Mechanism of Production of Hyperuricemia

The parent compound for uric acid is a purine base composed of a six-member pyrimidine ring fused to a five-member imidazole ring.[4,6,29,32,35] Purine nucleosides are composed of a purine base plus a pentose that is joined to the base by an N-glucosyl bond. Purine is synthesized by the conversion of phosphoribosylpyrophosphate (PRPP) to 5'-phosphoribsylamine, catalyzed by the enzyme amidophosphoribosyltransferase (amido PRT). The purine nucleosides are cleaved by a purine nucleoside phosphorylase, which results in the release of adenine, guanine, hypoxanthine, and xanthine. Adenine and guanine are actually helpful in that they decrease the production of uric acid, but hypoxanthine and xanthine are responsible for the production of uric acid. Hypoxanthine is oxidized to xanthine by xanthine oxidase and then further oxidized to uric acid, usually in the liver. Animals (except for the Dalmatian dog) have the ability to eliminate uric acid by action of uricase, which produces a benign material known as alantoin along with carbon dioxide. The breakdown of uric acid is essential to sufficiently diminish the concentration to avoid deposition of crystals in soft tissue, joints, and renal structures. Regrettably, humans cannot do that; as a result, if the concentration of uric acid rises, they are susceptible to the disorders known since very early days as gout.[4,6,29,32,33]

Once uric acid is formed in the liver, it is released into the circulation, where a small amount (< 4%) is bound to albumin or globulin. In males, the unbound urate pool is estimated at 1,200 mg, with a considerably lower value for females (< 600 mg). The turnover rate for males is approximately 700 mg/d. The values for patients with asymptomatic gout are considerably greater, with a range of 2,000 to 4,000 mg, but in patients with tophaceous gout this can be as high as 30,000 mg or more.[4,6,29] Clinical disorders that lead to increased purine synthesis or urate production include myeloproliferative disorders, polycythemia vera, malignant diseases, psoriasis, obesity, tissue hypoxia, alcoholism, purine-rich diet, excess Vitamin B12, cylotoxic drugs, and warfarin administration.[4,6,29,31,32,36-38,40,41,44,45] Decreased renal clearance of urates may result from renal failure, lead neuropathy, hypertension, dehydration, salt restriction, starvation, lactic acidosis, sarcoidosis, and several drugs, including diuretics, ethambutol, pyrazinamide, and cyclosporine.[4,6,29,32,45]

Histologic Images of Gout

The characteristic feature of gouty arthritis, tophaceous gout, or renal disease is uric acid crystals in the synovium, soft tissues, or kidney structure[4,6,13,29,52,53] (Figure 1). The urate crystals are needle-shaped and are sometimes clustered radially to form a "beach ball" appearance.[6,8] The presence of the crystals induces a sometimes severe synovitis and an inflammatory change in soft tissues or renal structure.[13,29,31,33,53] Within the joint, the articular cartilage can be damaged or destroyed and osteophytes produced that alter the anatomic structure.[4,6,32,33,52] Menisci in the knee joint sometimes contain islands of urate crystals. The kidney reaction characteristically appears as clusters of urates surrounded by granulation tissue and giant cells.[4,6,29,54]

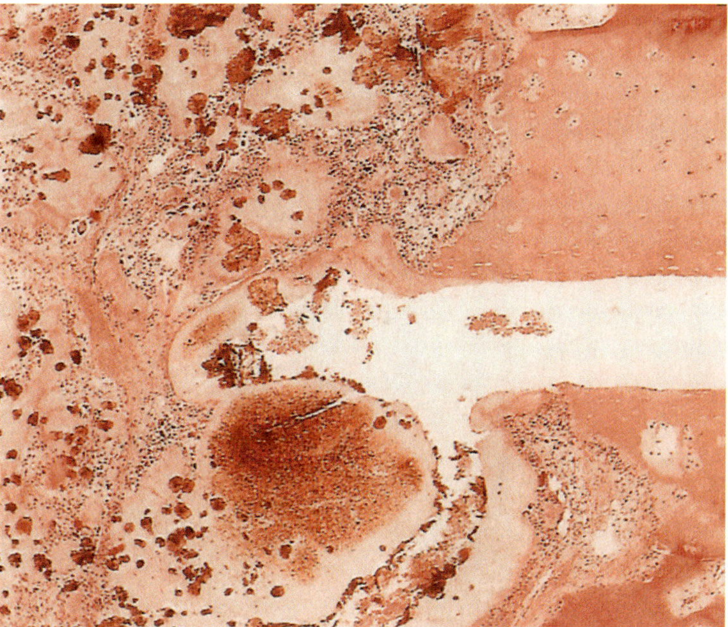

Figure 1
Histologic picture of a gouty tophus from the foot of an elderly patient. A very active inflammation is evident, and small segments of urate are present within the tissue.

Clinical Syndrome of Gout

As indicated above, there are several forms of gout; some are silent and of little concern to the patient, while others may become life-threatening. Asymptomatic hyperuricemia exists when the urate level is high but the symptoms have not occurred.[4,6,29,55] The disorder is most frequent in males and may be evident at puberty. Once developed, the disorder lasts for a lifetime. Asymptomatic hyperuricemia may be present in patients with chronic cardiac, renal, or pulmonary disorders and may be associated with greater cardiac risk.[4,6,32,33,54,56,57] Hyperuricemia is also precipitated in patients who take large amounts of medication that act to damage the purine-urate control system; diuretics are the most common such agents.[4,6,29]

Acute gouty arthritis is the second form of the disorder. Sydenham[9] described it beautifully, saying: "The patient goes to bed and sleeps quietly until about two in the morning when he is awakened by a pain which usually seizes his great toe, but sometimes the heel, ankle or instep. The pain resembles a dislocated bone and is associated with a chill and fever all of which grow more violent every hour." The acute attack lasts usually for a few days, but sometimes

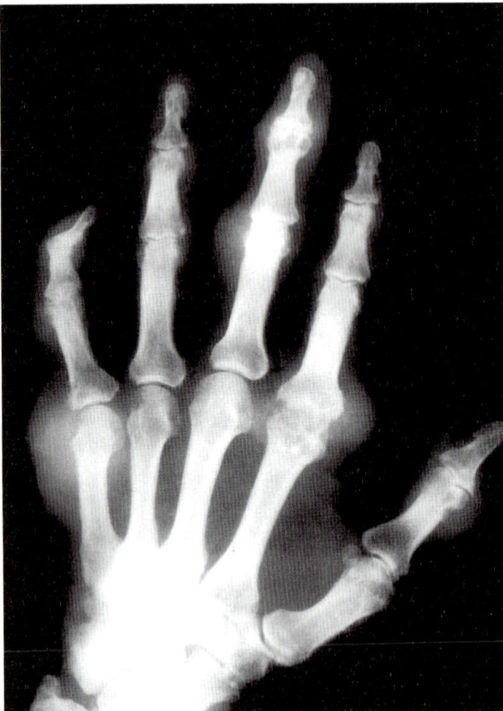

Figure 2
Radiograph of the hand of a patient with acute gouty arthritis showing multiple sites of inflammatory change in relation to the metacarpal and phalangeal joints.

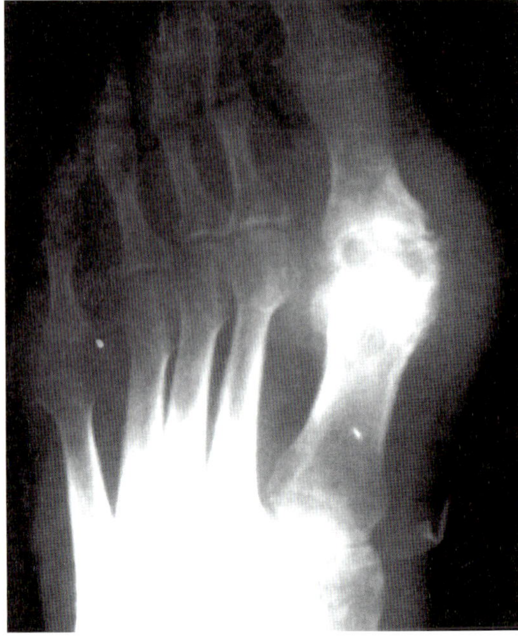

Figure 3
Highly destructive change in the metatarsophalangeal joint of the great toe of an elderly patient who had chronic gouty arthritis for many years. The joint is destroyed and clearly the source of great pain.

weeks. Full recovery frequently occurs. With multiple recurrences, however, polyarticular disease is noted with swelling, redness, and tenderness at the affected sites. If not treated, this disorder may lead to a chronic crippling arthritis.[4,6,29,32,33,52,55]

Chronic tophaceous gout is characterized by enlargement and sometimes marked deformity of the affected site, which is often tender, warm, and reddened.[3,4,6,29,33] The feet (especially the first metatarsophalangeal joint) and phalanges of the hands are most often affected, but other sites can be involved, including the knees, olecranon, or prepatellar bursae.[4,6] Occasionally the skin ulcerates over the site and a white crystalline material exudes. There is often profound limitation of motion, particularly for the hands. A common site for the presence of a sometimes large tophus is the helix of the ear, where the lesion appears as an irregular deposit of white crystalline material, poorly covered with skin.[4] Occasional ocular signs occur in patients with severe tophaceous gout.[58]

Radiographic Imaging of Gout

Early changes in joints and soft tissues show swelling and modest structural alteration on plain radiographs, CT, or MRI[4,6,29,33,45,59] (Figure 2). With advancing disease, the joints frequently show incipient arthritic change with edema of synovium, narrowing, and cartilaginous destruction of the joint tissues. Sharply punched out round or oval defects are characteristic for gout, as is meniscal calcification in the knee joint. With advancing disease, there may be osteophyte formation and increased density of the adjacent bones related to the structural alteration and pathologic fractures (Figure 3). The appearance of a tophus on imaging studies is sometimes characterized by bony "overhang" extending into the soft tissues.[4,6,29,59] In renal lesions, the stones are radiolucent, in contrast with other forms of calcified lesions in the kidneys or ureters.[4,6]

Treatment of Gout

The treatment of gout has a long history, with many approaches to dealing with the symptoms of the disorder, physiotherapy of affected parts, correction of uric acid accumulations, alterations of urate metabolism, and biologic approaches.

According to a remarkable description by Rodnan and Benedek[28] in 1963, the original approaches were those of prayer and saintly invocations by such individuals as Andrew the Apostle (1st century AD), Sebastian (3rd century), Placidus (5th century), Stapinus of Dourgne (8th century), and Albert of Messina (13th century). Paracelsus, in the 16th century, advised patients to take red myrrh, frankincense, vitra, and honey. In the 18th century, Boerhaave advocated warm fomentations and Rhenish wine. In the 19th century, acupuncture was introduced, along with drainage, bloodletting, and local cautery.

Treatment with an array of drugs began in the 20th century; the principal initial agent was colchicine, which appeared to be quite successful in relieving local gouty arthritis, although it caused gastrointestinal side effects in more than 50% of patients.[4,6,34] Indomethacin was introduced in 1963 and appears to be effective in dealing with acute episodes of gouty arthritis. Intra-articular glucocorticoids have also been proposed and are sometimes successful. Allopurinol is the drug of choice to reduce urate concentration in body fluids.[4,6,34] Several additional agents are now being tried, including febuxostat, probenecid, sulfinpyrazone, and raburicase, all of which are used to reduce urate or increase uricase activity.[6,35,60-63]

Surgical procedures were introduced by Benjamin Brodie in 1842,[64] and since then surgical treatment of badly arthritic joints has been advocated, especially for knees and hips but also for hands and feet. Removing tophi and sometimes fusing some of the small joints of the hands and feet reduce the suffering that some people have from extensive destructive gouty arthritis and tophaceous disease.

Conclusions

Hyperuricemia, asymptomatic gout, gouty arthritis, tophaceous gout, and renal gout lesions represent a major problem in rheumatology and orthopaedics. The disorder is clearly genetically related, both in terms of the people who have it and the sex-linked nature of the process. Although we have been able to establish the way that uric acid is formed, it is still not clear why we are unable to eliminate the material as do almost all other creatures in the world (except for the poor Dalmatian!). We have now managed to use drugs to reduce the urate concentrations and to make joint disease less symptomatic and painful, but are still not sure what to do about tophi or, for that matter, renal disease. The summary of Sydenham[9] still applies not only to gout, but to many other diseases that we treat: "As for a radical cure, one altogether perfect, and one whereby a patient might be freed from even the disposition to the disease—this lies, like Truth at the bottom of a well; and so deep is it in the innermost recesses of Nature, that I know not when or by whom it will be brought forward into the light of day." A spectacular comment that is unfortunately still very true. Even 325 years later, we cannot find the bottom of the well for gout and some other disorders.

References

1. Hippocrates: *The Genuine Works of Hippocrates,* Volumes I and II. Translated by Adams F. New York, NY, William Wood and Co, 1886.

2. Fraser KJ: William Stukeley and the gout. *Med Histo* 1992;36:160-186.

3. Rodnan GP: A gallery of gout: Being a miscellany of prints and caricatures from the 16th century to the present day. *Arthritis Rheum* 1961;4:27-46.

4. Wortmann RL, Kelley WN: Gout and hyperuricemia, in Ruddy S, Harris ED Jr, Sledge CB (eds): *Kelley's Textbook of Rheumatology,* ed 6. Philadelphia, PA, WB Saunders, 2001, pp 1339-1376.

5. Bennet T: *An essay on the gout: in which a method is propos'd to relieve the hereditary and to cure the acquir'd.* London, England, 1734.

6. Levinson DJ, Becker MA: Clinical gout and the pathogenesis of hyperuricemia, in McCarty DJ, Koopman WJ, eds: *Arthritis and Allied Conditions: A Textbook of Rheumatology,* ed 12. Philadelphia, PA, Lea and Febiger, 1993, pp 1773-1805.

7. Rush B: Observations upon the cause and cure of the gout, in *Medical Inquiries and Observations,* ed 3. Philadelphia, PA, Johnson and Warner, 1809, pp 245-322.

8. McCarty DJ: A historical note: Leeunwenhoek's description of crystals from a gouty tophus. *Arthritis Rheum* 1970;13:414-418.

9. Sydenham T: A treatise on gout and dropsy, in *The Works of Thomas Sydenham MD.* Translated by Latham RG. London. The Sydenham Society, 1850, pp 119-162.

10. Wollaston WH: On gouty and urinary concretions. *Philos Trans R Soc* 1797;87:386-400.

11. Garrod AB: *Treatise on Gout and Rheumatic Gout (Rheumatoid Arthritis)*, ed 3. London, England, Longman Green and Co, 1876.

12. Storey GD: Alfred Baring Garrod (1819-1907). *Rheumatology (Oxford)* 2001;40:1189-1190.

13. McCarty DJ, Hollander JL: Identification of urate crystals in gouty synovial fluid. *Ann Intern Med* 1961;54:452-460.

14. Appelboom T, Ehrlich GE: Historical note: The concept of gout in 1880. *Arthritis Rheum* 1998;41:1511-1512.

15. Ben-Noun L: What was the disease of the legs that afflicted King Asa? *Gerontology* 2001;47: 96-99.

16. Boonen A, van der Linden S: Case number 33: About being a famous European and suffering from gout. *Ann Rheum Dis* 2005;64:528.

17. Caughey DE: The arthritis of Constantine IX. *Ann Rheum Dis* 1974;33:77-80.

18. Espinoza R, Gonzalez C: The disease of Christopher Columbus. *Rev Med Chil* 1997;125:732-737.

19. Espinel CH: Michelangelo's gout in a fresco by Raphael. *Lancet* 1999;354:2149-2151.

20. Jeanselme E: La goutte a France. *Bull Soc Fr Hist Med* 1920;14:137-164.

21. Haslam F: Views from the gallery. *BMJ* 1995;311:1712-1713.

22. Kuehn W: Michelangelo's gouty knee. *Lancet* 2000;355:1104.

23. Lascaratos J: 'Arthritis' in Byzantium (AD 324-1453): Unknown information from non-medical literary sources. *Ann Rheum Dis* 1995;54:951-957.

24. Ring J: *A Treatise on the Gout: Containing the Opinions of the Most Celebrated Ancient and Modern Physicians on that Disease*. London, England, J Callow, 1811.

25. Rodnan GP, Benedek TG, Panetta WC: The early history of synovia (joint fluid). *Ann Intern Med* 1966;65:821-842.

26. Stukeley W: *An abstract of a treatise of the cause and cure of the gout*. London, England, 1740.

27. Weissmann G: Galileo's gout. *Pharos Alpha Omega Alpha Honor Med Soc* 2004;67:4-7.

28. Rodnan GP, Benedek TG: Ancient therapeutic arts in the gout. *Arthritis Rheum* 1963;6:317-340.

29. Agudelo CA, Wise CM: Gout: Diagnosis, pathogenesis and clinical manifestations. *Curr Opin Rheumatol* 2001;13:234-239.

30. Reginato AJ, Reginato AM: Diseases associated with deposition of pyrophosphate or hydroxyapatite, in Ruddy S, Harris ED Jr, Sledge CB (eds): *Kelley's Textbook of Rheumatology*, ed 6. Philadelphia, PA, WB Saunders, 2001, pp 1377-1390.

31. Suresh E: Diagnosis and management of gout: A rational approach. *Postgrad Med J* 2005;81:572-579.

32. Underwood M: Diagnosis and management of gout. *BMJ* 2006;332:1315-1319.

33. Wortmann RL: Gout and hyperuricemia. *Curr Opin Rheumatol* 2002;14:281-286.

34. Wortmann RL: Management of hyperuricemia, in McCarty DJ, Koopman WJ (eds): *Arthritis and Allied Conditions: A Textbook of Rheumatology*, ed 12. Philadelphia, PA, Lea and Febiger, 1993, pp 1807-1818.

35. Wortmann RL: Recent advances in the management of gout and hyperuricemia. *Curr Opin Rheumatol* 2005;17:319-324.

36. Baroletti S, Bencivenga GA, Gabardi S: Treating gout in kidney transplant recipients. *Prog Transplant* 2004;14:143-147.

37. Bruce IN, Schentag CT, Gladman DD: Hyperuricemia in psoriatic arthritis: Prevalence and associated features. *J Clin Rheumatol* 2000;6:6-9.

38. Choi HK, Atkinson K, Karlson EW, Curhan G: Obesity, weight change, hypertension, diuretic use and risk of gout in men: The health professionals follow-up study. *Arch Intern Med* 2005;165:742-748.

39. Choi HK, Atkinson K, Karlson EW, et al: Alcohol intake and risk of incident gout in men: A prospective study. *Lancet* 2004;363:1277-1281.

40. Lin HY, Rocher LL, McQuillan MA, et al: Cyclosporine-induced hyperuricemia and gout. *N Engl J Med* 1989;321:287-292.

41. Mikuls TR, Saag KG: New insights into gout epidemiology. *Curr Opin Rheumatol* 2006;18:199-203.

42. Nyhan WL: Lesch-Nyhan disease. *J Hist Neurosci* 2005;14:1-10.

43. Bingham C, Ellard S, van't Hoff WG, et al: Atypical familial juvenile hyperuricemic nephropathy associated with a hepatocyte nuclear factor-1beta gene mutation. *Kidney Int* 2003;63:1645-1651.

44. Bleyer AJ, Woodard AS, Shihabi Z, et al: Clinical characterization of a family with a mutation in the uromodulin (Tamm-Horsfall glycoprotein) gene. *Kidney Int* 2003;64:36-42.

45. Saag KG, Mikuls TR: Recent advances in the epidemiology of gout. *Curr Rheumatol Rep* 2005;7:235-241.

46. Turner JJ, Stacy JM, Harding B, et al: Uromodulin mutations cause familial juvenile hyperuricemic nephropathy. *J Clin Endocrinol Metab* 2003;88:1398-1401.

47. Rothschild BM, Tanke D, Carpenter K: Tyrannosaurs suffered from gout. *Nature* 1997;387:357-361.

48. Osborne CA, Bartges JW, Lulich JP, et al: Canine urolithiasis, in *Small Animal Clinical Nutrition*. Marceline, MO, Walsworth, 2000, pp 625-636.

49. Lawrence RC, Helmick CG, Arnett FC, et al: Estimates of the prevalence of arthritis and selected musculoskeletal disorders in the United States. *Arthritis Rheum* 1998;41:778-799.

50. Klemp P, Stansfield SA, Castle B, Robertson MC: Gout is on the increase in New Zealand. *Ann Rheum Dis* 1997;56:22-26.

51. Mody GM, Naidoo PD: Gout in South African blacks. *Ann Rheum Dis* 1984;43:394-397.

52. Parhami N, Greenstein N, Juozevicius JL: Erosive osteoarthritis and gout: Gout in 36 joints. *J Rheumatol* 1986;13:469-471.

53. Pascual E: Persistence of monosodium urate crystals and low grade inflammation of patients with untreated gout. *Arthritis Rheum* 1991;34:141-145.

54. Short R, Johnson R, Tuttle K: Uric acid, microalbuminuria and cardiovascular events in high-risk patients. *Am J Nephrol* 2005;25:36-44.

55. Poor G, Mituszova M: Saturnine gout. *Baillieres Clin Rheumatol* 1989;3:51-61.

56. Brand FN, McGee DL, Kannel WB, et al: Hyper-

uricemia as a risk factor for coronary artery disease: The Framingham study. *Am J Epidemiol* 1985;121:11-18.

57. Madsen T, Muhlestein J, Carlquist J, et al: Serum uric acid independently predicts mortality in patients with significantly angiographically defined coronary artery disease. *Am J Nephrol* 2005;25:45-49.

58. Ferry AP, Safir A, Melikian HE: Ocular abnormalities in patients with gout. *Ann Opthalmol* 1985;17:632-635.

59. McCarthy GM, Barthelemy CR, Veum JA, Wortmann RL: Influence of antihyperuricemic therapy on the clinical and radiographic progression of gout. *Arthritis Rheum* 1991;34:1489-1494.

60. Becker MA, Schumacher HR Jr, Wortmann RL, et al: Febuxostat compared with allopurinol in patients with hyperuricemia and gout. *N Engl J Med* 2005;353:2450-2461.

61. Bieber JD, Terkeltaub RA: Gout: On the brink of novel therapeutic options for an ancient disease. *Arthritis Rheum* 2004;50:2400-2414.

62. Pui CH: Raburicase: A potent uricolytic agent. *Expert Opin Pharmacother* 2002;3:433-442.

63. Schumacher HR Jr : Febuxostat: A non-purine, selective inhibitor of xanthine oxidase for the management of hyperuricaemia in patients with gout. *Exper Opin Investig Drugs* 2005;14:893-903.

64. Brodie BC: *Pathological and Surgical Observations on the Diseases of the Joints*, ed 4. Boston, MA, TR Marvin, 1842, pp 146-161.

Chapter 32

Hypophosphatasia

Rathbun's hypophosphatasia is a rare genetic disorder in which the patient has a defect in tissue-nonspecific alkaline phosphatase (TNSALP), which results in a disorder that in many ways resembles rickets and osteomalacia. It occurs in six forms: a perinatal intrauterine disease that almost always results in death of the fetus; an infantile disorder with rapidly evolving bony changes and a high death rate; a childhood form that progresses less rapidly but with marked bony changes, and a much milder adult presentation often associated with minimal bone changes; an odontohypophosphatasia syndrome that presents with often severe dental problems; and a peculiar very rare entity known as pseudohypophosphatasia, in which the alkaline phosphatase is normal but the patients have findings similar to those of the primary form of the disease. In all but the last-named form, the serum alkaline phosphatase is markedly reduced and urinary phosphoethanolamine is often increased. Hypercalcemia and hyperphosphatemia are often present as well, which helps distinguish this disorder from hypocalcemic or hypophosphatemic rickets. Although several treatments have been introduced, none as yet seems to be effective.

History and Nomenclature

The earliest report regarding hypophosphatasia was by Macey[1] in 1940. He described two brothers with "rickets" and multiple fractures but with a low alkaline phosphatase level. The first definition of the disease, however, was by John Campbell Rathbun[2] (1915-1972) of Toronto, Ontario, Canada in 1948. He described a 3-week-old male child with severe osteopenia, multiple fractures, and calvarial abnormalities who died after seizures developed. The patient's calcium and phosphate levels were both high but the alkaline phosphatase was low. Autopsy material showed a very low tissue alkaline phosphatase, and Rathbun introduced the term "hypophosphatasia." Fifty years later, the mother and father of the child were studied to determine the genetic nature of the problem, which provided important information regarding this very rare entity.[3] In 1960, Bethune and Dent[4] described two sisters in their 40s with a similarly diminished alkaline phosphatase level, and Pimstone and associates[5] described the dental problems in several patients in 1966. In 1966, Rupprecht and Doerfel[6] described six siblings with micromelia, microcephaly, and epiphyseal and metaphyseal alterations in the bones, including ribs and vertebrae. All of them had convulsions and two died. In subsequent years, valuable studies were published regarding these disorders;[3,7-35] however, the works of Michael P. Whyte[3,11-15,17,18,20-26] and Etienne Mornet[27-35] stand out for their very clear definition of the clinical, pathologic, and biologic nature of the diseases, as well as their contributions to our understanding of this very rare and at times terrifying clinical entity.

Hypophosphatasia has been described as consisting of six distinct presentations, ranging from intrauterine to adult; four are known as hypophosphatasia, one as odontohypophosphatasia, and one as pseudohypophosphatasia.[20] Adding the eponym provides the title of Rathbun's hypophosphatasia.[2] Another term occasionally used is phosphoethanolaminuria.[20] An abbreviation recently introduced for hypophosphatasia is HOPS.

Metabolic and Genetic Abnormalities

Alkaline phosphatase is a nonspecific metalloenzyme that hydrolyses many forms of phosphate esters at an alkaline pH, usually in the presence of magnesium and zinc.[36,37] There are several such enzymes, but the form present in the bone, liver, and kidney is produced by a specific gene.[20,38] In bone, the enzyme is produced by osteoblasts.[20,31,37] It is located in the Golgi vesicles formed by the endoplasmic reticulum, attached to the cell membrane, and anchored by glycophosphatidylinositol proteins.[11,20,31,36,37,39] The enzyme is also noted

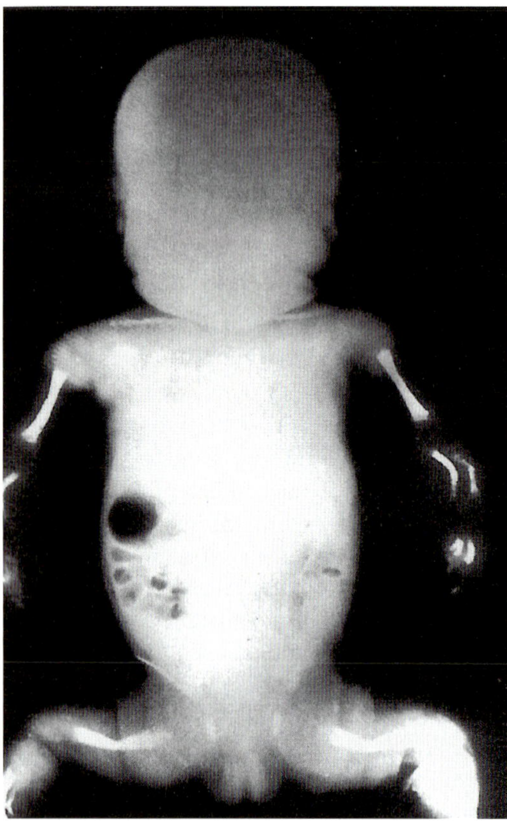

Figure 1

Type 1 hypophosphatasia in an infant. The radiographs show very poor bone structure with deformity. The survival rate is very low, regardless of treatment.

in matrix vesicles and tiny bone nodules, especially during the process of early calcification.[11,36] The serum and tissue levels for alkaline phosphatase increase in association with bone formation and decrease or are absent during bone destruction, and not found in relation to osteoclasts.[20,31,40] The normal substrates for alkaline phosphatase include phosphoethanolamine, inorganic pyrophosphate and pyridoxal 5'-phosphate.[19,20,23,31]

The cause of hypophosphatasia is a deficiency of the liver, bone, or kidney type of alkaline phosphatase otherwise known as TNSALP.[12,20,31] The TNSALP arises from the gene site 1p36.1-p34, which consists of 12 exons and 11 introns.[19,20,30,41] A vast array of errors has been described for this enzyme and approximately 65 have been identified.[14,21,27,28,32-35,38,42-47] The principal ones include 15 missense mutations, 2 nonsense mutations, and 2 nucleotide deletions. In addition, two mutations affecting splicing and a mutation at the transcription start site have been defined. Patients with a defect in the TNSALP gene may present with as many as six different forms of disorders, all known by the name hypophosphatasia, in which bone mineralization is diminished.[11,12,20] Because the alkaline phosphatase is reduced, the substrates phosphoethanolamine, inorganic pyrophosphate, and pyridoxyl 5'–phosphate levels are elevated in the serum or urine.[12,20,23,31,48]

Clinical Entities

There are five forms of clinical hypophosphatasia in which the patient's alkaline phosphatase is diminished and significant and sometimes fatal disorders develop as a result. In addition, there is another disorder known as pseudohypophosphastasia, which resembles the adult form of the disease but has different chemical characteristics.

Type 1: Perinatal Hypophosphatasia

This is a lethal condition that can be detected in utero by ultrasound studies and results in profound skeletal hypomineralization and deformity[20,43,44,49-52] (Figure 1). Polyhydramnios is frequent and most of the fetuses are dead at birth.[51,53] The limbs are short, markedly deformed, and peculiar bone spurs (Bowdler spurs) jut from the metaphyseal regions of the long bones and can traverse the skin.[50,51,53,54] Children who survive fail to gain weight, and seizures and periods of apnea develop. Severe chest deformity related to structural rib abnormalities compromises respiration and is typically fatal. It has recently become possible to diagnose the condition by prenatal genetic or ultrasound studies.[52,53,55] The disease is transmitted as an autosomal recessive trait, and sexes are equally affected.[20,51]

Type 2: Infantile Hypophosphatasia

This disorder is not identified in newborn infants but becomes apparent shortly thereafter, often appearing by 6 months of age.[40,41,56] Children are normal mentally and seem to do well initially, but soon show a failure to thrive and become hypotonic in association with increased calcium in the serum.[20,41,56] Severe rachitic changes in the skeleton develop and the fontanels of the cranium are widened and easily palpated[20,21,56,57] (Figure 2). Hypertelorism occurs, along with brachycephaly and increased intracranial pressure. Seizures and

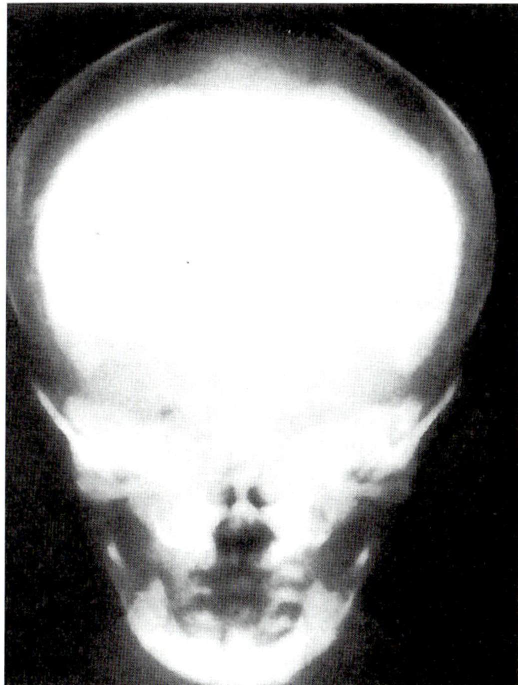

Figure 2
Radiograph of the skull in a patient with type 2 hypophosphatasia. The fontanels of the cranium are widened and easily palpated. Hypertelorism occurs, along with brachycephaly and increased intracranial pressure.

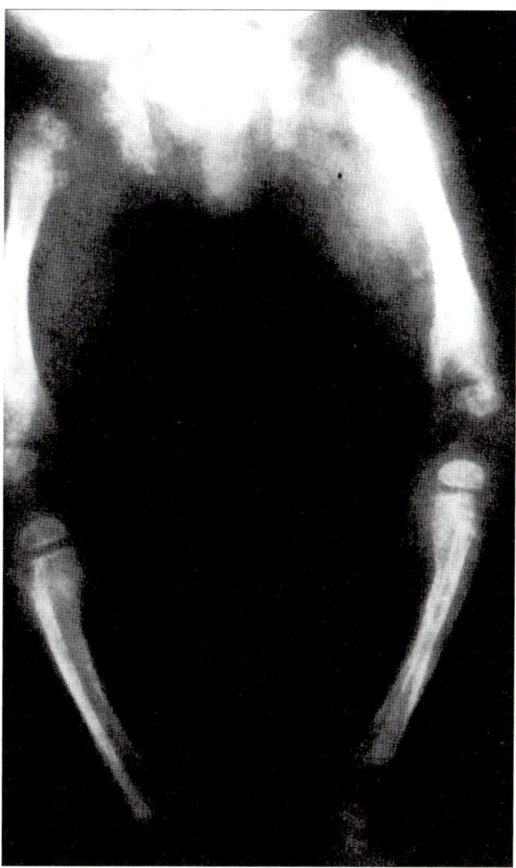

Figure 3
A child with type 3 hypophosphatasia. The bones are deformed and show changes consistent with rickets, including small fractures and irregular ossification of the bones.

periods of apnea may be present. Chest deformity is often marked and is the cause of respiratory impairment, pneumonia, and death in a high percentage of patients.[20,21,41,56] Like the perinatal form, this disorder appears to be transmitted as an autosomal recessive trait. Sexes are equally affected.

Type 3: Childhood Hypophosphatasia

These children seem to be in good health from birth until the age of 5 years, when they are noted to be of short stature and have mildly rachitic bone abnormalities[20] (Figure 3). The skull is moderately deformed, usually with frontal bossing, and one of the remarkable features is the hypoplasia or aplasia of dental cementum and loss of deciduous teeth.[5,57,58] Children are functional and walk reasonably well, but often with a waddling gait related to the presence of rachitic bowing or knock-knee deformities.[15,29,43] Most patients survive, however, in contrast with patients with type 1 and 2 disease. The mode of transmission for this disorder is unclear in that an autosomal dominant trait has been observed, par-

ticularly among inbred Mennonites in Canada.[29,43] The disease occurs with equal frequency in males and females.

Type 4: Adult Hypophosphatasia

This is a mild form of the disease and many patients or their physicians are unaware of any illness.[4,16,17,25,29] Patients are normal in height and have no real skeletal deformities evident on physical examination.[4,16,20] The principal problems are that the bones are impaired in a manner consistent with osteomalacia and fractures are frequent, sometimes without injury, through Looser's lines in the long bones.[13,16,20,24] Chondrocalcinosis can occur, and a form of pseudogout may be disabling.[20,24,59] Many patients have dental abnormalities and lose teeth at an early age.[5,16,25,58] This disorder has not been clearly defined in terms of genetic transmission or gender frequency.

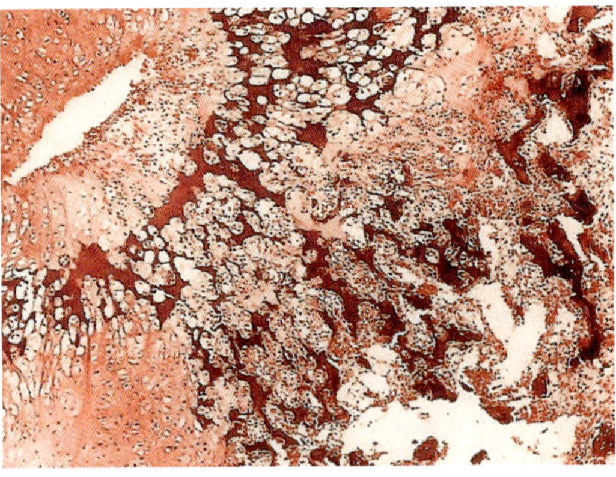

Figure 4
Histologic picture of the epiphyseal plate region in a patient with type 3 disease, showing gross distortion of the normal structure with highly irregular ossification in the lower portion of the epiphysis.

Type 5: Odontohypophosphatasia
These patients have no evidence of skeletal or systemic disease but have sometimes severe forms of dental abnormalities.[16,27,58,60] The disease is also very rare and has not been clearly defined in terms of genetic origin or frequency.

Type 6: Pseudohypophosphatasia
This is a very rare form of the disease in which patients' alkaline phosphatase concentrations are normal or even slightly elevated.[10,20] The disease may be severe and resemble type 2 or 3, but seems to result from a failure of the body to recognize TNSALP and then produce the characteristic changes. Serum calcium concentrations can be high.[20]

Laboratory and Imaging Studies
All patients, with the exception of those with pseudohypophosphatasia, have a diminished concentration of alkaline phosphatase (and especially TNSALP), both in the serum and in the body tissues.[12,16,18,20,25,29,40,48] The values may be 15% less than in normal individuals. All six forms of the disease may show hypercalcemia and hypercalcuria.[16,20,23] The other materials that are also increased include phosphoethanolamine, inorganic pyrophosphate, and pyridoxyl 5'-phosphate.[12,20,23,57] Phosphoethanolaminuria is a frequent finding, but not necessarily diagnostic.[12,20,57] Examination of tissue shows defective osseous mineralization that may vary based on the extent of the disease.[39,53] The changes in the epiphys-

eal and metaphyseal bones of children show rickettsial changes[7,9,51,54] (Figure 4). The skull in children shows marked abnormality in structure, with widening of sutures.[7,9,51,57] Examination of the dentition shows aplasia and hypoplasia, and impaired calcification of the tooth and the subjacent maxilla or mandible.[20,58] Enamel is not as affected.

Radiographic studies show an array of abnormalities depending on the type and extent of disease.[7,9,20,21,25,51,54,57] Imaging of the perinatal and infantile diseases shows failure of calcification of the cranial vault, with minimal calcification of the base and facial bones. The vertebrae are tiny and the ribs are filiform. Only small islands of osseous tissue are present in the pelvis and scapula. The bones are poorly ossified and deformed, and in the metaphyseal region are the laterally placed spurs that are sometimes quite large and can erode the skin.[54] Imaging studies of the childhood disease shows changes consistent with rickets. The epiphyseal plates are elongated and the metaphyseal bone shows poor ossification. The bones are short and often show fractures or Looser's lines. The skull is poorly ossified and sometimes deformed. The ribs are thin and the vertebrae are short and sometimes show a fairly marked scoliotic change.

The adult forms of the disease show bones that are relatively normal in structure, but have findings consistent with osteomalacia.[4,7,9,13,16,20,25,29,50,58] These include osteopenia, Looser's lines, fractures and deformities, and widened anterior aspects of the ribs. Many patients will show chondrocalcinosis of the joints.[39] The jaw changes are sometimes striking, with many absent teeth; those remaining are poorly structured and displaced.[20,46,58]

Treatment
Numerous treatments have been introduced for patients with these disorders. General supportive pediatric care has been minimally successful in caring for patients with perinatal and infantile disease.[56] None has been very effective. For the childhood and adult disorders, some therapies have been used that may for a period of time help the patients, but many of these ultimately are abandoned because of complications. Spe-

cifically, corticosteroids, nonsteroidal anti-inflammatory medications, calcitonin, chlorothiazide, and bisphosphonates have not greatly improved the patient's health or diminished the complications, and the problems that sometimes ensued have for the most part required that the treatment be stopped.[20,61-63] Despite the close resemblance of the disease to rickets and osteomalacia, the use of calcium or vitamin D is not only of no value but is dangerous to the patient.[20] Zinc and magnesium reduce the effect of the abnormal materials but are of limited value.[20] Of some interest is the attempt to provide serum from patients with Paget's disease, who have high levels of alkaline phosphatase, but the results thus far have been limited.[26] Bone marrow transplants from siblings without disease have a limited success.[22] With either of these approaches, there is a dangerous possibility that the other forms of alkaline phosphatase may be enhanced and result in renal, gastrointestinal, or liver abnormalities. The ideal treatment would consist of some form of genetic alteration, but at least at this point it has not been possible, mainly because the gene errors for these patients may be almost impossible to assess.

Dental care is sometimes a major problem for these patients. Frequently, damaged or deranged teeth must be removed and some form of corrective treatment instituted. Cardiac and pulmonary management will sometimes improve the patient's general health and increase survival. Orthopaedic care of fractures and crippling deformities is difficult because devices may not be effective in maintaining good alignment and they frequently cut out.[12,20]

It is sad to say that, at least at this point, the treatment approaches to these patients are of limited success and no single approach appears to have any great promise. A genetic modification would be ideal, but it is apparent that there are far too many errors to define the appropriate one for some sort of correction. There is also some danger in any form of treatment that the other forms of alkaline phosphatase that affect other organs may be sufficiently altered to cause difficulty for the patient. Fortunately, the entity is rare and at least the adult disease is seldom fatal or markedly disabling.

References

1. Macey JB: Multiple pseudofractures: Report of a case. *Proc Staff Meet Mayo Clinic* 1940;15:789-791.

2. Rathbun JC: Hypophosphatasia: A new developmental anomaly. *Am J Dis Child* 1948;75:822-831.

3. Mumm S, Jones J, Finnegan P, Whyte MP: Hypophosphatasia: Molecular diagnosis of Rathbun's original case. *J Bone Miner Res* 2001;16:1724-1727.

4. Bethune JE, Dent CE: Hypophosphatasia in the adult. *Am J Med* 1960;28:615-622.

5. Pimstone B, Eisenberg E, Silverman S: Hypophosphatasia: Genetic and dental studies. *Ann Intern Med* 1966;65:722-729.

6. Rupprecht E, Doerfel D: Enchondrolae dysostose Typ Nierhoff-Huebner bie. *Geschwistern Arch Kinderheilkd* 1966;172:64-73.

7. Currarino G, Neuhauser EB, Reyersbach GC, Sobel EH: Hypophosphatasia. *Am J Roentgenol Radium Ther Nucl Med* 1957;78:392-419.

8. Fraser D: Hypophosphatasia. *Am J Med* 1957;22:730-746.

9. Kozlowski K, Sutcliffe J, Barylak A, et al: Hypophosphatasia: Review of 24 cases. *Pediatr Radiol* 1976;5:103-117.

10. Scriver CR, Cameron D: Pseudohypophosphatasia. *N Engl J Med* 1969;281:604-606.

11. Anderson HC, Hsu HH, Morris DC, Fedde KN, Whyte MP: Matrix vesicles in osteomalacic hypophosphatasia bone contain apatite-like mineral crystals. *Am J Pathol* 1997;151:1555-1561.

12. Caswell AM, Whyte MP, Russell RG: Hypophosphatasia and the extracellular metabolism of inorganic pyrophosphate: Clinical and laboratory aspects. *Crit Rev Clin Lab Sci* 1991;28:175-232.

13. Coe JD, Murphy WA, Whyte MP: Management of femoral fractures and pseudofractures in adult hypophosphatasia. *J Bone Joint Surg Am* 1986;68:981-990.

14. Henthorn PS, Raducha M, Fedde KN, Lafferty MA, Whyte MP: Different missense mutations at the tissue–nonspecific alkaline phosphatase gene locus in autosomal recessively inherited forms of mild and severe hypophosphatasia. *Proc Natl Acad Sci USA* 1992;89:9924-9928.

15. Pauli RM, Modaff P, Sipes SL, Whyte MP: Mild hypophosphatasia mimicking severe osteogenesis imperfecta in utero: Bent but not broken. *Am J Med Genet* 1999;86:434-438.

16. Wendling D, Jeannin-Louys L, Kremer P, Fellmann F, Toussirot E, Mornet E: Adult hypophosphatasia: Current aspects. *Joint Bone Spine* 2001;68:120-124.

17. Weinstein RS, Whyte MP: Heterogeneity of adult hypophosphatasia: Report of severe and mild cases. *Arch Intern Med* 1981;141:727-731.

18. Weiss MJ, Ray K, Fallon MD, et al: Analysis of liver/bone/kidney alkaline phosphatase mRNA, DNA and enzymatic activity in cultured skin fibroblasts from 14 unrelated patients with severe hypophosphatasia. *Am J Hum Genet* 1989;44:686-694.

19. Weiss MJ, Ray K, Henthorn PS, Lamb B, Kadesch T, Harris H: Structure of the human liver/bone/kidney alkaline phosphatase gene. *J Biol Chem* 1988;263:12002-12010.

20. Whyte MP: Hereditary, metabolic and dysplastic skeletal disorders, in Coe FL, Favus MJ (eds): *Disorders of Bone and Mineral Metabolism.* New York, NY, Raven Press, 1992, pp 977-1026.

21. Whyte MP, Essmyer K, Geimer M, Mumm S: Homozygosity for TNSALP mutation 1348c>T (Arg433Cys) causes infantile hypophosphatasia manifesting transient disease correction and variably lethal outcome in a kindred of black ancestry. *J Pediatr* 2006;148:753-758.

22. Whyte MP, Kurtzburg J, McAlister WH, et al: Marrow cell transplantation for infantile hypophosphatasia. *J Bone Miner Res* 2003;18:624-636.

23. Whyte MP, Mahuren JD, Vrabel LA, Coburn SP: Markedly increased circulating pyridoxal-5'-phosphate levels in hyphophosphatasia: Alkaline phosphatase acts in vitamin B6 metabolism. *J Clin Invest* 1985;76:752-756.

24. Whyte MP, Murphy WA, Fallon MD: Adult hypophosphatasia with chondrocalcinosis and arthropathy: Variable penetrance of hyphophosphotasia in a large Oklahoma kindred. *Am J Med* 1982;72:631-641.

25. Whyte MP, Teitelbaum SL, Murphy WA, Bergfeld MA, Avioli LV: Adult hypophosphatasia: Clinical, laboratory, and genetic investigation of a large kindred with review of the literature. *Medicine (Baltimore)* 1979;58:329-347.

26. Whyte MP, Valdes R Jr, Ryan LM, McAlister WH: Infantile hypophosphatasia: Enzyme replacement therapy by intravenous infusion of alkaline phosphatase-rich plasma from patients with Paget bone disease. *J Pediatr* 1982;101:379-386.

27. Herasse M, Spentchian M, Taillandier A, et al: Molecular study of three cases of odontohypophosphatasia resulting from heterozygosity for mutations in the tissue non-specific alkaline phosphatase gene. *J Med Genet* 2003;40:605-609.

28. Hérasse M, Spentchian M, Taillandier A, Mornet E: Evidence of a founder effect of the tissue-nonspecific alkaline phosphatase (TNSALP) gene E174K mutation in hypophosphatasia patients. *Eur J Hum Genet* 2002;10:666-668.

29. Hu JC, Plaetke R, Mornet E, et al: Characterization of a family with dominant hypophosphatasia. *Eur J Oral Sci* 2000;108:189-194.

30. Mornet E: Hypophosphatasia: The mutations of the tissue-nonspecific alkaline phosphatase gene. *Hum Mutat* 2000;15:309-315.

31. Mornet E, Stura E, Lia-Baldini AS, Stigbrand T, Ménez A, Le Du MH: Structural evidence for a functional role of human tissue nonspecific alkaline phosphatase in bone mineralization. *J Biol Chem* 2001;276:31171-31178.

32. Mornet E, Taillandier A, Peyramaure S, et al: Identification of fifteen novel mutations in the tissue-nonspecific alkaline phosphatase (TNSALP) gene in European patients with severe hypophosphatasia. *Eur J Hum Genet* 1998;6:308-314.

33. Taillandier A, Lia-Baldini AS, Mouchard M: Twelve novel mutations in the tissue-nonspecific alkaline phosphatase gene (ALPL) in patients with various forms of hypophosphatasia. *Hum Mutat* 2001;18:83-84.

34. Taillandier A, Sallinen SL, Brun-Heath I, De Mazancourt P, Serre JL, Mornet E: Childhood hypophosphatasia due to de novo missense mutation in the tissue-nonspecific alkaline phosphatase gene. *J Clin Endocrinol Metab* 2005;90:2436-2439.

35. Taillandier A, Zurutuza L, Muller F, et al: Characterization of eleven novel mutations (M45L, R119H, 544delG, G145V, H154Y, C184Y, D289V, 862+5A, 1172delC, R411X, E459K) in the tissue-nonspecific alkaline phosphatase (TNSALP) gene in patients with severe hypophosphatasia: Mutations in brief no. 217. Outline. *Hum Mutat* 1999;13:171-172.

36. Bernard GW: Ultrastructural localization of alkaline phosphatase in initial intramembranous osteogenesis. *Clin Orthop Relat Res* 1978;135:218-225.

37. Kim EE, Wyckoff HW: Structure of alkaline phosphatase. *Clin Chim Acta* 1990;186:175-187.

38. Watanabe H, Goseki-Sone M, Orimo H, Hamatani R, Takinami H, Ishikawa I: Function of mutant (G1144A) tissue-nonspecific ALP gene from hypophosphatasia. *J Bone Miner Res* 2002;17:1945-1948.

39. Chuck AJ, Pattrick MG, Hamilton E, Wilson R, Doherty M: Crystal deposition in hypophosphatasia: A reappraisal. *Ann Rheum Dis* 1989;48:571-576.

40. Henthorn PS, Whyte MP: Infantile hypophosphatasia: Successful prenatal assessment by testing for tissue-non-specific alkaline phosphatase isoenzyme gene mutations. *Prenat Diagn* 1995;15:1001-1006.

41. Greenberg CR, Evans JA, McKendry-Smith S, et al: Infantile hypophosphatasia: Localization with chromosome region 1p36.1-34 and prenatal diagnosis using linked DNA markers. *Am J Hum Genet* 1990;46:286-292.

42. Brun-Heath I, Taillandier A, Sere JL, Mornet E: Characterization of 11 novel mutations in the tissue non-specific alkaline phosphatase gene responsible for hypophosphatasia and genotype-phenotype correlations. *Mol Genet Metab* 2005;84:273-277.

43. Greenberg CR, Taylor CL, Haworth JC, et al: A homoallelic Gly317→Asp mutation in ALPL causes the perinatal (lethal) form of hypophosphatasia in Canadian Mennonites. *Genomics* 1993;17:215-217.

44. Ito M, Amizuka N, Ozawa H, Oda K: Retention of the cis-Golgi and delayed degradation of tissue-non-specific alkaline phosphatase with an Asn153→Asp substitution, a cause of perinatal hypophosphatasia. *Biochem J* 2002;361:473-480.

45. Michigami T, Uchihashi T, Suzuki A, Tachikawa K, Nakajima S, Ozono K: Common mutations F310L and T1559del in the tissue-nonspecific alkaline phosphatase gene are related to distinct phenotypes in Japanese patients with hypophosphatasia. *Eur J Pediatr* 2005;164:277-282.

46. Orimo H, Shin YS, Shimada T: G317D mutation in the tissue-nonspecific alkaline phosphatase gene associated with childhood hypophosphatasia in a German family. *J Inherit Metab Dis* 2002;25:601-602.

47. Watanabe H, Takinami H, Goseki-Sone M, Orimo H, Hamatani R, Ishikawa I: Characterization of the mutant (A115V) tissue-nonspecific alkaline phosphatase gene from adult-type hypophos-

phatasia. *Biochem Biophys Res Commun* 2005;327:124-129.

48. Warshaw JB, Littlefield JW, Fishman WH, Inglis NR, Stolbach LL: Serum alkaline phosphatase in hypophosphatasia. *J Clin Invest* 1971;50:2137-2142.

49. Brock DJ, Barron L: First-trimester prenatal diagnosis of hypophosphatasia: Experience with 16 cases. *Prenat Diagn* 1991;11:387-391.

50. Comstock C, Bronsteen R, Lee W, Vettraino I: Mild hypophosphatasia in utero: Bent bones in a family with dental disease. *J Ultrasound Med* 2005;24:707-709.

51. Shohat M, Rimoin DL, Gruber HE, Lachman RS: Perinatal lethal hypophosphatasia: Clinical, radiologic and morphologic findings. *Pediatr Radiol* 1991;21:421-427.

52. Tongsong T, Pongsatha S: Early prenatal sonographic diagnosis of congenital hypophosphatasia. *Ultrasound Obstet Gynecol* 2000;15:252-255.

53. Vandevijver N, De Die-Smulders CE, Offermans JP, et al: Lethal hypophosphatasia, spur type: Case report and physiopathological study. *Genet Couns* 1998;9:205-209.

54. Oestreich AE, Bofinger MK: Prominent transverse (Bowdler) bone spurs as a diagnostic clue in a case of neonatal hypophosphatasia without metaphyseal irregularity. *Pediatr Radiol* 1989;19:341-342.

55. Watanabe A, Yamamasu S, Shinagawa T, et al: Prenatal genetic diagnosis of severe perinatal (lethal) hypophosphatasia. *J Nippon Med Sch* 2007;74:65-69.

56. Deeb AA, Bruce SN, Morris AA, Cheetham TD: Infantile hypophosphatasia: Disappointing results of treatment. *Acta Paediatr* 2000;89:730-733.

57. Morava E, Kárteszi J, Weisenbach J, Caliebe A, Mundlos S, Méhes K: Cleidocranial dysplasia with decreased bone density and biochemical findings of hypophosphatasia. *Eur J Pediatr* 2002;161:619-622.

58. Olsson A, Matsson L, Blomquist HK, Larsson A, Sjödin B: Hypophosphatasia affecting the permanent dentition. *J Oral Pathol Med* 1996;25:343-347.

59. O'Duffy JD: Hypophosphatasia associated with calcium pyrophosphate dihydrate deposits in cartilage: Report of a case. *Arthritis Rheum* 1970;13:381-388.

60. Eberle F, Hartenfels S, Pralle H, Käbisch A: Adult hypophosphatasia without apparent skeletal disease: "Odontohypophosphatasia" in four heterozygote members of a family. *Klin Wochenschr* 1984;62:371-376.

61. Fraser D, Laidlaw JC: Treatment of hypophosphatasia with cortisone. *Lancet* 1956;270:553.

62. Girschick HJ, Seyberth HW, Huppertz HI: Treatment of childhood hypophosphatasia with nonsteroidal antiinflammatory drugs. *Bone* 1999;25:603-607.

63. Wolfish NM, Heick H: Hyperparathyroidism and infantile hypophosphatasia: Effect of prednisone and vitamin K therapy. *J Pediatr* 1979;95:1079-1081.

Hypoparathyroidism, Pseudohypoparathyroidism, and Pseudopseudohypoparathyroidism

This chapter describes three rare disorders that are characterized by a biochemical alteration in calcium and phosphorus concentration based on problems in production or recognition of parathyroid hormone (PTH). The first of these, hypoparathyroidism, is an uncommon disorder that has many causes, some related to surgery or radiation and others that are metabolic, biochemical, or genetic in origin. All of these diseases are characterized by a decline in the production of PTH and resultant hypocalcemia and hyperphosphatemia. The disorders generally respond to administration of PTH or calcium. Pseudohypoparathyroidism is a genetic disorder that is quite similar in presentation, but the PTH levels are normal; the problem is that the body's target structures are unresponsive. Pseudopseudohypoparathyroidism is also genetic and similar to pseudohypoparathyroidism but is milder and has several different clinical and biochemical findings. The purpose of this presentation is to review the causes and metabolic and clinical presentations of all three of these rare disorders, and also to provide information regarding the treatments that are currently available.

History and Nomenclature

Recognition of the parathyroid glands and their activities is attributed to the comprehensive autopsy and histologic studies of Jakob Erdheim,[1] published in 1903. The history of the many forms of hypoparathyroidism is principally the result of the prodigious efforts of a famous endocrinologist, Fuller Albright (1900-1969), a clinical investigator who performed his studies on patients at the Massachusetts General Hospital (MGH). Beginning in 1929, Albright and his associates described a series of entities in several articles, which not only defined the nature of these rare disorders but added names to them as well.[2-6] He is responsible for defining the clinical characteristics and causes of hypoparathyroidism, pseudohypoparathyroidism, and pseudopseudohypoparathyroidism.[3,4] Other contributors to our understanding of these unusual disorders include Aub and associates,[7] Chase and associates,[8] Drezner and associates,[9,10] and, most recently, Michael Levine[11-15] of Johns Hopkins and John Potts, Harald Jüppner, and their associates at MGH.[16-19]

In terms of nomenclature, these disorders are also known as polyglandular autoimmune endocrinopathy, familial hypocalcemia, Albright hereditary osteodystrophy, calcium-sensing receptor hypocalcemia, and Seabright-Bantam syndrome.[3,14,15] In addition, several eponymic syndromes relate to these disorders and include the Kearns-Sayre syndrome,[20,21] Kenny-Caffey syndrome,[22-25] DiGeorge syndrome,[26-28] and Pearson marrow-pancreas syndrome.[29,30]

Biologic Actions of Parathyroid Hormone

There are four small parathyroid glands located on the posterior aspect of the thyroid gland. The cells in these glands are responsible for the production of PTH, a single-chain protein containing 84 amino acids.[17,19,31-33] The material is released from the cell in response to a G protein–coupled calcium-sensing receptor that is activated by a reduction in serum calcium concentration.[17,19,20,33,34]

Parathyroid hormone has several important functions principally related to mineral and bone metabolism. In the gastrointestinal cells responsible for absorbing calcium from dietary intake, PTH increases the production of adenyl-cyclase, which causes adenosine triphosphate (ATP) to be converted to cyclic adenosine monophosphate (cAMP), which is then responsible for opening up the cell membrane and allowing calcium ions to enter the cell.[31,35-38] With the aid of 1,25 dihydroxy vitamin D and calbindin, a calcium-binding protein, the calcium ions can then be transported into the serum.[31,35,36,39] Parathyroid hormone is also responsible for stimulating the reabsorption of calcium in the glomerulus and thus retaining the material in the serum.[17,35,40,41] In addition, however, PTH markedly decreases the tubular reabsorbtion of phosphate in the kidney, causing an increase in phosphaturia and a decrease in phosphatemia. Parathyroid hormone can also release calcium from osseous tissues in two ways: a process called "crystallysis," which consists of removing small amounts of calcium and phosphate that are attached or lie adjacent to the hydroxyapatite crystals; and second, as an activator of osteoclasts, which cause massive bone resorbtion and result in a major release of calcium and phosphate.[19,31,34,42-44] In the absence of excessive calcium or phosphate, by stimulating the activity of renal 1-alpha hydroxylase, PTH is also responsible for converting 25 hydroxy vitamin D to 1,25 dihydroxy vitamin D in the kidney, a material that is necessary to increase calcium absorption in the bowel and reabsorption in the kidney.[45-48] All of these actions result in two major effects—increasing the concentration of calcium in the serum, and decreasing the tubular reabsorption of phosphate as a protective action to prevent excessive body calcification.[31,40,49] Thus the chemical actions of PTH are to increase the serum calcium and reduce the serum phosphate in the serum, and the osseous action is to reduce the amount of bony substance principally by osteoclastic bone destruction.

Causes of Hypoparathyroidism

There are many causes for hypoparathyroidism—some destructive, some genetic, and some chemical.[5,17,20] The easiest to understand are those that result from damage to the parathyroid glands. Surgery for thyroid cancer or radiation of the neck may greatly damage the glands and markedly reduce their production of PTH.[20] Granulomatous infiltration, metal overload, or neoplastic invasion may also cause a reduced amount of the hormone.[17,20] Children born without parathyroid glands and patients with Addison's disease, type 1 diabetes, primary hypogonadism, thyroiditis, alcoholism, keratoconjunctivitis, pernicious anemia, hepatitis, candidiasis, and reduced magnesium have all been reported to occasionally have various degrees of hypoparathyroidism.[11,12,17,20,50]

Genetic problems are very rarely encountered but are quite striking, partly because they can also have other dramatic clinical characteristics. Congenital agenesis is either autosomal recessive or X-linked and has been mapped to Xq 26-q27.[11,12,17,20] It may be linked to thymic aplasia.[26] A second group of genetic decreases in PTH production have been labeled as the DiGeorge syndrome, which has multiple presentations and genetic errors, mostly in chromosome 22q11.[20,26-28,51] The syndrome includes distinctive facial features, cleft lip and palate, congenital heart disease, thymic hypoplasia, genital abnormalities, eye alterations, retarded growth, mental retardation, and renal disease.[20,27,28] The Kenny-Caffey syndrome is an autosomal recessive genetic disorder that is mapped to 1q42-q43.[20,22-24] For these patients, the hypoparathyroidism is associated with growth retardation, craniofacial anomalies, small hands and feet, and medullary stenosis of tubular bones.[20,22-24] The Kearns-Sayre syndrome is associated with a defect in mitochondrial DNA.[20,21] The clinical syndrome for these patients includes myopathy, dystonia, growth retardation, ophthalmoplegia, pigmentary retinal degeneration, cerebellar ataxia, and cardiac-conduction defects.[11,20,52] Patients with the fourth group, Pearson marrow-pancreas syndrome, have hypoparathyroidism associated with episodic crises, hepatic failure, lactic acidosis, neutropenia, anemia, and exoprine pancreatic dysfunction.[20,29,30]

Clinical Findings in Patients With Hypoparathyroidism

The onset of hypoparathyroidism for some patients with genetic variants may occur in infancy.[5,20,34-36,52] For patients with parathyroid destructive problems, it may occur considerably later. There are no identifiable ethnic or racial characteristics and for the most part the frequency is equal for males and females. Regardless of cause, patients with hypoparathyroidism are at risk for hypocalcemic disorders, including hyperreflexia, muscle spasm, tetany, nasal speech, and seizures.[12,17,20,28,34,36,52] Hypocalcemia may also cause a heart murmur, arrhythmia, and other cardiac problems, as well as airway obstruction.[17,20,36,52] Patients may show twitching of the facial muscles with tapping of the facial nerve in front of the ear (Chvostek sign).[20,53] They may also show carpopedal spasm, with inflation of a blood pressure cuff maintained at systolic pressure for several minutes (Trousseau sign).[20]

Parathyroid Hormone Resistance Syndromes (Pseudohypoparathyroidism and Pseudopseudohypoparathyroidism)

These two disorders are not only terminologically confusing, but quite clinically and metabolically unique. The earliest recognition of the disorders was by Albright and associates,[3,4] who named the disorders hereditary osteodystrophy or the Seabright-Bantam syndrome. In 1942, they identified the clinical characteristics and also indicated that patients have normal parathyroid glands.[3] The two forms, pseudohypoparathyroidism and pseudopseudohypoparathyroidism, are closely tied together. Both lesions are genetic in origin and patients have normal parathyroid glands and PTH production but display a remarkable target tissue unresponsiveness, which results in a failure of the normal action of autogenous or administered PTH on the bone or kidney.[9,11,12,14,54,55] In addition, there are some systemic findings, sometimes quite dramatic and disabling, seen in association with these syndromes.[11,12,15]

Pseudohypoparathyroidism has several forms. Type 1A appears to occur as a result of a defect in the adenyl-cyclase complex that produces cAMP in renal tubule cells.[8,54,56,57] Patients may show resistance to not only PTH, but also thyroid-stimulating hormone, gonadotrophins, and glucagons. Cellular elements from these patients show an approximately 50% reduction in expression of G2 alpha protein, which impairs the ability of PTH to activate adenyl-cyclase.[8,16,56-59] In addition, patients have physical changes as originally described by Albright, including short stature, round facies, obesity, subcutaneous ossification, mental retardation, and short fourth and fifth metatarsal and metacarpal bones.[14,60]

Pseudohypoparathyroidism type 1B appears to have a normal G2 alpha protein expression, but patients still have a defective nephrogenous cAMP response to PTH.[14,18,58,61] They may show increased density in the skeleton similar to that seen in hyperparathyroidism, which is in sharp contrast with the findings of hypoparathyroidism or pseudohypoparathyroidism type 1A.[14,16,18]

Pseudohypoparathyroidism type 2 is a heterogeneous disorder without a clear genetic or familial basis.[9,10,12,14,15] Renal resistance to PTH is manifested by a reduced phosphaturic response to administration of PTH, resulting in an increase in the serum phosphate[12,13] and, as a result, sometimes bony deposition.

Pseudopseudohypoparathyroidism describes patients who seem to respond to autogenous or exogenous PTH in a normal manner and have only limited biochemical abnormalities in relation to their calcium and phosphorus systems. The patients still have the same physical abnormalities seen in pseudohypoparathyroidism.[14,62] Pseudopseudohypoparathryroidism may be genetically related to pseudohypoparathyroidism type 1A.[14,60] Despite their normal calcium and phosphorus values, these patients are short of stature, obese, often mentally retarded, and have similar foot and hand disorders as those with pseudohypoparathyroidism.[60]

Diagnosis of the Hypoparathyroidism Syndromes

Patients with hypoparathyroidism have a reduced serum calcium concentration and an increased serum phosphorus concentration.[20] The level of PTH is usually low. Patients with pseudohypoparathyroidism and pseudopseudohypoparathyroidism also have a diminished concentration of serum calcium and phosphate but have a normal level of PTH.[11,12,14] Furthermore, neither of these entities respond to PTH when the agent is administered.[55] Genetic studies may be helpful both in the primary hypoparathyroidism group as well as in the

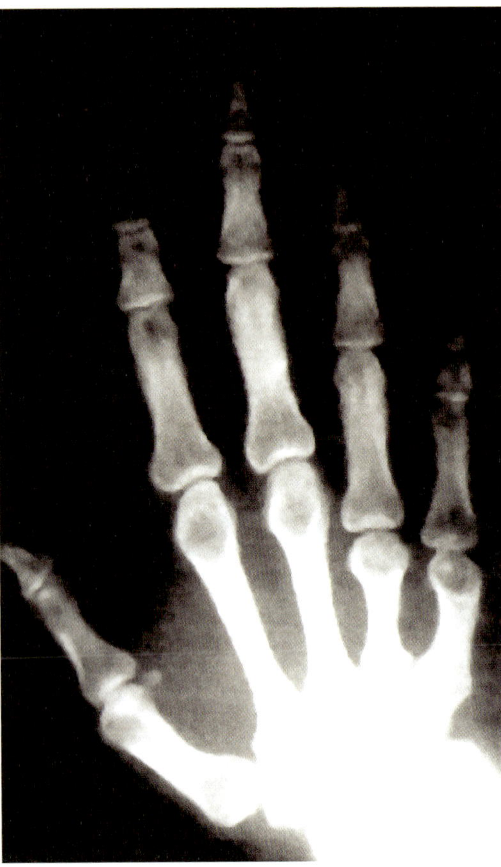

Figure 1
Radiograph of the hand of a patient with hypoparathyroidism, showing the characteristic shortening of the fourth and fifth metacarpals. The hand often has some limitations in function as a result.

pseudohypoparathyroidism and pseudopseudohypoparathyroidism groups. Distinguishing the two can often be performed by the Ellsworth-Howard test, in which synthetic PTH (1-34) peptide is administered and the blood measured for calcium and phosphate and the urine for cAMP and phosphate.[14,20,52] The response of hypoparathyroidism should be one of increased calcium and reduced phosphate and increased cAMP, and the response for the others much less specific, suggesting that the system is refractory.

Imaging studies of the hands and feet are often quite helpful because the pseudohypoparathyroidism and pseudopseudohypoparathyroidism forms of the disease often show rather remarkable and almost diagnostic changes in the third, fourth, and fifth metacarpals and metatarsals[60] (Figure 1). A recent report described bilateral slipped capital femoral epiphysis in a patient with pseudohypoparathyroidism.[63]

Treatment

The appropriate approach to treatment of hypoparathyroidism is to restore the calcium and phosphorus levels to normal.[20] This is most readily performed by administration of calcium and vitamin D. Recent use of PTH (1-34) is logical but patients have to be very carefully followed to avoid problems, particularly in the genetic disorders.[20] For patients with pseudohypoparathyroidism, use of calcium and vitamin D is appropriate and recently estrogen has been found to be useful in increasing the tissue response to autogenous PTH.[11,12] Orthopaedic problems include possible fractures of the weakened bones, which may be difficult to treat, partly because of the patient's cardiac or marrow-depleted status.[63] The small metacarpals and metatarsals may sometimes cause pain or limitation of hand motion; if that occurs, braces may be required.[60]

Conclusions

The hypoparathyroid disorders are rare and represent probably the least common of the metabolic bone disorders. Patients with rickets, osteomalacia, renal osteodystrophy, hyperparathyroidism, and osteoporosis are all encountered much more frequently by the pediatrician, endocrinologist, and especially the orthopaedic surgeon. Attempting to understand the causation of primary hypoparathyroidism and especially the rare genetic forms is far from the usual tasks of clinical practitioners. Most physicians are unlikely to be familiar with entities such as Kearns-Sayre, Kenny-Caffey, DiGeorge, or Pearson marrow-pancreas syndromes, and even less unlikely to have knowledge of the various forms of the Albright disorders. Pseudohypoparathyroidism and pseudopseudohypoparathyroidism are even more complex, particularly related to the fact that the concentration of PTH is normal. Because of genetic alterations, especially of the Gs alpha protein, the body doesn't recognize autogenous or even exogenous PTH and undergoes sometimes very problematic changes.

It seems quite clear that the future for these disorders is to eliminate them by genetic alteration, if that is possible. Some trials may include marrow transplant from genetically uninvolved siblings, stem-cell transplants, or developing a form of Gs alpha protein, which can be introduced into the body by some special techniques. In view of the infrequency of the disorders and the lack of current research, this may be far away in our future approaches to metabolic bone disorders. The fortunate aspect of the problem is that currently many patients respond to administration of calcium and vitamin D.

References

1. Erdheim J: Zur normalen and pathologischen histoligie der glandula thyreoidea, parathryreoidea and hypophysis. *Beitr Pathol Anat* 1903;33:158-236.

2. Albright F, Bauer W, Ropes M, Aub JC: Studies of calcium and phosphorus metabolism: IV. The effect of the parathyroid hormone. *J Clin Invest* 1929;7:139-181.

3. Albright F, Burnett CH, Smith PH: Pseudohypoparathyroidism: An example of "Seabright-Bantam syndrome". *Endocrinology* 1942;30:922-932.

4. Albright F, Forbes AP, Henneman PH: Pseudopseudohypoparathyroidism. *Trans Assoc Am Physicians* 1952;65:337-350.

5. Albright F, Reifenstein C: *The Parathyroid Glands and Metabolic Bone Disease.* Baltimore, MD, Williams & Wilkins, 1948.

6. Reifenstein EC Jr, Albright F, Wells SL: The accumulation, interpretation and presentation of data pertaining to metabolic balances, notably of calcium, phosphorus and nitrogen. *J Clin Endocrinol* 1945;5:367-395.

7. Aub JC, Tibbets DM, McLean R: The influence of parathyroid hormone, urea, sodium chloride, fat and intestinal activity upon calcium balance. *J Nutr* 1937;13:635-655.

8. Chase LR, Melson GL, Aurbach GD: Pseudohypoparathyroidism: Defective excretion of 3',5'-AMP in response to parathyroid hormone. *J Clin Invest* 1969;48:1832-1844.

9. Drezner MK, Hassler MR: Normocalcemic pseudohypoparathyoidism: Association with normal vitamin D3 metabolism. *Am J Med* 1979;66:503-508.

10. Drezner M, Neelon FA, Lebovitz HE: Pseudohypoparathyroidism type II: A possible defect in the reception of the cyclic AMP signal. *N Engl J Med* 1973;289:1056-1060.

11. Levine MA: Hypoparathyroidism and pseudohypoparathyroidism, in DeGroot LJ, Jameson JL, et al (eds): *Endocrinology*, ed 4. Philadelphia, PA, WB Saunders Company, 2001, pp 1133-1153.

12. Levine MA: Hypoparathyroidism and pseudohypoparathyroidism, in Avioli LV, Krane SM (eds): *Metabolic Bone Disease.* San Diego, CA, Academic Press, 1998, pp 501-529.

13. Levine MA, Germain-Lee E, Jan de Beur S: Genetic basis for resistance to parathyroid hormone. *Horm Res* 2003;60:87-95.

14. Levine MA: Parathyroid hormone resistance syndromes, in Favus MJ (ed): *Primer on the Metabolic Bone Diseases and Disorders of Mineral Metabolism*, ed 4. Philadelphia, PA, Lippincott, Williams & Wilkins, 1999, pp 230-253.

15. Levine MA: Pseudohypoparathyroidism: From bedside to bench and back. *J Bone Miner Res* 1999;14:1255-1260.

16. Jüppner H, Bastepe M: Different mutations within or upstream of the GNAS locus cause distinct forms of pseudohypoparathyroidism. *J Pediatr Endocrinol Metab* 2006;19:641-646.

17. Jüppner H, Brown EM, Kronenburg HM: Parathyroid hormone, in Favus MJ (ed): *Primer on the Metabolic Bone Diseases and Disorders of Mineral Metabolism*, ed 4. Philadelphia, PA, Lippincott Williams & Wilkins, 1999, pp 80-87.

18. Jüppner H, Schipani E, Bastepe M, et al: The gene responsible for pseudohypoparathyroidism type Ib is paternally imprinted and maps in four unrelated kindreds to chromosome 20q13.3. *Proc Natl Acad Sci USA* 1998;95:11798-11803.

19. Potts JT Jr, Jüppner JH: Parathyroid hormone and parathyroid hormone-related peptide in calcium homeostasis, bone metabolism, and bone development: The proteins, their genes and receptors, in Avioli LV, Krane SM (eds): *Metabolic Bone Disease.* San Diego, CA, Academic Press, 1998, pp 51-94.

20. Goltzman D, Cole DEC: Hypoparathyroidism, in Favus MJ (ed): *Primer on the Metabolic Bone Diseases and Disorders of Mineral Metabolism*, ed 4. Philadelphia, PA, Lippincott, Williams & Wilkins, 1999, pp 226-230.

21. Zeviani M, Moraes CT, DiMauro S, et al: Deletions of mitochondrial DNA in Kearns-Sayre syndrome: 1988. *Neurology* 1998;51:1525-1533.

22. Caffey J: Congenital stenosis of medullary spaces in tubular bones and calvaria in two proportionate dwarfs—mother and son; coupled with transitory hypocalcemic tetany. *Am J Roentgenol Radium Ther Nucl Med* 1967;100:1-11.

23. Diaz GA, Khan KT, Gelb BD: The autosomal recessive Kenny-Caffey syndrome locus maps to chromosome 1q42-q43. *Genomics* 1998;54:13-18.

24. Kenny FM, Linarelli L: Dwarfism and cortical thickening of tubular bones: Transient hypocalcemia in a mother and a son. *Am J Dis Child* 1966;111:201-207.

25. Parvari R, Hershkovitz E, Grossman N, et al: Mutation of TBCE causes hypoparathyroidism-retardation-dysmorphism and autosomal recessive Kenny-Caffey syndrome. *Nat Genet* 2002;32:448-452.

26. DiGeorge AM: *Congenital Absence of the Thymus and its Immunologic Consequences: Concurrence With Congenital Hypoparathyroidism.* White Plains, NY, March of Dimes–Birth Defects Foundations IV, 1968, pp 115-121.

27. Driscoll DA, Budarf ML, Emanuel BS: A genetic etiology for DiGeorge syndrome: Consistent deletions and microdeletions of 22q11. *Am J Hum Genet* 1992;50:924-933.

28. Minier F, Carles D, Pelluard F, Alberti EM, Stern L, Saura R: DiGeorge syndrome: A review of 52 patients. *Arch Pediatr* 2005;12:254-257.

29. Pearson HA, Lobel JS, Kocoshis SA, et al: A new syndrome of refractory sideroblastic anemia with vacuolization of marrow precursors and exocrine pancreatic dysfunction. *J Pediatr* 1979;95:976-984.

30. Seneca S, De Merleir L, De Schepper J, et al: Pearson marrow pancreas syndrome: A molecular study and clinical management. *Clin Genet* 1997;51:338-342.

31. Mankin HJ: Metabolic bone disease. *Instr Course Lect* 1995;44:3-29.

32. Rizzoli R, Ferrari LS, Pizurki L, Caverzasio J, Bonjour JP: Actions of parathyroid hormone and parathyroid hormone-related protein. *J Endocrinol Invest* 1992;15:51-56.

33. Segre GV: Secretion, metabolism and circulating heterogeneity of parathyroid hormone, in Favus ME (ed): *Primer on Metabolic Bone Diseases and Disorders of Mineral Metabolism.* Kelseyville, CA, American Society for Bone and Mineral Research, 1990, pp 43-44.

34. Broadus AE: Mineral balance and homeostasis, in Favus MJ (ed): *Primer on the Metabolic Bone Diseases and Disorders of Mineral Metabolism,* ed 4. Philadelphia, PA, Lippincott Williams & Wilkins, 1999, pp 74-80.

35. Bronner F: Current concepts of calcium absorption: An overview. *J Nutr* 1992;222:641-643.

36. Karbach U: Mechanism of intestinal calcium transport and clinical aspects of disturbed calcium absorption. *Dig Dis* 1989;7:1-18.

37. Lemann J Jr, Favus M: The intestinal absorption of calcium, magnesium and phosphate, in Favus MJ (ed): *Primer on the Metabolic Bone Diseases and Disorders of Mineral Metabolism,* ed 4. Philadelphia, PA, Lippincott Williams & Wilkins, 1999, pp 63-66.

38. Wasserman RH, Chandler JS, Meyer SA, et al: Intestinal calcium transport and calcium extrusion processes at the basolateral membrane. *J Nutr* 1992;122:662-671.

39. Wasserman RH, Brindak ME, Buddle MM, et al: Recent studies on the biological actions of vitamin D on intestinal transport and the electrophysiology of peripheral nerve and cardiac muscle. *Prog Clin Biol Res* 1990;332:99-126.

40. Bushinsky DA: Calcium, magnesium and phosphorus: Renal handling and urinary excretion, in Favus MJ (ed): *Primer on the Metabolic Bone Diseases and Disorders of Mineral Metabolism,* ed 4. Philadelphia, PA, Lippincott Williams & Wilkins, 1999, pp 67-73.

41. Friedman PA, Gesek FA: Calcium transport in renal epithelial cells. *Am J Physiol* 1993;264:F181-F198.

42. Boskey AL: Mineral-matrix interactions in bone and cartilage. *Clin Orthop Relat Res* 1992;281:244-274.

43. Broadus AE: Physiologic functions of calcium, magnesium and phosphorus, in Favus ME (ed): *Primer on Metabolic Bone Diseases and Disorders of Mineral Metabolism.* Kelseyville, CA, American Society for Bone and Mineral Research, 1990, pp 29-30.

44. Raisz LG: Mechanisms and regulation of bone resorption by osteoclastic cells, in Cole FL, Favus ME (eds): *Disorders of Bone and Mineral Metabolism.* New York, NY, Raven Press, 1992, pp 287-311.

45. Gross M, Kumar R: Physiology and biochemistry of vitamin D-dependent calcium binding proteins. *Am J Physiol* 1990;259:F195-F209.

46. Holick MF: Vitamin D, photobiology, metabolism, mechanism of action and clinical applications, in Favus M (ed): *Primer on the Metabolic Bone Diseases and Disorders of Mineral Metabolism,* ed 4. Philadelphia, PA, Lippincott Williams & Wilkins, 1999, pp 92-98.

47. Hollis BW, Clemens TL, Adams JS: Vitamin D metabolites, in Favus MJ (ed): *Primer on the Metabolic Bone Diseases and Disorders of Mineral Metabolism,* ed 4. Philadelphia, PA, Lippincott Williams & Wilkins, 1999, pp 124-127.

48. Kumar R: Vitamin D metabolism and mechanisms of calcium transport. *J Am Soc Nephrol* 1990;1:30-42.

49. Boden SD, Kaplan FS: Calcium homeostasis. *Orthop Clin North Am* 1990;21:31-42.

50. Laitinen K, Kamberg Allardt C, Tunninen R, et al: Transient hypoparathyroidism during acute alcohol intoxication. *N Engl J Med* 1991;324:721-727.

51. Saitta SC, Harris SE, McDonald-McGinn DM, et al: Independent de novo 22q11.2 deletions in first cousins with DiGeorge/velocardiofacial syndrome. *Am J Med Genet A* 2004;124A:313-317.

52. Guise TA, Mundy GR: Clinical review 69: Evaluation of hypocalcemia in children and adults. *J Clin Endocrinol Metab* 1995;80:1473-1478.

53. Hoffman E: The Chvostek sign: A clinical study. *Am J Surg* 1958;96:33-37.

54. Stirling HF, Darling JA, Barr DG: Plasma cyclic AMP response to intravenous parathyroid hormone in pseudohypoparathyroidism. *Acta Paediatr Scand* 1991;80:333-338.

55. Stone MD, Hosking DJ, Garcia-Himmelstine C, White DA, Rosenblum D, Worth HG: The renal response to exogenous parathyroid hormone in pseudohypoparathyroidism. *Bone* 1993;14:727-735.

56. Ahrens W, Hiort O: Determination of Gs alpha protein activity in Albright's hereditary osteodystrophy. *J Pediatr Endocrinol Metab* 2006;19:647-651.

57. De Sanctis L, Romagnolo D, Olivero M, et al: Molecular analysis of the GNAS1 gene for the correct diagnosis of Albright hereditary osteodystrophy and pseudohypoparathyroidism. *Pediatr Res* 2003;53:749-755.

58. Mantovani G, Maghnie M, Weber G, et al: Growth hormone-releasing hormone resistance in pseudohypoparathyroidism type Ia: New evidence for imprinting to the Gs-alpha gene. *J Clin Endocrinol Metab* 2003;88:4070-4074.

59. Weinstein LS, Chen M, Liu J: Gs(alpha) mutations and imprinting defects in human disease. *Ann N Y Acad Sci* 2002;968:173-197.

60. de Sanctis L, Vai S, Andreo MR, Romagnolo D, Silvestro L, de Sanctis C: Brachydactyly in 14 genetically characterized pseudohypoparathyroidism type Ia patients. *J Clin Endocrinol Metab* 2004;89:1650-1655.

61. Wu WI, Schwindinger WF, Aparicio LF, Levine MA: Selective resistance to parathyroid hormone caused by a novel uncoupling mutation in the carboxyl terminus of G alpha(s): A cause of pseudohypoparathyroidism type Ib. *J Biol Chem* 2001;276:165-171.

62. Lucky AW, Tsang R: Pseudopseudohypoparathyroidism, presenting with osteoma cutis. *J Bone Miner Res* 1997;12:995.

63. Agarwal C, Seigle R, Agarwal S, Bilezikian JP, Hyman JE, Oberfield SE: Pseudohypoparathyroidism: A rare cause of bilateral slipped capital femoral epiphysis. *J Pediatr* 2006;149:406-408.

Index